Clinical Nutrition of the Essential Trace Elements and Minerals

NUTRITION ◊ AND ◊ HEALTH
Adrianne Bendich, Series Editor

CLINICAL NUTRITION
OF THE ESSENTIAL TRACE
ELEMENTS AND MINERALS

THE GUIDE FOR HEALTH PROFESSIONALS

Edited by

JOHN D. BOGDEN, PhD

*Department of Preventive Medicine and Community
Health, University of Medicine and Dentistry
of New Jersey, New Jersey Medical School, Newark, NJ*

and

LESLIE M. KLEVAY, MD, SD IN HYG

*United States Department of Agriculture, Agricultural
Research Service, Grand Forks Human Nutrition Research
Center, Grand Forks, ND*

Foreword by

IRWIN ROSENBERG, MD

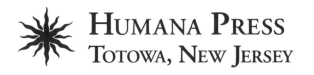

HUMANA PRESS
TOTOWA, NEW JERSEY

© 2000 Humana Press Inc.
999 Riverview Drive, Suite 208
Totowa, New Jersey 07512

Cover design by Patricia F. Cleary.

For additional copies, pricing for bulk purchases, and/or information about other Humana titles,
contact Humana at the above address or at any of the following numbers: Tel.: 973-256-1699;
Fax: 973-256-8341; E-mail: humana@humanapr.com or visit our website at http://humanapress.com

This publication is printed on acid-free paper. ∞
ANSI Z39.48-1984 (American National Standards Institute) Permanence of Paper for Printed Library Materials.

Photocopy Authorization Policy:

Printed in the United States of America.   10 9 8 7 6 5 4 3 2 1

Library of Congress Cataloging-in-Publication Data

Clinical nutrition of the essential trace elements and minerals: the guide for health
professionals / edited by John D. Bogden and Leslie M. Klevay.
      p.; cm. -- (Nutrition and health)
   Includes bibliographical references and index.
   ISBN 0-89603-407-0 (alk. paper)
   1. Trace elements in nutrition. 2. Trace element deficiency diseases. 3. Minerals in
nutrition. I. Bogden, John D. II. Klevay, Leslie M. III. Nutrition and health (Totowa,
N.J.)
   [DNLM: 1. Trace Elements. 2. Minerals. 3. Nutrition. QU 130.5 C641 2000]
   QP534.C585 2000
   612.3'924--dc21
   DNLM/DLC
   for Library of Congress   00-04979
                                                                              CIP

DEDICATION

J.D.B. dedicates this book to Doreen L. Bogden, Jennifer, and Kim for their encouragement and understanding, and to Donald B. Louria for his considerable advice and support.

L.M.K. dedicates this volume to Martha N. Klevay, Ann, Micheal, and Andrew for their support, and to Alfred E. Harper, Walter Mertz, and Henry A. Schroeder for their inspiration.

SERIES INTRODUCTION

The *Nutrition and Health* series of books have, as an overriding mission, to provide health professionals with texts that are considered essential because each includes 1) a synthesis of the state of the science, 2) timely, in-depth reviews by the leading researchers in their respective fields, 3) extensive, up-to-date fully annotated reference lists, 4) a detailed index, 5) relevant tables and figures, 6) identification of paradigm shifts and the consequences, 7) virtually no overlap of information between chapters, but targeted, inter-chapter referrals, 8) suggestions of areas for future research, and 9) balanced, data-driven answers to patient questions which are based upon the totality of evidence rather than the findings of any single study.

The series volumes are not the outcome of a symposium. Rather, each editor has the potential to examine a chosen area with a broad perspective, both in subject matter as well as in the choice of chapter authors. The international perspective, especially with regard to public health initiatives, is emphasized where appropriate. The editors, whose trainings are both research and practice oriented, have the opportunity to develop a primary objective for their book; define the scope and focus, and then invite the leading authorities from around the world to be part of their initiative. The authors are encouraged to provide an overview of the field, discuss their own research and relate the research findings to potential human health consequences. Because each book is developed de novo, the chapters can be coordinated so that the resulting volume imparts greater knowledge than the sum of the information contained in the individual chapters.

Clinical Nutrition of the Essential Trace Elements and Minerals, edited by John D. Bogden and Leslie M. Klevay, exemplifies the mission of the *Nutrition and Health* series. Drs. Bogden and Klevay provide the reader with a unique perspective and focused view of the importance of the essentiality of trace elements and minerals for optimal health as well as their requirements and functions in specific disease conditions. By including an extensive review of the basic concepts of mineral metabolism, consumption patterns over the history of Man, assessment tools, and safety issues, this text gains in importance as a valuable resource for students as well as those who are practicing health professionals. The text also includes critically important chapters that discuss the requirements of these essential nutrients during adolescence, pregnancy, and lactation, and in the elderly. Medically related professionals will certainly find the chapters related to the genetic diseases that affect mineral metabolism of particular importance to their practice. Additional chapters provide in-depth reviews of the functions of minerals and their roles in the endocrine, cardiovascular, gastrointestinal, immune, skeletal, and ocular systems of the body. This volume is of particular importance because it includes understandable chapters in highly technical areas written by the leading authorities of their fields of research. Thus, *Clinical Nutrition of the Essential Trace Elements and Minerals* represents a comprehensive, up-to-date resource for undergraduate, graduate, and medical students, nutrition and public health educators, practicing physicians, and other health care providers as well as clinical and laboratory researchers.

Adrianne Bendich, PhD
SmithKline Beecham Consumer Health Care
Parsippany, NJ

FOREWORD

As we cross from one century into another, a comprehensive and authoritative presentation of knowledge and science of the biology of trace elements and minerals not only fills a great need, but also represents growing recognition of the importance of nutrition science for its impact on health and policy. The first half of the last century was an era of discovery in nutrition with all of the vitamins discovered, culminating in the description of the structure of vitamin B12 in 1947. No less important was the elucidation of the biological and nutritional essentiality of many minerals leading to an appropriate place in our list of recommended nutrients for health. But it was in the second half of the 20th century that the definitions of essential nutrients and essential minerals underwent a most important change and even a paradigm shift as knowldge increased of the relationship between mineral nutrition and chronic degenerative disease. The history of mineral biology in the past three decades includes the important discoveries which have led to a virtual explosion in knowledge and understanding of the importance of these nutrients in health and disease as is so well documented in the second half of this timely text. The discovery of binding proteins which were regulatory in the metabolism of minerals, of cellular receptors, and of nuclear receptors, binding sites regulating the expression of macromolecules critical to human biology exerted by trace minerals, and the remarkable improvements in instrumentation and chemical measuring precision have put mineral nutrition research at the forefront of the nutritional/biological revolution. Now the promise of plant biotechnology adds further elements to the projection of beneficial changes in our food supply.

These enhancements in knowledge have permitted a much more science-based approach to some of the most important health problems in the world, including a better understanding of iron absorption and metabolism leading to better ways of preventing the most common nutritional deficiency in the world, iron deficiency. A better understanding of the role of zinc in growth and development and enzyme function and metabolism has permitted that mineral to take its place among those that are targeted for important interventions in worldwide problems of child undernutrition. A better understanding of the many functions of copper in biology and metabolism have permitted that nutrient to be added to the essential nutrients as a factor in our understanding of heart disease and diet–heart interactions.

Clinical Nutrition of the Essential Trace Elements and Minerals sets a high standard for presentation of the scientific bases for the importance of minerals in human biology and health and will thereby contribute in a major way to the appropriate application of science for improved public health and preventive nutrition. No less important will be its contribution to establishing the foundation for moving the science in this important field even further.

Irwin Rosenberg, MD
United States Department
of Agriculture, Human Nutrition
Research Center on Aging,
Tufts University, Boston, MA

PREFACE

There is widespread interest in nutrition among health professionals and the general public. Newspapers, general circulation magazines, television, and the internet are a daily source of nutrition information, but much of it is inaccurate and misleading. The public is frequently confused about specific nutrition issues, and many people turn to their health care providers as a source for accurate and up-to-date advice. However, physicians, nurses, registered dietitians, and other health care providers need sources of accurate, clinically relevant, and current information in order to provide sound guidance to their patients.

Perhaps the greatest need is for a comprehensive book on trace element and mineral nutrition. Recent confusion among both health care providers and the general public about the use of zinc lozenges to treat the common cold and chromium supplements to enhance muscle mass are two examples of the need for reliable information. The target audience for *Clinical Nutrition of the Essential Trace Elements and Minerals* is the health professional: physicians, registered dietitians, nurses, nutrition researchers, and college and university faculty who teach nutrition and/or medicine. However, it is also intended as a text for students in the health sciences. *Clinical Nutrition of the Essential Trace Elements and Minerals* has been written to provide up-to-date information, and should be useful as both a text and a reference for those in the field of nutrition.

Other books on this topic take an approach that disperses information about specific clinical topics throughout the text by element. In contrast, *Clinical Nutrition of the Essential Trace Elements and Minerals* employs a more practical and useful approach—discussing, within a chapter, all of the essential elements relevant to a specific condition or group of diseases.

Each chapter focuses on the clinical importance of the nine trace elements currently considered to be essential: chromium, copper, fluoride, iron, iodine, molybdenum, manganese, selenium, and zinc. The chapters also include discussion of the three major essential dietary minerals: calcium, magnesium, and phosphorus, where appropriate. Discussion of other trace elements and minerals is provided where relevant to a specific disease or condition. Each chapter is a review of current knowledge with an emphasis on human studies and clinical nutrition. Where useful, the authors include examples from their own research to explain key ideas and concepts. Tables and figures are used liberally to enhance learning by practitioners and students. The authors contributing to this volume are recognized as experts in their field as well as experienced teachers.

Clinical Nutrition of the Essential Trace Elements and Minerals consists of 21 chapters divided into four major sections. The first section contains seven chapters and discusses basic concepts, consumption, laboratory assessment, supplement safety, and deficiencies of the essential micronutrients and minerals. Unique features of this section are the inclusion of chapters on both prehistoric and current consumption of trace elements and minerals in food and the epidemiology of trace element and mineral deficiencies. The second section contains four chapters on trace element and mineral nutrition in healthy people, with chapters on pregnancy, lactation, adolescents, and older people. The third and largest section with ten chapters discusses trace element and mineral nutrition in various diseases, including: genetic, endocrine, skeletal, cardiovascular, kidney, gastrointestinal, infectious, surgical, and opthalmologic disorders. The final section contains an index and guide to the relevant literature.

As editors, we are very excited about each of the chapters and the breadth of the content of this book. We believe that this text can improve the teaching of trace element and mineral nutrition to students and health professionals and enhance their ability to provide sound dietary and medical advice to their clients and patients.

John D. Bogden
Leslie M. Klevay

CONTENTS

CONTRIBUTORS

GREGORY J. ANDERSON • *Iron Metabolism Laboratory, Queenland Institute of Medical Research, Brisbane, Queensland, Australia*

NANCY E. BADENHOP • *Departments of Physical Medicine and Rehabilitation, Medicine, and Nutrition, Bone and Mineral Metabolism Laboratory, Davis Medical Research Center, Ohio State University, Columbus, OH*

JOHN D. BOGDEN, PHD • *Department of Preventive Medicine and Community Health, University of Medicine and Dentistry of New Jersey, New Jersey Medical School, Newark, NJ*

GEORGE EDWIN BUNCE, PHD • *Virginia Polytechnic Institute and State University, Blacksburg, VA*

RONNI CHERNOFF, PHD, RD, FADA • *John L. McClellan Memorial Veterans Hospital, Geriatric Research Education and Clinical Center, Central Arkansas Veterans Healthcare System, Little Rock, AR*

SUSANNA CUNNINGHAM-RUNDLES, PHD • *The Immunology Research Laboratory, Division of Hematology/Oncology, Department of Pediatrics, The New York Hospital-Cornell University Medical Center, New York, NY*

RENATA D'INCÀ, MD • *Department of Surgical and Gastroenterological Sciences, University of Padua, Padua, Italy*

JOHN T. DUNN, MD • *Department of Medicine, University of Virginia Health Sciences Center, Charlottesville, VA*

S. BOYD EATON, MD • *Departments of Radiology and Anthropology, Emory University, Atlanta, GA*

STANLEY B. EATON III • *Departments of Radiology and Anthropology, Emory University, Atlanta, GA*

JOHN N. HATHCOCK, PHD • *Council for Responsible Nutrition, Washington, DC*

ROBERT P. HEANEY, MD, FACP, FAIN • *John A. Creighton University Professor, Creighton University, Omaha, NE*

JASMINKA Z. ILICH, PHD • *Departments of Physical Medicine and Rehabilitation, Medicine, and Nutrition, Bone and Mineral Metabolism Laboratory, Davis Medical Research Center, Ohio State University, Columbus, OH*

SAULO KLAHR, MD • *Department of Medicine, Barnes-Jewish Hospital, Washington University School of Medicine, St. Louis, MO*

LESLIE M. KLEVAY, MD, SD in Hyg • *United States Department of Agriculture, Agricultural Research Service, Grand Forks Human Nutrition Research Center, Grand Forks, ND*

ROBERTO MASIRONI, PHD • *Trace Element Institute for UNESCO, Lyon, France*

VELIMIR MATKOVIC, MD • *Departments of Physical Medicine and Rehabilitation, Medicine, and Nutrition, Bone and Mineral Metabolism Laboratory, Davis Medical Research Center, Ohio State University, Columbus, OH*

GORDON D. McLAREN, MD • *Division of Hematology/Oncology, Department of Medicine, and Chao Family Comprehensive Cancer Center, University of California, Irvine, CA*

CINZIA MESTRINER, MD • *Department of Surgical and Gastroenterological Sciences, University of Padua, Padua, Italy*

DAVID B. MILNE, PHD • *United States Department of Agriculture, Agriculture Research Service, Grand Forks Human Nutrition Research Center, Grand Forks, ND*

M. A. MOHIT-TABATABAI, MD • *Department of Surgery, University of Medicine and Dentistry of New Jersey, New Jersey Medical School, Newark, NJ*

FORREST H. NIELSEN, PHD • *United States Department of Agriculture, Agriculture Research Service, Grand Forks Human Nutrition Research Center, Grand Forks, ND*

JEAN A. T. PENNINGTON, PHD, RD • *Department of Nutrition Research, National Institutes of Health, Bethedsa, MD*

MARY FRANCES PICCIANO, PHD • *Department of Nutrition, The Pennsylvania State University, University Park, PA and Office of Dietary Supplements, National Institutes of Health, Bethesda, MD*

THOMAS M. REILLY, PHD • *Department of Primary Care, University of Medicine and Dentistry of New Jersey, School of Health Related Professions, Stratford, NJ*

THERESA O. SCHOLL, PHD, MPH • *Department of Obstetrics and Gynecology, University of Medicine and Dentistry of New Jersey-School of Osteopathic Medicine, Stratford, NJ*

ADRIA R. SHERMAN, PHD • *Department of Nutritional Sciences, Rutgers, The State University of New Jersey, New Brunswick, NJ*

GIACOMO CARLO STURNIOLO, MD • *Department of Surgical and Gastroenterological Sciences, University of Padua, Padua, Italy*

I   BASIC CONCEPTS, CONSUMPTION, DEFICIENCY, AND TOXICITY

1

The Essential Trace Elements and Minerals

Basic Concepts

John D. Bogden, PhD

1. THE ESSENTIAL MINERALS AND TRACE ELEMENTS

The objective of this introductory chapter is to discuss some basic ideas that can facilitate understanding of the nutriture of the essential trace elements and minerals. In depth discussion of individual nutrients in health and disease will be found in each of the next 20 chapters.

The most recent version of the Periodic Table contains 112 known elements, yet there is convincing evidence for essentiality for humans for only 21 of these. Of the latter, eleven are required in the diet in relatively large quantities. These are hydrogen, carbon, nitrogen, oxygen, sodium, potassium, magnesium, calcium, phosphorus, sulfur, and chlorine. Except for magnesium, calcium, and phosphorus, these elements will not be discussed in this book. They are essential as the major building blocks of lipids, nucleic acids, proteins, and carbohydrates, or in their roles as major intracellular and extracellular electrolytes. Hydrogen and oxygen are also of course the components of water. Though each of these 11 is essential, Recommended Dietary Allowances (RDAs) and/or Dietary References Intakes (DRIs) are established only for magnesium, calcium, and phosphorus. The challenge of establishing RDAs or DRIs for each of the other elements, for example carbon, is formidable, since they are major components of all cells and present in all foods at high concentrations. In addition, it would be of little practical value to do so; thus we do not have RDAs or DRIs for elements such as carbon, sulfur, and oxygen.

There are nine trace elements for which there is substantial evidence of essentiality: chromium, copper, fluorine (as fluoride), iodine, iron, manganese, molybdenum, selenium, and zinc (1). Cobalt is required only as a component of the vitamin B-12 molecule (2) and is thus not generally considered an essential trace element. For the other nine elements, RDAs or Estimated Safe and Adequate Daily Dietary Intakes (ESADDIs) were last established in 1989 (1). ESADDI were set for chromium, copper, fluoride, manganese, and molybdenum and RDAs for iodine, iron, selenium, and zinc, reflecting greater confidence in requirements for the latter than the former trace elements (*see* Table 2 in Chapter 4). The 1989 RDAs are being supplanted by the Dietary Reference Intakes (DRIs) (3). DRIs for minerals and trace elements have been established for calcium, magnesium, phosphorous, and fluoride (3) in conjunction with setting these values for the nutrients essential for bone health (*see* Chapter 14 and for selenium along with other antioxidants).

From: *Clinical Nutrition of the Essential Trace Elements and Minerals: The Guide for Health Professionals*
Edited by: J. D. Bogden and L. M. Klevay © Humana Press Inc., Totowa, NJ

However, the setting of dietary guidelines should be regarded as a dynamic situation. Reevaluation can result in changes in recommended intakes of nutrients already considered essential as well as the addition of other nutrients to the current list of essential trace elements. Chapter 2 focuses on the possibly essential trace elements, and these are the leading candidates for consideration for future addition to the list of essential nutrients.

The definition of the term trace element is somewhat arbitrary. Trace elements are generally present in most tissues at concentrations of less than 300 micrograms per gram (300 parts per million) or required in the daily diet in only microgram to low milligram quantities. For example, the trace element with the highest recommended daily intake is iron, with an RDA of 30 mg per day for pregnant women *(1)*. The lowest RDA is that of selenium — with a value of 55 µg per day for adult females *(1)*. Thus, the range of recommended intakes for the currently essential trace elements is from tens of micrograms to at most tens of milligrams per day, or about a range of three orders of magnitude *(4)*. Since recommended intakes for calcium, magnesium, and phosphorous are much higher, they are regarded as major minerals and not trace elements.

Worldwide, more than 2 billion people, (about 40% of the population of the globe) are at high risk for one or more trace element deficiencies *(5,6)*. The most common deficiencies, in order of prevalence, are iron (2 billion worldwide), iodine (1.5 billion worldwide), and zinc *(5,6)*, likely followed by selenium and copper *(see* Chapter 6).

2. SOME BASIC CONCEPTS

A number of factors can greatly influence micronutrient nutriture and their recognition can enhance our understanding of effects of trace elements on health. These factors include interactions between micronutrients, dose-response effects, oxidation state, binding to enzymes and other macromolecules, chelation, immutability, and bioavailability. In addition, compromised absorption and excretion can lead to trace element deficiency or toxicity. Distinguishing between cause and effect and the impact of a disease versus its treatment is also critical, as well as differentiating between correction of deficiency and the beneficial effects of pharmacologic doses of essential trace elements.

2.1. Interactions

Interactions among trace elements may greatly influence their clinical effects. For example, anemia due to copper deficiency may develop in people consuming high doses of zinc for an extended period of time *(7,8)*. An unanswered but important question is whether intakes of moderate doses of zinc in the range of 15–25 mg/day can also result in a more subtle compromise of copper nutriture *(9)* *(see* Chapter 15). Other interactions include the ability of dietary selenium to decrease the toxicity of mercury *(10)*. Small initial doses of the trace element cadmium are protective against subsequent large doses of cadmium or mercury. This results because cadmium induces the synthesis and storage in the liver and kidney of low molecular weight proteins (metallothioneins) which are rich in sulfur-containing amino acids, and can bind to subsequent doses of mercury or cadmium, thereby decreasing their toxicity *(11)*. High dietary intakes of calcium and magnesium decrease the gastrointestinal absorption of lead *(12,13)*, a beneficial effect, but calcium may also reduce iron and zinc absorption *(14,15)*. Molybdenum can reduce copper retention *(16)*. Numerous other examples of interactions have mandated their consideration in the establishment of the new DRIs. A key consideration is that interactions are not limited to inhibition of gastrointestinal absorption, but can occur at any step in the metabolism of an essential trace element *(17)*. However, a lack of adequate quantitative data will compromise our ability to use many of the known interactions in setting DRIs for the essential trace elements.

2.2. Dose-Response Effects

Dose-response effects must be considered in evaluation of the clinical implications of trace element nutrition. Each of the essential trace elements is toxic if the dose is high enough. For example zinc deficiency may develop as a result of inadequate intake, but an excessive intake can produce anemia and eventually death, as has occurred due to unrecognized zinc contamination of dialysis fluids in hemodialysis patients *(18)*. Cadmium in very small quantities has been found in one study to be essential for normal growth of rats, but larger quantities are quite toxic to the kidneys *(19)*.

2.3. Oxidation State

Oxidation state may also be a factor for some trace metals. Chromium is an essential micronutrient in the +3 oxidation state, as found in food *(1,20)*, and even high oral doses well above usual intakes are very well tolerated. However, the +6 oxidation state is not essential but actually quite toxic. In addition, chromates are well recognized lung carcinogens when inhaled *(21)*. Paradoxically, the cellular uptake and intracellular conversion of chromium in the very reactive +6 oxidation state to the +3 state is thought to be a key feature in the toxicity of the +6 state *(22)*. For other trace elements, for example zinc, only one oxidation state (+2) exists in vivo.

2.4. Enzymes and Hormones

Trace metals are essential in large part because they interact with and affect the function of enzymes. In addition, many enzyme molecules contain one or more atoms of an essential trace element. An example is ceruloplasmin, which contains 8 copper atoms per molecule and serves as a circulating copper transport protein. Binding of each copper atom is not identical, since an in vitro study demonstrated that the molecule contains copper bound in three different ways *(23)*. Other examples of metalloenzymes are alkaline phosphatase, carbonic anhydrase, alcohol dehydrogenase, RNA polymerase, and ALA dehydratase, which all contain zinc *(24)*. The presence of zinc in these and several dozen other enzymes very likely contributes to the numerous adverse effects of zinc deficiency, including its effects on growth and cellular immune function. Other copper containing enzymes besides ceruloplasmin are cytochrome-c-oxidase, lysyl oxidase, tyrosinase, and cytosolic superoxide dismutase *(25)*. The latter contains zinc in addition to copper, and is thus an example of an enzyme containing two different trace metals. Xanthine oxidase is a molybdenum enzyme, glutathione peroxidase contains selenium, and mitochrondrial superoxide dismutase has an atom of manganese *(15,26,27)*.

The role of trace elements in influencing enzyme function in part explains the in vivo activity exerted by very small quantities or concentrations of these elements. An atom of a trace element with an atomic weight of less than 100 can control the activity of an enzyme with a molecular weight that may be 100–1000 fold greater.

Trace elements may also influence hormone activity, for example the influence of iodine on thyroid hormones and chromium on insulin *(28)*.

2.5. Chelation

Chelation is a factor that may strongly influence trace element nutriture. A chelating agent is a molecule (ligand) that can bind to transition metals (e.g., iron, copper, chromium, molybdenum, manganese) with two or more bonds, thereby forming one or more ring structures. Chelating ligands can be bidentate, terdentate, quadridentate, quinquidentate, or multidentate depending on whether the number of bonds to a trace metal is 2, 3, 4, 5, or more. The bonds are usually between sulfur, nitrogen, and oxygen atoms of the chelating agent and the trace metal. Rings containing 5 or 6 atoms are very stable and their formation will be thermodynamically favored.

A number of enzymes and other macromolecules can behave as chelating agents since they are rich in oxygen, nitrogen, and sulfur atoms. Numerous drugs such as ethambutol, ethylenediamine-tetra acetate (EDTA), penicillamine, and isoniazid are chelating agents. When prescribing such drugs, the physician should be cognizant of their effects on the nutriture of essential metals. In addition, other health professionals should be aware of the potential effects of these drugs on trace element nutrition.

Chelating drugs tend to be nonspecific in their ability to bind to transition metals and usually can form very stable bonds with several essential metals. As an example, the drug penicillamine is a bidentate ligand that is highly effective in promoting excretion of excessive organ copper in Wilson's disease or lead in lead-poisoned children or adults, but can also cause excretion of enough zinc to produce symptomatic zinc deficiency *(29)*.

2.6. Immutability

A unique feature of trace elements and minerals is their immutability. Since they are elements they can neither be synthesized nor degraded in vivo unless, of course, they are radioactive. However, their sites of binding and/or oxidation state can change. In vivo, most trace elements are bound to the sulfur, nitrogen, and oxygen atoms of proteins. Thus, they are usually present in relatively large amounts in foods high in protein. However, there are numerous exceptions to this generalization. For example, tea has a high manganese content *(30)*.

Immutability is an advantage in analysis of biological tissues and fluids for trace elements since storage, even for a long period of time, cannot change the total quantity of a trace element or mineral present in the sample (assuming no net addition to or extraction from the sample by its container). This does not mean that the analysis of biological tissues and fluids for trace elements is not challenging, since there are numerous pitfalls that can compromise the analysis of samples for trace elements. A particular problem is the prevention of specimen contamination, since external sources can easily contain much more of a trace element than the biological sample to be analyzed. Contamination control has been an especially difficult problem for zinc, chromium, and lead (*see* Chapter 5). As an example, it is widely known that rubber stoppers of most vacutainers can hopelessly contaminate a blood sample with zinc *(31)*.

2.7. Bioavailability

Another factor that must be considered is that adequate dietary intake of a trace element or mineral does not guarantee adequate bioavailability. As an example, diets high in phytate interfere with gastrointestinal zinc absorption and may result in zinc deficiency even if the dietary zinc content appears to be sufficient *(32,33)*. Interactions between micronutrients (iron and vitamin C, copper and zinc) can also influence bioavailability.

2.8. Absorption and Excretion

In addition to compromised absorption, alterations in excretion can also result in a trace element deficiency or toxicity. An example of compromised absorption is hemochromatosis, a serious disorder of excessive organ iron accumulation that results from a failure of the normal control of iron absorption *(34–36)*. Liver disease patients with ineffective biliary excretion have developed serious and even fatal manganese toxicity since the bile is the major excretory route for this essential trace element *(37,38)*. These two diseases and Wilson's disease are examples of the substantial toxicity that can result when the usual homeostasis of an essential trace element is compromised, resulting in high organ metal concentrations and consequent cellular toxicity. (*see* Chapters 12 and 17)

2.9. Cause Versus Effect

An important clinical consideration is the distinguishing between cause versus effect. There is abundant evidence that severe zinc deficiency can cause a life-threatening impairment in cellular immune function *(39)*. In contrast, some diseases and conditions may themselves produce alterations in trace element metabolism. For example, alterations in copper metabolism are not a known cause of Hodgkins disease or non-Hodgkins lymphoma, but these diseases cause substantial changes in circulating copper concentrations that may be useful in monitoring responses to chemotherapy *(40)*. Pregnancy also alters the metabolism of a number of trace elements, including copper, zinc, and iron *(41,42)*. (*see* Chapter 8)

2.10. Treatment of a Disease

A related consideration is that the treatment of a disease, not the disease itself, may change trace element or mineral metabolism. Patients on total parenteral nutrition (TPN) can develop trace element deficiencies if the TPN fluids do not contain adequate quantities of these nutrients *(43,44)* (*see* Chapter 20). Ethambutol, a chelating drug used to treat tuberculosis, has been reported to decrease visual acuity due to its interaction with zinc *(45)*. As previously mentioned, penicillamine used to treat Wilson's disease may cause symptomatic zinc deficiency since it can promote the excretion of zinc as well as copper.

2.11. Pharmacologic Effects

A final consideration is that high doses of micronutrients may produce beneficial (or adverse) "pharmacologic" effects even in the absence of an underlying deficiency. For example, zinc at high doses well above the RDA can be effective in the treatment of Wilson's disease *(46,47)*, and high doses have also been reported to reduce the duration of symptoms of the common cold in some but not all studies *(48,49)*. These effects are not due to correction of an underlying deficiency.

A comparison to aspirin may aid in understanding this idea. Aspirin can be highly effective in a short period of time for treating pain or inflammation. It can also reduce the risk of a second heart attack in patients who take low doses daily. However, few would argue that these effects are due to correction of "aspirin deficiency."

The concepts briefly outlined in this chapter can be useful for understanding the clinical nutrition of the essential trace elements and minerals, as presented in detail in the subsequent chapters of this book.

ACKNOWLEDGMENT

This work was supported in part by a grant from the National Institutes of Health (HL56581).

REFERENCES

1. Subcommittee on the Tenth Edition of the RDAs, Food and Nutrition Board, National Research Council Recommended Dietary Allowances 10th Edition, National Academy Press, Washington D.C. 1989.
2. Mertz W. The essential trace elements. Science 1981;213:1332–1338.
3. Standing Committee on the Scientific Evaluation of Dietary Reference Intakes. Food and Nutrition Board. Institute of Medicine. Dietary Reference Intakes for Calcium, Phosphorus, Magnesium, Vitamin D, and Fluoride. National Academy Press, Washington, D.C. 1997.
4. Klevay LM. Teaching the recommended dietary allowances. Am J Clin Nutr 1970;23:1639–1641.
5. Underwood BA. From research to global reality: the micronutrient story. J Nutr 1998;128:145–151.
6. Ramalingaswami V. Challenges and opportunities – one vitamin, two minerals. Nutr Res 1998;18:381–390.
7. Hoffman HW, Phyliky RL, Fleming CR. Zinc-induced copper deficiency. Gastroenterol 1988;94:508–512.
8. Prasad AS, Brewer GJ, Schoomaker EB, Rabbani P. Hypocupremia induced by zinc therapy in adults. J Amer Med Assoc 1978;240:2166–2168.
9. Sandstead HH. Requirements and toxicity of essential trace elements illustrated by zinc and copper. Am J Clin Nutr 1995;61:621S–624S.
10. Shamberger RJ. Biochemistry of Selenium. Plenum Press, New York,1983, pp. 149–154.
11. Friberg L, Piscator M, Nordberg GF, Kjellström T. Cadmium in the Environment. CRC Press. Cleveland OH, 1974,54–55.
12. Bogden JD, Oleske JM, Louria DB. Lead poisoning: one approach to a problem that won't go away. Environ Health Perspect 1997;105:1284–1287.
13. Miller GD, Massaro TF, Massaro EJ. Interactions between lead and essential elements: a review. Neurotoxicology 1990;11:99–120.
14. Hallberg L, Brune M, Erlandsson M, Sandberg A, Russander-Holten L. Calcium: effect of different amounts on non-heme and heme-iron absorption in humans. Am J Clin Nutr 1991;53:112–119.
15. Argiratos V, Samman S. The effect of calcium-carbonate and calcium citrate on the absorption of zinc in healthy female subjects. Eur J Clin Nutr 1994;48:198–204.
16. Mills CF, Davis GK. Molybdenum in: Mertz W ed. Trace Elements in Human and Animal Nutrition, 5th ed. Academic Press, New York, 1986.pp. 429–463.
17. Davis GK. Microelement interactions of zinc, copper, and iron in mammalium species. Ann NY Acad Sci 1980;355:130–139.
18. Gallery ED, Blomfield J, Dixon SR. Acute zinc toxicity in hemodialysis. Br Med J 1972;4:331–333.
19. World Health Organization. Trace Elements in Human Nutrition and Health. World Health Organization Geneva, 1996, pp. 210–211.
20. Mertz W. Chromium occurrence and function in biological systems. Physiol Rev 1969;49:163–239.
21. Gad SC. Acute and chronic systemic chromium toxicity. Sci Total Environ 1989;86:149–157.
22. O'Flaherty EJ. A physiologically based model of chromium kinetics in the rat. Toxicol Appl Pharm 1996;138:54–64.
23. Vassiliev VB, Kachorin AM, Beltramini M, Roco GP, Salvato B, Gaitskhoki US. Copper depletion/repletion of human ceruloplasmin is followed by the changes in its spectral features and functional properties. J Inorgan Biochem 1997;65:167–174.
24. Hambidge KM, Casey CE, Krebs WF. Zinc, In: Mertz W, ed. Trace Elements in Human and Animal Nutrition – 5th Ed., Vol. 2. Academic Press, New York, 1986,pp. 1–137.
25. Davis GK, Mertz W. Copper, In: Mertz W, ed. Trace Elements in Human and Animal Nutrition – 5th Ed., Vol. 1. Academic Press, New York 1986,pp. 301–364.
26. Hurley LS, Keen CL. Manganese, In: Mertz W, ed. Trace Elements in Human and Animal Nutrition – 5th Ed. Vol. 1. Academic Press, New York ,1986, pp. 185–223.
27. Levander O. Selenium, In: Mertz W, ed. Trace Elements in Human and Animal Nutrition– 5th Ed. Academic Press, New York, 1986, pp. 209–219.
28. Klevay LM. Copper and other chemical elements that affect the cardiovascular system. In: Chang LW, ed. Toxicology of Metals. Lewis Publishers, New York, 1996, pp. 921–928.

29. Klingberg WG, Prasad AS, Oberleas D. Zinc deficiency following penicillamine therapy. In: Trace Elements in Human Health and Disease, Vol 1. Academic Press, New York, 1976, pp. 51–65.
30. Gillies ME, Birkbeck JA. Tea and coffee as sources of some minerals in the New Zealand diet. Amer J Clin Nutr 1983;38:936–942.
31. Bogden JD, Zadzielski E, Aviv A. Extraction of copper and zinc from rubber and silicone stoppers. J Toxicol Environ Health 1983;11:967–969.
32. Sandstrom B. Consideration in estimates of requirements and critical intake of zinc. Analyst 1995;120:913–915.
33. Larsson M, Rossander-Hulthen L, Sandstrom R, Sandberg AS. Improved zinc and iron absorption from breakfast meals containing malted oats with reduced phytate content. Br J Nutr 1996;76:677–688.
34. Rouault T. Hereditary hemochromatosis. J Amer Med Assoc 1993;269:3152–3154.
35. Bothwell TH. Overview and mechanisms of iron regulation. Nutr Rev 1995;53:237–345.
36. Lynch SR. Iron overload: prevalence and impact on health. Nutr Rev 1995;53:255–260.
37. Krieger D. Manganese and chronic hepatic encephalopathy. Lancet 1995;346:270–274.
38. Fell JM, Reynolds AP, Meadows N, Khan K, Long SG, Quaghebeur G, Taylor WJ, Milla DJ. Manganese toxicity in children receiving long-term parenteral nutrition. Lancet 1996;347:1218–1221.
39. Oleske JM, Westphal M, Shore S, Gorden D, Bogden J, Nahmias A. Zinc therapy of depressed cellular immunity in acrodermatitis enteropathica. Its correction. Amer J Dis Child 1979;133:915–918.
40. Gupta SK, Shukla VK, Gupta V, Gupta S. Serum trace elements and Cu/Zn ratio in malignant lymphoma in children. J Tropical Pediatr 1994;40:85–187.
41. Bogden JD, Thind IS, Kemp FW, Caterini H. Plasma concentrations of calcium, chromium, copper, iron, magnesium, and zinc in maternal and cord blood and their relationship to low birth weight. J Lab Clin Med 1978;92:455–462.
42. Bogden JD, Thind IS, Louria DB, Caterini H. Maternal and cord blood metal concentrations and low birth weight — a case-control study. Amer J Clin Nutr 1978;31:1181–1187.
43. Okadu A, Takagi Y, Nezu R, Sando K, Shenkin A. Trace element metabolism in parenteral and enteral nutrition. Nutrition 1995;11(Suppl 1),106–113.
44. Rudman D, Williams RJ. Nutrient deficiencies during total parenteral nutrition. Nutr Rev 1985;43:1–13.
45. Delacoux E, Moreau A, Godefroy A, Evstigneef T. Prevention of ocular toxicity of ethambutol: study of zincaemia and chromatic analysis. J Francois Ophthamol 1978;1:191–196.
46. Brewer GJ, Johnson U, Kaplan J. Treatment of Wilson's disease with zinc: XIV. Studies of the effect of zinc on lymphocyte function. J Lab Clin Med 1997;129:649–652.
47. Czlonkowska A, Gajda J, Rudo M. Effects of long-term treatment in Wilson's disease with D-penicillamine and zinc sulphate. J Neurol 1996;243:269–273.
48. Anonymous. Zinc lozenges reduce the duration of common cold symptoms. Nutr Rev 1997;55:82 85.
49. Mossad SB, Macknin ML, Medendorp SV, Mason D. Zinc gluconate lozenges for treating the common cold. Annals Intern Med 1996;125:81–88.

2   Possibly Essential Trace Elements

Forrest H. Nielsen, PhD

1. INTRODUCTION

An ever expanding number of mineral elements have received attention as being of possible importance in the prevention of disease with nutritional roots, or for the enhancement of health and longevity. Because of some promising physiological or clinical finding, most often in an animal model or a special human situation, these elements are promoted by the supplement industry, some authors of health books and newsletters, and other merchants of "health-promoting" materials whose objective is financial gain by taking advantage of the desire "to live better and to live longer." It is not difficult for the public to get authoritative reports by apparently well-qualified individuals expounding the nutritional or health benefits of some element; most often the benefit involves avoiding some of life's most feared diseases such as cancer, heart disease, and loss of cognitive function. Health and nutrition professionals will have many of these mineral elements brought to their attention by their clients. Ignoring the questions or dismissing the claims without providing sound reasons is unlikely to counteract an "authoritative" report that often gives disparaging statements about authentic health professionals. Additionally, several of these mineral elements apparently have health benefits that are now only being discovered or defined; some of these benefits might be the result of unrecognized essential functions. Being aware of these benefits could be of use in providing information that could promote health and well-being. Thus, it is appropriate that these possibly essential trace elements be discussed in a clinical nutrition text such as this book.

At least 15 elements could be considered possibly essential; these are aluminum, arsenic, boron, bromine, cadmium, chromium, fluorine, germanium, lead, lithium, nickel, rubidium, silicon, tin, and vanadium. The key characteristic of these elements is that, although there is circumstantial evidence suggesting essentiality, they do not have a defined specific biochemical function in higher animals. The quality of circumstantial evidence for nutritional essentiality varies widely for these elements. As indicated in this chapter, the evidence is substantial for arsenic, boron, chromium, nickel, silicon, and vanadium. The evidence for essentiality for the other listed elements is more limited in nature, often includes apparent deficiency findings in experimental animals that were not very marked or not necessarily indicative of a suboptimal biological function, or were obtained under less than satisfactory experimental conditions.

From: *Clinical Nutrition of the Essential Trace Elements and Minerals: The Guide for Health Professionals*
Edited by: J. D. Bogden and L. M. Klevay © Humana Press Inc., Totowa, NJ

2. DEFINITION OF ESSENTIALITY

2.1. Early Definitions of Essentiality

According to the Food and Nutrition Board *(1)*, the concept of essential nutrients was well established by 1940. Nutrients were defined as chemical substances found in food that are necessary for life, and tissue growth and repair; those that the body cannot synthesize were called essential (or indispensable). Essential nutrients were identified when dietary deficiency led to disease or failure to grow. The use of animal growth models to identify essential nutrients and to quantify requirements was the foundation of early experimental nutrition. In the 1960s and 1970s, the criteria for establishing essentiality of mineral elements that could not be fed at dietary concentrations low enough to cause death or to interrupt the life cycle (interferes with growth, development, or maturation such that procreation is prevented) usually included the following *(2–6)*:

1. The element must react with biological material or form chelates.
2. The element must be ubiquitous in sea water and the earth's crust. In other words, it had to be present during evolution of organisms so it could be incorporated when essential functions developed which required the element.
3. The element must be present in a significant quantity in animals.
4. The element should be toxic to animals only at relatively high intakes in comparison to nutritional intakes.
5. Homeostatic mechanisms must exist for the element so that it is maintained in the body in a rather consistent amount during short term variations in intake.
6. Finally, and most importantly, a dietary deficiency must consistently and adversely change a biological function from optimal, and this change is preventable or reversible by physiological amounts of the element.

Eventually, this criterion by itself became a definition of essentiality *(7,8)*.

2.2. Current Acceptance of Definitions of Essentiality

In the 1980s and 1990s, establishing essentiality on the basis of the above criteria began to receive resistance when a large number of elements was suggested to be essential based on some small change in a physiological or biochemical variable. The use of criterion number six above seemed to be too liberally applied to changes found in experimental animals that were supposedly fed a diet deficient in some element. Many of these changes were questioned as to whether they were necessarily the result of a suboptimal function, and sometimes were suggested to be the consequence of a pharmacological or toxicological action in the body, including an effect on intestinal microorganisms. As a result of this questioning, if the lack of an element can not be shown to cause death or to interrupt the life cycle, many scientists, probably a majority, now do not consider an element essential unless it has a defined biochemical function. However, there still are scientists that base essentiality on the older criteria. Thus, there is no universally accepted list of trace elements that are considered essential. This explains why, in other chapters of this book, the elements chromium and fluoride are considered essential, but based on the apparently more generally accepted definition of essentiality today, probably should be considered only possibly essential. Furthermore, because chromium and fluoride were considered before pre-1980 criteria for essentiality began to receive considerable challenge, the Food and Nutrition Board of the National Academy of Sciences established estimated safe and adequate daily dietary intakes (ESADDI) for these elements in 1980 *(9)* which were continued in 1989 *(10)*. New dietary reference intakes for fluoride were established in 1997 *(11)*.

2.3. Other Terms Used to Describe Nutritional Effects

2.3.1. CONDITIONAL ESSENTIALITY

Recently the term "conditional essential nutrient" has appeared in the nutritional literature. In 1993, Harper *(12)* defined this term as nutrients, ordinarily dispensable, that become indispensable under certain pathologic conditions. Conditional essential nutrients also have been defined as nutrients that must be provided in the diet for maintenance of health for certain people, or at specific ages, stages, or pathologic conditions *(13)*. This term has been applied to several of the possibly essential trace elements because they have been shown to have essential-type actions when an animal is exposed to an environmental, nutritional, physiological, or hormonal stressor. However, the term conditionally essential seems to be applicable mainly to organic substances (e.g., glutamine, carnitine) with known biochemical functions and normally synthesized by the body, but under certain situations, not produced in sufficient quantities so that an endogenous source is needed. Thus, the term does not apply well to the possibly essential mineral elements.

2.3.2. PHARMACOLOGICALLY BENEFICIAL

In 1985, Nielsen *(14)* described concerns about some of the findings used to suggest essentiality for some trace elements. One concern was that "control animals" used for comparison with "deficient animals" often were fed very high amounts of an element under investigation; the amounts were 10 to 1000 times the suggested requirement. It was suggested that some of the differences between control and deficient animals were caused by toxicological or pharmacological actions of the trace element. Pharmacological action was defined as the ability of a dietary intake of a substance to alleviate a condition other than the nutritional deficiency of that substance, or to alter biochemical function(s) or biological structure(s) in a therapeutic way. In 1994, the Food and Nutrition Board *(1)* stated that for pharmacological effects, doses greatly exceeding the amount of a nutrient present in foods are usually needed to obtain a therapeutic response; the specificity of the pharmacological action is often different from the physiological function; and chemical analogs of the nutrient that are often most effective pharmacologically may have little or no nutritional activity. Examples of well-established pharmacologically beneficial elements include fluoride, which has the ability to protect against pathological demineralization of calcified tissues, and lithium which has antimanic properties.

2.3.3. NUTRITIONALLY BENEFICIAL

Another term that has been used recently for the possibly essential trace elements is nutritionally beneficial elements. This term has not been defined but the signal characteristics that differentiate it from the term pharmacologically beneficial are the amount of the element needed to produce a biological action in vivo and the nature of the effect (restorative rather than therapeutic). The amount supplemented to a control animal is usually less than 10 times that in the diet of the deficient animal. Because they do not take dosage into consideration, some people consider pharmacologically beneficial and nutritionally beneficial to be synonymous. Nutritionally beneficial differs from conditionally essential in that it applies to substances without a defined biochemical function. Because I have promoted the term nutritionally beneficial, a definition seems appropriate here. An element is nutritionally beneficial if it has health restorative effects, when compared to animals fed an apparent deficient intake of that element, at intakes that are found with normal diets; these health restorative effects can be amplified by nutritional, physiological, hormonal, or metabolic stressors. This definition implies that the change caused by a low intake of the element eventually has detrimental consequences and thus a certain intake is desirable.

The use of stressors to demonstrate nutritionally beneficial effects is a concept that helps in the delineation of situations in which an element is important. The basis for this concept is the formula *(15)*:

$$\text{Pathological effects} = \text{stress} \times \text{organic vulnerability}$$

This formula states that pathological effects are likely to be minor if the low dietary intake of an element is not multiplied by some significant stressor. Similarly, an organism probably can handle a specific stressor easily if there is no organic vulnerability (e.g., low intake of some trace element, disease) that alters mechanisms used to deal with the stressor. But, the multiplication of a subnormal intake of a nutritionally important element times the presence of a stressor enhancing the need for that element most likely will lead to pathological consequences.

Examples of nutritionally beneficial elements whose health restorative effects have been shown to be amplified by a stressor are boron, whose effects can be amplified by a marginal vitamin D_3 deficiency *(16,17)*; arsenic, whose effects apparently can be amplified by an amino acid imbalanced diet (high in arginine and/or low in methionine) *(18)*; and, vanadium whose effect can be amplified by deficient or luxuriant dietary iodine *(19,20)*.

3. NUTRITIONAL IMPORTANCE BEYOND ESSENTIALITY

Although the elements discussed in this chapter do not meet the current strict definition of essentiality, the other aforementioned definitions indicate that they can be of nutritional importance. It is well known that diet is linked to risks leading to chronic disease that are disabling and terminate life prematurely. Moreover, dietary components other than essential nutrients, or essential nutrient (e.g., selenium) intakes beyond those that prevent deficiency pathology, have been found to promote health and reduce the risks leading to chronic disease. As a result the Food and Nutrition Board *(1)* concluded that the reduction in the risk of chronic disease is a concept that should be included in the formulation of future Recommended Dietary Allowances (which are now being called Dietary Reference Intakes [DRI]) where sufficient data for efficacy and safety exist *(11)*. In other words, a new paradigm is emerging in which the dominating role of the concept of deficiency in the determination of nutritional requirements is being complemented by the concern for the total health effects of a nutrient *(21)*. For nutrients that are given dietary intake recommendations that exceed those required to prevent deficiency pathology, this includes the determination of an upper safe level of intake. Moreover, the new paradigm includes making recommendations for substances that are not considered nutritionally essential. Because several of the possibly essential trace elements have been found to have nutritionally beneficial effects that indicate they may be useful in reducing the risks leading to chronic disease, they probably deserve a set of dietary intake recommendations; that is, even though conclusive evidence for essentiality remains to be determined, some possibly essential trace elements are nutritionally important.

Another reason that DRIs need to be considered for some of the possibly essential trace elements is that regulatory agencies, which still routinely adhere to the paradigm of elements being divided into essential and toxic categories, often use the reports of the Food and Nutrition Board to establish which elements are essential and not essential. The reports are also used for setting toxic thresholds. As a result, elements for which emerging evidence suggests nutritional and health benefits are subjected to risk assessments and given toxicological standards that may be in conflict with amounts apparently beneficial to health.

4. CATEGORIZATION OF THE POSSIBLY ESSENTIAL TRACE ELEMENTS

Circumstantial evidence used to support the contention that a trace element is essential generally fits into four categories. These are:

1. A dietary deprivation in some animal model consistently results in a changed biological function, body structure, or tissue composition that is preventable or reversible by an intake of an apparent physiological amount of the element in question.
2. The element fills the need at physiological concentrations for a known in vivo biochemical action to proceed in vitro.
3. The element is a component of known biologically important molecules in some life form.
4. The element has an essential function in lower forms of life.

In this discussion, an element is considered to have strong circumstantial support for essentiality if it has all four types of evidence, and limited or weak circumstantial support if it has only one or two types of evidence. Through the use of these criteria, one can conclude from the following discussion that there is strong circumstantial evidence for the essentiality of arsenic, boron, chromium, nickel, silicon, and vanadium, and limited circumstantial evidence for the essentiality of aluminum, bromine, cadmium, fluorine, germanium, lead, lithium, rubidium, and tin.

5. EVALUATION OF THE CLINICAL NUTRITIONAL IMPORTANCE OF THE POSSIBLY ESSENTIAL TRACE ELEMENTS

5.1. Aluminum

The circumstantial evidence for the essentiality of aluminum is limited. A dietary deficiency of aluminum in goats reportedly results in increased abortions, incoordination and weakness in hind legs, and decreased life expectancy (22,23). Aluminum deficiency also has been reported to depress growth in chicks (24). Additionally, aluminum in vitro has been described as being required for the activation of the guanine nucleotide-binding regulatory component of adenylate cyclase by fluoride (25); being able to stimulate DNA synthesis in quiescent cultures of Swiss 3T3 and 3T6 cells (26); and being able to stimulate osteoblasts to form bone through activating a putative G-protein coupled sensing system (27).

In the popular media and with the general public, aluminum essentiality does not receive much attention; it is mostly directed toward aluminum toxicity because at one time it was suggested that this could be a cause of Alzheimer's disease (28,29). Although ingestion of high dietary amounts of aluminum is questioned as a cause of Alzheimer's disease (30,31), toxicity still is the major clinical or nutritional concern for aluminum. High intakes of aluminum from such sources as buffered analgesics and antacids by susceptible individuals (e.g., those with impaired kidney function (see Chapter 16), including the elderly and low-birth-weight infants) may lead to pathological consequences and thus should be avoided *(32)*. Aluminum toxicity is of most concern when contaminated solutions are used for parenteral feeding or for kidney dialysis *(32,33)*; this has led to neurotoxicity and adverse skeletal changes. Severe neurotoxicity, called dialysis dementia, is characterized by speech disturbances, disorientation, seizures, and hallucinations. Aluminum skeletal toxicity is characterized by bone pain and fractures.

Aluminum toxicity or deficiency should not be of concern if dietary intakes are near those in a typical well-balanced diet. The typical daily dietary intake of aluminum is 2 to 25 mg. Rich sources of aluminum include baked goods prepared with chemical leavening agents (e.g., baking powder), processed cheese, grains, vegetables, herbs, and tea *(34)*.

5.2. Arsenic

The circumstantial evidence to support arsenic essentiality is somewhere between strong and limited. Arsenic deprivation has been induced in chickens, hamsters, goats, pigs, and rats *(18,35–37)*. In the goat, pig, and rat, the most consistent signs of arsenic deprivation were depressed growth and abnormal reproduction characterized by impaired fertility and increased perinatal mortality. Other notable signs of deprivation in goats were depressed serum triglyceride concentrations and death during lactation. Myocardial damage also occurred in lactating goats. Other reported signs of arsenic deprivation include changes in mineral concentrations in various organs, including exacerbation of kidney calcification in female rats fed diets conducive to calcification *(38)*. The response to arsenic deprivation can be changed and enhanced by nutritional stressors that affect sulfur amino acid or labile methyl-group metabolism *(18)*.

Arsenic has been shown to activate some enzymes in vitro *(35)*, probably by acting as a substitute for phosphate. Other in vitro actions of arsenic include the induction of certain proteins known as heat shock or stress proteins in isolated cells *(39)*; increased methylation of the p53 promoter, or DNA, in human lung cells *(40)*; and enhancement of DNA synthesis in unsensitized human lymphocytes and in those stimulated by phytohemagglutinin *(41)*. The most important biochemical forms of arsenic are those that contain methyl groups. Methylation of inorganic oxyarsenic anions occurs in organisms ranging from microbial to mammalian. The methylated endproducts include arsenocholine, arsenobetaine, dimethyarsinic acid, and methylarsonic acid *(42,43)*. Arsenolipids and arsenosugars are found in a variety of marine life *(43)*.

A biochemical function for arsenic has not been identified in lower forms of life, although a microorganism designated MIT-13 reduces As^{5+} to As^{3+} to gain energy for growth *(44)*. However, there are enzymes that methylate arsenic with S-adenosylmethionine as the methyl donor *(45)*. Arsenite methyltransferase is the enzyme that methylates arsenite. Methylation of the monomethylarsenic acid by monomethylarsenic acid methyltransferase yields dimethyarsinic acid, the major form of arsenic in urine.

Although the attention of the media is directed toward the toxicity of arsenic, the evidence for essentiality suggests that this element may be of nutritional importance. Results of numerous epidemiological studies suggest an association between chronic arsenic overexposure and the incidence of some forms of cancer, particularly skin cancer; however, the role of arsenic in carcinogenesis, especially at low intakes, remains controversial *(46)*. Arsenic does not seem to act as a primary carcinogen and is either an inactive or extremely weak mitogen. In contrast, it has been suggested that arsenic could play an essential role in humans because injuries of the central nervous system, vascular diseases, and cancer were correlated with markedly decreased serum arsenic concentrations *(47)*.

Arsenic deprivation possibly predisposes an animal or human to cancer because deprivation decreases the S-adenosylmethionine/S-adenosylhomocysteine ratio in some tissues *(36)*; such a decreased ratio has been associated with DNA hypomethylation, and this is associated with some types of cancer *(48,49)*. Regardless of the final outcome in the determination of the nutritional role of arsenic, it is important to recognize that arsenic most likely is essential for humans. Thus, the belief that any form or amount of arsenic is unnecessary, toxic, or carcinogenic is unrealistic, if not potentially harmful.

Based on data obtained from animal studies, a possible arsenic requirement for humans was determined to be about 12–25 µg daily *(50)*. Because of differences in the means by which they determine the safe intake of arsenic, toxicologists and nutritionists have arrived at different values. A reference dose (RfD), which is an amount of exposure in a lifetime that is unlikely to cause adverse effects, of 0.3 µg/kg body weight/d (21 µg/d for a 70 kg person) has been suggested for arsenic *(51)*. Nutritionists have suggested that a safe upper limit of arsenic intake could well be 140–250 µg/d *(50)*. Reports from various parts of the world indicate that the average daily intake of arsenic is in the range of 12–60 µg *(50,52)*. In the United States, the individual mean total arsenic intake from all food, excluding shellfish, has been estimated to be 30 µg/d *(52)*. Fish, grain, and cereal products contribute the most arsenic to the diet.

5.3. Boron

Although boron is categorized here as an element with strong circumstantial evidence for essentiality, it probably should be considered as an established essential nutrient for higher animals because it has recently been found that boron is required to complete the life cycle of fish *(53)* and frogs *(54)*. This is complemented by the fact that boron is essential for plants to complete their life cycle *(55)*. Naturally occurring boron-containing biological compounds include antibiotics synthesized by various bacteria *(56)*, and a bis (rhamnogalacturonan-II)-borate complex in plant cell walls *(57)*. Boron influences the activity of a number of enzymes in vitro *(56)*. This has led to the hypothesis that boron acts as a metabolic regulator by complexing with a variety of substrate or reactant compounds that have hydroxyl groups in favorable positions *(16)*. Because this complexing usually results in competitive inhibition of enzymes in vitro, the regulation is hypothesized to be mainly negative.

A large number of responses to boron deprivation have been found. These responses suggest that boron deprivation impairs calcium metabolism, brain function, and energy metabolism *(58)*. Recent studies also suggest that boron deprivation impairs immune function and exacerbates adjuvant-induced arthritis in rats *(59,60)*. As often happens with the possibly essential elements, a lack of response of experimental animals to lower dietary boron has been reported. The experimental conditions used in these reports need to be closely evaluated for shortcomings. For example, one report suggested that boron supplementation compared to boron deprivation may actually be detrimental to bone calcification in ovariectomized rats fed a diet marginal in magnesium *(61)*. However, the boron supplementation used was 40 mg/kg diet, an amount at least 40 times that considered adequate and thus was not nutritional, and may even have amplified the marginal magnesium deficiency. This made it difficult to detect changes caused by low dietary boron.

Boron is the only element discussed in this chapter that has findings derived from a controlled deprivation of humans. In two studies, men over the age of 45, postmenopausal women, and postmenopausal women on estrogen therapy were fed a low-boron diet (about 0.25 mg/2000 kcal) for 63 d and then fed the same diet supplemented with 3.0 mg of boron/day for 49 d *(62)*. The major differences between the two experiments were the intakes of copper and magnesium; in one experiment they were marginal or inadequate, in the other, they were adequate. Some findings from these two experiments are summarized in Table 1. Boron supplementation after depletion also enhanced the elevation in serum 17β–estradiol and plasma copper caused by estrogen ingestion *(63)*, altered encephalograms to suggest improved behavioral activation (e.g., less drowsiness) and mental alertness, and improved psychomotor skills and the cognitive processes of attention and memory *(64)*.

An unsuccessful attempt to induce a response to low dietary boron in humans has been reported *(65)*, which might have resulted in negative impressions about the nutritional importance of boron. Several aspects of the experimental design of this attempt, however, almost assured lack of success, and thus make the study ill-suited for making a nutritional assessment of boron. For example, the subjects were only equilibrated on the experimental diet for two days before starting on the low dietary regimen, and this regimen lasted only 21 d. The data presented from only six subjects suggests that they were still adjusting from their self-selected diets to the experimental diet, and thus to changes in other nutrient intakes when they began receiving boron supplementation. Moreover, 21 d is an extremely short period of deprivation for an adult organism when the diet is only marginally deficient and statistical power is limited by a small number of subjects. In the successful experiments, 14 subjects were equilibrated to the experimental diet for 14 d, and the first 21 d of boron deprivation were not included in the analysis *(62)* because only minimal responses occurred during this time.

Within 3 months of the first report *(66)* describing findings from nutritional experiments with humans, boron supplements were being marketed. Shortly thereafter, numerous health claims for boron began to appear in tabloids, magazines, advertisements, and so on; these included boron preventing and/or curing osteoporosis, being an ergogenic aid, preventing or curing arthritis, stopping memory loss and keeping motor skills sharp. These health claims generally were the result of overzealous extrapolation of the findings from humans *(67)*, but have since moderated markedly in tone and manifestation. Nonetheless, health claims for boron still appear with some regularity.

Although probably not to the extent that one would be led to believe by the marketers of boron, there may be some validity to the suggestion that boron is of practical nutritional importance. An analysis of both human and animal data resulted in the suggestion that an acceptable safe range of population mean intakes of boron for adults could well be 1 to 13 mg/d *(68)*. Based on recent analysis of foods and food products, estimations of daily intakes of various age and sex groups have been made. There are reports indicating that many people are consuming much less than 1 mg/d *(69,70)*. Foods of plant origin, especially fruits, leafy vegetables, nuts, and legumes, are rich sources of boron *(71)*, while meat, fish, and dairy products are poor sources.

At present, there is no clinical disorder that can be conclusively attributed to suboptimal boron nutriture. Nonetheless, because boron is a biologically dynamic element at physiological concentrations in higher animals, it would not be surprising to find that it could influence the occurrence or severity of some disorders with uncertain or multiple causes (e.g., osteoporosis, arthritis, urolithiasis). Thus, there is an urgent need to identify the specific biochemical roles of boron to facilitate the determination of its clinical and nutritional importance.

Table 1
Responses of Boron-Deprived (0.25 mg/2,000 kcal for 63 Days) Men Over
Age 45, Postmenopausal Women, and Postmenopausal Women on Estrogen
Therapy to a 3.0 mg Boron/Day Supplement for 49 Days[a]

Metabolism affected	Evidence for effect
Macromineral and electrolyte	Increased serum 25-hydroxycholecalciferol
	Decreased serum calcitonin[b]
Energy	Decreased serum glucose[b]
	Increased serum triglycerides[c]
Nitrogen	Decreased blood urea nitrogen
	Decreased serum creatinine
	Increased urinary hydroxyproline excretion
Oxidative	Increased erythrocyte superoxide dismutase
	Increased serum ceruloplasmin
Erythropoiesis/hematopoiesis	Increased blood hemoglobin[c]
	Increased mean corpuscular hemoglobin content[c]
	Decreased hematocrit[c]
	Decreased platelet number[c]
	Decreased red cell number[c]

[a] Compiled by Nielsen [62]. n = 5 men, 4 postmenopausal women, and 5 postmenopausal women on estrogen therapy in each of two experiments.
[b] Found when dietary copper was marginal and magnesium was inadequate.
[c] Found when dietary copper and magnesium were adequate.

5.4. Bromine

Only limited circumstantial evidence exists to support the essentiality of bromine. It has been reported that a dietary deficiency of the bromide anion results in depressed growth, fertility, hematocrit, hemoglobin, and life expectancy, and in increased milk fat and abortions in goats (72,73). Also, insomnia exhibited by some hemodialysis patients has been associated with bromide deficiency (74). Bromide was found to alleviate growth retardation caused by hyperthyroidism in mice and chicks, and to substitute for part of the chloride requirement of chicks (75–77). There has been a report describing the isolation of a bromine-containing compound from human cerebrospinal fluid, with properties corresponding to 1-methyl heptyl-γ-bromoacetoacetate (78); this compound has been shown to provoke paradoxical sleep when administered intravenously to cats (79).

Bromine has received very little attention as an element with some health consequence. However, before barbiturates were used, doctors prescribed bromide for sleep. The bromide anion has a low order of toxicity; thus, it is not of toxicological concern in nutrition. The typical daily intake of bromide is 2 to 8 mg. Rich sources of bromide are grains, nuts, and fish (80).

5.5. Cadmium

The circumstantial evidence for the essentiality of cadmium is very limited. Cadmium deficiency reportedly depresses the growth of goats (81), and rats (82); these findings were obtained in experiments with some shortcomings (8). Cadmium has transforming growth factor activity and stimulates the growth of cells in soft agar *(83)*. It is a consistent component of metallothionein, a high-sulfhydryl-containing protein apparently involved in regulating cadmium distribution in the body *(84)*. Although there is a possibility that cadmium is an essential element at very low intakes, it is of more concern because of its toxic properties *(84)*. Cadmium is a potent antagonist of several essential minerals, including zinc, copper, iron, and calcium. It has a long half-life in the body and thus it does not take much of an elevation in intake to result in an accumulation that could lead to damage to some organs, especially the kidney. In addition to renal dysfunction, high cadmium intakes have been associated with hypertension, some types of cancer, and osteomalacia. The World Health Organization has set 70 µg/d for a 70 kg person as an upper safe intake of cadmium *(85)*. The typical daily dietary intake of cadmium is 10 to 20 µg. Sources of cadmium include shellfish, grains (especially those grown on high-cadmium soils), and leafy vegetables *(84)*.

5.6. Chromium

The circumstantial evidence for chromium is strong. In fact, preliminary reports suggest that a defined biochemical function has been identified for chromium *(86)*, thus it probably should be considered an established essential element. The nutritional and clinical importance of chromium is described elsewhere in this book (*see* Chapters 1, 4, 7–9, 11, 13 and 20).

5.7. Fluorine

Only limited circumstantial evidence exists to support fluorine essentiality. It has been reported that fluoride deficiency in rats depressed growth *(87)* and in goats decreased life expectancy and caused pathological histology in the kidney and endocrine organs *(88,89)*. This report is complemented by the finding that pharmacological doses of fluoride improve fertility, hematopoiesis, and growth of iron-deficient mice and rats *(90)*; prevent phosphorus-induced nephrocalcinosis *(91)*, and can prevent pathological demineralization of bones and teeth *(90)*. About 99% of fluorine in the body exists in mineralized tissues as fluoroapatite *(90)*. Fluoride in vitro activates some enzymes of which the best known is adenylate cyclase *(90)*.

In clinical nutrition, the importance of high intakes of fluoride in the prevention of dental caries is well known and well established *(92)*. In the lay media, the suggestion that high intakes of fluoride may be useful in increasing bone density and thus preventing osteoporosis occasionally appears. Although the use of pharmacologic amounts of fluoride to prevent bone loss is still being investigated, its usefulness in this regard seems limited in comparison to estrogen or calcium *(93)* (*see* Chapter 14).

The popular media also has given some attention to notions that fluoridation of water poses some health risks such as increasing the risk of contracting AIDS, cancer, Down's syndrome, heart disease, kidney disease, and osteoporosis. But the evidence from numerous reports by reputable scientists has discredited these notions as having essentially no scientific basis. However, because fluoride accumulates in bone, chronic high exposure to this element through food or water results in crippling fluorosis characterized by osteomalacia, osteoporosis, and/or osteosclerosis; areas of the world where this is prevalent include India, China, South Africa, and Tanzania *(94)*.

Although fluoride is not generally considered an essential element for humans, it is still considered a pharmacologically beneficial element. Thus, the Food and Nutrition Board

(11) has established Adequate Intakes (AI) and Tolerable Upper Levels (UL) for fluoride. For adults, the AI for females is 3.8 mg/d and for males is 3.1 mg/d. The UL for adults is 10 mg/d. The major source of dietary fluoride in the United States is drinking water; about 52% of the population uses water with a fluoride concentration adjusted between 0.7 and 1.2 mg/L *(95)*. There are also many people whose drinking water contains naturally high fluoride concentrations. The richest dietary sources of fluoride are tea and marine fish that are consumed with their bones. Fluoride is ubiquitous in foodstuffs, but similar products can vary greatly with source. Foods marketed in different parts of the United States contribute about 0.3 to 0.6 mg to the daily intake of fluoride *(10)*.

5.8. Germanium

The circumstantial evidence for the essentiality of germanium is very limited. In the rat, a low germanium intake alters the mineral composition of bone and liver, and decreases tibial DNA concentrations *(96)*. Germanium also reverses some changes in rats caused by silicon deprivation *(96)* and some organic germanium compounds have antitumor activity in animal models *(97)*. In plants, germanium supplementation can delay boron deficiency signs *(98)*.

In recent years, organic germanium compounds, such as carboxyethyl germanium sesquioxide (Ge-132) and lactate-citrate-germanate have been marketed as nutritional supplements with immune enhancing or anticancer properties. These organic germanium supplements were promoted by a series of lay-directed monographs that began to appear in 1987 *(97)*. These publications failed to indicate that the amounts of germanium used to get responses in animal models were pharmacological, not nutritional. They also did not mention that high intakes of inorganic germanium, which is more toxic than organic forms of germanium, cause kidney damage *(97)*. Some individuals consuming high amounts of organic germanium supplements contaminated with inorganic germanium have died from kidney failure *(97)*.

Germanium should not be of deficiency or toxicologic concern if dietary intakes are near those in a typical well-balanced diet. The typical daily dietary intake of germanium is 0.4 to 1.5 mg. Wheat bran, vegetables, and leguminous seeds are high in germanium *(80)*.

5.9. Lead

The circumstantial evidence for the essentiality of lead is limited to findings that an apparent dietary deprivation results in changes in experimental animal models. A large number of those findings have come from one research group which found that a low dietary intake has adverse effects in pigs and rats *(99–102)*. Apparent deficiency signs found include depressed growth; anemia; elevated serum cholesterol, phospholipids, and bile acids; disturbed iron metabolism; decreased liver glucose, triglycerides, LDL-cholesterol and phospholipid concentrations; increased liver cholesterol; and altered blood and liver enzymes. This work is complemented by the finding that lead supplementation improved development of suboptimally growing rats *(103)*, and alleviated iron deficiency signs in young rats *(104)*; these later findings have been suggested to be pharmacological in nature. Lead in vitro can affect biochemical systems because it binds with a variety of anionic ligands, including sulfhydryl, imidazole, carboxyl, and phosphate groups. The usual result of lead binding to enzymes is inhibition, although lead can substitute in vitro for other metals with the retention of some activity, e.g., alkaline phosphatase *(105)*. These in vitro findings do not provide strong support for lead essentiality. Lead is not known to be essential for lower forms of life, or to be a component of some important biological molecule in some life form.

In the popular media and with the general public, lead essentiality does not receive much credence; attention is mainly directed as it should be toward lead toxicity. Lead is considered a major environmental pollutant because of past use of lead-based paints and combustion of fuels containing lead additives. Because of environmental pollution, current body lead burdens are 2 to 3 orders of magnitude greater than those of our preindustrial ancestors *(106)*. Lead toxicity *(105,107)* results in anemia, kidney damage, and central nervous system abnormalities ranging from subtle IQ deficits to ataxia and stupor to coma and convulsions. Ingestion of high amounts of lead from the environment by children has been associated with reduced intelligence and impaired motor function. Lead toxicity is enhanced by iron and calcium deficiencies *(105)*.

The possibility that lead is essential cannot be dismissed. However, if it is essential, any requirement is likely to be very small and easily achieved. In other words, in clinical nutrition, lead intakes that are too high are the major concern. A safe intake probably is a typical daily intake of lead with a balanced diet; such intakes are probably in the range of 5 to 50 μg/d. Foods relatively high in lead include seafood and plant foodstuffs grown in soils with high lead concentrations *(108)*.

5.10. Lithium

Lithium is an element difficult to categorize. There is no question that it is a pharmacologically beneficial element because of it antimanic properties *(109)*. Its ability to affect mental function perhaps explains the findings that the incidence of violent crimes is higher in areas with low-lithium drinking water concentrations *(110)*, and aggression was greater in lithium-supplemented than rats with low lithium intakes *(111)*. However, lithium is not known to be essential for lower forms of life, or be an integral part of some important biological molecule in any life form. The circumstantial evidence for essentiality comes from its effects at nutritional amounts in experimental animals. Lithium deficiency reportedly results in depressed fertility, birth weight, and life span and in altered activity of several liver and blood enzymes in goats *(112,113)*. In rats, lithium deficiency apparently depresses fertility, birth weight, litter size, and weaning weight *(114,115)*. Low dietary lithium also has been associated with decreased aggression, and delayed wheel-running activity with decreased amplitude in rats *(111)*. Lithium has been shown to stimulate growth of some cultured cells *(116)*. Another pharmacologic action of lithium is that it has insulin mimetic properties *(117)*.

In contrast to its antidiabetogenic action indicated above, therapeutic amounts of lithium for treatment of mental disorders can cause nephrogenic diabetes insipidus *(118)*. In fact, the principal disadvantage in the use of lithium for psychiatric disorders is the narrow safety margin between therapeutic and toxic doses. Mild lithium toxicity results in gastrointestinal disturbances, muscular weakness, tremor, drowsiness, and a dazed feeling *(109)*. Severe toxicity results in coma, muscle tremor, convulsions, and even death *(109)*.

Having some lithium in the diet is apparently beneficial. The typical daily dietary intake of lithium of 200 to 600 μg probably is close to amounts that are beneficial but yet safe. Rich sources of lithium include eggs, processed meat, fish, milk, milk products, potatoes, and vegetables *(113)*.

5.11. Nickel

The circumstantial evidence for the essentiality of nickel is substantial. The reported signs of nickel deprivation for six animal species — chicken, cow, goat, pig, rat, and sheep — are extensive and have been listed in several reviews *(119–122)*. Unfortunately, many of the reported signs may have been misinterpreted manifestations of pharmacologic actions of nickel *(14,123)*. However, recent studies with rats and goats indicate that nickel deprivation depresses growth, reproductive performance, and plasma glucose and alters the distribution of other elements in the body, including calcium, iron, and zinc *(124)*. As with other ultratrace elements, the nature and severity of signs of nickel deprivation are affected by diet composition. For example, both vitamin B_{12} and folic acid affect the response to nickel deprivation *(125–127)*. Nickel is essential for enzymatic hydrogenation, desulfurization, and carboxylation reactions in mostly anaerobic microorganisms *(128,129)*, and in a tightly bound form is required for the activity of urease, an enzyme found in both plants and microorganisms *(130,131)*. In higher animals and in vitro, nickel can complex, bind, or chelate with many substances of biologic interest, and is found in a blood macroglobulin called nickeloplasmin *(132)*. In vitro, nickel can activate numerous enzymes.

Because nickel has not been associated with any chronic disease, it has not received much attention in the lay media or from the supplement industry. However, this could change if it is confirmed that nickel has an effect on the function of vitamin B_{12} or folic acid. These vitamins are receiving attention because each has an influence on the concentration of homocysteine in blood which, in high concentrations, has been associated with an increased risk of cardiovascular disease *(133)*. Moreover, increased folic acid intake has been associated with decreased neural tube defects in newborns *(134)*.

Life threatening toxicity of nickel through oral intake is unlikely. Because of excellent homeostatic regulation, nickel salts exert their toxic action mainly by gastrointestinal irritation and not by inherent toxicity *(135)*. However, nickel may have adverse effects in humans at relatively low intakes. An oral dose in water as low as 0.6 mg as nickel sulfate, which is well absorbed, given to fasting subjects produced a positive skin reaction in some individuals with nickel allergy *(136)*. That dose is only a few times higher than the human daily nickel requirement postulated on the basis of results from animal studies.

Based on intake data and extrapolation from animal experiments, a dietary requirement for humans of 25 to 35 μg/d has been suggested for nickel *(137)*. An upper safe intake is difficult to determine because of the nickel allergy finding described above, and, because of this, probably should be lower than 600 μg/d. Total dietary nickel intakes of humans vary greatly with the amounts and proportions of foods of animal (nickel-low) and plant (nickel-high) origin consumed. Rich sources of nickel include chocolate, nuts, dried beans, peas, and grains *(137,138)*; diets high in these foods could supply more than 900 μg nickel/d. Conventional diets, however, often provide less than 150 μg daily, and some much less than 100 μg daily.

5.12. Rubidium

The circumstantial evidence supporting rubidium essentiality is limited. Rubidium deficiency in goats reportedly results in depressed food intake, growth, and life expectancy and increased spontaneous abortion *(139)*. These findings with goats are complemented by earlier reports that rubidium can possibly act as a nutritional substitute for potassium in some functions, especially in lower forms of life *(80)*, and can affect some neurophysiological functions such as turnover of brain norepinephrine *(140)* and electroencephalogram activation *(141)*. Rubidium has not been described as essential for lower forms of life and has not been identified as an integral part of some biologically important molecule. Rubidium is relatively nontoxic and thus not of toxicologic concern.

Because rubidium is not of toxicologic concern and has not been associated with any chronic disease, it has not received any attention from the lay media or the supplement industry. Nonetheless, rubidium has been shown to have positive effects under certain situations in some living organisms and thus could be beneficial for higher animals. The typical daily dietary intake of rubidium of 1 to 5 mg probably can be considered safe and, if essential, adequate. Good sources of rubidium include coffee, black tea, fruits, vegetables (especially asparagus), and poultry *(142)*.

5.13. Silicon

There is strong circumstantial evidence indicating silicon is an essential nutrient. Signs of silicon deficiency in chickens and rats demonstrate aberrant metabolism of connective tissue and bone *(143–145)*. Silicon-deprived chicks exhibited structural abnormalities of the skull and longbone abnormalities characterized by small poorly formed joints, defective endochondral growth and depressed contents of articular cartilage, water, hexosamine, and collagen *(143–146)*. Rats fed a diet low in calcium and silicon and high in aluminum accumulated high amounts of aluminum in the brain; silicon supplements prevented the accumulation *(147)*. In bone tissue culture, silicon is required for maximal prolylhydroxylase activity *(148)*. Silicon is essential for some lower classes of organisms (diatoms, radiolarians, and sponges), in which silica serves a structural role *(144)*. In animals, silicon is consistently found bound in collagen and glycosaminoglycans, but the chemical nature of the binding has not been rigorously defined. Silicon has been suggested to be present as a silanolate, an ether or ester derivative of silicic acid *(145)*.

Silicon is essentially nontoxic when taken orally. Magnesium trisilicate, an over-the-counter antacid, has been used by humans for more than 40 yr without obvious deleterious effects. Other silicates are food additives used as anticaking or antifoaming agents *(149)*.

As early as 1911, researchers *(150)* suggested that silicon might have antiatheroma activity. In the 1970s, reports appeared suggesting that inadequate dietary silicon may contribute to some cases of atherosclerosis and hypertension, in addition to some bone disorders, Alzheimer's disease, and the aging process *(146,151)*. Since then, reports have periodically appeared that give further support for silicon being nutritionally important in preventing some chronic diseases associated with aging. Surprisingly, these reports seem to have been generally ignored by media personnel or the supplement industry. However, if further evidence indicates that silicon nutriture affects macromolecules such as glycosaminoglycans, collagen and elastin, and thus is needed for healthy bones, brains, and blood vessels *(146)*, this may change. Thus, dietary recommendations are probably appropriate for silicon.

Postulating a silicon requirement is difficult because only limited data are available. Rats fed about 4.5 mg silicon/kg diet, mostly as the very available sodium metasilicate, do not differ from rats fed about 35 mg silicon/kg diet; both prevent, equally well, silicon deficiency signs exhibited by rats fed about 1.0 mg silicon/kg diet *(146)*. Thus, if dietary silicon is highly available, as animal data suggest, the human requirement for silicon is quite small, perhaps in the range of 2 to 5 mg/d. However, much of the silicon found in most diets probably is not absorbable or as available as sodium metasilicate; significant amounts probably occur as aluminosilicates and silica, from which silicon is not readily available. Thus, the recommended intake of silicon probably should be higher than the estimated requirement. On the basis of balance data, a silicon intake of 30 to 35 mg/d was suggested for athletes, which was 5 to 10 mg higher than that for nonatheletes *(152)*. Average daily intakes of silicon apparently range from about 20 to 50 mg *(153)*. The best sources of silicon are unrefined grains of high fiber content and cereal products *(154,155)*.

5.14. Tin

Tin is another element for which there is only limited evidence to support essentiality. A dietary deficiency of tin has been reported to depress growth, response to sound, and feed efficiency; to alter the mineral composition of several organs; and to cause hair loss in rats *(156,157)*. Tin has been found in high concentrations in thymus and thus has been suggested to be of importance in immune function *(158)*. On the other hand, tin has not been found essential for lower forms of life, nor has it been found to be a component of a biologically important molecule in any life form.

Inorganic tin is relatively nontoxic. However, routine consumption of foods packed in unlacquered tin-plated cans may result in excessive exposure to tin, which could adversely affect the metabolism of other trace elements including zinc and copper *(159)*.

Tin has not received much attention from the lay media or supplement industry. This is probably appropriate because of its uncertain nutritional importance, and because it has not been shown to have any marked beneficial action in higher animals. Nonetheless, the possibility of essentiality cannot be ignored. An appropriate daily intake probably is that found in the typical diet, or 1 to 40 mg. Canned foods often are high in tin *(159)*.

5.15. Vanadium

The circumstantial evidence for the essentiality of vanadium is substantial. However, the statement made by Schroeder et al. *(160)* in 1963 that "no other trace metal has so long had so many supposed biological activities without having been proved to be essential" still remains true today. Signs of apparent vanadium deficiency have been described for goats *(161)* and rats *(19)*. For goats, the signs included an elevated abortion rate and depressed milk production. About 40% of kids from vanadium-deprived goats died between days 7 and 91 of life, with some deaths preceded by convulsions; only 8% of kids from vanadium-supplemented goats died during the same time. Also, skeletal deformations were seen in the forelegs, and forefoot tarsal joints were thickened *(161)*. Vanadium-deprived rats exhibited altered thyroid hormone metabolism *(19,20)*, especially when stressed with high or low iodine intakes. Supporting the suggestion that vanadium is essential for higher animals is the finding of functional roles for vanadium in lower forms of life. Algae, lichens, fungi, and bacteria all have enzymes that require vanadium for activity *(162–164)*. These enzymes include haloperoxidases, which catalyze the oxidation of halide ions by hydrogen peroxide, thus facilitating the formation of a carbon-halide bond. Some bacteria have a vanadium-containing nitrogenase, which reduces nitrogen gas to ammonia *(165)*.

Numerous biochemical and physiological functions for vanadium have been suggested on the basis of its in vitro actions on cells and pharmacological actions in animals. These actions include insulin-mimetic properties, numerous stimulatory effects on cell proliferation and differentiation, effects on cell phosphorylation-dephosphorylation, effects on glucose and ion transport across the plasma membrane, and effects on oxidation-reduction processes *(166–169)*.

Vanadium is receiving a fair amount of attention from the lay media and the supplement industry because of its ability to mimic insulin. The antidiabetic effects of vanadium have been investigated in animal models of type I and II diabetes *(170)*. In type II diabetic models, vanadium prevented the depletion of insulin stores, lowered plasma insulin concentrations, and improved tolerance to glucose loads. These improvements developed through correction of the poor sensitivity to insulin of peripheral tissues, particularly muscles. Recent research indicates that vanadium improves glucose metabolism by improving the transport of glucose into the cell where it can be metabolized. Because these findings suggest that vanadium could have an anabolic effect on skeletal muscle and other tissues through insulin promotion of amino acid uptake and protein synthesis while retarding protein degradation, vanadium salts alone, or in combination with other nutrients, herbs, and amino acids in the form of tablets, capsules, powders, and beverages have been put on the market as muscle and strength enhancers. The amounts of vanadium in these nutritional supplements and formulations are not nutritional, but are pharmacological, and potentially toxic.

The amounts of vanadium used in animals to show insulin-mimetic actions were extremely high to the point of being toxic. Poor appetite, poor growth, diarrhea, and death have commonly occurred in some studies because of the high dosages of vanadium given *(170)*. It should be noted that long term high vanadium supplementation induced hypertension in rats *(171)*. Moreover, vanadium pentoxide, vanadyl sulfate, and sodium metavanadate have been shown to be genetoxic in various bacterial systems, and mouse and human cell lines; thus, high vanadium intakes may be potentially carcinogenic *(172)*. However, no increase in the incidence of cancer was observed in the few studies that have addressed this question in whole animals.

Experiments have been performed in which small doses of vanadyl sulfate (100 mg/d), or sodium metavanadate (125 mg/d) were administered to diabetic patients for two to three weeks *(173–176)*. The "small doses" are an order of magnitude greater than possible nutritional needs indicated below, but they were about 100-fold lower than those used in most studies of diabetic animal models. Type I diabetic patients showed no consistent glycemic control response, but their daily insulin requirements decreased; in type II diabetic patients, insulin sensitivity increased during vanadium treatment. Although these results look promising, concern needs to be directed to evidence indicating that the threshold level for human vanadium toxicity is about 10 to 20 mg/d, or about one-fifth the doses that had these mildly beneficial effects *(177)*. These findings demonstrate that there are no nutritional bases to tout vanadium as an antidiabetic or anabolic agent, and that it is dangerous to attempt to use it in therapeutic amounts in diabetes.

If vanadium is essential for humans, its requirement most likely is very small. The diets used in animal deprivation studies contained only 2 to 25 µg vanadium/kg diet; these amounts often did not markedly affect the animals. Vanadium deficiency has not been identified in humans, yet diets generally supply less than 30 µg vanadium daily and most supply only 15 µg daily *(138,178,179)*. Thus, a daily dietary intake of 10 µg vanadium probably will meet any postulated requirement. Suggesting an upper safe nutritional intake for vanadium is difficult because humans apparently are more tolerant of high vanadium intakes than experimental animals such as rats, and there are only limited human toxicological data on which to base a suggestion. There are findings indicating an

Table 2
Summary of Some Characteristics of Mineral Elements Suggested to be Essential but Lacking a Defined Biochemical Function

Element	Evidence for Essentially	Apparent Deficient Intake Per Kg/Diet (Species)	Typical Human Daily Dietary Intake	Major Clinical Nutritional Concern
Aluminum	Limited; deficiency signs reported for two species; positive in vitro biochemical actions.	160 µg (goat)	2–10 mg	High intakes by individuals with impaired kidney function could lead to pathology.
Arsenic	Strong; deficiency signs reported for several species; enzymes exist for metabolizing arsenic; epidemiological evidence indicating beneficial or essential effects in humans.	<25 µg (chicks) 35 µg (goat) <15 µg (hamster) <30 µg (rat)	12–60 mg	Both low (<12 µg/day) or high (>250 µg/day) intakes possibly enhance susceptibility to some forms of cancer (bladder, kidney, liver, lung, skin).
Boron	Strong; deficiency signs reported for several species including humans; essential for plants, affects enzyme action in vitro.	<0.3 mg (chick) 0.25–0.35 mg/day (human) <0.3 mg (rat)	0.5 –3.5 mg	Deficient intakes might impair calcium metabolism, brain function and energy metabolism.
Bromine	Limited; nonspecific deficiency signs reported only for one species; supportive findings probably caused by pharmacologic action, or substitution for essential elements.	0.8 mg (goat)	2–8 mg	No major clinical concern at present.
Cadmium	Limited; depressed growth main deficiency sign reported; component of metallothionein	<5 µg (goat) <4 µg (rat)	10–20 mg	High intakes which can lead to kidney damage, and possibly result in hypertension, osteomalacia, and some types of cancer. Accumulative in cigarette smokers. Upper safe intake set by World Health Organization is 70 µg/day for 70 kg person.

Table 2, continued
Summary of Some Characteristics of Mineral Elements Suggested to be Essential but Lacking a Defined Biochemical Function

Element	Evidence for Essentiality	Apparent Deficient Intake Per Kg/Diet (Species)	Typical Human Daily Dietary Intake	Major Clinical Nutritional Concern
Chromium	Strong; deficiency signs reported for several species including humans; epidemiologic and supplementation studies show beneficial or essential actions.	<20 μg/ day (humans) <100 μg (rat)	25–50 μg	Low intakes resulting in impaired insulin action in metabolizing glucose, decreased stores with age.
Fluorine	Limited; depressed growth main deficiency sign reported; most reported beneficial effects are the result of pharmacologic action.	<0.3 mg (goat) <0.45 mg (rat)	Fluoridated areas, 1–3 mg; Nonfluoridated areas, 0.3–0.6 mg	Phamacologically beneficial in preventing caries; high intakes result in tooth mottling and crippling skeletal fluorosis.
Germanium	Limited; deficiency signs reported only for one species, may have some beneficial pharmacologic action.	0.7 mg (rat)	0.4–3.4 mg	High intakes of inorganic supplements resulting in kidney failure.
Lead	Moderate but controversial; numerous deficiency signs reported for two species; can be pharmacologically beneficial to iron-deficient animals.	<32 μg (pig) <45 μg (rat)	15–50 μg	High intakes which could result in anemia, kidney damage and central nervous system abnormalities including IQ deficits.
Lithium	Moderate; deficiency signs reported for two species; in vitro and epidemiologic evidence of beneficial or essential action; beneficial pharmacologic actions.	<1.5 mg (goat) <15 μg (rat)	200–600 μg	Pharmacologically beneficial for treating mania; narrow safety margin between therapeutic and toxic doses.

Table 2, continued
Summary of Some Characteristics of Mineral Elements Suggested to be Essential but Lacking a Defined Biochemical Function

Element	Evidence for Essentially	Apparent Deficient Intake Per Kg/Diet (Species)	Typical Human Daily Dietary Intake	Major Clinical Nutritional Concern
Nickel	Strong; deficiency signs reported for several species; functional roles (mainly an essential component of specific enzymes) exist for nickel in lower forms of life; activates numerous enzymes in vitro.	<100 µg (goat) <20 µg (rat)	70–260 µg	High intakes possibly exacerbate nickel allergy.
Rubidium	Limited; nonspecific deficiency signs only for one species.	180 µg (goat)	1–5 mg	No major clinical concern at present.
Silicon	Strong; deficiency signs reported for two species; functional roles exist in lower form of life; beneficial effects with high intakes under certain conditions.	<2.0 mg (chick) <4.5 mg (rat)	20–50 mg	No major clinical concern at present; low intakes possibly enhance susceptibility to some chronic diseases associated with aging.
Tin	Limited; deficiency signs reported for one species.	<20 µg (rat)	1–40 mg	No major clinical concern at present; high intakes could adversely affect the metabolism of other trace elements.
Vanadium	Strong; deficiency signs reported for at least three species; numerous pharmacologic and in vitro actions; functional role (essential for enzme activity) in lower forms of life.	<10 µg (goat) <2 µg (rat)	10–30 µg	Potentially toxic intakes through supplement use; more needs to be known about the consequences of chronic intakes one order of magnitude greater than hypothesized requirement.

intake of more than 10 mg daily can result in toxicity. However, much lower amounts of vanadium have been found to have pharmacological actions in humans; this suggests that amounts near these may have toxic manifestations under certain conditions. Most mineral elements at intakes 100 times their nutritional requirement show some toxicity. This suggests that a safe daily intake for vanadium is under 1.0 mg/d and might be 100 µg or less/d. Foods rich in vanadium include shellfish, mushrooms, parsley, dill seed, and some prepared foods *(178,180)*. Beverages, fats and oils, and fresh fruits and vegetables contain the least vanadium (less than 5 ng/g).

6. CONCLUDING STATEMENT

An ever expanding number of mineral elements receive attention as being of possible importance in the prevention of disease with nutritional roots, or for the enhancement of health and longevity. Health and nutrition professionals will have many of these mineral elements brought to their attention because their potential health benefits are often promoted by the lay media and the supplement industry. In addition to the established essential mineral elements, there are at least 15 other elements that have been suggested to be essential; some of these elements are also receiving attention because of their toxic or pharmacologic properties that can affect health and well-being. These elements, whose characteristics are summarized in Table 2 are aluminum, arsenic, boron, bromine, cadmium, chromium, fluorine, germanium, lead, lithium, nickel, rubidium, silicon, tin, and vanadium. The key characteristic of these elements is that, although there is circumstantial evidence suggesting essentiality, they do not have a specific defined biochemical function, or their deficiency has not been shown to interrupt the life cycle in higher animals including humans. Thus, they are usually considered possibly essential; other terms applied to these elements are conditionally essential, pharmacologically beneficial, and nutritionally beneficial. Emerging evidence indicates that two of these elements will soon fit in the category of clearly essential elements. These elements are boron, because it has been shown to interrupt the life cycle of some higher animals, and chromium because of findings of a specific biochemical function. Regardless of whether they meet the strict definition of essentiality, several of the possibly essential elements have effects at physiological or pharmacological amounts that suggest a reduction in risks leading to chronic disease. Furthermore, a new paradigm is emerging in which the dominating role of the concept of deficiency for giving dietary advice, is being complemented or replaced by the concern for the total health effect of a dietary substance. Thus, many of these elements probably deserve a set of dietary recommendations to help people make appropriate decisions that will enable them to achieve the often stated goal of "living longer and better."

REFERENCES

1. Food and Nutrition Board. How Should the Recommended Dietary Allowances Be Revised? National Academy Press, Washington DC, 1994.
2. Schroeder HA, Balassa JJ, Tipton IH. Abnormal trace metals in man-nickel. J Chron Dis 1961;15:51–65.
3. Cotzias GC. Importance of trace substances in environmental health as exemplified by manganese. Trace Sub Environ Health 1967;1:5–19.
4. Underwood EJ. Introduction. In: Underwood EJ, ed. Trace Elements in Human and Animal Nutrition 3rd ed. Academic Press, New York, NY,1971, pp. 1–13.
5. Mertz W. Some aspects of nutritional trace element research. Fed Proc 1970;29:1482–1488.
6. Nielsen FH. Essentiality and function of nickel. In: Hoekstra WG, Suttie JW, Ganther HE, Mertz W, eds. Trace Element Metabolism in Animals-2. University Park Press, Baltimore, MD, 1974,pp. 381–395.

7. Mertz W. The essential trace elements. Science 1981;213:1332–1338.
8. Nielsen FH. Ultratrace elements in nutrition. Annu Rev Nutr 1984;4:21–41.
9. Food and Nutrition Board. National Research Council. Recommended Dietary Allowances 9th ed; National Academy Press, Washington, DC, 1980.
10. Food and Nutrition Board. National Research Council. Recommended Dietary Allowances 10th ed. National Academy Press, Washington, DC, 1989.
11. Food and Nutrition Board. Dietary Reference Intakes for Calcium, Phosphorus, Magnesium, Vitamin D, and Fluoride. National Academy Press, Washington, DC, 1997.
12. Harper AE. Evaluating the concept of nutritional essentiality. Nutritional essentiality: Historical perspective. In: Roche AF, Gussler JD, Silverman E, Redfern DE, eds. Nutritional Essentiality: A Changing Paradigm, Report of the Twelfth Ross Conference on Medical Research. Ross Products Division, Abbott Laboratories, Columbus, OH, 1993,pp.3–11.
13. McCormick DB. The meaning of nutritional essentiality in today's context of health and disease. In: Roche AF, Gussler JD, Silverman E, Redfern DE, eds. Nutritional Essentiality: A Changing Paradigm, Report of the Twelfth Ross Conference on Medical Research. Ross Products Division, Abbott Laboratories, Columbus, OH, 1993,pp.11–15.
14. Nielsen FH. The importance of diet composition in ultratrace element research. J Nutr 1985;115:1239–1247.
15. Tapp WN, Natelson BH. Consequences of stress: a multiplicative function of health status. FASEB J 1988;2:2268–2271.
16. Hunt CD. The biochemical effects of physiologic amounts of dietary boron in animal nutrition models. Environ Health Perspect 1994;1029 (Suppl 7):35–43 .
17. Bai Y, Hunt CD. Dietary boron enhances efficacy of cholecalciferol in broiler chicks. J Trace Elem Exp Med 1996;9:117–132.
18. Uthus EO. Evidence for arsenic essentiality. Environ Geochem Health 1992;14:55–58.
19. Uthus EO, Nielsen FH. Effect of vanadium, iodine and their interaction on growth, blood variables, liver trace elements and thyroid indices in rats. Magnesium Trace Elem 1990;9:219–226.
20. Nielsen FH. Dietary vanadium affects carbohydrate and thyroid metabolism in the BB rat. North Dakota Acad Sci Proc 1998;52:43.
21. Mertz W. Essential trace metals: New definitions based on new paradigms. Nutr Rev 1993;51:287–295.
22. Anke M, Groppel B, Müller M, Regius A. Effects of aluminum–poor nutrition in animals. In: Pais I, ed. Proceedings of the 4 International Trace Element Symposium. New Results in the Research of Hardly Known Trace Elements and Their Importance in the International Geosphere-Biosphere Programme, University of Horticulture and Food Industry, Budapest, 1990,pp.303–324.
23. Angelow L, Anke M, Groppel B, Glei M, Müller M. Aluminum: an essential element for goats. In: Anke M, Meissner D, Mills CF, eds. Trace Elements. Man and Animals–TEMA 8.Verlag Media Touristik, Gersdorf, 1993,pp.699–704.
24. Carlisle EM, Curran MJ. Aluminum: an essential element for the chick in Trace Elements. In: Anke M, Meissner D, Mills CF, eds. Trace Elements. Man and Animals–TEMA 8. Verlag Media Touristik, Gersdorf, 1993,pp.695–698.
25. Sternweis PC, Gilman AG. Aluminum: a requirement for activation of the regulatory component of adenylate cyclase by fluoride. Proc Natl Acad Sci USA 1982;79:4888–4891.
26. Smith JB. Aluminum ions stimulate DNA synthesis in quiescent cultures of Swiss 3T3 and 3T6 cells. J Cell Physiol 1984;118:298–304.
27. Quarles LD, Hartle JE II, Middlcton JP, Zhang J, Arthur JM, Raymond JR. Aluminum-induced DNA synthesis in osteoblasts: Mediation by a G-protein coupled cation sensing mechanism. J Cell Biochem 1994;56:106–117.
28. Crapper McLachlan DR, Farnell BJ. Aluminum and neuronal degeneration. In: Gabay S, Harris J, Ho BT, eds. Metal Ions in Neurology and Psychiatry Alan R Liss, New York, 1985,pp.69–87.
29. Crapper McLachlan DR, Lukiw WJ, Kruck TPA. Aluminum altered transcription and the pathogenesis of Alzheimer's disease. Environ Geochem Health 1990;12:103–114.
30. Glenner GG. The pathobiology of Alzheimer's disease. Ann Rev Med 1989;40:45–51.
31. Joshi JG, Dhar M, Clauberg M, Chauthaiwale V. Iron and aluminum homeostasis in neural disorders. Environ Health Perspect 1994;102(Suppl 3):207–213.
32. Van De Vyver FL, Visser WJ. Aluminum accumulation in bone. In: Priest ND, Van De Vyver FL, eds. Trace Metals and Fluoride in Bones and Teeth. CRC Press, Boca Raton, FL,1990,pp.41–81.
33. Alfrey AC. Aluminum. In: Mertz W, ed. Trace Elements in Human and Animal Nutrition, Vol 2. Academic Press, Orlando, 1986,pp.399–413.
34. Greger JL. Aluminum metabolism. Ann Rev Nutr 1993;13:43–63.

35. Nielsen FH, Uthus EO. Arsenic. In: Frieden E, ed. Biochemistry of the Essential Ultratrace Elements. Plenum, New York, 1984,pp.319–340.
36. Uthus EO. Arsenic essentiality and factors affecting its importance. In: Chappell WR, Abernathy CO, Cothern CR, eds. Arsenic: Exposure and Health. Science and Technology Letters, Northwood,1994,pp.199–208.
37. Anke M. Arsenic. In: Mertz W, ed. Trace Elements in Human and Animal Nutrition, Vol 2. Academic Press, Orlando. 1986;pp:347–372.
38. Uthus EO. Diethyl maleate, an in vivo chemical depletor of glutathioine affects the response of male and female rats to arsenic deprivation. Biol Trace Elem Res 1994;46:247–259.
39. Desrosiers R, Tanguay RM. Further characterization of the posttranslational modifications of core histones in response to heat and arsenite stress in Drosphilia: Biochem Cell Bio 1986;64:750–757.
40. Wang L, Roop BC, Mass MJ. Arsenic hypermethylates the p53 promotor in human lung cells. Fund Appl Toxicol Toxicologist 1996;30:87.
41. Meng Z, Meng N. Effects of inorganic arsenicals on DNA synthesis in unsensitized human blood lymphocytes in vitro. Biol Trace Elem Res 1994;42:201–208.
42. Vahter M. Metabolism of arsenic. In: Fowler BA, ed. Biological and Environmental Effects of Arsenic. Elsevier, Amsterdam, 1983;pp,171–198.
43. Phillips DJH. The chemical forms of arsenic in aquatic organisms and their interrelationships. In: Nriagu JO, ed. Arsenic in the Environment, Part I: Cycling and Characterization. Wiley & Sons, New York, 1994,pp.263–288.
44. Ahmann D, Roberts AL, Krumholz LR, Morel FMM. Microbe grows by reducing arsenic. Nature 1994;371:750.
45. Aposhian HV. Enzymatic methylation of arsenic species and other new approaches to arsenic toxicity. Annu Rev Pharmacol Toxicol 1997;37:397–419.
46. Mushak P. Arsenic and human health: some persisting scientific issues. In: Chappell WR, Abernathy CO, Cothern CR, eds. Arsenic: Exposure and Health. Science and Technology Letters, Northwood, 1994,pp.305–318.
47. Mayer DR, Kosmus W, Pogglitsch H, Mayer D, Beyer W. Essential trace elements in humans. Serum arsenic concentrations in hemodialysis patients in comparison to healthy controls. Biol Trace Elem Res 1993;37:27–38.
48. Dizik M, Christman JK, Wainfan E. Alternatives in expression and methylation of specific genes in livers of rats fed a cancer promoting methyl-deficient diet. Carcinogenesis 1991;12:1307–1312.
49. Zapisek WF, Cronin GM, Lyn-Cook BD, Poirier LA. The onset of oncogene hypomethylation in the livers of rats fed methyl-deficient amino acid-defined diets. Carcinogenesis 1992;13:1869–1872.
50. Uthus EO. Estimation of safe and adequate daily intake for arsenic. In: Mertz W, Abernathy CO, Olin SS, eds. Risk Assessment of Essential Elements. ILSI Press, Washington, DC, 1994,pp.273–282.
51. Abernathy CO, Dourson ML. Derivation of the inorganic arsenic reference dose. In: Chappell WR, Abernathy CO, Cothern CR, eds. Arsenic: Exposure and Health. Science and Technology Letters, Northwood, 1994,pp.295–303.
52. Adams MA, Bolger PM, Gunderson EL. Dietary intake and hazards of arsenic. In: Chappell WR, Abernathy CO, Cothern CR, eds. Arsenic Exposure and Health. Science and Technology Letters, Northwood, 1994,pp.41–49.
53. Rowe RI, Eckhert CD. Boron is essential for zebrafish embryogenesis. FASEB J 1998;12:A205.
54. Forte DJ, Propst TL, Schetter T, Stover EL, Strong PL, Murray FJ. Adverse development and reproductive effects of insufficient boron in Xenopus: Building a case for nutritional essentiality. FASEB J 1998;12:A205.
55. Lovatt CJ, Dugger WM. Boron. In: Frieden E, ed. Biochemistry of the Essential Ultratrace Elements. Plenum, New York, 1984,pp.389–421.
56. Hunt CD. Biochemical effects of physiological amounts of dietary boron. J Trace Elem Exp Med 1996;9:185–213.
57. Power PP, Wood WG. The chemistry of boron and its speciation in plants. Plant and Soil 1997;193:1–13.
58. Nielsen FH. Evidence for the nutritional essentiality of boron. J Trace Elem Exp Med 1996;9:215–229.
59. Bai Y, Hunt CD. Dietary boron alleviates adjuvant-induced arthritis (AIA) in rats. FASEB J 1995;9:A576.
60. Bai Y, Hunt CD. Dietary boron (B) increases serum antibody concentrations in rats immunized with heat-killed mycobacterium tuberculosis (MT). FASEB J 1996;10:A819.
61. Beattie JH, MacDonald A. Effect of boron on bone metabolism in rats. In: Momcilovic B, ed. Trace Elements in Man and Animals–7. IMI, Zagreb, 1991,pp.26:29–26:30.
62. Nielsen FH. Biochemical and physiologic consequences of boron deprivation in humans. Environ Health Perspec 1994;102(Suppl 7):59–63.
63. Nielsen FH, Gallagher SK, Johnson LK, Nielsen EJ. Boron enhances and mimics some effects of estrogen therapy in postmenopausal women. J Trace Elem Exp Med 1992;5:237–246 .

64. Penland JG. Dietary boron: brain function and cognitive performance. Environ Health Perspect 1994;102(Suppl 7):65–72.
65. Beattie JH, Peace HS. The influence of a low-boron diet and boron supplementation on bone, major mineral and sex steroid metabolism in postmenopausal women. Br J Nutr 1993;69:871–884.
66. Nielsen FH. Boron - an overlooked element of potential nutritional importance. Nutr Today 1988;23:4–7.
67. Nielsen FH. Facts and fallacies about boron. Nutr Today 1992;27:6–12.
68. WHO/FAO/IAEA. Trace Elements in Human Nutrition and Health, World Health Organization, Geneva, 1996,pp.175–179.
69. Nielsen FH. Dietary supplementation of physiological amounts of boron increases plasma and urinary boron of perimenopausal women. Proc ND Acad Sci 1996;50:52.
70. Rainey CJ, Christensen RE, Nyquist LA, Strong PL, Coughlin JR. Boron daily intake from the American diet. FASEB J 1996;10:A785.
71. Anderson DL, Cunningham WC, Lindstrom TR. Concentration and intakes of H, B, S, K, Na, Cl, and NaCl, in foods. J Food Comp Anal 1994;7:59–82.
72. Anke M, Regius A, Groppel B, Arnhold W. Essentiality of the trace element bromine. Acta Agron Hung 1990;39:297–303.
73. Anke M, Groppel B, Angelow L, Dorn W, Drusch S. Bromine: an essential element for goats. In: Anke M, Meissner D, Mills CF, eds. Trace Elements in Man and Animals–TEMA 8. Verlag Media Touristik, Gersdorf, 1993,pp.737–738.
74. Oe PL, Vis RD, Meijer JH, van Langevelde F, Allon W, Meer Cvd, Verheul H. Bromine deficiency and insomnia in patients on dialysis. In: Howell JMcC, Gawthorne JM, White CL, eds. Trace Element Metabolism in Man and Animals, TEMA–4. Australian Academy of Science, Canberra, 1981,pp.526–529.
75. Huff JW, Bosshardt DK, Miller OP, Barnes RH. A nutritional requirement for bromine. Proc Soc Exp Biol Med 1956;92:216–219.
76. Bosshardt DK, Huff JW, Barnes RH. Effect of bromine on chick growth. Proc Soc Exp Biol Med 1956;92:219–221.
77. Leach RM Jr, Nesheim MC. Studies on chloride deficiency in chicks. J Nutr 1963;81:193–199.
78. Yanagisawa I, Yoshikawa H. A bromine compound isolated from human cereobrospinal fluid. Biochim Biophys Acta 1973;329:283–294.
79. Torii S, Mitsumori K, Inubushi S, Yanagisawa I. The REM sleep-inducing action of a naturally occurring organic bromine compound in the encéphale isolé cat. Psychopharmacologia 1973;29:65 75.
80. Nielsen FH. Other elements: Sb, Ba, B, Br, Cs, Ge, Rb, Ag, Sr, Sn, Ti, Zr, Be, Bi, Ga, Au, In, Nb, Sc, Te, Tl, W. In: Mertz W, ed. Trace Elements in Human and Animal Nutrition, Vol 2. Academic Press, Orlando, 1986,pp.415–463.
81. Anke M, Hennig A, Groppel B, Partschefeld M, Grün M. The biochemical role of cadmium. In: Kirchgessner M, ed. Trace Element Metabolism in Man and Animals-3. Tech Univ Munchen, Freising–Weihenstephen, 1978,pp.540–548.
82. Schwarz K, Spallholz JE. The potential essentiality of cadmium. In: Bolck F, Anke M, Schneider H-J, eds. Kadmium-Symposium. Friedrich-Schiller Universitat, Jena, 1979,pp.188–194.
83. Barham SS, Tarara JE, Enger MD. Cadmium as a transforming growth factor. Fed Proc 1985;44:520.
84. Kostial K. Cadmium. In: Mertz W, ed. Trace Elements in Human and Animal Nutrition, Vol 2. Academic Press, Orlando, 1986,pp.319–345.
85. World Health Organization. Evaluation of Certain Food Additives and Contaminants. 33rd Report of the Joint FAO/WHO Expert Committee on Food Additives 776. World Health Organization, Geneva, 1989,pp.28–31.
86. Vincent JB. Mechanism of chromium action. In: International Symposium on the Health Effects of Dietary Chromium Abstracts. Dedham, MA, 1998,pp.16 .
87. Schwarz K, Milne DB. Fluorine requirement for growth in the rat. Bioinorg Chem 1972;1:331–338.
88. Anke M, Groppel B, Krause U. Fluorine deficiency in goats. In: Momcilovic B, ed. Trace Elements in Man and Animals-7. IMI, Zagreb, 1991,pp. 26:28–26:29.
89. Avtsyn AP, Anke M, Zhavoronkov AA, Groppel B, Kaktursky LV, Mikhaleva LM, Lösch E. Pathological anatomy of the experimentally-induced fluorine deficiency in she-goats. In: Anke M, Meissner D, Mills CF, eds. Trace Elements in Man and Animals-TEMA 8. Verlag Media Touristik, Gersdorf, 1993,pp.745–746.
90. Messer HH. Fluorine. In: Frieden E, ed. Biochemistry of the Essential Ultratrace Elements. Plenum, New York, 1984,pp.55–87.
91. Fransbergen AJ, Lemmens AG, Beynen AC. Dietary fluoride, unlike bromide or iodide, counteracts phosphorus–induced nephrocalcinosis in female rats. Biol Trace Elem Res 1991;31:71–78.
92. Jenkins GN. The metabolism and effects of fluoride. In: Priest ND, Van De Vyver FL, eds. Trace Metals and Fluoride in Bones and Teeth. CRC Press, Boca Raton, FL, 1990,pp.141–173.

93. Kleerekoper M, Balena R. Fluorides and osteoporosis. Annu Rev Nutr 1991;11:309–324.
94. Krishnamachari KAVR. Fluorine. In: Mertz W, ed. Trace Elements in Human and Animal Nutrition, Vol 1. Academic Press, San Diego, CA, 1987,pp:365–415 .
95. Phipps KR. Fluoride. In: Ziegler EE, Filer LJ Jr, eds. Present Knowledge in Nutrition, 7th ed. ILSI Press, Washington, DC, 1996,pp:329–333.
96. Seaborn CD, Nielsen FH. Effects of germanium and silicon on bone mineralization. Biol Trace Elem Res 1994;42:151–164.
97. Schauss AG. Nephrotoxicity and neurotoxicity in humans from organogermanium compounds and germanium dioxide. Biol Trace Elem Res 1991;29:267–280.
98. Loomis WD, Durst RW. Chemistry and biology of boron. Biofactors 1992;3:229–239.
99. Kirchgessner M, Reichlmayr-Lais AM. Lead deficiency and its effects on growth and metabolism. In: Howell JMcC, Gawthorne JM, White CL, eds. Trace Element Metabolism in Man and Animals, TEMA-4. Australian Academy of Science, Canberra 1981,pp.390–393.
100. Reichlmayr-Lais AM, Kirchgessner M. Newer research on lead essentiality. In: Mills CF, Bremner I, Chesters JK, eds. Trace Elements in Man and Animals-TEMA 5. Commonwealth Agricultural Bureaux, Farnham Royal, 1985,pp.283–286.
101. Reichlmayr-Lais AM, Kirchgessner M. Lead - an essential trace element. In: Momcilovic B, ed. Trace Elements in Man and Animals 7. IMI, Zagreb, 1991,pp.35:1–35:2.
102. Kirchgessner M, Plass DL, Reichlmayr-Lais AM. Lead deficiency in swine. In: Momcilovic B, ed. Trace Elements in Man and Animals 7. IMI, Zagreb, 1991,pp.11:20–11:21.
103. Schwarz K. Potential essentiality of lead. Arh Hig Rada Toksikol 1975;26(Suppl):13–28.
104. Uthus EO, Nielsen FH. Effects in rats of iron on lead deprivation. Biol Trace Elem Res 1988;16:155–163.
105. Quarterman J. Lead. In: Mertz W, ed. Trace Elements in Human and Animal Nutrition, Vol 2. Academic Press, Orlando, 1986,pp:281–317.
106. Patterson C, Ericson J, Manca-Krichten M, Shirahara H. Natural skeletal levels of lead in Homo sapiens sapiens uncontaminated by technological lead. Sci Total Environ 1991;107:205–236.
107. Goyer RA. Lead. In: Bronner F, Coburn JW, eds. Disorders of Mineral Metabolism, Vol I. Academic Press, New York,1981,pp.159–199.
108. Müller M, Anke M, Thiel C, Hartmann E. Exposure of adults to lead from food estimated by analysis and calculation-comparison of methods. In: Anke M, Meissner D, Mills CF, eds. Trace Elements in Man and Animals-TEMA 8. Verlag Media Touristik, Gersdorf, 1993,pp.241–242.
109. Birch NJ. Lithium in medicine. In: Berthon G, ed. Handbook of Metal-Ligand Interactions in Biological Fluids. Bioinorganic Medicine, Vol 2. Marcel Dekker, New York, 1995,pp.1274–1281.
110. Schrauzer GN, Shrestha KP. Lithium in drinking water and the incidence of crimes, suicides, and arrests related to drug addictions. Biol Trace Elem Res 1990;25:105–113.
111. Klemfuss H, Schrauzer GN. Effects of nutritional lithium deficiency on behavior in rats. Biol Trace Elem Res 1995;48:131–139.
112. Anke M, Grün M, Groppel B, Kronemann H. The biological importance of lithium. In: Anke M, Schneider H-J, eds. Mengen-und Spurenelemente. Karl–Marx- Universitat, Leipzig, 1981,pp:217–239.
113. Anke M, Arnhold W, Groppel B, Krause U. The biological importance of lithium. In: Schrauzer GN, Klippel K-F, eds. Lithium in Biology and Medicine. VCH Publishers, Weinheim, 1990,pp.148–167.
114. Patt EL, Pickett EE, O'Dell BL. Effect of dietary lithium levels on tissue lithium concentrations, growth rate and reproduction in the rat. Bioinorg Chem 1978;9:299–310.
115. Pickett EE, O'Dell BL. Evidence for dietary essentiality of lithium in the rat. Biol Trace Elem Res 1992;34:299–319.
116. Rybak SM, Stockdale FE. Growth effects of lithium chloride in BALB/c 3T3 fibroblasts and Madin-Darby canine epithilial cells. Exp Cell Res 1981;136:263–270.
117. Rossetti L, Giaccari A, Klein-Robbenhaar E, Vogel LR. Insulinomimetic properties of trace elements and characterization of their in vivo mode of action. Diabetes 1990;39:1243–1250.
118. Amdisen A. Serum level monitoring and clinical pharmacokinetics of lithium. Clin Pharmacokinet 1977;2:73–91.
119. Nielsen FH. Nickel. In: Frieden E, ed. Biochemistry of the Essential Ultratrace Elements. Plenum, New York, 1984,pp.293–308.
120. Kirchgessner M, Roth-Maier DA, Schnegg A. Progress of nickel metabolism and nutrition research. In: Howell JMcC, Gawthorne JM, White CL, eds. Trace Element Metabolism in Man and Animals, TEMA-4. Australian Academy of Science, Canberra 1981,pp.621–624.
121. Anke M, Groppel B, Kronemann H, Grün M. Nickel - an essential element. In: Sunderman FW, ed. Nickel in the Human Environment. International Agency for Research of Cancer, Lyon, 1984,pp.339–365.

122. Spears JW. Nickel as a "newer trace element" in the nutrition of domestic animals. J Anim Sci 1984;59:823–835.
123. Nielsen FH, Shuler TR, McLeod TG, Zimmerman TJ. Nickel influences iron metabolism through physiologic pharmacologic and toxicologic mechanisms in the rat. J Nutr 1984;114:1280–1288.
124. Nielsen FH. Individual functional roles of metal ions in vivo. Beneficial metal ions. Nickel, In: Berthon G, ed. Handbook of Metal-Ligand Interactions in Biological Fluids. Bioinorganic Medicine, Vol I. Marcel Dekker, New York, 1995, pp.257–260.
125. Nielsen FH, Zimmerman TJ, Shuler TR, Brossart B, Uthus EO. Evidence for a cooperative metabolic relationship between nickel and vitamin B_{12} in rats. J Trace Elem Exp Med 1989;2:21–29.
126. Nielsen FH, Uthus EO, Peollot RA, Shuler TR. Dietary vitamin B_{12} sulfur amino acids and odd-chain fatty acids affect the response of rats to nickel deprivation. Biol Trace Elem Res 1993;37:1–15.
127. Uthus EO, Poellot RA. Dietary folate affects the response of rats to nickel deprivation. Biol Trace Elem Res 1996;52:23–35.
128. Przybyla AE, Robbins J, Menon N, Peck HD, Jr. Structure-function relationships among the nickel-containing hydrogenases. FEMS Microbiol Rev 1992;88:109–136.
129. Hausinger RP. Nickel enzymes in microbes. Sci Tot Environ 1994;148:157–166.
130. Andrews RK, Blakely RL, Zerner B. Urease - a Ni (II) metalleonzyme. In: Lancaster JR Jr, ed. The Bioinorganic Chemistry of Nickel. VCH, New York, 1988,pp.141–165.
131. Mobley HL, Island MD, Hausinger RP. Molecular biology of microbiol ureases. Microbiol Rev 1995;59:451–480.
132. Nomoto S, Sunderman FW Jr. Presence of nickel in alpha-2 macroglobulin isolated from human serum by high performance liquid chromatography. Ann Clin Lab Sci 1988;18:78–84.
133. Malinow MR. Plasma homocyst(e)ine: A risk factor for arterial occlusive diseases. J Nutr 1996;126:1238S–1243S.
134. Oakley GP Jr, Adams MJ, Dickinson CM. More folic acid for everyone now. J Nutr 1996;126:751S–755S.
135. Nielsen FH. Nickel toxicity. In: Goyer RA, Mehlman MA, eds. Advances in Modern Toxicology: Toxicology of Trace Elements, Vol 2. Wiley, New York 1977;pp.129–146.
136. Cronin E, DiMichiel AD, Brown SS. Oral challenge in nickel-sensitive women with hand eczema. In: Brown SS, Sunderman FW Jr, eds. Nickel Toxicology. Academic Press, New York, 1980,pp:149–152.
137. Anke M, Angelow L, Müller M, Glei M. Dietary trace element intake and excretion of man. In: Anke M, Meissner D, Mills CF, eds. Trace Elements in Man and Animals-TEMA 8. Verlag Media Touristik, Gersdorf 1993,pp:180–188.
138. Pennington JAT, Jones JW. Molybdenum, nickel, cobalt, vanadium, and strontium in total diets. J Am Diet Assoc 1987;87:1644–1650.
139. Anke M, Angelow L, Schmidt A, Gürtler H. Rubidium: an essential element for animal and man? In: Anke M, Meissner D, Mills CF, eds. Trace Elements in Man and Animals-TEMA 8. Verlag Media Touristik, Gersdorf 1993,pp. 719–723.
140. Stolk JM, Nowack WJ, Barchas JD, Platman SR. Brain norepinephrine: enhanced turnover after rubidium treatment. Science 1970;168:501–503.
141. Meltzer HL, Nowack WJ, Barchas JD, Platman SR. Rubidium: A potential modifier of affect and behaviour. Nature (London) 1969;223:321–322.
142. Anke M, Angelow L. Rubidium in the food chain. Fresenius J Anal Chem 1995;352:236–239.
143. Carlisle EM. Silicon in bone formation. In: Simpson TL, Volcani BE, eds. Silicon and Siliceous Structures in Biological Systems. Springer, New York, 1981,pp.69–94.
144. Carlisle EM. Silicon. In: Frieden E, ed. Biochemistry of the Essential Ultratrace Elements. Plenum, New York, 1984,pp.257–291.
145. Schwarz K. Recent dietary trace element research exemplified by tin, fluorine, and silicon. Fed Proc 1974;33:1748–1757.
146. Seaborn CD, Nielsen FH. Silicon: A nutritional beneficence for bones, brains, and blood vessels? Nutr Today 1993;28:13–18.
147. Carlisle EM, Curran MJ. Effect of dietary silicon and aluminum on silicon and aluminum levels in the rat brain. Alzheimer Dis Assoc Disorders 1987;1:83–89.
148. Carlisle EM, Berger JW, Alpenfels WF. A silicon requirement for prolyl hydroxylase activity. Fed Proc 1981;40:886.
149. Villota R, Hawkes JG. Food applications and the toxicological and nutritional implications of amorphous silicon dioxide. CRC Crit Rev Food Sci Nutr 1986;23:289–321.
150. Gouget MA. Athérome expérimental et silicate de soude. La Presse Medicale 1911;97:1005–1006.
151. Carlisle EM. Silicon as an essential element. Fed Proc 1974;33:1758–66.

152. Nasolodin VV, Rusin VY, Vorob'ev VA. Zinc and silicon metabolism in highly trained athletes under hard physical stress (in Russian). Vopr Pitan 1987;4:37–39.
153. Kelsay JL, Behall KM, Prather ES. Effect of fiber from fruits and vegetables on metabolic responses of human subjects. II. Calcium, magnesium, iron, and silicon balances. Am J Clin Nutr 1979;32:1876–1880.
154. Bowen HJM, Peggs A. Determination of the silicon content of food. J Sci Food Agric 1984;35:1225–1229.
155. Pennington JAT. Silicon in foods and diets. Foods Addit Contam 1991;8:97–118.
156. Schwarz K, Milne DB, Vinyard E. Growth effects of tin compounds in rats maintained in a trace element-controlled environment. Biochem Biophys Res Commun 1970;40:22–29.
157. Yokoi K, Kimura M, Itokawa Y. Effect of dietary tin deficiency on growth and mineral status in rats. Biol Trace Elem Res 1990;24:223–231.
158. Cardarelli N. Tin and the thymus gland: A review. Thymus 1990;15:223–231.
159. Greger JL. Tin and aluminum. In: Smith KT, ed. Trace Minerals in Foods. Marcel Dekker, New York, 1988,pp.291–323.
160. Schroeder HA, Balassa JJ, Tipton IH. Abnormal trace metals in man - vanadium. J Chronic Dis 1963;16:1047–1071.
161. Anke M, Groppel B, Gruhn K, Langer M, Arnhold W. The essentiality of vanadium for animals. In: Anke M, Baumann W, Bräunlich H, Bruckner C, Groppel B, Grün M, eds. 6th International Trace Element Symposium, Vol 1. Friedrich-Schiller-Universitat, Jena, 1989,pp.17–27.
162. Vilter H. Vanadium-dependent haloperoxidases. In: Sigel H, Sigel A, eds. Metal Ions in Biological Systems, Vol 31, Vanadium and Its Role in Life. Marcel Dekker, New York, 1995,pp,325–362.
163. Wever R, Krenn BE. Vanadium haloperoxidases. In: Chasteen ND, ed. Vanadium in Biological Systems, Physiology and Biochemistry. Kluwer Academic, Dordrecht, Netherlands, 1990,pp.81–97.
164. van Schijndel JWPM, Vollenbroek EGM, Wever R. The chloroperoxidase from the fungus *Curvularia inaequalis;* a novel vanadium enzyme. Biochim Biophys Acta 1993;1161:249–256.
165. Eady RR. Vanadium nitrogenases of Azotobacter. In: Sigel H, Sigel A, eds. Metal Ions in Biological Systems, Vol 31, Vanadium and Its Role in Life. Marcel Dekker, New York, 1995,pp.363–405.
166. Boyd DW, Kustin K. Vanadium: a versatile biochemical effector with an elusive biological function. Adv Inorg Biochem 1984;6:311–365.
167. Nechay BR. Mechanisms of action of vanadium. Annu Rev Pharmacol Toxicol 1984;24:501–524.
168. Willsky GR. Vanadium in the biosphere. In: Chasteen ND, ed. Vanadium in Biological Systems, Physiology and Biochemistry. Kluwer Academic, Dordrecht, Netherlands, 1990,pp.1–24.
169. Stern A, Yin X, Tsang S-S, Davison A, Moon J. Vanadium as a modulator of cellular regulatory cascades and oncogene expressions. Biochem Cell Biol 1993;71:103–112.
170. Orvig C, Thompson KH, Battell M, McNeill JH. Vanadium compounds as insulin mimics. In: Sigel H, Sigel A, eds. Metal Ions in Biological Systems, Vol 31, Vanadium and Its Role in Life. Marcel Dekker, New York, 1995,pp.575–594.
171. Carmignani M, Boscolo P, Ripanti G, Porcelli G, Volpe AR. Mechanisms of the vanadate-induced arterial hypertension only in part depend on the levels of exposure. In: Anke M, Meissner D, Mills CF, eds. Trace Elements in Man and Animals - TEMA 8. Verlag Media Touristik, Gersdorf, 1993,pp.971–975.
172. Agency for Toxic Substances and Disease Registry (ASTDR). Toxicological Profile for Vanadium, US Department of Health and Human Services, Public Health Service, Atlanta, GA, 1992.
173. Cohen N, Halbertstam M, Shlimovich P, Chang CJ, Shamoon H, Rossetti L. Oral vanadyl sulfate improves hepatic and peripheral insulin sensitivity in patients with non-insulin-dependent diabetes mellitus. J Clin Invest 1995;95:2501–2509.
174. Goldfine AB, Simonson DC, Folli F, Patti M-E, Kahn R. Metabolic effects of sodium metavanadate in humans with insulin-dependent and noninsulin-dependent diabetes mellitus in vivo and in vitro studies. J Clin Endocrinol Metab 1995;80:3311–20.
175. Halbertstam M, Cohen N, Shlimovich P, Rossetti L, Shamoon H. Oral vanadyl sulfate improves insulin sensitivity in NIDDM but not in obese nondiabetic subjects. Diabetes 1996;45:659–666.
176. Boden G, Chen X, Ruiz J, van Rossum GDV, Turco S. Effects of vanadyl sulfate on carbohydrate and lipid metabolism in patients with non-insulin-dependent diabetes mellitus. Metabolism 1996;45:1130–35.
177. Nielsen FH. Other Trace Elements. In: Ziegler EE, Filer LJ Jr, eds. Present Knowledge in Nutrition. ILSI Press, Washington, DC, 1996,pp.353–376.
178. Byrne AR, Kosta L. Vanadium in foods and in human body fluids and tissues. Sci Total Environ 1978;10:17–30.
179. Myron DR, Zimmerman TJ, Shuler TR, Klevay LM, Lee DE, Nielsen FH. Intake of nickel and vanadium by humans. A survey of selected diets. Am J Clin Nutr 1978;31:527–531.
180. Myron DR, Givand SH, Nielsen FH. Vanadium content of selected foods as determined by flameless atomic absorption spectroscopy. Agric Food Chem 1977;25:297–300.

3

Consumption of Trace Elements and Minerals by Preagricultural Humans

Stanley B. Eaton III and S. Boyd Eaton, MD

1. INTRODUCTION

The existing human genome reflects evolutionary experience of human and prehuman ancestral species extending ultimately to the origin of life on earth. Comparative studies reveal that over 98% of our genes are shared by chimpanzees and gorillas (*1*) so that most of our genetic makeup must antedate the hominid-pongid split when the ancestors of humans and chimpanzees diverged, perhaps five million years ago. Early hominine evolution, dominated by successive Ardipithecine and Australopithecine species, produced characteristics, including hairlessness and erect posture, which set our ancestors apart from other primates. However, it was the Pleistocene, the 2.5 million years preceding agriculture, during which the defining characteristics of contemporary humans were selected: our resting metabolic rate, body proportions, sexual dimorphism, daily foraging range (which became more like that of carnivores and less primate-like) and brain size (*2,3*). Under certain circumstances genetic evolution can be "rapid." For example, significant changes in large mammal (e.g., red deer, mastodon, bison) body size have occurred in just a few thousand years. However, recent conditions have not been conducive to human evolutionary innovation. Increased population size and greater mobility have led to the conclusion that, ". . . never ever, in the history of any species, have conditions been less propitious for the fixation of evolutionary novelties" (*4 - see* also *5,6*). So, while genetic evolution has continued since the appearance of agriculture, it is not hyperbole to maintain that from the standpoint of our genes all humans living in the present are still Stone Agers — well over 99% identical, genetically, to our ancestors of 15,000 years ago. Our biochemistry and physiology remain adapted for the lifestyle which existed then, not that of the present.

Experiential factors during the Pleistocene, known in human context as the Paleolithic or Old Stone Age, included physical exertion, psychosocial interactions, exposures to toxins and allergens, reproductive experience, microbial encounters, and nutrition. All of these exerted important selective influences on the genetic makeup which still

From: *Clinical Nutrition of the Essential Trace Elements and Minerals: The Guide for Health Professionals*
Edited by: J. D. Bogden and L. M. Klevay © Humana Press Inc., Totowa, NJ

characterizes contemporary humans, but in each case experience in current affluent nations differs greatly from what it was during almost all of human evolution. The time course for change has been variable; for example, the most important alterations in physical exertion and reproduction have occurred only recently, chiefly in the last century. In contrast, human nutrition changed drastically in the earliest days of agriculture: cereal grains, previously used only in times of severe shortage, became the dominant source of food energy, an innovation unprecedented in primate experience (7). The extraordinary dietary perturbations of the twentieth century have further distanced human nutrition from what it was during the evolution of our species.

2. THE DISCORDANCE HYPOTHESIS

To an astonishing degree risk factors for chronic degenerative illnesses, established by clinical and epidemiological investigations, restate differences between ancestral human experiences and those of current humans. Furthermore, preventive recommendations tend to recapitulate major features of the Paleolithic lifestyle. These observations underlie the discordance hypothesis: human biology has been selected for the biobehavioral circumstances of life in the Stone Age and deviations from that paradigm promote the chronic degenerative diseases which have been termed "afflictions of affluence" (8).

The discordance hypothesis places great value on correctly assessing preagricultural human experience and on appreciating how life in the present has come to differ from what it was. In a very real sense the past can serve as a guide for biomedical science generally and for human nutrition in particular. The evolutionary paradigm may eventually become one of the bases for nutritional recommendations; in the present it can serve as a source of novel research initiatives. Furthermore, orthodox investigations sometimes yield results that are hard to interpret or difficult to reconcile with findings from other studies; in such cases the evolutionary benchmark holds potential for improved understanding, a reference standard against which to measure and appreciate the contributions of current, conventional investigative effort.

3. PALEOLITHIC NUTRITION

There was no one standardized nutritional pattern during the 2.5 million years between the emergence of the first Homo species, Homo habilis, and the appearance of agriculture, beginning about 10,000 years ago. Ancestral diets varied according to geographical location, season, climatic conditions, and cultural development. Similar caveats apply to all aspects of experience during this period — including psychosocial development. Evolutionary psychologists have addressed this issue by introducing a concept, the "environment of evolutionary adaptedness" to encompass the broad spectrum of biobehavioral environmental circumstances which occurred during our evolution. The effect is to create a time-weighted statistical composite broadly representative of conditions which influenced past genetic selection (9).

The same principle can be applied to recreating ancestral diets. The "diet of evolutionary adaptedness" (10) is also a temporally and geographically weighted statistical composite integrating subsistence patterns of recent hunter-gatherers from multiple geographical locations, the nutritional makeup of uncultivated plant foods and wild game animals (see data source references), and archeological data concerning the eating patterns of humans during the Paleolithic.

3.1. Basic Considerations

For ancestral humans wild plant foods and game animals provided the overwhelming majority of daily subsistence. Since they had no domesticated animals, there were no dairy products of any sort for humans after they were weaned, typically at about age three. Preagricultural humans presumably knew that cereal grains could be used as food. However, processing costs — the time and energy needed to mill grains into digestible form using technologically primitive methods — were sufficiently great to prohibit their routine use *(11)*. In the earliest agricultural communities grinding grain to a digestible state took four hours each day (for a family of four) and, over time, produced severe arthritic changes in the spines, knees, and toes of those doing the grinding *(12)*. Not surprisingly, cereals remained an emergency ration, consumed chiefly in times of shortage when other foods were largely unavailable.

Animal:plant subsistence ratios for Paleolithic humans varied widely with rainfall, altitude, stage of cultural development, population density, and, especially, latitude. In colder, chiefly Northern, climates, the proportion of animal foods increased whereas in more equatorial regions plants made up a majority of the intake. Time weighting is important in this regard. If the "Out of Africa" scenario is correct, as currently seems likely, the ancestors of all current humans lived in Africa until about 100,000 years ago *(13)*. This means a low latitude, warm climate, relatively high plant food subsistence pattern would have prevailed until fairly recently (in evolutionary context), with few human ancestors reaching really cold environments until 50,000–30,000 years ago. Based on this reasoning, paleoanthropologists and hunter-gatherer specialists have commonly accepted a 35:65 animal:plant subsistence pattern as that typical for preagricultural humans *(14)*. This data has been derived from weighing the food consumed, not by directly assessing contribution to energy intake.

Another consideration of importance involves total energy consumption. Obligatory physical exertion in the Stone Age much exceeded that in present day industrial nations. Furthermore, their skeletal remains show that preagricultural humans were as tall as or slightly taller than we are today. The diminutive stature of most recently studied hunter-gatherers reflects their displacement into areas unsuitable for agriculture and hence generally less fruitful than those that were available to Paleolithic humans. The combination of large stature and obligatory physical exertion means that ancestral humans generally consumed more energy per day than do the more sedentary citizens of current affluent nations — probably half again as much, say 3000 kcal/d (~12MJ/d) for them and 2000 kcal/d (~8MJ/d) for ourselves, on average *(15)*.

3.2. Method

Proximate analyses for both wild game animals (85 species) and unaccultured fruits and vegetables (255 species) have been collected from the literature *(16)*. Averaging nutrient values for these foods is straightforward, but using the averages to reconstitute ancient nutritional patterns involves assumptions which are subject to varying degrees of dispute. The choice of subsistence ratio, degree of selective butchering (i.e., preferential use of organ meats, marrow, and fatty tissue vs muscle tissue), and usage pattern for plant items (fruits/roots/surface vegetables vs nuts and seeds, and so on) all affect the nutrient mix ancestral humans are likely to have enjoyed. However, when these variables have been systematically assessed, the importance of varying preagricultural intake patterns on Paleolithic human nutrition has been found to be far less than the differences which obtain between any given Paleolithic dietary regimen and that typical for affluent Western nations *(17,18)*. The dramatic differences between the range of current diets and those for preagricultural humans appear to result from introduction of food categories "new" in evolutionary context: cereal grains, dairy products, separated fats, alcohol, fatty meat, refined flours, sugar, and other sweeteners. Such foods, some providing relatively "empty calories," (Table 1) now comprise two-thirds or more of our daily energy; they were not a part of ancestral human diets.

Given mean energy values for wild plant foods and game (112 and 129 kcal/100 g, respectively), a simple model *(16)* allows calculation of average daily intake:

$$A(C^aX)+B(C^vX) = \text{Daily Energy Intake}$$

where A and B are the mean energy content (kcal/100g) of animal and vegetable foods, respectively; C^a and C^v are the proportions of animal and vegetable foods (say 35% and 65%, although any complimentary values can be substituted) and X is the total number of food grams necessary to provide a given amount of daily energy — such as 3000 kcal.

When both the gross amounts (814 g meat and 1741 g vegetable foods per day (d) in this instance) and the mean nutrient concentrations in game and wild vegetal items have been estimated, the amounts of individual nutrients as amount/day or amount/1000 kcal can be calculated readily by multiplying the amount of meat or vegetable food per day times the nutrient concentration. For example, $(8.14 \times 100\text{g meat/d}) \times (5.57 \text{ mg iron/100g meat}) = 45.3$ mg iron/d from meat.

3.3. Results Overview

Maximum and minimum estimates for daily intakes of selected minerals for which data on unacculturated plant and wild game nutrient content are available are listed in Table 2. In all cases (except for sodium) Paleolithic intake would have exceeded that in the present, usually by twofold or more, whether the data be presented as intake/d or intake/1000 kcal. These estimates for mineral consumption parallel those presented elsewhere for vitamins *(16)*, whose preagricultural intake also ranged from 2 to 8 times higher than that of present day Westerners. Three factors probably contribute to the striking disparity. Firstly, ancestral humans consumed almost no "empty" calories — energy intake without associated nutrients. The closest Stone Age parallel, honey as found in a nonagricultural setting, has far higher nutrient content (including minerals) than do sugars and other current sweeteners (Table 3). Secondly, uncultivated plants (Table 4) and wild game (Table 5) generally have more nutrients per unit energy than do analogous commercial foods available in the present. For example, the mean iron content of 85 wild game species is 5.57 mg/100 kcal whereas the average of four meat items (T-bone steak, hamburger, frankfurter, and pork sausage) commonly consumed at present is only 0.615 mg/100 kcal. Thirdly, Stone Agers generally consumed more energy per day than do most current humans. Of course, this factor would have affected only the total nutrient intake per day, not nutrient intake per 1000 kcal, but it nevertheless contributes to significant differences. Demand for essential nutrients increases with physical activity far less than the elevation in energy output would seem to warrant *(19)*. Hence Paleolithic nutrient intake would have provided a reserve or extra quota, above currently established requirements. This consideration may impact controversy regarding "optimal" versus "minimal" nutrient requirements and/or recommendations.

Table 1
Nutrient Values of Some Foods "New" in Evolutionary Context
vs Comingled Game and Wild Plant Foods

	Alcoholic Beverages	Carbonated Beverages	Separated Fats	Sugar & Other Sweeteners	Comingled Nutrient Values: 35% Game 65% Wild Plant
			mg/1000kcal		
Iron	1.4	2.67	?	0.16	31.2
Calcium	36.41	103.45	18.2	5.98	540.59
Phosphorus	84.03	181.03	22.53	5.98	1074.14
Magnesium	53.22	34.48	1.3	2.99	407.77
Copper	0.14	0.47	?	0.08	4.06
Zinc	0.42	1.64	0.12	0.07	11.97
Manganese	1.76	0.83	?	0.14	4.43

Alcoholic beverages include beer, red wine, gin, rum, vodka, and whiskey
Carbonated beverages include cola, diet cola, ginger ale, and lemon-lime soda
Separated fats include butter, mayonnaise, and olive oil
Sweeteners include sugar and corn syrup
Data sources (32–34)

4. INDIVIDUAL MINERALS AND TRACE ELEMENTS

4.1. Calcium

Because Paleolithic humans had no dairy foods after weaning it is surprising that their calcium intake generally exceeded present levels. The explanation lies in the high mean calcium content of uncultivated vegetable foods which nearly equals that of milk (20). Except in high latitudes, vegetable intake for Stone Agers made up a very sizable proportion of total energy consumption, so intake of calcium from this source was considerable. Cereal grains, which displaced vegetables and fruits as the major dietary staple with the advent of agriculture, are poor sources of calcium. (Table 4) At present the trade off: high intake of uncultivated vegetable foods vs cereal grains plus dairy foods operates to the detriment of calcium intake. On the other hand, the greater bioavailability of calcium in dairy foods relative to that in some vegetables presumably offsets this differential to an undetermined degree.

4.2. Phosphorus

Paleolithic intake of phosphorus must have varied with the proportion of animal foods in the diet, but in virtually all cases would have exceeded that at present. At lower latitudes, where subsistence depended more heavily on vegetable foods, the ratio between dietary phosphorus and calcium would have approached contemporary levels (~1.6:1), but in colder locations, where animal foods predominated, the amount of phosphorus provided by the diet relative to its calcium content (~4.5:1) would have been substantially higher.

4.3. Iron

The greater dietary iron intake of preagricultural humans reflects the importance of meat in their diets. For an animal-vegetable subsistence ratio of 35:65, iron intake is

Table 2
Paleolithic and Current Mineral Intake

	Fe	Ca	P	Mg	Cu	Zn	Mn
Number of Data Points	193	173	126	153	129	121	49
Subsistence Ratio							
Animal:Plant			Intake, mg/d				
20:80	85.3	1925	2917	1380	13.9	30.9	16.1
35:65	93.6	1622	3223	1223	12.2	35.9	13.3
50:50	101.9	1318	3528	1066	10.4	40.9	10.4
65:35	110.2	1015	3833	909	8.6	46.0	7.6
Paleolithic Intake							
Minimum	85.3	1015	2917	909	8.6	30.9	7.6
Maximum	110.2	1925	3833	1380	13.9	46.0	16.1
Current Intake	18.3	920	1510	320	~1.2	12.3	3.0
Paleolithic:Current							
Intake Ratio							
Minimum	4.7	1.1	1.9	2.8	7.2	2.5	2.5
Maximum	6.0	2.1	2.5	4.3	11.6	3.7	5.4

Data sources (32–37,39–42)

estimated at eight times the current level. At extreme high-latitudes, iron intake must have been higher still, especially since selective butchering emphasizing organ meats would probably have occurred in such environments (21). Humans living in the south central Siberian mammoth steppe between 30,000 and 10,000 years ago were probable examples of such a population and are likely ancestors of Mongoloid peoples who make up the majority of today's human population (22,23). At intake levels of this magnitude, potential toxicity becomes an important consideration, and experimental investigations designed to evaluate effects of the nutrient mix most probable for ancient populations living in such circumstances could be highly instructive.

The experience of nonhuman primates may bear on this topic. Wild howler monkey iron consumption averages 5470 μg/kg/d (nearly all from plant food) whereas the RDA is 227 μg/kg/d. Of course, bioavailability considerations mitigate the differential, but the disparity of such a closely related species is nevertheless sobering (24,25).

4.4. Copper and Zinc

It seems likely that in the Paleolithic both these elements would have been consumed in amounts exceeding those at present. Nutritionists often assess the dietary contribution of these nutrients in terms of the zinc-copper ratio, because excessive zinc can adversely affect absorption and utilization of copper (and iron). The zinc-copper ratio for American diets is approx 7.5; for typical Paleolithic diets this ratio would have been closer to 3.0.

4.5. Cobalt, Selenium, and Iodine

For these trace elements (and others such as chromium) there are too few nutrient analyses of wild foods, either plant or animal, to allow formal estimates of Paleolithic intake. However, certain speculative observations may nevertheless be valid. Cobalt is biologically important because it is a constituent of vitamin B_{12}, cobalamin. This essen-

Table 3
"Paleolithic-Style" Honey Contrasted with Currently Available Sweeteners

	Wild Honey[*]	Domestic Honey	Corn Syrup	Granulated Sugar
		mg/100 g		
Iron	2.05	0.50	0.05	0.01
Calcium	218.50	5.00	3.00	1.00
Phosphorus	21.46	6.00	2.00	2.00
Magnesium	33.79	3.00	2.00	0.00

[*] Three varieties consumed by Tanzanian Hadza (hunter-gatherers). All contained honeycomb and bee larvae - as would the honey eaten by preagricultural humans.

Data sources *(32,35–37)*

Table 4
Nutrients in Uncultivated Fruits and Vegetables as Contrasted with Cereal Grains

	Uncultivated Fruits and Vegetables		Cereal Grains[*]	
	mg/100 g	mg/1000 kcal	mg/100 g	mg/1000 kcal
Iron	2.770	24.760	3.520	9.830
Calcium	87.000	776.600	24.100	67.300
Phosphorus	94.000	837.000	299.000	835.000
Magnesium	59.400	530.000	118.700	331.100
Copper	0.608	5.429	0.451	1.258
Zinc	0.901	8.049	2.607	7.271
Manganese	0.744	6.641	2.401	6.695

[*] Includes barley, corn, millet, oats, rice, rye, and wheat.

Data sources *(16,35)*; reference *38* can serve as an independent cross-check on mineral content in wild plant foods.

Table 5
Nutrients in Wild Game and Commercial Meats

	Wild Game		Commercial Meats[*]	
	mg/100 g	mg/1000 kcal	mg/100 g	mg/1000 kcal
Iron	5.570	43.170	1.340	5.700
Calcium	13.200	102.200	10.300	43.700
Phosphorus	195.000	1515.000	178.000	755.000
Magnesium	23.300	180.900	21.900	93.000
Copper	0.195	1.508	0.085	0.360
Zinc	2.482	19.243	2.859	12.157
Manganese	0.042	0.322	0.019	0.080

[*] Includes pork, beef, hamburger, turkey, chicken, veal, and lamb.

Data sources *(16,39–42)*

tial nutrient is available only from animal foods, so the substantial contribution of game to preagricultural diets — greater than that of animal foods at present — should have provided vitamin B_{12} at higher levels than those common for contemporary humans. The best sources of selenium are meats, especially organ meats, and cereal grains. In this light both current and ancestral diets represent tradeoffs: the greater contribution of game and organ meats for Stone Agers being balanced against the far greater importance of cereal grains in the present. Because there is substantial geographical variability in soil and hence in plant selenium concentrations, it may prove impossible to estimate whether or not preagricultural selenium intake was generally greater or less than at present unless proximate analyses of wild plant foods and game from multiple regions where Stone Agers lived become available. It seems likely that iodine intake also varied according to geographical region as it did for many humans living before iodized salt became generally available in the early twentieth century. Although relatively recent Stone Agers maintained trading and/or gift exchanging networks, these were for luxury items such as shells, amber, carnivore teeth, and exotic stones, not for foods. Because of their nomadism, preagricultural humans may have minimized the adverse impacts of geography on iodine (and selenium) availability relative to subsequent agriculturalists whose yearly travel patterns were far more restricted. Still the general problem must have been significant, at least in some areas. Lack of iodine is probably the main example of a nutritional deficiency encountered by humans before the epipaleolithic.

4.6. Sodium and Potassium

The sodium intake of Paleolithic humans was far less than that at present. Current food processing, preparation, and flavoring practices account for 90% of the sodium consumed in contemporary nations. Only 10% of the sodium now consumed is intrinsic to the foods themselves. In contrast, potassium appears to be leached out of food by the same processes which add sodium. Daily preagricultural electrolyte intake is estimated at Na+ 768 mg, K+ 10,500 mg (K+/Na+ ratio = 13.7) whereas comparable estimates for Americans are Na+ 4000 mg and K+ 2950 mg (K+/Na+ ratio = 0.7) *(16)*. The fact that contemporary humans are the only free-living, terrestrial mammals to consume more sodium than potassium and the only mammals to commonly develop essential hypertension shows how far discordance has progressed.

5. NUTRIENT INTERACTIONS

It is important to stress that the "high" Paleolithic intake patterns for minerals should not be considered in isolation; these nutrients interacted with each other and with other components of the preagricultural diet — especially protein and fiber. Protein intake varied directly and fiber intake inversely with latitude, but for both, typical consumption during the Stone Age would have substantially exceeded that in the present: on average protein probably provided 30—35% of the total energy while dietary fiber likely approx 100 g/d *(16)*. High levels of protein can induce hypercalciuria while, by reducing gastrointestinal absorption, elevated fiber intake can exert significant effects on calcium, zinc, and iron metabolism. Complex interactions between zinc and copper and also between phosphorus and calcium have been described. Availability of certain vitamins can affect mineral physiology, for example, ascorbic acid facilitates absorption of nonheme iron. That vitamin C intake was six times greater for Paleolithic humans than in the present is therefore of potential significance *(16)*. These and other nutrient-nutrient interactions must all be integrated in order to achieve a full understanding of Paleolithic nutrition generally and macromineral/trace element metabolism in particular.

6. LEAD

Although tangential to the main thrust of this volume, it should be noted that differences in mineral availability for preagricultural and current human populations are affected by processes other than nutrition: interactions with lead afford a telling example. Glacial ice cores obtained in Greenland, Switzerland, and elsewhere contain microscopic air bubbles, in effect fossilized air. The deeper the bubble, the older the air and samples from nearly 8,000 years ago have been analyzed. These reveal that atmospheric lead levels in current urban settings are 20,000 times those which obtained before metallurgy *(26)*. Even the air now present in remote rural areas has 400 times the lead found in preagricultural air samples *(27)*.

These differences are reflected in skeletal lead levels which are now 500–1000 times those found in preagricultural bony remains *(27)*. Extrapolating Paleolithic blood levels from skeletal lead content suggests an average of 0.016 µg/dL; in contrast fully 17% of American children have blood lead levels exceeding 15 µg/dL, over 900 times greater *(28)*! Blood lead levels considered "high" by current standards exert adverse effects on brain development which can be measured by differences in cognitive index, today's politically correct term for intelligence quotient. For example, an Australian study of four-year-old children showed that a threefold difference in blood lead level is associated with a 7% difference in cognitive index *(29)*. The several hundred-fold difference between the blood lead levels of current and preagricultural children has sobering potential implications for human intelligence in the present relative to that in the past.

7. CONCLUDING OVERVIEW

Reconstructions of human nutrition during the evolutionary experience of our genus must necessarily be inexact; readers need to remember that where this chapter cites specific figures they are merely the results generated by a model — not the findings of assessment by dietary histories or food frequency questionnaires. But despite its shortcomings, the evolutionary view of human dietary requirements offers unique and valuable insights. There is increasing recognition that contemporary humans remain very similar genetically to our Stone Age ancestors of 20,000 years ago *(4–6)* and it follows that our biochemistry, physiology, and nutritional needs relate to the circumstances of the past as much or more than to those of the present.

With regard to mineral/trace element nutriture our ancestors consumed more each day (generally 2–3X, but up to 8–9X for certain nutrients). Sodium is the obvious and solitary exception because current processing, preparation, and flavoring practices artificially increase its consumption. Lack of iodine was probably the only mineral deficiency commonly encountered by preagricultural humans. In addition to gross differences in mineral intake, there were also intriguing variations in the dietary ratios of certain constituents. Two deserve particular comment: it appears our ancestors consumed more phosphorus relative to calcium than do humans at present, especially at higher latitudes. And the zinc:copper ratio of ancestral diets appears to have been about 50% lower in the past than presently. The high apparent intake of certain minerals, especially iron, challenges current toxicity concepts. However, the excess iron stores found in many older Americans apparently result from accumulation over a lifetime *(30)*. Because relatively few Stone Agers reached advanced ages (about 9% of the Kung San attained age 60 or beyond) *(31)* age-related micronutrient toxicity may have been primarily a theoretical problem for preagricultural humans

The dietary differences discussed in this chapter reflect interaction of multiple factors including:

1. the near complete absence of "empty" calories,
2. the higher nutrient:energy ratio of most wild plant and animal foods relative to their contemporary analogs,
3. the introduction of foods "new" in evolutionary perspective; these have displaced a sizable fraction of the foods which fueled human evolution, and
4. the higher energy requirement of ancestral humans whose lives involved substantially greater energy expenditure.

Determining the character of ancestral human nutrition should not be viewed as a challenge to existing nutritional recommendations. Rather it should generate investigational initiatives designed to assess the impact of Paleolithic dietary practices in the present. By definition, Stone Age nutrition fueled the multimillion year evolution of our genus and species; its thoughtful study by nutrition scientists seems both logical and important.

REFERENCES

1. Lewin R. Principles of human evolution. Blackwell, Oxford, 1998,pp.192.
2. Leonard WR, Robertson ML. Evolutionary perspectives on human nutrition: the influence of brain and body size on diet and metabolism. Am J Hum Biol 1994;6:77–88.
3. Ruff CB, Trinkaus E, Holliday TW. Body mass and encephalization in Pleistocene Homo. Nature 1997;387:173–176.
4. Tattersall I. Becoming human. Evolution and human uniqueness. Harcourt Brace, New York, 1998,pp.239.
5. Johansen D. Reading the minds of fossils. Sci Amer 1998;278(3):102–103.
6. Neel JV. Physician to the gene pool. Wiley, New York 1994,pp. 315.
7. Milton K. Diet and primate evolution. Sci Amer 1993;269(Aug):86–93.
8. Eaton SB, Eaton SB. The evolutionary context of chronic degenerative diseases. In: Stearns SC, ed. Evolution in Health and Disease. Oxford University Press, Oxford. 1998, pp. 251–259.
9. Tooby J, Cosmides L. The past explains the present. Emotional adaptations and the structure of ancestral environments. Ethology and Sociobiology 1990;11:375–424.
10. Eaton SB, Eaton SB. Evolutionary aspects of diet: the diet of evolutionary adaptedness. In: Proceedings of the 16th International Congress of Nutrition. Canad Fed Biol Sciences, Ottowa, Canada,1999 in press.
11. Bettinger RL. Hunter-gatherers Archaeological and evolutionary theory. New York, Plenum Press,
12. Molleson T. The eloquent bones of Abu Hureyra. Sci Amer 1994;(Aug):70–75.
13. Stringer C, McKie R. African Exodus. The Origins of Modern Humanity. Henry Holt, New York, 1996, pp. 11.
14. Lee RB. What hunters do for a living or how to make out on scarce resources. In: Lee RB, DeVore I eds. Man the Hunter. Chicago, Aldine, 1968, pp. 30–48.
15. Cordain L, Gotshall RW, Eaton SB. Evolutionary aspects of exercise. World Rev Nutr Dietet 1997;81:49–60.
16. Eaton SB, Eaton SB, Konner M. Paleolithic nutrition revisited: a twelve-year retrospective on its nature and implications. Eur J Clin Nutr 1997;51:207–216.
17. Eaton SB, Konner M. Paleolithic nutrition A consideration of its nature and current implications. N Engl J Med 1985;312:283–289.
18. Eaton SB, Eaton SB, Sinclair AJ, Cordain L, Mann NJ. Dietary intake of long chain polyunsaturated fatty acids during the Paleolithic. World Rev Nutr Dietet 1998;83:12–23.

19. Åstrand PO. Whole body metabolism. In: Horton ES, Terjung RL, eds. Exercise Nutrition and Energy Metabolism. Macmillan, New York, 1988,pp. 1–8.

20. Eaton SB, Nelson DA. Calcium in evolutionary perspective. Am J Clin Nutr 1991;54:281S–287S.

21. Speth JD. Early hominid hunting and scavenging: the role of meat as an energy source. J Hum Evol 1989;18:329–343.

22. Guthrie RD. The mammoth steppe and the origins of Mongoloids and their dispersal. In: Akazawa T, Szathmary EJE, eds. Prehistoric Mongoloid Dispersals. Oxford University Press, Oxford, 1996,pp.172–186.

23. Nei M, Roychoudhury AK. Evolutionary relationships of human populations on a global scale. Mol Biol Evol 1993;10:927–943.

24. Nagy K, Milton K. Energy metabolism and food consumption by howler monkeys. Ecology 1979;60:475–80.

25. Nagy K, Milton K. Aspects of dietary quality, nutrient assimilation and water balance in wild howler monkeys. Oecologia 1979;30:249–258.

26. Patterson CC. Contaminated and natural lead environments of man. Arch Environ Health 1965;11:344–360.

27. Patterson C, Ericson J, Manea-Krichten M, Shirahata H. Natural skeletal levels of lead in Homo sapiens sapiens uncontaminated by technological lead. Sci Total Environ 1991;107:205–236.

28. Flegal AR, Smith DR. Lead levels in preindustrial humans. N Engl J Med 1992;326:1293–1294.

29. Baghurst PA, McMichael AJ, Wigg NR, Vimpani GV, Robertson EF, Roberts RJ, Tong SL. Environmental exposure to lead and childhood intelligence at the age of seven years. The Port Pirie cohort study. N Engl J Med 1992;327:1279–1284.

30. Wood RJ, Fleming DJ, Jacques PF, Wilson PWF. Iron status of the elderly Framingham heart study cohort: an iron-replete population with a high prevalence of elevated iron stores. FASEB J 1998;12:A 846.

31. Howell N. Demography of the Dobe !Kung New York: Academic Press, 1979.

DATA SOURCES

32. Cutrufelli R, Pehrsson PR. Composition of Foods: Snacks and Sweets. Agriculture Handbook 8-19. US Dept of Agriculture, Washington, DC, 1991,pp. 319,326.

33. Reeves JB, Wehrauch JL. Composition of Foods: Fats and Oils. Agriculture Handbook 8-4. US Dept of Agriculture, Washington, DC, 1979,pp. 16,36,115.

34. Cutrufelli R, Matthews RH. Composition of Foods: Beverages. Agriculture Handbook 8-14. US Dept of Agriculture, Washington, DC, 1986,pp. 21,42,52,57,59,61,66.

35. Drake DL. Composition of Foods: Cereal Grains and Pasta. Agriculture Handbook 8-20. US Dept of Agriculture, Washington, DC, 1989,pp. 22,31,48,50,66,77,86.

36. Watt BK, Merrill AL. Composition of Foods. Agriculture Handbook 8. US Dept of Agriculture, Washington, DC, 1963,pp. 34,152.

37. Unpublished material collected in Tanzania by Woodburn J. and analyzed by Southgate, D.A.T. 1964.

38. Brand Miller JC, Holt SHA. Australian aboriginal plant foods: a consideration of their nutritional composition and health implications. Nutr Res Rev 1998;11:5–23.

39. Anderson BA. Composition of Foods: Pork Products. Agriculture Handbook 8-10. US Dept of Agriculture, Washington, DC, 1983,pp. 22.

40. Anderson BA, Lauderdale JL, Hoke IM. Composition of Foods: Beef Products. Agriculture Handbook 8–13. US Dept of Agriculture, Washington, DC, 1986,pp. 35,339.

41. Anderson BA. Composition of Foods: Lamb Veal and Game Products. Agriculture Handbook 8-17. US Dept of Agriculture, Washington, DC, 1989,pp. 31,120,176–211.

42. Anderson BA. Composition of Foods: Poultry Products. Agriculture Handbook 8-5. US Dept of Agriculture, Washington, DC, 1983,pp. 37,193

4

Current Dietary Intakes of Trace Elements and Minerals

Jean A. T. Pennington, PhD, RD

1. INTRODUCTION

The purpose of this chapter is to summarize what is known about current dietary intakes of trace elements and minerals. The trace elements and minerals discussed in this chapter are calcium (Ca), chromium (Cr), copper (Cu), fluoride (F), iron (Fe), iodine (I), magnesium (Mg), manganese (Mn), molybdenum (Mo), phosphorus (P), selenium (Se), and zinc (Zn). The information about dietary intakes of these trace elements and minerals was obtained primarily from government surveys and studies. Table 1 provides a listing of food consumption surveys conducted by the United States Department of Agriculture (USDA) and the National Center for Health Statistics (NCHS), Centers for Disease Control (CDC), Department of Health and Human Services (DHHS) since the 1970s. Table 1 indicates the years these surveys were conducted, the methods for obtaining the food consumption information, and the trace elements and minerals evaluated in each survey.

In addition to the surveys conducted by the USDA and the NCHS, estimates of daily trace element and mineral intakes have also been made by the US Food and Drug Administration (FDA) through the Total Diet Study (TDS) *(1,2)*. From 1973 to 1982, the TDS estimates of trace element and mineral intakes were based on the analysis of food group composites. Since 1982, the TDS trace element and mineral intake estimates have been based on a core food model that allows 200–300 core foods to be purchased quarterly and analyzed in FDA laboratories for minerals and other food components including pesticide residues, radionuclides, industrial chemicals, and heavy metals. The last published TDS data for daily trace element and mineral intakes were for 1982 through 1991 *(3)*. The trace elements and minerals in that TDS report include Ca, Cu, Fe, I, Mg, Mn, P, Se, and Zn (Table 1). The core food model used in the TDS is based on the food consumption data from USDA and NCHS surveys. The "overlapping" trace elements and minerals in the TDS and in the USDA and NCHS surveys are Ca, Cu, Fe, Mg, P, and Zn. This chapter presents dietary intake data for Ca, Cu, Fe, Mg, P, and Zn from the 1994–1996 CSFII and the first three years (1988–1991) of the NHANES III and dietary intake data for I, Mn, and Se from the 1982–1991 TDS.

Information on Cr intake was obtained from a USDA study *(4)*. TDS data from work in the 1970s at the University of Minnesota provided data on daily F intakes *(5–8)*. A TDS

From: *Clinical Nutrition of the Essential Trace Elements and Minerals: The Guide for Health Professionals*
Edited by: J. D. Bogden and L. M. Klevay © Humana Press Inc., Totowa, NJ

Table 1.
US government nutrition surveys and studies

Survey/study Name	Years conducted	Methods used	Trace Elements/ Minerals Included
NHANES I	1971-74	24-hour recall	Ca, Fe, Mg, P
NHANES II	1976-80	24-hour recall	Ca, Fe, Mg, P
HHANES	1982-84	24-hour recall	Ca, Cu, Fe, Mg, P, Zn
NHANES III	1988-94	24-hour recall	Ca, Cu, Fe, Mg, P, Zn
NFCS	1977-78	24-hour recall + 2-day diary	Ca, Fe, Mg, P
CSFII	1985-86	six 1-day intakes	Ca, Cu, Fe, Mg, P, Zn
CSFII	1989-91	24-hour recall + 2-day diary	Ca, Cu, Fe, Mg, P, Zn
CSFII	1994-96	two 24-hour recalls	Ca, Cu, Fe, Mg, P, Zn
TDS	1973	food composite analysis	Se, Zn
TDS	1974-75,78-79	food composite analysis	Ca, Fe, I, P, Se, Zn
TDS	1976	food composite analysis	Ca, Cu, Fe, I, Mg, Mn, P, Se, Zn
TDS	1977	food composite analysis	Cu, Fe, Mg, Mn, Se, Zn
TDS	1980-81	food composite analysis	Cu, Fe, I, Mg, Mn, Se, Zn
TDS	1982-91	core food analysis	Ca, Cu, Fe, I, Mg, Mn, P, Se, Zn
TDS	1992-present	core food analysis	Ca, Cu, Fe, Mg, Mn, P, Se, Zn

CSFII = Continuing Survey of the Food Intake of Individuals, United States Department of Agriculture (USDA).

HHANES = Hispanic Health and Nutrition Examination Survey, National Center for Health Statistics (NCHS), Centers for Disease Control (CDC), Department of Health and Human Services (DHHS).

NFCS = Nationwide Food Consumption Survey, USDA.

NHANES = National Health and Nutrition Examination Survey, NCHS, CDC, DHHS.

project in the mid-1980s allowed for evaluation of daily intakes of Mo and some other trace elements (aluminum, cobalt, nickel, strontium, vanadium) in US diets *(9)*. Additional information about dietary intake estimates for Cr, F, and Mo are provided from other published studies.

2. ASSESSMENT OF DIETARY INTAKE OF TRACE ELEMENTS AND MINERALS

Assessment of dietary status with respect to trace elements and minerals requires that the daily intake in milligram (mg) or microgram (mcg) amounts for specified age and sex groups be compared to recommended standards of intake. The dietary standards used in the US are the Recommended Dietary Allowances (RDAs) and the Estimated Safe and Adequate Daily Dietary Intakes (ESADDIs) established by the Food and Nutrition Board of the National Academy of Sciences (NAS) *(10)*. Comparison of dietary survey data with RDAs and ESADDIs is useful to determine nutritional adequacy of populations groups and to identify groups by demographic variables (e.g., age, sex, race, income level) that might be vulnerable to nutrient deficiencies or toxicities. Table 2 presents the 1989 RDAs for Ca, Fe, I, Mg, P, Se, and Zn and the ESADDIs for Cr, Cu, F, Mn, and Mo *(10)*.

In 1997, the NAS published new intake standards, termed Dietary Reference Intake Values (DRIs) for Ca, F, Mg, and P *(11)*. The four sets of DRIs include RDAs, Estimated Average Requirements (EARs), Adequate Intakes (AIs), and Tolerable Upper Intake

Table 2
Recommended Dietary Allowances (RDAs) for Ca, Fe, I, Mg, P, Se, and Zn and Estimated Safe
and Adequate Daily Dietary Intakes (ESADDIs) for Cr, Cu, F, Mn, and Mo *(10)*

Group, age (yr)	Ca (mg)	Fe (mg)	I (mcg)	Mg (mg)	P (mg)	Se (mcg)	Zn (mg)
Infants							
0.0–0.5	400	6	40	40	300	10	5
0.5–1.0	600	10	50	60	500	15	5
Children							
1–3	800	10	70	80	800	20	10
4–6	800	10	90	120	800	20	10
7–10	800	10	120	170	800	30	10
Females							
11–14	1,200	15	150	280	1,200	45	12
15–18	1,200	15	150	300	1,200	50	12
19–24	1,200	15	150	280	1,200	55	12
25–50	800	15	150	280	800	55	12
51+	800	10	150	280	800	55	12
Pregnant	1,200	30	175	320	1,200	65	15
Lactating							
1st 6 mo	1,200	15	200	355	1,200	75	19
2nd 6 mo	1,200	15	200	340	1,200	75	16
Males							
11–14	1,200	12	150	270	1,200	40	15
15–18	1,200	12	150	400	1,200	50	15
19–24	1,200	10	150	350	1,200	70	15
25–50	800	10	150	350	800	70	15
51+	800	10	150	350	800	70	15

Group, age (yr)	Cr (mcg)	Cu (mg)	F (mg)	Mn (mg)	Mo (mcg)
Infants					
0–0.5	10–40	0.4–0.6	0.1–0.5	0.3–0.6	15–30
0.5–1	20–60	0.6–0.7	0.2–1.0	0.6–1.0	20–40
Children and adolescents					
1–3	20–80	0.7–1.0	0.5–1.5	1.0–1.5	25–50
4–6	30–12	1.0–1.5	1.0–2.5	1.5–2.0	30–75
7–10	50–20	1.0–2.0	1.5–2.5	2.0–3.0	50–150
11+	50–20	1.5–2.5	1.5–2.5	2.0–5.0	75–250
Adults	50–20	1.5–3.0	1.5–4.0	2.0–5.0	75–250

Levels (ULs). The 1997 NAS report provides AIs for Ca and F; AIs for Mg and P for infants; and EARs and RDAs for Mg and P for other age/sex groups. The criterion for each RDA, EAR, and AI is specified. There are ULs for all four trace elements/minerals. Intake standards for other trace elements and minerals will be revised by NAS in subsequent reports. Assessments of dietary intakes of trace elements and minerals from nutrition surveys and studies will vary depending upon which sets of standards are used to evaluate them. Assessments presented in this chapter are based on the 1989 RDAs and ESADDIs as these were the standards that were in place when the surveys/studies were conducted and these are the standards used in the consulted references *(12–14)*.

3. ACCURACY OF CURRENT DATA
ON TRACE ELEMENT AND MINERAL INTAKES

The accuracy and reliability of information on trace element and mineral intakes is dependent on the accuracy and reliability of food intake information collected from survey participants and on the accuracy and reliability of the food composition database that specifies the levels of each trace element or mineral in each food. Each national survey attempts to improve upon the techniques for collecting information about what people eat, and each survey is accompanied by enlarged and updated food composition databases. Other concerns with regard to the accuracy of dietary intakes of trace elements and minerals are the bioavailablity of the trace elements/minerals; the need to confirm dietary status findings with clinical and biochemical status measures on the same individuals; and trace element/mineral intakes from dietary supplements.

3.1. Food Intake Information

The main problems with methods to assess food intake are the memory and honesty of the subjects and the effects of the methods (e.g., 24-h recalls and food diaries) on usual food intake patterns. Keeping food records tends to restrain the usual eating patterns of survey participants. Participants may be intimidated by questions about their dietary patterns and may not respond accurately, especially about consumption of alcohol, desserts, or other high-fat foods. Based on results from doubly-labeled water techniques, it appears that methods used to assess food intakes, especially those methods used in surveys, underestimate total food (and hence total energy/calorie) intake *(15–19)*. The level of underestimation may vary according to age, gender, and other demographic variables. Martin et al. *(17)* reported a 20% caloric underestimation for adult females. Trace element and mineral intakes are probably underestimated as well, and this needs to be considered when trace element/mineral intakes are compared with dietary standards. Actual trace element/mineral intakes may be higher than results from national food consumption surveys indicate.

3.2. Food Composition Databases

Food composition databases generally present a single value for the level of a trace element or mineral in a food per 100 g or per serving portion of the food. Improvements in analytical techniques and methods may produce more accurate levels of trace elements/ minerals in foods that may differ from those previously reported. Also, the trace element/ mineral composition of mixed dish foods may change with new ingredients or formulations. Databases need to be continuously updated to incorporate new foods and new values.

The levels of trace elements/minerals in foods vary according to inherent, environmental, and processing factors. The single value for a trace element/mineral in a food found in a food composition database does not represent the variability of the trace element/mineral in the food. Even if the variability is represented (by a range or standard deviation), this variability cannot be factored into the daily dietary intake of the trace element/mineral. Daily food intake records usually include about 15–20 different foods, each with their own trace element/mineral variabilities.

3.3. Bioavailability

Assessment of daily intakes of trace elements/minerals does not usually address the bioavailability of trace elements/minerals from foods, mixed diets, or the gastrointestinal tract. Current knowledge and methodology are not sophisticated enough to factor in the bioavailability of different valence states such as ferric vs ferrous iron; the bioavailability of various mineral salts such as ferrous sulfate vs ferrous phosphate; the interference with mineral absorption caused by the presence of phytic acid (phytate) or oxalic acid (oxalate) in foods; mineral-mineral interactions (e.g., Cu-Zn interactions) which may inhibit absorption; or competition of minerals for absorption sites in intestinal cells (e.g., Ca and lead (Pb) competition). In addition, the absorption of some trace elements/minerals (e.g., Ca and Fe) is dependent on body stores, i.e., percent absorption decreases if body stores are high and increases if body stores are low.

3.4. Confirmation with Biochemical and Clinical Data

Dietary surveys are quick, inexpensive tools for monitoring the dietary status of populations and population subgroups. Such data may identify potential problems relating to trace element/mineral deficiency or toxicity. However, to determine if individuals or populations have nutrient deficiences or toxicities, the dietary findings need to be confirmed with data from biochemical and/or clinical measures. Ideally the clinical and biochemical data will be obtained from the same individuals who provide dietary information. The NHANES I-III and HHANES have dietary, clinical, and biochemical information from each survey participant.

3.5. Use and Potency of Mineral Supplements

At least 35–40% of Americans took dietary supplements between 1988 and 1991 *(13)*. Females were more likely to take supplements than males, and non-Hispanic whites and older adults were more likely to take supplements than non-Hispanic blacks and younger adults *(13)*. In 1986, more than 70% of all supplements used by adults and children were taken daily *(13)*. The supplements most commonly used by adults were vitamin-mineral combinations and single vitamins and minerals (specifically, vitamin C and Ca), whereas for children 2–6 yr of age, the most commonly used supplements were multivitamins *(13)*.

Assessment of daily intakes of trace elements/minerals by individuals or population groups requires information on the extent of use and potency of trace element/mineral supplements. A single trace element/mineral supplement may contain 100% or more of the RDA or ESADDI for one or more trace elements/minerals. Because trace element/mineral intakes from supplements can overwhelm trace element/mineral intakes from food, it is best to separate the dietary intake data for survey participants who use trace element/mineral supplements from those who do not. (This is especially important if one is trying to relate trace element/mineral intake to clinical and biochemical measures.) It could be misleading to determine average trace element/mineral intakes for a population if some people are using supplements. The average intake could be biased on the high side, and specific problems with high or low trace element/mineral intakes could be overlooked. The data presented here from the 1994–1996 CSFII and the 1988–1991 NHANES III represent only trace elements/minerals derived from foods; they do not include trace elements/minerals obtained from dietary supplements.

4. PUBLIC HEALTH MEASURES TO IMPROVE TRACE ELEMENT/MINERAL STATUS

Public health measures in the US that include a focus on dietary trace element/mineral intakes are the DHHS/USDA *Dietary Guidelines for Americans (20)*, the USDA Food

Guide Pyramid, the FDA Nutrition Facts on food labels, and the National Cancer Institute's (NCI) 5 A Day Program. *The Dietary Guidelines for Americans (20)* encourage variety in food choices and emphasize consumption of grain products, vegetables, and fruits. They promote the Food Guide Pyramid and note the importance of meat, fish, and poultry for Fe and Zn and milk for Ca. The Dietary Guidelines provide cautions about mineral levels in vegetarian diets; note that women and adolescent girls need Ca-rich foods and that young children, teenage girls, and women of childbearing age need Fe-rich foods; provide information on sources of Ca and Fe; and provide a sample label for lowfat milk that shows the importance of milk for providing Ca.

The graphic and accompanying educational materials for the Food Guide Pyramid indicate that minerals are obtained primarily from grain group (Fe); dairy group (Ca, Mg, P), meat group (Fe, Zn); and vegetable group (Ca, Fe, Mg). The Nutrition Facts Panel on food labels requires that the percent Daily Value (DV) per serving for Ca and Fe be listed. This allows consumers to determine if foods are sources of these minerals. The DV for Ca used on food labels is 1,000 mg (1 g), and the DV for Fe is 18 mg. Food manufacturers may also voluntarily list the percent DV for other trace elements/minerals on food labels. If a trace element/mineral is added to a food as a source of enrichment or fortification, the percent DV for that trace element/mineral must be listed on the Nutrition Facts Panel. The NCI's 5 A Day Program encourages consumption of at least five servings per day of fruits and vegetables, some of which are good sources of some trace elements/minerals (e.g., Ca, Fe, and Mg in dark green leafy vegetables).

5. TRACE ELEMENT AND MINERAL INTAKES

The following presents information on the dietary intakes and food sources of 12 trace elements/minerals. Trace element/mineral consumption data from the 1994–1996 CSFII for Ca, Cu, Fe, Mg, P, and Zn are presented in Table 3 (as mg or mcg per day) and in Table 4 (as percent of the 1989 RDAs) *(12)*. The *Third Report on Nutrition Monitoring in the United States* (TRONM) *(13)* provides median daily intakes of Ca, Cu, Fe, Mg, P, and Zn from the 1988–1991 NHANES III data as percent of 1989 RDAs for ethnic and race groups (i.e., non-Hispanic whites, non-Hispanic blacks, and Mexican-Americans). Some of these data are reproduced in Table 5. It appears that the percent RDAs for trace elements/ minerals in Table 4 (1994–1996 CSFII data) are higher than those in Table 5 (1988–1991 NHANES III data). It is possible that there might have been some changes (i.e., improve-ments) in US dietary patterns regarding trace element/mineral intakes between 1988–1991 and 1994–1996; however, some of the differences may also be explained by the following: 1) different survey methods, techniques, personnel, and databases between the two surveys; 2) the CSFII data are based on average intakes and the NHANES III data are based on median intakes; and 3) the data from the two surveys are presented by different age and ethnic/racial groupings.

Table 6 provides information on dietary sources of Ca, Cu, Fe, Mg, P, and Zn from the US food supply *(14,21)*. Tables 7 and 8 provide dietary intake information and food source information, respectively, for I, Mn, and Se based on 1982–1991 TDS data *(3,22)*.

5.1. Calcium (Ca)

Ca is a high profile mineral that has been included in every US national food consumption survey (Table 1) and in the TDS. Ca has been the focus of many nutrition

Table 3

Average trace element/mineral intakes per day by sex and age, 1 day, CSFII, 1994–1996 *(12)*

Sex and age (yr) Females and males	Ca (mg)	Cu (mg)	Fe (mg)	Mg (mg)	P(mg)	Zn (mg)
under 1	664	0.7	15.7	98	526	6.4
1–2	848	0.7	10.5	186	961	7.4
3–5	819	0.8	12.4	200	1,027	8.6
Females						
6–11	857	0.9	13.7	218	1,131	9.5
12–19	771	1.0	13.8	223	1,108	9.9
20–29	701	1.1	13.5	229	1,090	9.5
30–39	661	1.1	12.9	234	1,048	9.7
40–49	634	1.1	13.2	237	1,014	9.3
50–59	630	1.1	12.5	244	1,023	8.9
60–69	604	1.0	12.4	230	957	8.5
≥70	584	1.0	12.4	225	918	8.3
Males						
6–11	970	1.0	16.6	245	1,275	11.2
12–19	1,145	1.4	19.8	311	1,633	14.5
20–29	990	1.5	19.5	335	1,619	14.8
30–39	951	1.6	19.8	344	1,581	15.5
40–49	876	1.5	18.2	329	1,467	13.3
50–59	791	1.5	17.1	318	1,386	13.2
60–69	796	1.3	17.4	311	1,315	12.4
>70	746	1.3	16.3	283	1,198	11.3

CSFII = Continuing Survey of the Food Intake of Individuals, USDA.

* There were 16,103 participants in the 1994–1996 CSFII. Participants recalled food intake information for 2 separate days. Data on mean intakes and mean percentages are based on respondents' intakes on the first surveyed day. The day 1 response rate was 80.0%, and the day 2 response rate was 76.1%. The data are national probability estimates for the US population. The results were weighted to adjust for differential rates of sample selection and for nonresponse. The sample sizes for each age/sex group provide a sufficient level of precision to ensure statistical reliability of the estimates. Breast–fed children were excluded from these data.

research studies, and its food sources (milk, yogurt, cheese, other dairy products, and some vegetables) are well known (Table 6). Inadequate dietary intakes of calcium are associated with osteoporosis; however, this relationship is complicated as the disease takes years to develop and is related to race/ethnic group, estrogen levels, and intakes of other nutrients (vitamin D and P) (*see* Chapter 14). Those most vulnerable to osteoporosis are middle-aged and older white women of northern European derivation. Some racial/ethnic groups (Asian and Black) seem to have much lower requirements for Ca than other groups. It is also of interest that lactose intolerance (and hence, lower Ca intakes) is most common in Asians and Blacks. There is much research interest in the relationship of calcium intake with hypertension, i.e., that hypertension in some individuals may be associated with a low calcium intake. (Reference *23*, pages 355–356, 551–553 provides a summary of research studies on calcium intake and hypertension.)

Table 4
Average trace element/mineral intakes as percent of the 1989 RDA by sex
and age, 1 day, CSFII, 1994–1996 (12)[*]

Sex and age (years) Males and females	Ca (%)	Fe (%)	Mg (%)	P (%)	Zn (%)
Under 1	132	197	189	129	128
1–2	106	105	232	120	**74**
3–5	102	124	193	128	86
Females					
6–11	101	129	128	133	92
12–19	**64**	91	77	92	82
20–29	**71**	87	80	110	76
30–39	81	85	83	128	79
40–49	79	87	85	126	77
50–59	79	120	87	128	**74**
60–69	75	124	82	120	**71**
≥70	**73**	124	80	115	**69**
Males					
6–11	114	160	144	150	105
12–19	95	169	92	136	97
20–29	103	195	96	169	98
30–39	119	198	98	198	103
40–49	109	182	94	183	88
50–59	99	171	91	173	88
60–69	99	174	89	164	82
≥70	93	163	81	150	76

RDA=Recommended Dietary Allowance (10).
CSFII=Continuing Survey of the Food Intake of Individuals,USDA.
[*]Intakes less than 75% RDA are bolded.

Average dietary intakes of Ca for 19 age and sex groups from the 1994–1996 CSFII are presented in Table 3. Intakes ranged from 584 mg Ca per day for women 70 yr and over to 1,145 mg/day for 12–19 yr-old males. Average Ca intake declined for females after 6–11 yr and for males after 12–19 yr. Mean Ca intakes as percent RDA for the 1994–1996 CSFII (Table 4) were less than 75% for females in the age ranges of 12–19 yr, 20–29 yr, and 70 yr and over. Average Ca intakes for males ranged from 93 to 119% RDA.

Median daily intakes of Ca as percent 1989 RDA from the 1988–1991 NHANES III (Table 5) were 66% RDA or less for females 12–15 yr and 16–19 yr. Ca intakes as percent 1989 RDA were higher for men than for women. Intakes for non-Hispanic whites were higher than those for non-Hispanic Blacks and were generally higher than those for Mexican-Americans.

5.2. Chromium (Cr)

There is probably less information about Cr intake and Cr in foods than for any of the other essential trace elements or minerals. The reason for this may be the many problems associated with the analyses of foods for Cr. Cr may be a contaminant on analytical equipment and utensils. Leaching of Cr from stainless steel blender blades into foods and

Table 5
Median daily intakes* of Ca, Cu, Fe, Mg, P, and Zn as percent of 1989 RDAs, NHANES III+ (13)

Females and males	2–11 mo			1–2 yr			3–5 yr		
	NHW	NHB	MA	NHW	NHB	MA	NHW	NHB	MA
Ca	139	121	131	102	82	97	103	84	80
Cu	144	154	152	91	97	96	79	97	100
Fe	176	204	176	85	87	79	101	109	108
Mg	222	194	212	220	208	218	162	163	166
P	139	119	133	114	104	113	123	121	126
Zn	111	122	120	**61**	**63**	**58**	**69**	78	**74**

Females	6–11 yr			12–15 yr			16–19 yr			20–59 yr			≥60 yr		
	NHW	NHB	MA	NHW	NHB	MA	NHW	NHB	MA	NHW	NHB	MA	NHW	NHB	MA
Ca	103	86	111	**62**	**51**	**66**	**66**	**52**	**56**	80	**62**	79	77	**50**	**62**
Cu	86	92	88	**67**	**62**	**59**	**63**	**66**	**67**	**70**	**59**	**68**	**65**	**55**	**56**
Fe	107	107	108	**67**	**65**	**68**	**63**	**69**	**68**	**74**	**66**	**72**	103	96	84
Mg	115	116	128	**64**	**70**	**74**	**62**	**58**	**66**	85	**66**	85	83	**67**	**65**
P	134	128	142	87	81	94	88	87	90	130	113	134	116	96	102
Zn	77	81	81	**67**	**71**	**72**	**70**	78	**72**	**70**	**65**	**70**	**62**	**55**	**54**

Males	6–11 yr			12–15 yr			16–19 yr			20–59 yr			≥60 yr		
	NHW	NHB	MA	NHW	NHB	MA	NHW	NHB	MA	NHW	NHB	MA	NHW	NHB	MA
Ca	124	95	123	90	**60**	85	103	76	79	113	**74**	103	90	**62**	82
Cu	101	99	101	81	76	79	93	87	84	100	82	97	81	**59**	79
Fe	132	122	125	128	110	119	146	119	114	161	139	152	140	102	127
Mg	137	119	144	103	85	97	78	**68**	**70**	95	**74**	96	83	**58**	**74**
P	154	138	162	118	97	114	141	126	122	188	155	196	152	121	148
Zn	90	92	93	77	**59**	**70**	90	**32**	80	87	75	84	**72**	**57**	**55**

NHW = non–Hispanic whites, NHB = non–Hispanic Blacks, MA = Mexican Americans, RDA = Recommended Dietary Allowance (10), NHANES III = Third National Health and Nutrition Examination Survey, NCHS, CDC.

* Intakes less than 75% RDA are bolded.

+ NHANES III was a six–year study with data collected in two phases, 1988–1991 and 1991–1994. A nationally representative sample was used for each phase. The sampled population was civilian, noninstitutionalized, 2 months of age and older. There was oversampling of non–Hispanic Blacks and Mexican Americans, children < 6 years of age, and adults aged ≥ 60 yr. The dietary data included one 24–hour recall and a food frequency. Two additional 24–hour recalls were obtained for participants ≥ 50 yr. Also obtained were socioeconomic and demographic information, biochemical analyses of blood and urine, physical examination, body measurements, blood pressure measurements, bone densitometry, dietary and health behaviors, and health conditions.

Table 6
Nutrient Content of the US Food Supply, by Food Group, 1990 *(14,21)*

	Ca (%)	Cu (%)	Fe (%)	Mg (%)	P (%)	Zn (%)
Dairy products	74.5	3.5	2.1	17.6	33.7	19.0
Grain products	4.4	22.7	48.9	23.7	19.0	16.9
Meat, poultry, fish	3.4	15.6	18.5	13.6	26.5	43.7
Vegetables	6.2	20.6	11.9	14.4	7.3	7.0
Legumes, nuts, soy	3.7	16.6	7.3	12.0	5.2	5.8
Fruits	2.5	7.0	2.9	6.2	1.7	1.3
Eggs	1.7	0.3	2.4	0.9	3.6	2.8
Sugars and sweeteners	0.8	4.4	1.1	0.9	0.3	0.5
Fats and oil	0.1	0.1	0.1	0.0	0.1	0.1
Miscellaneous foods	2.6	9.4	5.5	10.8	2.6	3.0
Total	99.9	100.2	100.7	100.1	100.0	100.1

beverages has been documented *(24)*. Some of the older (and usually higher) published values for Cr in foods may be overestimated due to contamination during laboratory analysis. Inorganic Cr compounds are poorly (1–2%) absorbed, while organic Cr compounds are absorbed at a higher level (10–25%).

Currently, there are no reliable food composition databases for Cr from which to calculate dietary Cr intake from diet records. Therefore, dietary Cr intake must be measured more directly, as with the duplicate portion technique. A few estimates of daily Cr intake are available from the literature. Reported Cr intakes have decreased in past decades due primarily to increased awareness of Cr contamination, recent use of standard reference materials, and improved analytical instrumentation and procedures *(24)*. Pi-Sunyer and Offenbacher *(25)* estimated an intake of 5–150 mcg/d in US diets. Recent, well-controlled studies suggest that dietary Cr intake is approx 50 mcg/d or less in Finland, Canada, England, and the US *(4,26–28)*. Values for dietary Cr intake for Canada *(27)* were slightly above 50 mcg, while the daily dietary Cr intake for the other three countries was approx 30 mcg/d. Average intakes of 25 mcg/d for adult females and 33 mcg/d for adult males from self-selected diets in Beltsville, MD on diets containing 1,600 and 2,300 kcal, respectively, were reported from the USDA study by Anderson and Kozlovsky *(4)*.

Anderson *(29)* found that from a daily intake of 29.1 mcg of Cr, about 6.8 mcg comes from fruits, vegetables, and nuts (70% from fruits); 6.6 mcg from beverages (mostly beer, wine, and soft drinks); 6.2 mcg from dairy products (85% from milk); 5.2 mcg from meat (55% from pork); with lesser amounts from cereal products (3.7 mcg); and negligible amounts (0.6 mcg) from fish and seafood. Some brands of beer may contain 20 mcg per 12 fl oz, but other brands have much lower concentrations *(30)*.

The NAS *(10)* set 50–200 mcg of Cr per day as a safe and adequate level for adolescents and adults and 10–120 mcg for infants and children based "on the absence of signs of chromium deficiency in the major part of the US population consuming an average of 50 mcg/d." The average intakes reported above are less than the levels set by the NAS as safe and adequate. More knowledge and information is needed about Cr in foods and in daily diets.

Table 7
Average daily intakes and percent RDA/ESADDI of I, Mn and Se, TDS,
1982–1991 *(3)*

	I mcg (%RDA)	Mn mg (%ESADDI)[*]	Se mcg (%RDA)
Females and males			
6–11 mo	170 (340)	1.07 (178)	18 (120)
2 yr	261 (373)	1.47 (147)	46 (228)
Females			
14–16 yr	312 (208)	1.79 (90)	68 (136)
25–30 yr	248 (165)	2.21 (111)	71 (129)
60–65 yr	227 (151)	2.29 (115)	64 (116)
Males			
14–16 yr	332 (498)	2.76 (138)	104 (207)
25–30 yr	386 (257)	2.85 (143)	111 (159)
60–65 yr	311 (207)	2.66 (133)	92 (131)

RDA = Recommended Dietary Allowance *(10)*.
ESADDI = Estimated Safe and Adequate Daily Dietary Intake *(10)*.
TDS = Total Diet Study, FDA.
[*]Percent of lower end of ESADDI range.

5.3. Copper (Cu)

Cu has been included in the TDS and in USDA and NCHS surveys (Table 1) since the early 1980s. Table 3 indicates that Cu intakes from the 1994–1996 CSFII ranged from 0.7 mg/d for infants and children 1–2 yr of age to 1.6 mg/d for 30–39 year-old males. Cu intakes for adolescent females and males and for adult females were less than the 1.5+ mg/d recommended by NAS (Table 2). Median Cu intakes from NHANES III ranged from 50–80% RDA for females (age 12 yr and over) and 59–100% RDA for males (age 12 yr and over) (Table 5). (LSRO *(13)* used the lower end of the Cu ESADDI range to calculate percent RDAs.) Thus, dietary intakes of Cu appear low compared with standards. Klevay *(31)* and Klevay and Medeiros *(32)* recommend that RDAs for Cu should be established based on copper depletion experiments with consideration for losses during pregnancy, the potential relationship of low copper to cholesterolemia, and the effects of diets high in iron and zinc on copper nutriture.

5.4. Fluoride (F)

There is little information about current levels of F in foods or in daily dietary intakes of population groups. Because F is added to many local water supplies, daily intakes depend on the amount of local water that is consumed. Information on local water intake and the use of local water to make beverages (coffee, tea, juices, and juice drinks) is not captured in national food consumption surveys. Currently, there is a large market in bottled water and in prepared beverages that may or may not be made with fluoridated water. Bottled water does not usually contain added F. The variability in dietary F in both fluoridated and nonfluoridated areas appears to be due to the varying F content of water used in the preparation of processed foods *(33)*, so that the dietary F content may even be relatively high in nonfluoridated areas. In addition to fluoridated water (and products made with it), the few foods naturally high in F include

Table 8
Contributions of food groups to I, Mn, and Se intakes, TDS,
1982–1991 *(22)*

	I (%)[*]	Mn (%)[*]	Se (%)[*]
Fruits	1	6	0
Vegetables	9	17	1
Nuts	0	4	0
Grain products	32	34	28
Milk and cheese	18	0	3
Eggs	5	0	9
Animal flesh	13	2	48
Mixed dishes and soups	8	7	9
Desserts	10	6	2
Fats	1	0	0
Sweeteners	2	1	0
Beverages	4	26	0
Total	103	103	100

TDS = Total Diet Study, FDA.
[*] Average contribution of food groups to the diets of 25–30 yr–old women
and men and of 60–65 yr–old women and men.

tea *(34)* and seafood *(35)*. Other sources of F are fluoridated toothpaste and mouthwash and F treatments provided in dentists' offices.

Some estimates of dietary F intake are available from studies reported in the 1970s. Spencer et al. *(36)* reported F intakes of 3.4 mg/d, and Kramer et al. *(37)* reported 0.8–3.4 mg/d. F analyses of diets used for metabolic studies at a Chicago hospital averaged 1.2 mg F/d, exclusive of the F in drinking water, and ranged from 1.6–1.9 mg/d with drinking water *(38)*.

San Filippo and Battistone *(39)* analyzed TDS food collections for young adult males in 1967–1968 and reported that the dietary F intake ranged from 2.09 to 2.34 mg/d, including beverages and fluoridated drinking water. Estimated F intakes from Singer et al. *(7,8)* and Ophaug et al. *(5,6)* were also based on analysis of TDS food composites. Singer et al. *(7)* reported that F intakes of adults ranged from 0.85 to 1.44 mg/d, exclusive of the F content of beverages, and from 1.46 to 2.57 mg/d including beverages. The F intake of four 1975 TDS collections for young male adults were 0.912, 0.988, 1.215, and 1.720 mg/d *(8)*. Another TDS collection for young adult males in 1977 yielded a daily F intake of 1.636 mg/d *(8)*. F intakes for two-year old children in four TDS collections were 0.315, 0.410, 0.554, and 0.610 mg/d *(5)*. Daily F intakes for 6-mo-old children from four TDS collections were 0.207, 0.272, 0.354, and 0.541 mg/d *(6)*. Major sources of F for all three age-sex groups were beverages and drinking water. These F intakes from analysis of TDS foods are in line with NAS recommended intakes (Table 2).

5.5. Iron (Fe)

Fe, like Ca, is another high profile mineral that is included in national food consumption surveys and the TDS (Table 1) and is emphasized in dietary guidance materials (i.e., the *Dietary Guidelines for Americans (20)*, the Food Guide Pyramid, and the Nutrition Facts Panel). The importance of iron during pregnancy and infancy is so well known, that pregnant women are routinely given iron supplements, and infants are given iron drops (as supplements to breast feeding) or iron-fortified infant formula (*see* chapters 8 and 9). Other groups that do not routinely meet their recommended intakes for iron are women of child-bearing age and young children (*see* Tables 4 and 5). Women of child-bearing age have an Fe RDA of 15 mg/ d, which is considerably higher than the 10 mg/d required for men or for older women.

Average Fe intakes from 1994–1996 CSFII (Table 3) range from 10.5 mg/d for children 1–2 yr to 19.8 mg/d for males 12–19 yr and 30–39 yr of age. Average Fe intakes for females ages 6 yr and over ranged from 12.4 for the older age groups (60 yr and over) to 13.8 mg/d for 12–19 yr-olds. Mean Fe intakes as percent of the 1989 RDA (Table 4) appeared adequate for all but the women of childbearing age. However, median daily Fe intakes as percent of 1989 RDAs for NHANES III ranged from only 63 to 74% for females 12 to 59 yr. Fe intakes for men in NHANES III were adequate at 110–152% RDA.

The main dietary sources for iron are grain products; meat, poultry, and fish; and vegetables (Table 6). Vegetable sources of Fe include legumes (beans and peas) and dark, green leafy vegetables, like spinach and kale. Iron is present naturally in whole grain products and is present as an enrichment nutrient in many refined grain products (e.g., white flour and products made from it, white rice, and corn meal). If a grain product has been enriched with iron, the food label will list iron (usually as a ferrous compound) on the ingredient panel.

5.6. Iodine (I)

I has not been included in national food consumption surveys, but it was included in the TDS from the mid-1970s until 1991 (Table 1). Average I intakes are generally high compared to RDAs, ranging from 151 to 498% RDA (Table 7). The main food sources of I are grain products; milk and cheese; animal flesh (especially fish), and desserts made with milk (Table 8). I is present in milk because it is added to dairy cattle feed supplements and because iodophors are used extensively in the dairy industry to clean the cattle prior to milking and to clean and disinfect the milking equipment. Thus, the I in milk comes primarily as an unintentional food additive.

Other sources of I are iodized salt and other foods to which I compounds have been added as direct food additives. I has been added to table salt in the US since 1946, when it was first used to prevent widespread cases of goiter in the midwestern states. Salt is available in both the iodized and noniodized forms. The salt used in restaurants and by food manufacturers in the making of processed food is usually noniodized. Iodized salt contains about 400 mcg I per 5 g (teaspoon). The RDA for I for adults is 150 mcg/d (Table 2). I is present in baked products made with iodate dough conditioners and foods containing the red food coloring, FD&C Red No. 3 (erythrosine). Erythrosine is about 47% I on a weight basis, and the I from this source is about 2–5% bioavailable. Erythrosine is permitted in many foods, and is found in some red-colored breakfast cereals, candies, and pastries.

Results from the 1982–1991 TDS (Table 7) indicate that average I intakes ranged from 170 mcg/d for infants to 386 mcg/day for 25–30 yr-old men. Average intakes for the more recent (1990–1991) TDS, were somewhat lower, 117 mcg/d for infants to 317 mcg/d for 14–16 yr-old males, and there seems to have been a declining trend in I intake from 1982 to 1991 *(3)*. I intakes are well above RDAs without including I from discretionary salt (that added during home cooking or at the table). The TDS estimates of I intake will be underestimated for individuals using iodized salt.

Estimates of dietary iodine intakes in other countries are found in Pennington *(40)*. That paper also summarizes reports of adverse effects of iodine from foods, dietary supplements, oral drugs, topical medications, and injected solutions.

5.7. Magnesium (Mg)

Mg has been included in national food consumption surveys and the TDS (Table 1), and results from the 1994–1996 CSFII (Table 3) indicate that intakes range from 98 mg/d for infants to 344 mg/d for men 30–39 yr of age. Intakes compared with RDAs (Table 4) appear adequate (all 80% or more RDA). Median daily intakes as percent RDA from the NHANES III (Table 5) are lower. Intakes for females 12–19 yr range from only 58 to 74% RDA. Intakes for males are higher, 68–103% RDA for the 12–19 yr group. However, there are no clear indications of Mg deficiency symptoms in the US population or in the groups that have the lower intakes of this mineral. Food sources of Mg include grain products; dairy products; vegetables; meat, poultry, and fish; and legumes, nuts, and soy products (Table 6).

5.8. Manganese (Mn)

Although Mn has not been included in national food consumption surveys, it has been included in the TDS. Estimates of Mn intake from the 1982 to 1991 TDS (Table 7) ranged from 1.07 mg/d for infants to 2.85 mg/d for 25–30 yr-old men. These average intakes appeared adequate meeting 90 to 178% of the lower end of the ESADDI range. The major food sources of Mn are grain products, beverages, and vegetables (Table 8).

5.9. Molybdenum (Mo)

Along with Cr, there is little information about the levels of Mo in the food supply or in daily diets. Pennington and Jones *(9)* summarized 16 reports, published between 1966 and 1985, with estimates of Mo intakes and provided additional information on Mo intake from a TDS project. A TDS quarterly food collection from 1984 was analyzed for Mo and several other trace minerals. The results indicated an average intake of 76 and 109 mcg Mo/day for adult females, and males, respectively. Of the 234 foods analyzed, Mo was found to be highest in legumes, grain products, and nuts. The TDS results were higher than those of Tsongas et al. *(41)*, who analyzed 40 foods for Mo and estimated intakes for 21 age/sex groups based on US food consumption data. They estimated Mo intakes to be 120 to 240 mcg/d with an average of about 180 mcg/d. Tsongas et al. *(41)* reported that foods that contributed the most Mo to the diet were milk, beans, breads, and cereals.

5.9. Phosphorus (P)

P, along with Ca and Fe has been evaluated in national food consumption surveys and the TDS (Table 1). P is widely distributed in the food supply and appears to be consumed in adequate amounts by all age-sex groups evaluated. Average P intakes from the 1994–1996 CSFII (Table 3) ranged from 526 mg/d for infants to 1,633 mg/d for 12–19 yr-old males. P intakes expressed as percent 1989 RDAs (Table 4) ranged from 92% (for 12–19 yr-old females) to 198% for 30–39 yr-old males. Median daily intakes as percent 1989 RDAs from the NHANES III were lower (Table 5), but still appear quite adequate. Food sources of P (Table 6) include milk and other dairy products; meat, poultry, and fish; and grain products.

5.11. Selenium (Se)

Information about dietary Se is provided primarily from the TDS (Tables 7 and 8). Intakes appear adequate, ranging from 18 mcg/d for infants to 111 mcg/d for 25–30 yr-old men. Average Se intakes met 116 to 228% RDA for the eight age-sex groups included in the 1982–1991 TDS. Thus, there is little concern about Se deficiency in the US. Major dietary sources (Table 8) are animal flesh and grain products. These two sources provide about 76% of daily Se intake. It should, however, be noted that the Se content of foods is variable and this variability can be a problem when attempting to estimate average daily dietary intakes.

There are some concerns about Se toxicity in areas where the soil and water are particularly high and where residents consume locally-grown foods, use the local water supply, and/or consume local wildlife (primarily fish and birds). Thus, there are pockets of concern in the US about Se intake. Local officials in these selected areas have attempted to post warning signs to hunters and to inform local inhabitants about the potential dangers of locally-grown or locally-raised foods. There have also been a few cases of dangerous side effects from Se taken in the form of supplements.

5.12. Zinc (Zn)

Zn is routinely evaluated in national food consumption surveys and the TDS (Table 1). Average Zn intakes reported from the 1994–1996 CSFII (Table 3) ranged from 6.4 mg/d for infants to 15.5 mg/d for 30–39 yr-old men. Zn intakes expressed as percent 1989 RDA (Table 4) indicate several values less than 75%, notably children 1–2 yr of age and women age 50 yr and older. Median intakes of Zn expressed as percent 1989 RDAs from the NHANES III reveal even lower values for females 12–19 yr and 60 yr and over and for males 60 yr and over (Table 5). These may be the groups vulnerable to low Zn intakes. No specific deficiency symptoms appear in the US population with regard to Zn, and no general recommendations have been made by government agencies or by NAS (23) regarding Zn intake. Dietary sources of Zn (Table 6) include meat, poultry, and fish; dairy products, and grain products.

6. CURRENT KNOWLEDGE ABOUT TRACE ELEMENT AND MINERAL INTAKES

Table 9 provides a brief summary of intake levels of trace elements/minerals (from foods, not including dietary supplements) based on the information available from government surveys and studies and the other studies mentioned here. The TRONM (13) provides the following conclusions regarding trace element/mineral intakes in the US:

1. Many Americans are not getting the Ca they need to maintain optimal bone health and prevent age-related bone loss. Many people, particularly adolescents, adult females, and elderly people across racial/ethnic groups and non-Hispanic Black adult males, consumed less than the recommended amount of calcium from food in 1988–1991. Median Ca intakes from food were below recommended values for non-Hispanic Black children 1–11 yr of age, all adolescents except non-Hispanic white males 12–15 yr of age, all females aged 20 years and older, non-Hispanic Black males 20–59 yr of age, and all males 60 years of age and older.

2. Data on the dietary intakes of pregnant women in 1988–1991 indicate that mean intakes from food were lower than recommended levels for several key nutrients including Ca, Fe,

Table 9
Average daily intakes of trace elements and minerals in US diets

	All ages (<1–≥70 yr)	Adult females (20–≥70 yr)	Adult males (20–≥70 yr)	based on 1994–1996 CSFII data (12)
Ca (mg)	584–1,145	584–701	746–990	
Cu (mg)	0.7–1.6	1.0–1.1	1.3–1.6	
Fe (mg)	10.5–19.8	12.4–13.5	16.3–19.8	
Mg (mg)	98–344	225–244	283–344	
P (mg)	526–1,633	918–1,090	1,198–1,619	
Zn (mg)	6.4–15.5	8.3–9.7	11.3–15.5	
	8 age–sex groups	Adult females 25–30 yr	Adult males 25–30 yr	based on TDS data
I (mcg)	170–386	248	386	1982–1991 (3)
Mn (mg)	1.07–2.85	2.21	2.85	1982–1991 (3)
Se (mcg)	18–111	71	111	1982–1991 (3)
Mo (mcg)		76	109	1984 (9)
F (mg)	0.206–2.57*		0.912–2.57	1975, 1977 (5,6,8)
				based on USDA data
Cr (mcg)		25	33	(4)

*Ranges for F intakes of 6–m–old infants, 2–yr–old children, and young adult males.

Zn, and Mg. This was evident across racial/ethnic groups. Pregnant non-Hispanic Black females had a mean Ca intake that was lower than that of non-Hispanic white and Mexican-American pregnant females. The intake data did not include dietary supplements.
3. Median intakes of Zn and Cu from food were below recommended values for most age, sex, and racial/ethnic subgroups.
4. Median Fe intakes from food were below recommended values for children 1–2 yr of age, female adolescents 12–19 yr of age, and female adults 20–59 yr of age across racial/ethnic groups.
5. Median intakes of Mg from food were below recommended values for all adolescents and adults except adolescent males 12–15 yr of age.

According to the TRONM (13), Ca and Fe are classified as "current public health issues"; Cu, F, Mg, P, Se, and Zn are classified as "potential public health issues for which further study is required"; and I is classified among the nutrients that are "not current public health issues." The TRONM did not include evaluation of data on Cr, Mn, or Mo. The "recommended research action" for Ca, Cu, Fe, Mg, P, Se, and Zn is to "develop interpretive criteria to link monitoring data to functional outcomes or health outcomes" (13). For P, the recommendation is specific to determining the effects of high phosphorus and high protein on bone density when Ca intakes are low. In addition, there are recommendations to improve food composition data for Cu and to improve biochemical assays for Zn.

7. CURRENT KNOWLEDGE ABOUT TRACE ELEMENT/MINERAL INTAKES AND HEALTH

Information from Diet and Health. Implications for Reducing Chronic Disease Risk (23) summarizes what is known (or what was known as of 1989) about the evidence supporting relationships of nutrients (including trace elements and minerals) to chronic diseases. This NAS report included a review of national surveys, research studies, and epidemiologic studies concerning diet, health, and disease. A summary of the conclusions and recommendations of this report concerning trace elements and minerals is listed below. The six conclusions concern, Ca, F, Se, and Cu, and the two recommendations concern Ca and F.

Conclusions:

1. Epidemiologic, clinical, and animal studies suggest that sustained low calcium intake is associated with a high frequency of fractures in adults, but the role of dietary calcium in the development of osteoporosis and the potential benefits of calcium supplements — in amounts that exceed the RDAs — in decreasing the risk of osteoporosis are unclear.
2. Some epidemiologic studies have shown an association between calcium intake and blood pressure, but a causal association between low calcium intake and high blood pressure has not been established.
3. A few data from epidemiologic and animal studies suggest that a high calcium intake may protect against colon cancer, but the evidence is preliminary and inconclusive.
4. Unequivocal evidence from epidemiologic and clinical studies indicates that fluoridation of drinking water supplies at a level of 1 ppm protects against dental caries. Such concentrations are not associated with any known adverse health effects, including cancer.
5. Low selenium intake in epidemiologic and animal studies and low selenium levels in human sera have been associated with an increased risk of several cancers. Moreover, some studies in animals suggest that diets supplemented with large doses of selenium offer protection against certain cancers. These data should be extrapolated to humans with caution, however, because high doses of selenium can be toxic.
6. The data on most trace elements examined in this report (e.g., Cu) are too limited or weak to permit any conclusions about their effects on chronic disease risk.

Recommendations:

1. Maintain adequate Ca intake.
2. Maintain an optimal intake of F, particularly during the years of primary and secondary tooth formation and growth.

8. NEXT STEPS

The current and future needs to provide better data for estimating daily intakes of trace elements and minerals and assessing the dietary status of trace elements and minerals are:

1. improved methods for assessing usual food intakes, especially to prevent underestimation of total food and energy (calorie) intakes;
2. better data (i.e., accurate data on more foods) on food composition;
3. information and ways to measure and calculate trace element and mineral bioavailability;
4. accurate data on the trace element and mineral levels in dietary supplements (including botanicals) and about the intakes of such supplements in the population and population subgroups; and
5. methods to correlate trace element/mineral dietary intake data with clinical and biochemical measures of trace element/mineral deficiency and toxicity.

Fortunately, research and progress are being made in all of these areas and the next few years should bring us closer to estimating dietary trace element and mineral intakes with more accuracy and reliability.

It appears that efforts to increase Ca and Fe intakes for some population groups and to monitor the intakes of all trace elements and minerals should continue. In addition, efforts are needed to determine if reported low intakes of Cu, Mg, and Zn are compromising health and if public health efforts are warranted to try to increase intakes of these trace elements/minerals. It needs to be determined if dietary intakes of Cu, Mg, and Zn are really low, as current surveys indicate, or if intakes are underestimated by current survey methods and/or if intakes from dietary supplements compensate for low intakes from foods. It will not be possible to correlate dietary intakes of trace elements/minerals with clinical and biochemical data on trace element/mineral status until the inaccuracies caused by dietary underestimation and lack of information about the intake of trace elements/minerals from supplements are corrected.

REFERENCES

1. Pennington JAT, Gunderson EL. History of the Food and Drug Administration's Total Diet Study – 1961 to 1987. J Assoc Off Anal Chem 1987;70:772–782.
2. Pennington JAT, Capar SC, Parfitt CH, Edwards CW. History of the Total Diet Study (Part II). J AOAC Intl 1996;79:163–170.
3. Pennington JAT, Schoen SA. Total Diet Study: Dietary Intakes of Nutritional Elements 1982–1991. Intl J Vit Nutr Res 1996;66:350–362.
4. Anderson RA, Kozlovsky AS. Chromium intake absorption and excretion of subjects consuming self-selected diets. Am J Clin Nutr 1985;41:1177–1183.
5. Ophaug RH, Singer L, Harland BF. Estimated fluoride intake of average two-year-old children in four dietary regions of the United States. J Dental Res 1980;59:777–781.
6. Ophaug RH, Singer L, Harland BF. Estimated fluoride intake of 6-month-old infants in four dietary regions of the United States. Am J Clin Nutr 1980;33:324–327.
7. Singer L, Ophaug RH, Harland BF. Fluoride content of adult foods. J Dent Res AADR Progr & Abst 1978;57:No 1044 .
8. Singer L, Ophaug RH, Harland BF. Fluoride intake of young male adults in the United States. Am J Clin Nutr 1980;33:328–332.
9. Pennington JAT, Jones JW. Molybdenum nickel cobalt vanadium and strontium in total diets. J Am Diet Assoc 1987;87:1644–1650.
10. National Academy of Sciences (NAS) Subcommittee on the Tenth Edition of the RDAs, Food and Nutrition Board Commission on Life Sciences, National Research Council. Recommended Dietary Allowances, 10th Edition, National Academy Press, Washington, DC, 1989.
11. National Academy of Sciences (NAS) Standing Committee on the Scientific Evaluation of Dietary Reference Intakes, Food and Nutrition Board, Institute of Medicine. Dietary Reference Intakes for Calcium, Phosphorus, Magnesium, Vitamin D, and Fluoride. National Academy Press, Washington, DC,1997 .
12. United States Department of Agriculture (USDA), Agricultural Research Service. Data tables: Results from USDA's 1994–96 Continuing Survey of Food intakes by Individuals and 1994–96 Diet and Health Knowledge Survey. Riverdale, MD,1997.
13. Life Sciences Research Office (LSRO) Federation of American Societies for Experimental Biology (FASEB). Third Report on Nutrition Monitoring in the United States, Volume I, Chapter 6. Food Consumption and Nutrient Intake Prepared for the Interagency Board for Nutrition Monitoring and Related Research. Superintendent of Documents, US Government Printing Office, Washington, DC,1995.
14. Life Sciences Research Office (LSRO) Federation of American Societies for Experimental Biology (FASEB). Third Report on Nutrition Monitoring in the United States, Volume II, Appendix V. Supporting data tables and figures. Prepared for the Interagency Board for Nutrition Monitoring and Related Research. Superintendent of Documents, US Government Printing Office, Washington, DC,1995.
15. Clark D, Tomas F, Withers RT, Chandler C, Brinkman M, Phillips J, Berry M, Ballard FJ, Nestel P. Energy metabolism in free-living 'large eating' and 'small-eating' women: studies using $^{2}H_{2}{}^{18}O$. Br J Nutr 1994;72:21–31.
16. Johnson RK, Driscoll P, Goran MI. Comparison of multiple-pass 24-hour recall estimates of energy intake with total energy expenditure determined by the doubly labeled water method in young children. J Am Diet Assoc 1996;96:1140–1144.

17. Martin LJ, Su W, Jones PJ, Lockwood GA, Tritchler DL, Boyd NF. Comparison of energy intakes determined by food records and doubly labeled water in women participating in a dietary-intervention trial. Am J Clin Nutr 1996;63:483–490.

18. Sawaya AL, Tucker K, Tsay R, Willett W, Saltzman E, Dallal GE, Roberts SB. Evaluation of four methods for determining energy intake in young and older women: comparison with doubly labeled water measurements of total energy expenditure. Am J Clin Nutr 1996;63:491–499.

19. Warwick PM, Baines J. Energy expenditure in free-living smokers and nonsmokers: comparison between factorial intake-balance and doubly labeled water measures. Am J Clin Nutr 1996;63:15–21.

20. Department of Health and Human Services/United States Department of Agriculture (DHHS/USDA). Dietary Guidelines for Americans, 3rd edition. Home and Garden Bulletin No. 232. Washington, DC,1995.

21. Gerrior SA, Zizza C. Nutrient Content of the US Food Supply, 1909-1990. Home Economics Research Report No. 52. USDA, Washington, DC, 1994.

22. Pennington JAT, Schoen SA. Contribution of food groups to element intakes: Results from the FDA Total Diet Studies, 1982–91. Intl J Vit Nutr Res 1996;66:342–350.

23. National Academy of Sciences (NAS) Committee on Diet and Health, Food and Nutrition Board, Commission on Life Sciences, National Research Council. Diet and Health Implications for Reducing Chronic Disease Risk. National Academy Press, Washington, DC, 1989.

24. Anderson RA. Chromium. In: Smith KT, ed. Trace Minerals in Foods. Marcel Dekker, New York and Basel, 1988, pp. 231–247.

25. Pi-Sunyer FX, Offenbacher EG. Chromium. In: Olson RE, Broquist HP, Chichester CO, Darby WJ, Kolbye AC, Stalvey RM, eds. Nutrition Reviews' Present Knowledge in Nutrition. Nutrition Foundation, Washington, DC, 1984, pp. 571–586.

26. Koivistoinen P. Mineral element composition of Finnish foods: N, K, Ca, Mg, P, S, Fe, Cu, Mn, Zn, Mo, Co, Ni, Cr, F, Se, Si, Rb, Al, B, Br, Hg, As, Cd, Pb, and ash. Acta Agric Scand, 1980;Suppl 22,Stockholm.

27. Gibson RS, Scythes CA. Chromium, selenium and other trace element intakes of a selected sample of Canadian premenopausal women. J Biol Trace Element Res 1984;6:105–116.

28. Bunker W, Lawson MS, Delves HT, Clayton BE. The uptake and excretion of chromium by the elderly. Am J Clin Nutr 1984;39:717–802.

29. Anderson RA. Chromium requirements and needs in the elderly. In: Watson RR, ed. Handbook of Nutrition in the Aged. CRC Press Inc., Boca Raton, FL, 1985,pp. 137–144.

30. Anderson RA, Bryden NA. Concentration insulin potentiation and absorption of chromium in beer. J Agric Food Chem 1983;31:308–311.

31. Klevay LM. Lack of a Recommended Dietary Allowance for copper may be hazardous to your health. J Am College Nutr 1998;17:322–326.

32. Klevay LM, Medeiros D M. Deliberations and evaluations of the approaches endpoints and paradigms for dietary recommendations about copper. J Nutr 1996;124:2419S–2426S.

33. Shannon IL, Wescott WB. Fluoride levels in drinking water. N Carolina Dent J 1975;58:15.

34. McClure FJ. Fluoride in foods-survey of recent data. Pub Health Rep 1949;64:1061.

35. McClure FJ, Mitchell HH, Hamilton TS, Kinser CA. Balances of fluorine ingested from various sources in food and water by five young men. J Indust Hyg Toxicol 1945;27:159.

36. Spencer H, Lewin I, Wiatrowski E, Samachson J. Fluoride metabolism in man. Am J Med 1970;49:807–813.

37. Kramer L, Osis D, Wiatrowski E, Spencer H. Dietary fluoride in different areas in the United States. Am J Clin Nutr 1974;27:590–594.

38. Osis D, Kramer L, Wiatrowski E, Spencer H. Dietary fluoride intake in man. J Nutr 1974;104:1313–1318.

39. San Filippo FA, Battistone GC. The fluoride content of a representative diet of the young adult male. Clin Chim Acta 1971;31:453–457.

40. Pennington JAT. A review of iodine toxicity reports. J Am Diet Assoc 1990;90:1571–1581.

41. Tsongas TA, Meglen RR, Walravens PA, Chappell WR. Molybdenum in the diet: an estimate of average daily intake in the United States. Am J Clin Nutr 1980;33:1103–1107.

5   Laboratory Assessment of Trace Element and Mineral Status[1,2]

David B. Milne, PhD

1. INTRODUCTION

Few entirely satisfactory laboratory methods have been established for the clinical evaluation of the status of most trace elements or minerals in humans. Measurements of metalloenzyme activities have been proposed as useful assessment tests because plasma or serum trace metal concentrations are often affected by factors not related to the whole-body mineral element status. A simultaneous battery of tests involving body tissue or fluid elemental determinations, metalloenzyme assays, and functional-morphological indices provides the most reliable assessment of mineral element status. However, in a clinical diagnostic setting it is most practical to assess trace mineral status by analysis of a single blood specimen. The use of hair mineral content as an indicator of status is somewhat limited. Whereas low metal concentration in hair may be indicative of metal depletion, "normal" or high amounts do not necessarily preclude depletion or indicate toxic amounts *(1)*, because of hair's susceptibility to environmental contamination and other problems. Further investigations are needed to establish the clinical value of whole blood, platelet, leukocyte, erythrocyte, saliva, skin, and fingernail analyses as indices of trace mineral nutriture.

1.1. Sample Collection and Testing

Accurate determination of trace elements in biological specimens requires special precautions and presents special analytical difficulties. Sampling procedures must be carefully considered because heterogeneity of trace element distributions in tissues is the rule rather than the exception. Analysis of apparently homogeneous samples such as blood, sweat, or saliva can be significantly affected by sampling and processing procedures. For example, hemolysis or microhemolysis of a sample can lead to erroneously high plasma or serum values for iron, zinc, and manganese because red blood

[1]Mention of a trademark or proprietary product does not constitute a guarantee of warranty of the product by the United States Department of Agriculture and does not imply its approval to the exclusion of other products that may also be suitable.
[2]U.S. Department of Agriculture, Agricultural Research Service, Northern Plains Area is an equal opportunity/ affirmative action employer and all agency services are available without discrimination.

From: *Clinical Nutrition of the Essential Trace Elements and Minerals: The Guide for Health Professionals*
Edited by: J. D. Bogden and L. M. Klevay © Humana Press Inc., Totowa, NJ

cell concentrations are 10-fold or more greater than those in plasma for these elements *(2)*. Zinc concentrations are 5 to 15 percent higher in serum than plasma because of the release of zinc from erythrocytes and platelets during clotting. Conversely, the choice of anticoagulant affects plasma values by osmotic influences on fluid shifts from blood cells.

1.2. Sample Contamination

The primary analytical problem encountered in trace element analysis is external contamination. Many trace elements are present in the laboratory environment in nanogram and even microgram amounts. Thus, a significant portion of an analytical value may be the result of contamination unless extraordinary measures are taken. This is a major reason for the wide variation of reported reference values, particularly for mineral elements present in the parts per billion range. A laboratory contemplating trace element analysis must be prepared to take precautions, to a point of fanaticism, for all sampling, preparation, and analytical procedures to assure that contamination is minimized.

Major sources of contamination in the laboratory include dust, rubber, paper products, wood, metal surfaces, skin, dandruff, and hair. Plastic and borosilicate glass are best suited for trace element analysis. Of these, fluorocarbon, polyethylene, and polypropylene plastics are generally the best. Prior to use, glassware should be cleaned of surface trace metal contamination by soaking overnight in dilute nitric acid or diluted commercial metal-scavenging solutions, followed by a thorough rinsing with deionized water. Water should meet, or exceed American Chemical Society specifications for type I water with greater than 14 $M\Omega/cm^2$ resistance. All anticoagulants and reagents used should be checked for trace element content prior to use. Only disposable plastic syringes with stainless steel needles should be used for blood collection. Stainless steel needles are not suitable for blood collection for chromium, nickel, and possibly other ultratrace metals unless they are siliconized, since stainless steel has a high chromium and nickel content. Evacuated blood collection tubes specified for trace metal analysis are also suitable if tops are removed after collection and the sample is not allowed to come in contact with the stopper. Leaching of metals from the stoppers of these and other types of tubes may contaminate the specimen.

1.3. ANALYTICAL METHODS

Any analytical method used for the determination of trace and ultratrace mineral elements in biological specimens must be sensitive, specific, precise, accurate, and relatively fast. Analytical sensitivity is extremely important because concentrations of trace or ultratrace elements in most biological samples are in the nanogram to microgram per gram range. The choice of analytical technique is dependent on the sample type and the element to be determined, because method requirements are not the same for all mineral elements or specimens.

The most popular techniques currently used for the determination of trace elements in biological specimens include photometry, atomic absorption spectrophotometry (AAS), and emission spectroscopy, which includes inductively coupled plasma emission spectroscopy (ICPES). Other techniques include inductively coupled plasma mass spectrometry, neutron activation analysis, X-ray fluorescence spectrometry, and electrochemical techniques. The most practical for use in most clinical settings are AAS and ICPES techniques. ICPES provides simultaneous multielement detection.

AAS is the method of choice for most routine trace mineral element analyses. Methods that involve diluted serum or plasma being aspirated directly into the AAS flame are effective for the determination of elements such as magnesium, zinc, and copper. Electrothermal, or flameless, AAS micromethods using as little as 10 μL of sample are used for many of the ultratrace elements or limited volume samples. Background correction using Zeeman or deuterium arc techniques is often necessary with electrothermal AAS methods to overcome matrix interferences. Matrix modifiers, reagents added to the serum or plasma sample to reduce background signals, may also be used. The sensitivities of the AAS techniques for determining the various elements depend upon the element of interest, sample, and on the technique used. The flame AAS technique is simpler and less tedious to perform than the flameless mode and is less subject to matrix interferences. Generally, if analyte concentrations of a specimen are below 50 ng/g, flameless techniques are necessary.

The ICPES technique is a rapidly developing multielement method and is replacing even AAS as the method of choice for many trace element applications. ICPES provides time savings because of simultaneous multielement determinations over a wide analytical range. Several useful reviews are available that discuss the principals of AAS and ICPES and their applications to biological and clinical samples (2–5).

1.4 Quality Assurance

Effective quality control measures must be incorporated into trace analysis schemes because methods for trace element analysis are not standardized and are subject to matrix effects and contamination problems. An effective quality assurance program for trace or ultratrace element analyses requires the incorporation of the following into each batch of analyses:

1. reagent blanks,
2. replicate analyses to assess precision,
3. calibrators of the elements of interest in the expected concentration range of the specimens to be analyzed, and
4. a control or reference solution with known or certified concentrations of the trace elements to be determined to assess accuracy and batch to batch precision.

The reference material should be of the same matrix type and contain approximately the same amounts of analytes as the specimens. A wide variety of control or reference materials are available from several sources, for example, the National Institute of Standards and Technology. Recovery studies of elements from samples containing known quantities of added analyte are useful at regular intervals and when developing a method for assessing accuracy and linearity (Table 1).

2. CALCIUM AND PHOSPHOROUS

Calcium and phosphorous are the major mineral components of the body. These minerals occur in combination with organic and inorganic compounds and as free ions. Their two major roles are structural components of bone and regulatory agents in body

Table 1
Adult Reference Ranges for Selected Mineral Elements in Plasma (P) or Serum (S)

Analyte	Reference Interval	Factors Affecting Concentration
Total Calcium (S) Ionized Calcium (S)	8.6–10.2 mg/dL 4.64–5.28 mg/dL	↑Hyperparathyroidism, alkaline antacids, some cancers, vitamin D toxicity ↓ hypoparathyroidism, vitamin D deficiency, Mg deficiency, chronic renal failure.
Chromium (S)	<0.05–0.5 µg/L	↓Diabetic children, pregnancy
Copper (S)	♀80–190 µg/dL ♂70–140 µg/dL	↑pregnancy, estrogen, birth control pills, infection, inflamation ↓Wilson's disease, Menkes' syndrome, protein malnutrition, cystic fibrosis.
Iron (S)	♀ 50–70 µg/dL ♂65–165 µg/dL	↑Hemochromatosis, acute leukemia, acute hepatitis, thalassemia, excessive Fe therapy. ↓Iron deficiency anemia, infection, hypothyroidism, kwashiorkor
Magnesium (S)	1.6–2.6 mg/dL	↑Dehydration, renal insufficiency, hypothyroidism. ↓Inadequate Mg intake/absorption, kwashiorkor, chronic alcoholism, hypercalcemia, pregnancy.
Manganese (S, P) (Whole Blood)	0.4–1.1 µg/L 7.7–12.1 µg/L	↑Industrial exposure, myocardial infarction, acute hepatitis. ↓Seizure disorders, phenylketonuria.
Molybdenum (S, P) (Whole Blood)	0.1–3.0 µg/L 0.8–3.3 µg/L	
Selenium (S, P) (Whole Blood)	7–160 µg/L 58–234 µg/L	↑Industrial toxicity. ↓Cardiomyopathy (Keshans Disease), GI cancer, pregnancy, cirrhosis, hepatitis.
Zinc (P)	70–150 µg/dL	↑Coronary heart disease, arteriosclerosis. ↓Estrogens, oral contraceptives, acute infections, acrodermatitis enteropathica, leukemias, pregnancy.

fluids. Bone also serves as a reservoir for these minerals. Calcium and phosphorous exist in the bones mostly as calcium hydroxyapatite and octacalcium phosphate.

2.1. Calcium

Calcium is the most abundant mineral in the body. More than 99 % of body calcium occurs in bone. The remainder, located in body tissues and extracellular fluids, is involved in several metabolic processes, such as blood coagulation, muscle contractibility, enzyme activation, nerve transmission, hormone function, and membrane transport. Calcium exists in three physiochemical states in plasma. Approximately 50 % of plasma calcium is free or ionized, whereas about 40 % is bound to plasma proteins, chiefly albumin; its binding is pH dependent. Approximately 20 % of protein-bound calcium in serum is bound to the globulins. In some patients with multiple myeloma, the high concentrations of serum globulin may bind sufficient calcium to cause an increase in the total serum calcium concentration. The remaining 10 % of plasma calcium is complexed with small diffusable anions, including bicarbonate, lactate, citrate, and phosphate. Calcium can be redistributed among the three pools, acutely, or chronically, thus affecting the quantities of ionized and total calcium in the serum.

2.1.1. Methods for Assessing Calcium Status

The method most commonly used for assessing calcium is either total or ionized (or free) calcium. Ionized calcium is considered to be more useful than total calcium as an indication of calcium status because it is biologically active and is tightly regulated by calcium-regulating hormones. Because calcium is bound to serum proteins, total calcium concentrations are greatly influenced by protein concentrations, especially albumin (6).

2.1.1.1. Total Serum Calcium. Although many methods have been used to determine total calcium in biological fluids, only three are in use today. These include photometric analysis, titration of a fluorescent calcium complex with EDTA or ethylene glycol tetraacetic acid (EGTA), or AAS. AAS has been approved by the National Committee for Clinical Laboratory Standards as the reference method for measuring serum concentrations of calcium (7). AAS provides better accuracy and precision than widely used spectrophotometric methods.

Total serum calcium is determined by AAS after diluting the specimen 1 to 50 with a solution of lanthanum-HCl ($LaCl_3$, 10 mmol/L; HCl, 50 mmol/L). The lanthanum is used to prevent interference by phosphate. The diluted sample is aspirated into an air-acetylene flame. Detailed procedures for the determination of calcium in serum and reviews of this method have been published (8).

2.1.1.2. Serum Ionized Calcium Concentrations. Serum ionized calcium makes up approx 50 % of the calcium in serum and is the physiologically active form of calcium in the blood. Reductions in ionized calcium concentrations occur in hypoparathyroidism and vitamin D deficient rickets, and result in neuromuscular irritability. Elevated ionized calcium concentrations indicate functional hypercalcemia, and occur in patients with hyperparathyroidism or receiving chronic renal dialysis. Total serum calcium may be normal under these conditions.

Several factors affect the measurement of serum ionized calcium concentrations. These include changes in pH of the specimen, high concentrations of magnesium and sodium, and the presence of EDTA or heparin. Physiological anions such as citrate, phosphate, oxalate, and sulfate form complexes with free calcium and may lower its apparent concentration. Because most anticoagulants act by binding calcium, serum is the preferred specimen for the measurement of ionized, or free calcium. Standards that contain sodium and magnesium in the approximate concentration range of the sample will minimize the impact of these ions on the outcome. The binding of calcium by protein and small anions is affected by pH both in vivo and in vitro. Ideally, specimens should be analyzed at the pH of the patients blood because of the inverse relationship between pH and free, or ionized, calcium. Anaerobic conditions should be maintained because specimens lose carbon dioxide and become more alkaline on exposure to air. In addition, samples need to be handled so as to minimize metabolism by red and white blood cells, which produce acids and reduce pH.

2.1.1.3. Calcium Reference Intervals. Serum calcium concentrations in healthy adults range from 8.6 to 10.2 mg/dL [2.15–2.55 mmol/L] *(8)*. Concentrations decrease with age in men and females have slightly lower concentrations than males. Serum ionized calcium concentrations range between 4.64 to 5.28 mg/dL [1.16–1.32 mmol/L] in healthy adults. The reference interval for ionized calcium should be determined for a specific instrument, specimen type, and collection protocol. Ionized calcium values have been reported to vary between capillary blood and venous blood, and serum because of differences in pH. Correction to pH 7.4 eliminated the differences. Differences in reference intervals between laboratories are primarily a result of differences in sample handling and instrumentation.

2.2. Phosphorous

Phosphorous is the second most abundant mineral in the body. About 85 % of phosphorous in the adult body is present in the skeleton as either hydroxyapatite or as calcium phosphate. The remainder in cells and extracellular fluid is present as inorganic phosphate or in nucleic acids, phosphoproteins, phospholipids, and high energy compounds involved in cellular integrity and energy metabolism. Phosphorous is an essential factor in most of the energy-producing reactions of cells.

Phosphorous depletion results in low intracellular concentrations of phosphoglycerate and other energy-rich phosphate esters, failure of muscle contractility, impairment of oxygen delivery, severe muscular weakness, and cardiac and respiratory failure. Phosphorous depletion may occur in patients receiving long term total parenteral nutrition not supplemented with phosphorous, and in patients with keto-acidosis treated with insulin and unsupplemented with phosphorous. Suboptimal phosphorous status may also arise in people with prolonged and excessive intakes of antacids containing aluminum hydroxide or aluminum carbonate, because absorption of phosphate is impaired by high intakes of aluminum and other cations that form insoluble complexes with phosphate.

2.2.1. METHOD FOR ASSESSING PHOSPHOROUS STATUS

Serum phosphorous, measured as phosphate, is used most frequently to assess phosphorous status. Phosphate in serum exists both as the monovalent and divalent anion. The ratio of $H_2PO_4^-$: $HPO_4^=$ varies from 1:1 in acidosis to 1:4 at pH 7.4 and 1:9 in alkalosis. Approximately 55% of the phosphate in serum is free; 35% is complexed with sodium, calcium, and magnesium, and 10% is protein bound. Serum phosphorous concentrations are generally measured colorimetrically by a modification of the molybdenum blue method of Fiske and Subbarow *(9)*. Serum is the specimen of choice for phosphorous determinations because many anticoagulants, such as citrate, oxylate, and EDTA interfere with formation of the phosphomolybdate complex. It is important to separate the cells from the serum as soon as possible because high concentrations of organic phosphate esters in the cells may be hydrolyzed to inorganic phosphate during storage.

2.2.2. PHOSPHOROUS REFERENCE INTERVALS

Reference intervals for serum phosphate concentrations vary considerably with age. Concentrations are about 50 % higher in infancy and decline throughout childhood until adult concentrations are reached. Serum phosphate, expressed as phosphorous, ranges from 2.5 to 4.5 mg/dL [0.81 to 1.45 mmol/L] in healthy adults, and 4.0 to 7.0 mg/dL [1.29 to 2.26 mmol/L] in children.

3. MAGNESIUM

Magnesium is the fourth most abundant cation in the body; within the cell it is second only to potassium. The adult human body (70 kg) contains 21 to 28 g of magnesium. Of this, about 60% is in bone, 20% in skeletal muscle, 19% in other cells, and about 1% in extracellular fluid.

There are two major roles for magnesium in biological systems: (1) it can compete with calcium for binding sites on proteins and membranes, and (2) it can form chelates with important intracellular ligands, notably adenosine triphosphate (ATP). Magnesium catalyzes or activates more than 300 enzymes in the body. Magnesium acts as an essential cofactor for enzymes concerned with cell respiration, glycolysis, and transmembrane transport of other cations.

The best defined manifestation of magnesium deficiency is impairment of neuromuscular function; examples are hyperirritability, tetany, convulsions, and electrocardiographic changes. Hypertension, preeclampsia, myocardial infarction, cardiac dysrhythmias, coronary vasospasm, and premature atherosclerosis have also been linked to magnesium depletion. Reviews that further detail the biochemical and clinical aspects of human magnesium nutrition are available (10–11).

3.1. Methods for Magnesium Assessment

Assessing magnesium status in humans is problematic because there is no simple, rapid, and accurate laboratory test to indicate total body magnesium status. For the past several decades, clinical chemistry laboratories have offered two tests to assess magnesium status: total serum magnesium concentration and urinary magnesium excretion. These two tests do not provide meaningful information about intracellular magnesium status, but only address the throughput of magnesium. Several other tests that may be of value in assessing magnesium status may be organized into three groups: tissue magnesium, ionized magnesium, and physiologic assessment of magnesium status.

3.1.1. Serum or Plasma Magnesium Concentration

Serum magnesium is the most frequently used index of magnesium status. However, the serum or plasma magnesium concentration provides only an approximate guide to the presence or absence of magnesium deficiency. Hypomagnesemia reliably indicates magnesium deficiency, but its absence does not exclude significant magnesium depletion. The concentration of magnesium in serum has not been shown to correlate with any other tissue pools of magnesium except interstitial fluid (12).

Serum is preferred rather than plasma because an additive such as an anticoagulant may be contaminated with magnesium or affect the assay procedure. Because the magnesium content of erythrocytes is three times as great as serum, it is important to prevent hemolysis and to harvest the serum promptly. Magnesium concentrations in serum are determined directly by flame AAS after diluting 50-fold with a lanthanum chloride or oxide diluent.

3.1.2. Ionized Magnesium Concentration

Magnesium in serum exists in several forms, protein bound (19–34% of total), as the free Mg^{2+} ion (61–67% of the total), and complexed to certain anions (5.5–14% of the total) (13). It is believed that free or ionized magnesium is the metabolically active form (14). The technology for measuring ionized magnesium in serum with ion specific electrodes has only recently been made available. Thus, more research is needed before the importance of this test is fully realized. Ionized magnesium location and concentrations in tissues may be estimated by the use of flourescent probes or by nuclear magnetic resonance spectroscopy. At present these techniques are limited to the research laboratory, but may have a future use in diagnosing disturbances in magnesium status and metabolism.

3.1.3. Magnesium Concentration in Muscle

Muscle contains approx 27% of the total body magnesium. Thus, it is an important tissue for magnesium status assessment. Needle biopsy has been used to determine the magnesium concentration in muscle, but this procedure is invasive, requires special skills, and the assay is tedious *(12)*.

3.1.4. Magnesium Concentration in Blood Cells

The mononucleated white cell (MNC) magnesium concentration has been proposed as a possible index of intracellular magnesium. In humans, magnesium concentrations in MNCs do not correlate with serum or erythrocyte concentrations. However, several studies show a correlation between the MNC magnesium concentration and muscle magnesium *(15)*. The magnesium content of MNCs is reportedly a better indicator of cardiac arrhythmias associated with magnesium deficiency than is serum magnesium concentration *(16)*.

As with serum, the erythrocyte magnesium concentration has not been shown to correlate significantly with other tissue pools of magnesium. Genetic regulation of this pool has been documented *(17)*. Thus, the usefulness of determining erythrocyte magnesium in clinical medicine is unclear, even though changes in total erythrocyte magnesium have been linked to hypertension, premenstrual syndrome, and chronic fatigue syndrome *(14)*.

3.1.5. Magnesium Retention After Acute Administration

Oral and intravenous magnesium loading tests have been described and are more widely used in clinical practice for diagnostic purposes than intracellular measurements. Normal individuals in magnesium balance excrete most (75–100%) injected magnesium in the urine within 24 to 48 h after administration, whereas individuals with a magnesium deficit retain a significant fraction of the injected magnesium. Patients who are to undergo this test should have normal kidney function, not be taking medication that affects kidney function and not have disturbances in cardiac conduction or advanced respiratory insufficiency.

3.2. Magnesium Reference Intervals

Total magnesium concentrations in healthy adults, as determined by AAS, range from 1.6–2.6 mg/dL (0.66–1.07 mmol/L) *(7)*. Serum concentrations in newborns are slightly lower than in adults. Infants older than 5 mo, children, and adolescents have concentrations essentially the same as adults. Concentrations do not change appreciably throughout the day.

4. CHROMIUM

Chromium functions in the control of glucose and lipid metabolism. Studies have demonstrated that chromium is a potentiator of insulin action. Insulin resistance may be a consequence of chromium deficiency; insulin apparently is ineffective as a glucose regulator without chromium. Few definitive studies of human chromium deficiency have been carried out mainly because of analytical difficulties in determining ultratrace amounts of chromium in tissue. Evidence of human chromium deficiency is mostly indirect, based on the improvement of insulin-resistant glucose tolerance after supplementation with chromium-containing compounds. Reviews that detail the biochemical and clinical aspects of chromium nutrition are available (18,19).

4.1. Methods for Chromium Assessment

No laboratory tests that reliably define body chromium status have been established as the determination of chromium in human tissues and fluids is one of the most difficult of trace metal determinations. Reported serum and urine chromium concentrations have been grossly overestimated in the past. As method sensitivity has improved, the capability of identifying and eliminating exogenous chromium contamination has resulted in substantially decreased estimates of chromium concentrations in biological specimens.

AAS with a graphite furnace and Zeeman background correction is the preferred method for estimating chromium in biological material (20). Strict avoidance of even brief contact with any metal surface by the sample must be avoided. Even stainless steel needles used for blood collection should be avoided unless they are siliconized.

4.2. Chromium Reference Intervals

The present accepted adult reference range for the chromium concentration in serum is <0.05–0.5 μg/L [1–10 nmol./L]. The presently established urinary excretion of chromium is between 100 and 200 ng/24 h. This may vary, depending upon recent chromium intake or the use of supplements.

5. COPPER

Copper is an integral component of many metalloenzymes, including ceruloplasmin, superoxide dismutase, dopamine-β-hydroxylase, ascorbate oxidase, lysyl oxidase, and tyrosinase. The major functions of copper metalloproteins involve oxidation-reduction reactions. Most known copper-containing enzymes bind and react directly with molecular oxygen.

A number of pathological conditions have been attributed to the loss of cuproenzyme activity. Failure of pigmentation has been attributed to the depressed tyrosinase activity required in the first step in the biosynthesis of melanin. A variety of connective tissue cross-linking defects (cardiac, vascular, and skeletal) are believed to be caused by a loss of amine oxidase activity, particularly that of lysyl oxidase. Ataxia may result from depressed cytochrome c oxidase activity in motor neurons. Depressed dopamine-β-hydroxylase activity may result in abnormal catecholamine conversions.

Reviews that discuss in detail the biochemical and clinical aspects of copper are available in this volume and elsewhere (20–24).

5.1. Methods for Copper Assessment

The assessment of copper nutriture in adult humans has not been perfected (25). However, there are a number of indices that are useful in the diagnosis of human copper deficiency.

5.1.1. SERUM OR PLASMA COPPER CONCENTRATIONS

Serum or plasma copper provides a relatively routine test for the clinical assessment of copper nutriture; low concentrations may be indicative of severely depleted copper stores. However, plasma copper concentrations are a poor indicator of short-term marginal copper status in humans. Plasma copper concentrations are regulated by strong homeostatic mechanisms and are maintained within a relatively narrow range within an individual; plasma copper falls only after stores are severely depleted *(26)*. Circulating copper concentrations are sensitive to factors which may not be directly related to copper nutriture. Women generally have higher plasma or serum copper concentrations than men, and estrogen increases plasma copper concentrations in both younger women taking oral contraceptives and postmenopausal women on estrogen therapy *(27)*. Other conditions that result in increased plasma copper concentrations include pregnancy, infections, inflammation, and rheumatoid arthritis *(28)*. Increased serum copper has also been reported in patients with dialated cardiomyopathy and immediately following myocardial infarction *(29–30)*. Conversely, corticosteroid and corticotropin tend to decrease plasma copper concentrations *(28)*. Thus, conditions that elevate serum copper may obscure changes in copper status, even during copper deprivation. Conditions that decrease plasma copper also need to be ruled out before a proper assessment may be made.

AAS after direct dilution with deionized water is the method of choice for determining serum or plasma copper concentrations. Hemolysis is not a great concern for copper determinations because concentrations of copper in plasma and erythrocytes are nearly equal.

5.1.2. CERULOPLASMIN

Most of the changes observed in plasma copper concentrations are associated with changes in the cuproprotein, ceruloplasmin (EC 1.16.3.1); over 70–80% of the plasma copper is associated with ceruloplasmin. Both the enzyme activity of ceruloplasmin and the immunoreactive ceruloplasmin protein respond in a similar manner to age, gender, and hormone use. They are also both elevated in pregnancy, and as a result of inflammatory responses. Enzymatically measured ceruloplasmin has been shown to be a sensitive indicator of copper status in several species of animals and has been found to be depressed in some men and women during copper deprivation studies *(31)*.

Serum ceruloplasmin may be measured immunochemically or by its oxidase activity. It is likely that a copper-depleted apoceruloplasmin is present in normal and copper-deficient serum *(32)*. Thus, assays of its oxidase activity may be preferred to immunological methods. Recent studies of experimental copper deprivation demonstrated that the specific activity of ceruloplasmin, defined as the ratio of the enzyme activity to the immunoreactive protein, is a better indicator of copper status than either the enzyme activity or immunoreactive protein alone *(31)*. Ceruloplasmin specific activity is sensitive to copper status and is inversely related to the autonomic blood pressure response in young women *(33)*. It is not affected by age, gender, or hormone use *(27)*.

5.1.3. SUPEROXIDE DISMUTASE ACTIVITY

Erythrocyte copper-zinc superoxide dismutase (EC 1.15.1.1) activity is depressed during copper deficiency in several animal species and in humans. It has also been shown to be sensitive to changes in copper status in several studies of experimental copper deprivation *(31)*. In contrast to plasma copper or ceruloplasmin, erythrocyte copper-zinc superoxide dismutase activity does not seem to be affected by age, gender, or hormone use *(27)*. Recent studies, however, have suggested that some conditions that produce oxidative stress may increase copper-zinc superoxide dismutase activity, even during periods of low copper intake; erythrocyte superoxide dismutase activity was elevated in competitive swimmers during training, presumably as a functional adaptation to increased oxygen utilization during aerobic training *(34)*.

Most available assays are based on the indirect measurement of activity that consists of a superoxide generating system and a superoxide indicator that is measured spectrophotometrically *(35)*. Addition of copper-zinc superoxide dismutase inhibits the absorption change. However many of these assays are prone to interferences. A method based on the autoxidation of pyrogallol *(36)* is probably the method of choice and seems to be relatively free of interferences.

A major disadvantage related to the measurement of superoxide dismutase is the lack of a standard assay. In spite of the plethora of methods that provide apparently different numbers and definitions of "units," analysis of copper-zinc superoxide dismutase in erythrocytes can provide clinically useful data if reference ranges are established in each laboratory and conditions used for analysis are carefully maintained.

5.1.4. CYTOCHROME C OXIDASE ACTIVITY

Depressed tissue cytochrome c oxidase (EC 1.9.3.1) activity is an early and consistent sign of copper deficiency in animals. Defects in cytochrome c oxidase activity can cause neurological, cardiac, and muscle defects when the activity is only about 50% of normal *(37)*. Markedly lower leukocyte cytochrome c oxidase activity has also been reported in patients with Menkes disease *(38)* *(see* Chapter 12). Platelet and leukocyte cytochrome c oxidase activity was reduced in young women on a low copper intake *(32)*. Platelet cytochrome c oxidase activity was the most sensitive indicator of changes in copper status in a recent study with postmenopausal women *(39)*. Studies with rats demonstrated that both platelet and leukocyte cytochrome c oxidase activity is sensitive to copper status *(40,41)*; the cytochrome c oxidase activity in platelets correlates with liver copper, an established marker of copper status in animals.

Most methods for determining cytochrome c oxidase activity in tissues and blood cells are based on the spectrophotometric analysis of the oxidation of ferricytochrome c *(20)*. A microassay has been described that utilizes a coupled reaction between cytochrome c and 3,3'-diaminobenzidine tetrachloride in microwell plates *(42)*.

Platelet and mononuclear leukocyte cytochrome c oxidase activities are higher in older adults than in young adults, but are not affected by gender or hormone use *(27)*. However, there seems to be large subject to subject variation, the enzyme is fairly labile, and cytochrome c oxidase assays are sensitive to minor variations in technique.

5.1.5. OTHER POTENTIAL COPPER INDICATORS

Other potential indices of copper status, which have not been well investigated or are too tedious for routine use, include platelet, erythrocyte or leukocyte copper content, skin lysyl oxidase activity, and measurements of copper retention and turnover.

5.2. Copper Reference Intervals

Serum copper concentrations are higher in women of child bearing age, 80 to 190 µg/dL [12.6 to 24.4 µmol./L] than in men, 70 to 140 µg/dL [11 to 22.0 µmol./L]; serum copper is highest in pregnant women, 118 to 302 µg/dL [18.5 to 47.4 µmol./L]. The reference interval for infants is 20 to 70 µg/dL [3.1 to 11.0 µmol./L] and 80 to 190 µg/dL [12.6 to 29.9 µmol./L] in children 6 to 12 yr of age *(7)*.

6. IRON

Iron deficiency is the most prevalent micronutrient deficiency in both industrialized and developing countries *(see* Chapter 6). It is particularly common in children and pregnant women. Severe iron deficiency results in anemia, which may be accompanied by loss of energy, anorexia, increased susceptibility to infection, abnormalities in thermogenesis and behavior, and reductions in intellectual performance and work capacity. Iron overload is also a problem that occurs most frequently with idiopathic hemochromatosis, a potentially fatal hereditary disease characterized by a progressive accumulation of iron in tissues, and may contribute to heart disease (*see* Chapter 12). Iron overload also may result from excessive intakes of dietary or medicinal iron, injections of therapeutic iron, or blood transfusions.

Iron functions mainly in the transport of oxygen from the environment to the terminal oxidases. Iron is also involved in electron transport and in oxidation-reduction reactions in the body. Reviews that detail the biochemical and clinical aspects of iron nutrition are available *(43–45)*.

6.1. Methods for Iron Assessment

The iron status of humans can range from dangerous iron overload to severe iron-deficiency anemia. Thus, many different methods have been used to assess the iron status of an individual. These include hemoglobin, hematocrit, mean cellular hemoglobin, mean cell volume, free erythrocyte protoporphyrin, bone marrow iron stain, serum iron, total iron binding capacity, serum transferrin, transferrin saturation, serum ferritin, and more recently, serum transferrin receptors. These methods vary in their specificity and sensitivity.

6.1.1. Hemoglobin and Hematocrit

Measurement of hemoglobin concentration in whole blood probably is the most widely used screening test for iron deficiency anemia. However, it is relatively insensitive and has low specificity. Concentrations fall only in the third stage of iron deficiency, and considerable overlap exists between iron deficient and normal nonanemic individuals. Hemoglobin concentrations also are altered by several conditions, such as dehydration, cigarette smoking, chronic inflammation, infection, protein energy malnutrition, pregnancy, folic acid deficiency, and vitamin B_{12} deficiency. Hemoglobin can be measured spectrophotometrically in whole blood, anticoagulated with EDTA or heparin, and after conversion to cyanmethemoglobin.

The hematocrit falls after hemoglobin production has become impaired. It is also relatively insensitive and nonspecific because hematocrit is affected by the same factors that affect hemoglobin, including changes in plasma volume.

6.1.2. Ferritin

There is a close correlation between serum ferritin concentration and storage iron *(46)*. In a controlled study of young women depleted of iron by a diet low in iron and phlebotomy, then repleted with iron, serum ferritin was the most sensitive measured indicator of changes in iron status and stores *(47)*. Concentrations of less than 12 µg/L are believed to indicate depletion of body stores, while concentrations above 300 µg/L indicate iron overload. Elevated serum ferritin concentrations also occur with both acute and chronic inflammations, vitamin B_{12} and folic acid deficiencies, liver disease, leukemia, hyperthyroidism, and Hodgkin's Disease *(46)*. Serum ferritin concentrations are determined by immunological techniques. A number of commercial kits are available.

6.1.3. Serum Iron, Total Iron-Binding Capacity, Transferrin, and Transferrin Saturation

Serum iron and total iron binding capacity reflect the iron in transit from the reticuloendothelial system to the bone marrow. Transferrin, the serum transport protein, is about one-third saturated with iron in normal circumstances. Transferrin may be measured immunologically, but is often determined as total iron binding capacity. The most useful measure of iron transport is transferrin saturation, the ratio of serum iron and total iron binding capacity, because plasma iron and total iron binding capacity move in reciprocal fashion in both iron deficiency and overload. A transferrin saturation below 16 % is indicative of an under supply of iron to the body, whereas saturation of over 55 % is diagnostic of iron overload or hemochromatosis.

Serum or plasma iron may be measured by using chromogens such as ferrozine or bathophenanthroline sulphonate. Total iron binding capacity is determined by saturating the serum with excess iron, followed by the addition of magnesium carbonate, which removes all of the iron not bound to transferrin. Determination of serum iron by AAS is not advisable because, unlike the colorimetric procedure, AAS will also measure the heme iron released from hemolysed erythrocytes.

6.1.4 TRANSFERRIN RECEPTOR

Transferrin receptors are transmembrane proteins present on the surface of most cells. Studies have shown that serum concentrations of transferrin receptors increase in iron-deficiency anemia, thus making it a useful marker in diagnosing microcytic anemias *(48)*. Circulating transferrin receptor concentrations increase in tissue iron deficiency; this reflects the degree of iron deficiency in the erythroid precursors in the marrow. In a controlled study *(49)*, serum transferrin receptors declined as iron stores were depleted. Circulating transferrin receptor concentrations increased only after iron stores were depleted, but before changes in other markers of iron deficiency, such as transferrin saturation, mean red cell volume, and erythrocyte protoporphryrin concentrations. The ratio of transferrin receptor to ferritin displays an inverse relationship to iron status, covering the spectrum from usual iron stores in health to substantial iron deficiency *(49)*. Thus, this ratio may be a useful indicator of preanemic iron status. Unlike ferritin, transferrin receptor concentrations are not significantly affected by inflammation or by liver disease *(50)*. Transferrin receptor concentrations can be determined by enzyme immunoassay systems that are now available.

6.1.5. FREE ERYTHROCYTE PROTOPORPHYRIN AND ZINC PROTOPORPHYRIN

Free erythrocyte protoporphyrin and zinc protoporphyrin concentrations have been shown to be sensitive indices of iron-deficient erythropoiesis. In iron deficiency, porphyrins accumulate in the erythrocytes because the lack of iron decreases the rate of heme synthesis *(51)*. Changes in free erythrocyte protoprophyrin or zinc protoporphyrin are relatively insensitive to acute changes in iron status because iron stores must be depleted before heme synthesis is affected, and because of the relatively slow turnover of erythrocytes *(47)*. Porphyrins also increase in lead poisoning because lead interferes with several enzymes involved with heme synthesis. Free erythrocyte protoporphyrin and zinc protoporphyrin concentrations are measured spectrofluorometrically *(44)*.

6.2. Iron Reference Intervals

Serum iron concentrations range from 65 to 165 µg/dL [11.6 to 31.3 µmol./L] in men and 50 to 170 µg/dL [9.0 to 30.4 µmol./L] in women *(7)*. Total serum iron binding capacity in healthy adults ranges between 250 and 425 µg/dL [44.8 and 76.1 µmol./L]. Serum ferritin concentrations range from 20 to 250 µg/L in men and 10 to 120 µg/L in women. Ferritin concentrations below 10 µg/L are indicative of depleted iron stores, whereas concentrations above 300 µg/L indicate iron overload.

7. MOLYBDENUM

The essentiality of molybdenum for animals and humans is based on molybdenum being an essential component of three metalloenzymes: xanthine oxidase, aldehyde oxidase, and sulfite oxidase. Xanthine oxidase participates in the degredation of purines into uric acid. Aldehyde oxidase catalyzes the oxidation of aldehydes, and sulfite oxidase catalyzes the final stage of sulfur amino acid oxidation.

No well-defined cases of dietary human molybdenum deficiency have been reported. However, a single case was reported *(53)* of a patient on prolonged parenteral nutrition with a syndrome characterized by hypermethionemia, hypouricemia, hyperoxypurinemia, hypouricosuria, and low urinary sulfate excretion that was corrected by molybdenum. A possible congenital defect in molybdenum metabolism was suggested for an infant who showed feeding difficulties, mental retardation, skull asymmetry, and biochemical defects in xanthine and sulfite oxidase activities *(52)*. Reviews that detail the biochemical and clinical aspects of molybdenum nutrition are available *(53,54)*.

7.1. Methods for Molybdenum Assessment

Current methods for determining molybdenum in biological specimens are inadequate. The methods have mostly employed emission spectroscopy, neutron activation, and AAS techniques. Use of a nitrous oxide-acetylene flame has been suggested for molybdenum determinations by flame AAS. However, concentrations in biological specimens are so low that preconcentration or prior extraction is necessary prior to analysis.

7.2. Molybdenum Reference Intervals

Reported reference intervals for molybdenum in healthy adults range from 0.8 to 3.3 µg/L [8.3 to 34.4 nmol./L] for whole blood, 0.1 to 3.0 µg/L [1.0 to 34.4 nmol./L] for serum or plasma, and 8 to 34 µg/L [83 to 354 nmol./L] for urine excretion.

8. MANGANESE

Manganese is associated with the formation of connective and bony tissue, with growth and reproductive functions and with carbohydrate and lipid metabolism. Important manganese-containing enzymes include arginase, pyruvate carboxylase, and manganese superoxide dismutase in mitochondria. Manganese can also act as an enzyme activator by binding to a substrate (such as ATP) or directly to the protein, causing conformational changes. Enzymes that are specifically activated by manganese include glycosyltransferases, glutamine synthetase, and phosphoenolpyruvate carboxykinase.

Manganese is accepted as essential for humans mainly on the basis of its proven role in manganese-dependent enzymes and on the production of manganese deficiency in experimental animals rather than on direct evidence of human deficiency. Although manganese deficiency has not been documented in humans consuming natural diets, some disease states have been linked to possible disturbances in manganese metabolism. Low blood and tissue manganese concentrations have been reported in children with seizure disorders without head trauma and in children with maple syrup disease and phenylketonuria *(55)*. Additionally, manganese deficiency was suggested as an underlying factor in the development of hip abnormalities, joint disease, and congenital malformations *(56)*. Serum manganese concentrations are increased following industrial exposure, acute hepatitis and other liver diseases, and myocardial infarction. Increased erythrocyte concentrations have been reported in patients with rheumatoid arthritis. Manganese toxicity is a problem in manganese miners in Chile and other countries and in liver disease patients *(see* Chapter 17), due to the prominent role of biliary excretion in manganese homeostasis. Reviews that detail the biochemical and clinical aspects of manganese nutrition are available *(55,56)*.

8.1. Methods for Manganese Assessment

Laboratory tests that reliably assess body manganese status have not been established. The most common method for estimating changes in manganese metabolism and status is to measure its concentration in whole blood or serum. It is likely that whole-blood manganese, or manganese in blood cells, may best reflect manganese stores in tissue. Recent evidence indicates that the manganese concentration and manganese superoxide dismutase activity in lymphocytes are sensitive to changes in manganese status *(57,58)*. Widely varying concentrations for manganese in blood have been reported, up to a 35-fold range for serum. This large variation in reported manganese concentrations can be partly attributed to sample contamination during collection or processing, and the use of older, relatively insensitive and nonspecific analytical methods.

Because of the low concentrations of manganese in blood, hair, and urine, AAS with Zeeman background correction is the method of choice for manganese determinations. Instrumental parameters, pitfalls, and references to published methods for the flameless AAS determination of manganese have been reviewed *(59,60)*.

8.2. Manganese Reference Intervals

Current acceptable adult reference intervals for blood manganese are 0.4 to 1.1 µg/L [7.0 to 20.0 nmol./L] for serum or plasma and 7.7 to 12.1 µg/L [140 to 220 nmol./L] for whole blood *(59,60)*.

9. SELENIUM

Selenium helps defend the body against oxidant stress and is involved in the metabolism of thyroid hormones *(see* Chapter 13). The existence of a number of selenoproteins has been demonstrated. However, four different glutathione peroxidases and three different iodothyronine deiodinases are the only characterized selenoproteins with clearly defined functions. Selenoprotein P, isolated from plasma, may transport selenium between tissues and is an extracellular antioxidant defense protein. Selenoprotein W, found in muscle, may be involved in the pathogenesis of muscular degeneration seen in combined selenium and vitamin E deficiencies. All of the above proteins and enzymes are significantly decreased in selenium deficiency.

Selenium deficiency has been associated with two diseases of childhood in China. Keshan disease is an endemic cardiomyopathy that affects primarily children and women of child bearing age in areas of China with low soil selenium concentrations. Kashin-Beck disease, an endemic osteoarthritis that occurs during adolescent and preadolescent years, is another disease linked to low selenium status in China. In both instances, most indicators of selenium status are 30 to 40% lower than controls. Selenium supplementation has been shown to prevent or control these diseases. Other factors, in addition to selenium, may also be involved in the etiology of these diseases. Patients who were intravenously fed preparations not supplemented with selenium exhibited low selenium status, and some developed cardiomyopathy and skeletal muscle weakness. The relation of selenium to human health and disease has been reviewed (61–63).

9.1. Methods for Selenium Assessment

The determinations of urinary and blood selenium are useful measures of human selenium status. Plasma or serum concentrations may be a more sensitive indicator of selenium status than whole blood concentrations. In China, hair selenium concentrations were found to correlate with blood concentrations of selenium and were used to assess risk of selenium deficiency. Assay of erythrocyte glutathione peroxidase activity has been shown to correlate with blood selenium and is useful as a functional test of selenium status. The determination of selenoprotein P, the major selenium-containing protein in plasma, is also a useful and sensitive test for selenium nutritional status.

Recommended methods for determining selenium in biological specimens are flameless AAS, with either deuterium arc (64) or Zeeman effect background correction (65), and spectrofluorometry. The capability of selenium in forming covalent organocompounds impacts on its analytical determination in two ways: (1) the organo-selenium forms are likely to be quite volatile and therefore can be lost in certain sample preparation steps such as high temperature ashing; and (2) the facile reduction of sample selenium to the volatile hydride form allows the determination of selenium by the AAS hydride generation technique.

9.2. Selenium Reference Intervals

Reported selenium concentrations from healthy adults range from 58 to 234 µg/L in whole blood, 75–240 µg/L in erythrocytes, 46 to 143 µg/L in serum or plasma, 7 to 160 µg/L excretion in urine, and 0.2 to 1.4 µg/g in hair (66). Blood and tissue selenium contents vary with the selenium status of the particular geographic area.

10. ZINC

The essentiality of zinc for growth and well-being of both plants and animals is well established. The metabolic functions of zinc are based largely on its presence in over 300 metalloenzymes involved in virtually all aspects of metabolism. Important zinc-containing enzymes in humans include carbonic anhydrase, alkaline phosphatase, RNA and DNA polymerases, thymidine kinase, carboxypeptidases, and alcohol dehydrogenase. Zinc also plays a major role in protein synthesis and has an important function in gene expression; the involvement in gene expression is both a structural role and an enzymatic role. For detailed information on the metabolic interactions of zinc refer to recent reviews (67–69).

Nutritional zinc deficiency in humans is fairly prevalent throughout the world; it was first documented in 1961 in Egyptian and Iranian males as being the result of a low zinc diet in which a high fiber content decreased the availability of zinc for intestinal absorption. As zinc deficiency progresses, the clinical manifestations exist as a spectrum. In mild zinc deficiency, oligospermia, weight loss, hyperammonemia and lowered alcohol tolerance have been observed (67). Moderate zinc deficiency is characterized by growth retardation in adolescents and children, hyopgonadism in adolescent males, mild dermatitis, poor appetite, delayed wound healing, mental lethargy, impaired immune responses, and abnormal dark adaptation. Manifestations of severe zinc deficiency, as in the disease acrodermatitis enteropathica, include bullous-pustular dermatitis, alopecia, diarrhea, weight loss, recurrent infection, neuropsychiatric disorders, and ultimately death if not treated.

10.1. Methods for Zinc Assessment

Laboratory tests for assessing zinc status can be classified into two groups: those involving analysis of zinc in a body tissue or fluid and those testing a zinc-dependent function. Useful tests in the first category include determinations of the zinc content of the plasma or serum, blood cells, urine, and saliva. Functional tests include measurements of activities of zinc-containing enzymes and assessment of taste acuity. Other tests that are either too complex for routine diagnosis or not well investigated include measurement of changes of plasma zinc during exercise, blood ethanol clearance, zinc balance, ^{65}Zn uptake by erythrocytes, and ^{65}Zn retention and turnover.

Although the above tests have been shown to be related to zinc depletion in humans and animals, no single test has been proven to be a definitive indicator of zinc status *(20)*. Test results must be interpreted with caution because they may be confounded by clinical conditions unrelated to the subjects' zinc status *per se*.

10.1.1. PLASMA OR SERUM ZINC

Although the zinc concentration in plasma or serum has often been shown to indicate human zinc deficiency, it does not reflect whole-body zinc status in all cases. Other conditions that depress plasma zinc without causing deficiency include nonfasting states, infection, inflammation, administration of steroids, pregnancy, and hypoalbuminemic conditions, such as hepatic cirrhosis and malnutrition.

The determination of plasma or serum zinc concentrations by AAS is the simplest and, analytically, most reliable test for the routine assessment of zinc nutriture. An AAS method using a fivefold diluted plasma, and standards in 5% glycerol matrix are recommended for plasma or serum zinc determination *(70)*. Hemolysis must be avoided during sample acquisition and preparation because erythrocytes contain at least ten times more zinc than plasma.

10.1.2. HAIR ZINC CONCENTRATION

Low hair zinc concentrations have been documented in zinc-deficient, Egyptian dwarfs, in zinc deficient US infants and children, and in conditions associated with zinc deficiency, such as sickle cell anemia, acrodermatitis enteropathica, and celiac disease. However, in some cases of severe zinc deficiency, above normal hair zinc concentrations were attributed to zinc accumulation in hair whose growth rate was decreased as a result of the deficiency. Environmental contamination can also lead to apparently high hair zinc concentrations. Correlations between hair zinc and blood or tissue zinc are usually poor. Thus hair zinc is unreliable as a measure of zinc status.

10.1.3. URINARY ZINC EXCRETION

Decreased urinary zinc excretion usually accompanies human zinc deficiency. However, conditions associated with zinc depletion, such as hepatic cirrosis, high alcohol intake, sickle cell anemia, total parenteral nutrition, and postsurgical periods, often result in increased urinary zinc excretion.

10.1.4. ZINC IN LEUKOCYTES

Studies have indicated reductions in the apparent zinc content of peripheral leukocytes in experimental zinc depletion and other conditions related to zinc deficiency *(71)*. However, other investigators using different cell separation techniques were unable to confirm these findings *(72)*. The apparent changes in zinc content of the leukocyte fractions apparently were related to the degree of contamination by blood platelets.

10.1.5. ZINC-CONTAINING ENZYME ACTIVITIES

Several zinc-dependent enzymes such as alkaline phosphatase, carbonic anhydrase, nucleoside phosphorylase, and ribonuclease are useful indicators of zinc deficiency. Depression of alkaline phosphatase activity in either serum or neutrophils has been observed in a number of human zinc-deficient conditions. A study of zinc-deficient patients supplemented with zinc showed increases in alkaline phosphatase activity that parallelled the degree of zinc repletion. However, as with serum zinc, alkaline phosphatase activities are nonspecific and are affected by conditions unrelated to zinc status. In patients with sickle cell anemia whose zinc nutriture was impaired, carbonic anhydrase and nucleoside phosphorylase activities were related to zinc status and responded to zinc supplementation *(71)*. Zinc metalloenzyme assay methods that require zinc in the reagents are not suitable tests for zinc status.

10.1.6. OTHER POTENTIAL ZINC INDICES

Metallothionein I concentration in plasma or erythrocytes was proposed as a potentially useful index of zinc status; it was related to zinc status in some human and animal studies *(73)*. However, questions have been raised about the effects of other minerals on this measurement *(74)*. Recent studies have also suggested that serum extracellular superoxide dismutase, thymulin, and plasma 5' nucleotidase may also be sensitive to zinc deprivation. However, more rigorous evaluation is needed before these can be accepted as specific indicators of zinc status.

10.2. Zinc Reference Intervals

The accepted reference interval for zinc in plasma is 70 to 150 µg/dL [10.7 to 22.9 µmol/L]. Serum zinc concentrations are generally 5 to 15 % higher than plasma because of osmotic fluid shifts from blood cells when various anticoagulants are used. A fasting morning sampling is important for zinc determination because plasma zinc exhibits both circadian and postprandial fluctuations.

11. OTHER ELEMENTS

Arsenic, boron, nickel, vanadium, and silicon are considered possibly essential trace or ultratrace elements with tissue concentrations in the nanogram per gram amounts. These elements are most likely essential to animals and thus may be essential to humans. However, no well-defined cases of deficiency of these elements have been described in humans. Several publications review the evidence for essentiality and proposed functions of these elements *(54,75)* including Chapter 2 of this book.

11.1. Methods for Assessment

Currently there are no well defined methods for evaluating the nutritional status of these elements in humans. Several methods have been described for measuring these elements in biological specimens.

11.1.1. Arsenic

Techniques that have been commonly used to determine arsenic in biological specimens are mass spectrometry, neutron activation analysis, emission spectroscopy, and AAS. For most laboratories, AAS may be the most practical technique. Hydride generation AAS methods are required for arsenic determination in most situations because organo-arsenic forms may be quite volatile.

11.1.2. Boron

The boron content of human tissues and body fluids is poorly documented mainly because of contamination and methodological problems associated with earlier methods of analysis. A technique involving low-temperature wet ashing of specimens in Teflon containers and measurement of boron by ICPES shows promise for use in the clinical setting *(76)*. Use of borosilicate glass apparatus should be avoided.

11.1.3 Nickel

Sensitive techniques are required for the determination of the ultratrace amounts of nickel in biological specimens. Flameless AAS is recommended. Instrumental parameters and published methods for AAS determination of nickel in biological samples have been summarized *(3)*. Contact of specimens with stainless steel must be avoided.

11.1.4 Vanadium

Current analytical techniques for vanadium in biological specimens are inadequate. The techniques most commonly employed are neutron activation analysis and flameless AAS *(54)*.

11.1.5. Silicon

The techniques that have been used for determining silicon concentrations in biological materials include mass spectrometry, ICPES, and AAS *(54)*.

11.2. Reference Intervals

Because of the low concentrations and tentative nature of many of the analytical techniques, there are no reliable or established reference ranges for these elements in human fluids and tissues except for toxic levels of arsenic. Compilations of reported concentrations and comments on the reliability of the data are found in several references *(77,78)*.

REFERENCES

1. Klevay LM, Bistran BR, Flemming CR, Newman CG. Hair analysis in clinical and experimental medicine. Am J Clin Nutr 1987;46:233–236.
2. Sunderman FW, Jr. Atomic absorption spectrometry of trace metals in clinical pathology. Hum Pathol 1973;4:549.
3. Sunderman FW, Jr. Electrothermal atomic absorption spectrometry of trace metals in biological fluids. Ann Clin Lab Sci 1975;5:421.
4. Abercrombie FN, Silvester MD, Cruz RB. Simultaneous multielement analysis of biologically related samples with RF–ICP in Ultratrace Metal Analysis. In: Risby TH, ed. Biological Sciences and Environment. American Chemical Society, Washington, DC, 1979,pp.10–26
5. Chaudhri MA, Hannaker P. Reliability of the ICP–AES for trace elements studies of biological materials. Biol Trace Elem Res 1987;13:417.
6. Kragh-Hansen U, Vorum H. Quantitative analysis of the interaction between calcium ions and human serum albumin. Clin Chem 1993;39:202–208.

7. National Committee for Clinical Laboratory Standards. Status of Certified Reference Materials Definitive Methods and Reference Methods for Analytes. National Reference for the Clinical Laboratory 7-CR, Villanova, PA, 1985.
8. Bowers GN, Jr, Rains TC. Measurement of total calcium in biological fluids: Flame atomic absorption spectrometry. Methods Enzymol 1988;158:302–319.
9. Garber CC, Miller RC. Revision of the 1963 semidine HCL standard method for phosphorous. Clin Chem 1983;29:184–188.
10. Shils ME. Magnesium. In: Ziegler EE, Filer LJ, Jr Eds. Present Knowledge in Nutrition, 7th ed. ILSI Press, Washington, DC, 1996,pp. 256–264.
11. Ryan MF. The role of magnesium in clinical biochemistry: an overview. Ann Clin Biochem 1991;28:19–26.
12. Elin RJ. Assessment of magnesium status. Clin Chem 1987;33:1965–1970.
13. Altura BT, Altura BM. A method for distinguishing ionized complexed and protein-bound Mg in normal and diseased subjects. Scand J Clin Lab Invest 1994;54(Suppl 217):83–87.
14. Elin RJ. Magnesium: the fifth but forgotten electrolyte. Am J Clin Pathol 1994;102:616– 622.
15. Elin RJ. Status of the mononuclear blood cell magnesium assay. J Am Coll Nutr 1987;6:105–107.
16. Cohen L, Kitzes R. Magnesium and digitalis-toxic arrhythmias. J Am Med Assoc 1983;249:2808–2810.
17. Darlu P, Rao DC, Henrotte JG, Lalouel JM. Genetic regulation of plasma and red blood cell magnesium concentration in man. I. Univariant and bivariant path analyses. Am J Hum Genet 1982;34:874–887.
18. Stoeker BJ. Chromium. In: Ziegler EE, Filer LJ, Jr, Eds. Present Knowledge in Nutrition, 7th ed. ILSI Press, Washington, DC, 1996,pp.344–352.
19. Anderson RA. Recent advances in the role of chromium in human health and disease. In: Prasad AS, ed. Essential and toxic trace elements in human health and disease. Alan R. Liss, New York 1988,pp. 189–197.
20. Milne DB. Trace elements. In: Burtis CA, Ashwood ER, eds. Tietz Textbook of Clinical Chemistry, 2nd ed. WB Saunders, Philadelphia, PA, 1994,pp. 1317–1353.
21. Danks DM. Copper deficiency in humans. Ann Rev Nutr 1988;8:235–257.
22. O'Dell BL. Copper. In: Brown ML, ed. Present Knowledge in Nutrition, 6th ed. ILSI, Washington, DC, 1990,pp. 261–267.
23. Strain JJ. Newer aspects of micronutrients in chronic disease: copper. Proc Nutr Soc 1994;53:583–598.
24. Linder MC. Copper. In: Ziegler EE, Filer LJ, eds. Present Knowledge in Nutrition, 7th ed. ILSI, Washington, DC, 1996,pp.307–319.
25. Milne DB. Assessment of copper nutritional status. Clin Chem 1994; 40:1479–1484.
26. Milne DB Johnson PE, Klevay LM, Sandstead HH. Effect of copper intake on balance absorption and status indices of copper in men. Nutr Res 1990;10:975– 986.
27. Milne DB, Johnson PE. Assessment of copper status: effect of age and gender on reference ranges in healthy adults. Clin Chem 1993;39:883–887.
28. Solomons NW. On the assessment of zinc and copper nutriture in man. Am J Clin Nutr 1979;32:856–871.
29. Versieck J, Barbier F, Speecke A, Hoste J. Influence of myocardial infarction on serum manganese, copper, and zinc concentrations. Clin Chem 1975;21:578– 581.
30. Oster O. Trace element concentrations (Cu, Zn, Fe) in sera from patients with dilated cardiomyopathy. Clin Chim Acta 1993;214:209–218.
31. Milne DB. Copper intake and assessment of copper status. Am J Clin Nutr 1998;67:10415–10455.
32. Milne DB, Klevay LM, Hunt JR. Effects of ascorbic acid supplements and a diet marginal in copper on indices of copper nutriture in women. Nutr Res 1988;8:865–873.
33. Lukaski HC, Klevay LM, Milne DB. Effects of copper on human autonomic cardiovascular function. Eur J Appl Physiol 1988;58:74–80.
34. Lukaski HC, Hoverson BS, Gallagher S, Bolonchuk WW. Physical training and copper, iron, and zinc status of swimmers. Am J Clin Nutr 1990;51:1093–1099.
35. Flohé L and Ötting F. Superoxide dismutase assays. Methods in Enzymology 1984;105:93–104.
36. Marklund S, Marklund G. Involvement of the superoxide anion in the autoxidation of pyrogallol and a convenient assay for superoxide dismutase. Eur J Biochem 1974;47:469–474.
37. DiMauro S, Bonilla E, Zevani M, Nakagawa M, DeVivo DC. Mitochondrial myopathies. Ann Neurol 1985;17:521–538.
38. Garnica AD, Frias JL, Rennert OM.; Menkes' kinky hair syndrome: is it a treatable disorder? Clin Genet 1977;11:154–161.
39. Milne DB, Nielsen FH. Effects of a diet low in copper on copper status indicators in postmenopausal women. Am J Clin Nutr 1996;63:358–364.

40. Ralston NVC, Milne DB. Effect of dietary copper on platelet volume and cytochrome c oxidase in platelets. FASEB J 1989;3:A357 (abstract).
41. Johnson WT, Dufault SN, Thomas AC. Platelet cytochrome c oxidase is an indicator of copper status in rats. Nutr Res 1993;13:1153–1162.
42. Chrzanowska-Lightowlers ZMA, Turmbull DM, Lightowlers RN. A microtiter plate assay for cytochrome c oxidase in permablized whole cells. Anal Biochem 1993;214:45–49.
43. Dallman PR. Biochemical basis for the manifestations of iron deficiency. Ann Rev Nutr 1986;6:13–40.
44. Fairweather-Tait S. Minerals: iron. Intl J Vit Nutr Res 1993;63:296–301.
45. Beard JL, Dawson H, Piñero J. Iron metabolism: a comprehensive review. Nutr Rev 1996;54:295–317.
46. Lipschitz DA, Cook JD, Finch CA. A clinical evaluation of serum ferritin as an index of iron stores. N Engl J Med 1974;290:1213–1216.
47. Milne DB, Gallagher SK, Nielsen FH. Response of various indices of iron status to acute iron depletion produced in menstruating women by low iron intake and phlebotomy. Clin Chem 1990;36:487–491.
48. Kondo Y, Niitsu Y, Kondo H, Kato J, Sasaki K, et al. Serum transferrin receptor as a new index of erythropoiesis. Blood 1987;70:1955–1958.
49. Skikne BS, Flowers CH, Cook JD. Serum transferrin receptor: a quantitative measure of tissue iron deficiency. Blood 1990;75:1870–1876.
50. Skikne BS. Circulating transferrin receptor assay - coming of age. Clin Chem 1998;44:7–8.
51. Langer EE, Haining RG, Labbé RF, et al. Erythrocyte protoporphyrin. Blood 1972;40:112–127.
52. Duran M, Beemer FA, Van der Heiden C, et Al. Combined deficiency of sulfite oxidase and xanthine oxidase: a defect of molybdenum metabolism or transport? Proc 16th Ann Meeting of the Society of Inborn Errors of Metabolism.1978, p 165.
53. Rajagopalan KV. Molybdenum: an essential trace element in human nutrition. Ann Rev Nutr 1988;8:401–427.
54. Nielsen FH. Other trace elements. In: Ziegler EE, Filer LJ Jr, eds. Present Knowledge in Nutrition, 7th ed. ILSI Press, Washington, DC, 1996,pp. 353–377.
55. Keen CL, Zidenberg–Cherr S, Lönnerdal B. Nutritional and toxicological aspects of manganese intake: an overview. In: Mertz W, Abernathy CO, Olin SS, eds. Risk assessment of essential elements. ILSI Press, Washington, DC, 1994,pp. 221–235.
56. Keen CL, Zidenberg-Cherr S. Manganese. In: Ziegler EE, Filer LJ, eds. Present Knowledge of Nutrition, 7th ed. ILSI Press, Washington DC, 1996, pp. 334– 343.
57. Davis CD, Greger JL. Longitudinal changes of manganese-dependent superoxide dismutase and other indexes of manganese and iron status in women. Am J Clin Nutr 1992;55:747–752.
58. Matsuda A, Kimura M, Takeda T, Kataoka M, Sato M. Changes in manganese content of mononuclear blood cells in patients receiving total parenteral nutrition. Clin Chem 1994;40:829 832.
59. Milne DB, Sims RL, Ralston NVC. Manganese content of the cellular components of blood. Clin Chem 1990;36:450–452.
60. Néve J, Leclercq N. Factors affecting the determinations of manganese in serum by atomic absorption spectrometry. Clin Chem 1991;37:723–728.
61. Levander OA, Burk RF. Selenium. In: Ziegler EE, Filer JF, Jr, eds. Present knowledge in Nutrition, 7th ed. ILSI Press, Washington, DC, 1996,pp. 320 328.
62. Stadtman TC. Selenium biochemistry. Ann Rev Biochem 1990;59:111–127.
63. Arthur JR, Beckett GJ. New metabolic roles for selenium. Proc Nutr Soc 1994;53:615–624.
64. Jacobson BE, Lockitch G. Direct determination of selenium in serum by graphite furnace atomic absorption spectrometry with deuterium background correction and a reduced palladium modifier: age specific reference ranges. Clin Chem 1988;34:709–714.
65. Morisi G, Patriarca M, Menotti A. Improved determination of selenium in serum by Zeeman atomic absorption spectrometry. Clin Chem 1988;34:127–130.
66. Tietz NW, ed. Clinical Guide to Laboratory Tests, 3rd ed. WB Saunders, Philadelphia, 1995.
67. Prasad AS. Clinical manifestations of zinc deficiency. Ann Rev Nutr 1985;341–363.
68. Mills CF, ed. Zinc in Human Biology Springer-Verlag, Berlin, 1989.
69. Cousins RJ. Zinc. In: Ziegler EE, Filer FF, Jr, eds. Present Knowledge in Nutrition, 7th ed. ILSI Press, Washington, DC, 1996, pp.293–306.
70. Smith JC, Jr, Butrimovitz GP, Purdy WC. Direct measurement of zinc in plasma by atomic absorption spectroscopy. Clin Chem 1979;25:1487–1492.
71. Prasad AS. Laboratory diagnosis of zinc deficiency. J Am Coll Nutr 1985;4:591– 598.
72. Milne DB, Ralston NVC, Wallwork JC. Zinc content of blood cellular components: cell separation and analysis methods evaluated. Clin Chem 1985;31:65–69.

73. Grider A, Bailey LB, Cousins RJ. Erythrocyte metallothionein as an index of zinc status in humans. Proc Natl Acad Sci 1990;87:1259–1262.
74. Thompson RPH. Assessment of zinc status. Proc Nutr Soc 1991;50:19–28.
75. Nielsen FH. Nutritional requirements for boron, silicon, vanadium, nickel, and arsenic: current knowledge and speculation. FASEB J 1991;5:2661.
76. Hunt CD, Shuler TR. Open vessel wet-ash low-temperature digestion of biological materials for inductively coupled argon plasma emission spectroscopy (ICAP) analysis of boron and other elements. J Micronutrient Anal 1989;6:161–166.
77. Iyengar GV, Kollmer WE, Bowen HJM. The elemental composition of human tissues and body fluids. Verlag Chemie, Weinheim, 1978.
78. Iyengar V, Wolttiez J. Trace elements in human clinical specimens: evaluation of literature data to identify reference values. Clin Chem 1988;34:474–481.

6   The Epidemiology of Trace Element Deficiencies

Roberto Masironi, PhD

1. INTRODUCTION

Both excesses and deficiencies in trace element intakes may cause diseases in individuals and populations. Many studies have been carried out on the role of several trace elements either individually or in combination/antagonism in the pathogenesis and etiology of various diseases. Excesses of heavy metals are the domain of toxicology and will not be considered here. In the present review emphasis is placed on diseases associated with widespread nutritional deficiencies in essential trace elements, often reflecting geo-environmental factors.

According to the World Health Organization (WHO) and the Food and Agriculture Organization (FAO) of the United Nations, trace element deficiencies are a public health problem in many countries particularly in the developing ones. Many poverty-stricken areas of the world are affected by starvation and malnutrition and by deficiency of several essential trace elements. In addition, parasitic infections and blood losses, heavy transpiration such as occurs in tropical countries and, in women, menstruation, frequent pregnancies, and prolonged lactation increase trace element requirements and losses. Children and the elderly are especially at risk (1).

The epidemiology of trace element deficiencies and related diseases is not as clear-cut as that of many other diseases and disease agents. Except for iodine and iron deficiencies which give rise to well-defined pathologies in deficient areas, for other elements the deficiency symptoms are not specific enough and many other underlying factors could mimic the effects of trace element deficiency. Also, the analytical methodologies are rather complex and expensive for certain trace elements (see Chapter 5), and this is a problem for laboratories in developing countries. This may explain why, except for iodine and iron, research on trace element nutrition has generally had low priority in developing countries.

Blood, hair, and urine, the human samples usually analyzed, may not indicate possible cause-effect relationships of marginal deficiencies on health, and may only reflect preceding dietary intakes, whereas autopsy specimens may only indicate changes in element concentrations which have occurred in tissues after death. Despite these limitations, laboratory results can be very useful for defining the epidemiology of trace element deficiencies.

From: *Clinical Nutrition of the Essential Trace Elements and Minerals: The Guide for Health Professionals*
Edited by: J. D. Bogden and L. M. Klevay © Humana Press Inc., Totowa, NJ

Examples of environmental deficiencies of essential trace elements affecting human health are known, e.g., iodine deficiency and goiter or cretinism, and fluoride deficiency and dental caries. The opposite is also known: fluorine excess and skeletal fluorosis. Several studies have shown associations between trace element deficiencies and higher mortality rates from cardiovascular diseases (*see* Chapter 15). Other diseases have been studied including various forms of cancer and Alzheimer disease, but the evidence is not fully established.

Iron and iodine deficiencies are particularly widespread and are the most extensively studied. The mechanisms of action are known and clinical and dietary intervention are effective.

2. IRON

Iron (Fe) could be considered to be on the borderline between a major mineral and a trace element. The latter are contained in the body at the 0.0001% level, equivalent to a few to tens of milligrams whereas the average iron content in the human body is about 3–4 g. Compared to the much larger amounts of major minerals such as calcium, this is a small quantity but is vital.

Iron deficiency is quite common and is a cause of widespread ill health in practically all parts of the world. Anemias of nutritional origin are common in both developed and developing countries. Body losses of Fe amount to only about 1 mg daily through excretion and sweat. The dietary requirements are small, but increase in menstruating, pregnant and lactating women, and growing children. Iron-deficiency anemias are not always of dietary origin. Although iron is widely present in food, its absorption and bioavailability may be limited as phytates, tannins and phosphates present in food, especially in vegetables, interfere with its absorption. Best bioavailability is from heme iron as contained in meat. Vegetarian diets are a poor source of iron. This is a widespread health problem in many countries and individuals where socio-cultural, economic, climate, and religious factors play important roles in promoting daily use of vegetarian, and often poor, diets. Populations that drink considerable amounts of tea may also experience decreased iron absorption due to the tannins present in tea. Thus it is important for most people to eat at least some meat and fish daily, as these types of food enhance iron absorption.

Iron deficiency is more pronounced in women owing to losses through menstrual blood, lactation and pregnancy, and in growing children. In tropical countries, blood and intestinal losses because of parasite infections as well as heavy sweating contribute to iron losses. Anemia is thus prevalent in tropical and other developing areas of the world.

According to FAO *(1,2)* more than 2 billion people can be considered to be iron deficient even if not all of them are frankly anemic. In many population groups, as many as 40–60 % are affected. Iron deficiency affects about 1. 6 billion people in Asia and the Pacific, 200 million in Africa, almost 100 million in the Americas, 150 million in North Africa and Near East, and only 27 million in Europe (2).

3. IODINE

FAO/WHO estimate that, more than 20 % of the world's population lives in iodine-deficient (I) areas. Dietary iodine deficiency is the most important cause of mental retardation, reproductive failure, goiter, and increased mortality and morbidity in general (*see* Chapter 13). Iodine is present in soil and foods in varying amounts. It is highly prevalent in mountainous areas where soils are leached by streams and rain water and iodine ends up usually in oceans. In coastal areas where shellfish and fish are rich in iodine, deficiency is less prevalent. There are also "goitrogenic" foods like cabbage, rape, cassava, turnip and other, the consumption of which as staple food may be related to the occurrence of endemic goiter *(2)*. As for other nutrient deficiencies, children and women are more vulnerable to deficiency. Iodine deficiency affects about 685 million people in Asia and the Pacific, 150 million in Africa, almost 55 million in the Americas, 33 million in North Africa and Near East, and 82 million in Europe. Goiter affects about 200 million people world-wide. About 26 million people have some degree of brain damage and mental retardation and six million are affected by cretinism because of iodine deficiency *(1–3)*. Whereas prevalence rates of 5–20% are considered mild, in certain communities in Africa, Asia, and Latin America more than 60% of the people have goiter *(3)*. Not only are humans affected by dietary iodine deficiency, but also farm animals which then exhibit stunted growth and poor reproduction *(2)*. It is now widely accepted that the best way to prevent and control iodine deficiency on a population basis is the use of iodized table salt.

4. ZINC

Marginal zinc (Zn) deficiency is fairly common in both developed and developing countries. It is not detected in early stages because symptoms are not very evident or specific. In developing countries heavy transpiration losses, frequent pregnancies, and prolonged lactation contribute to Zn losses. Environmental pollution e.g., high exposure to lead (Pb) in the diet can interfere with zinc absorption. In many developing countries, like India, daily intake may be as low as 5–7 mg/d, which is less than half the recommended dietary allowances *(3)*.

Zinc deficiency is a cause of growth retardation in Iran, Tunisia, Egypt, and other developing countries, and impairs the immune system *(4)*. The adverse effects of dietary Zn deficiency were first reported in the 1960s by Prasad and Sandstead, who noted numerous cases of dwarfism, and stunted skeleton and sexual development in Iran and Egypt *(5)*. The authors believed that use of unleavened bread as a staple food reduced zinc absorption because of the presence of phytates in this type of bread. Diets deficient in zinc may also impair fetal development during pregnancy and neonatal growth (*see* Chapter 8).

5. SELENIUM

Considered a carcinogenic element several decades ago, selenium (Se) was not even allowed to be fed to cattle (the so-called Delaney clause in the US) in spite of the fact that it was considered essential for the animals. Cattle develop wasting muscular disorders (white muscle disease) and cardiac necrosis if grazing on selenium-poor soils *(6)*. Selenium has now instead become a very attractive element for human use for its antioxidant properties that protect cells from the adverse action of free radicals.

The effects on human health of Se present in the geo-ecosystem were first revealed in China. Two Se-deficiency related pathologies — reversed by Se supplementation — are widespread in China and other Asiatic countries *(6)*. Kashin-Beck disease (so-called from the names of its discoverers in 1859 and 1906) is highly prevalent in large Se-poor areas of China, Central Asia, and Siberia. Its etiology is still unclear and it manifests itself as an osteoarthropathy with enlarged joints, short fingers and toes, and sometimes dwarfism, affecting mainly children. In China, hair Se levels in children in nonaffected areas range from 93 to 2965 ppb but in affected areas they are much lower: 44 to 165 ppb. Oral administration of Sodium selenite as aqueous solution, 0.5 to 2.0 mg/wk depending on child age, together with vitamin E, was effective in improving the condition.

Selenium deficiency in soil, vegetables, and the staple cereal foods of those populations was reported to also be the cause of a widespread disease in large Se-poor areas of China (6,7). The pathology was called "Keshan disease" from the name of the area where it was first discovered in 1935. The disease is a form of cardiomegaly, often lethal, including acute and chronic cardiac insufficiency, electrocardiographic abnormalities, and congestive heart failure. Sometimes the disease remains in the latent state. The disease affected mostly children in farming families who ate primarily locally grown vegetables with practically no intake of food of animal origin. Although other, still unidentified factors besides Se deficiency may play a role, nevertheless preventive oral administration of sodium selenite 1–2 mg/wk to children in table salt and as tablets and better dietary habits have greatly improved the situation and the pathology is now seldom reported.

In China both diseases have a similar geographic distribution forming a wide belt running from North-east to South-west China, where low Se was also found in foods and feeds. It is a large area covering a major part of the country including the provinces of Sichuan, Yunnan, Heilonjiang, Jilin, and parts of Inner Mongolia. Rocks, soil, water, foodgrains, staple cereals, vegetables, and also human blood and hair were all low in selenium. The two diseases occurred in the Se low (0.005–0.018 ppm in cereals) areas but never in the Se adequate areas (cereals: 0.024–0.087 ppm). Selenium levels in topsoils of affected areas are less than 125 ppb, and less than 3 ppb are water soluble. Se-deficiency diseases of farm animals (so-called white muscle disease in New Zealand where it is widespread) are also endemic in these areas (6).

In the US, cardiovascular effects on humans were detected in the early 1970s by R. Shamberger (8) as an inverse association between Se concentrations in locally grown forage crops and death rates from hypertension. Similarly, Salonen first reported that low Se levels in wheat in Finland were a contributing cause to the high rates of cardiovascular diseases, (the highest in Europe at that time). Low Se levels were also detected in human serum. The deficiency was brought under control when Se rich wheat began to be imported.

Masironi (7) hypothesized that countries of northern Europe, where cardiovascular death rates are significantly higher than in other areas of Europe, are underlain by geologically very old rocks of the pre-Cambrian era (more than 600 million years ago). These rocks and soils have lost most of their trace minerals through weathering, except for insoluble silicates. This is typical in e.g., Finland and Sweden relative to other countries in central and southern Europe, where cardiovascular rates are lower. Waters in those northern areas are "soft," i.e., demineralized. Selenium levels in staple foods and in human body fluids were also low.

Cancer mortality also seems to be correlated with environmental Se levels and dietary intake. An inverse association was evident in several US counties between mortality for cancer of the GI tract, lung, and breast and Se levels in locally grown forage crops. Likewise, a multicountry survey revealed an inverse correlation between average per capita Se intake and overall cancer mortality. In Finland, mean serum Se concentrations were reported to be significantly lower in cancer patients than in noncancer controls. In conclusion, although the nature of a causal relationship is not clear yet, the evidence is consistent with the findings that people living in high-Se areas have lower cancer mortality rates than those from low-Se areas (6).

Keshan disease and goiter, cardiovascular and cerebrovascular diseases including hypercholesterolemia and atherosclerosis were the pathologies most extensively studied from the clinical, etiologic, and epidemiological aspects *(10)*. They provided numerous and relatively consistent results, but the mechanisms of action are still hypothetical. As to other diseases including various types of cancer, Alzheimer disease, neurological and other conditions, results are inconsistent.

6. OTHER TRACE ELEMENTS

Deficiencies of other trace elements like manganese, chromium, and copper may also be a significant health problem but only in certain circumstances. Deficiencies in copper and manganese are not common. They have been reported, but their public health importance is not well established *(1)*. Copper (Cu) deficiency seems to be a cause of anemia in cattle but this is not reported in humans. Klevay *(11)* carried out substantive research on the possibility that Cu deficiency is related to atherosclerosis and cardiac infarction by mechanisms still poorly understood (*see* Chapter 15).

Epidemiological studies indicate that low chromium (Cr) levels may be indirectly related to glucose intolerance *(12)*, and indirectly to diabetes and cardiovascular diseases *(13)* in industrialized countries. In these populations tissue chromium levels decrease markedly with age and are associated with higher cardiovascular mortality rates, a condition which does not occur among Africans and Orientals. Chromium depletion in industrial countries may be because of excessive consumption of refined and industrially prepared food which has lost much of its chromium and other trace elements. The mechanisms of action of chromium are not clear yet, and it is thought to play a role in maintaining normal glucose tolerance *(13)*.

Years ago a well known controversy raged concerning soft, mineral-poor, and hard, mineral-rich waters, and cardiovascular or cerebrovascular disease epidemiology. Several studies were later carried out in the US and showed negative statistical associations between "hard," mineralized waters and cardiovascular diseases and hypertension. Noncardiovascular diseases did not show such associations.

The statistical association with the cardiovascular diseases was reported not only with municipal drinking water but also with raw river water, and this suggested a broader factor, the geochemical environment. Populations living in areas served by soft water practically always showed significantly higher death rates by cardiovascular or cerebrovascular diseases as compared to the hard-water areas *(14)*. This was found in Japan, in the US, in the UK, in Sweden, in South Africa, and in other countries where the studies were carried out. Even at present, studies continue to show this trend. A causal role for the water factor could never be proved, but not disproved either, and more recent reports *(15–16)* coincide with, and support, older ones *(12)*.

7. CONCLUSIONS

The importance of trace elements was stressed at the International FAO/WHO International Conference on Nutrition that was held in Rome in 1992 *(1)*. The Conference emphasized that deficiencies in micronutrients like I, Fe, Se, Zn, and Cu have significant health impacts on populations. The Conference emphasized that "Zn and Se are two essential trace elements whose deficiencies are known to present substantial public health problems to large population groups. Se deficiency is associated with Keshan disease, a cardiomyopathy affecting mainly children and women. Deficiencies of Mo, Cu, and Cr have been described, but their public health importance is not well defined."

The Conference determined that "Preventing specific micronutrient deficiencies" is one of the nine strategies and actions for "protecting and promoting nutritional well-being for all." Such actions include better dietary education, food fortification and micronutrient supplementation when needed.

In industrial countries widespread deficiencies are less frequent as food is usually abundant and varied so as to ensure adequate intake of trace elements. Usually food is also fortified with some micronutrients in these countries. But in many developing countries instead, food is often limited and monotonous, and diets are often based on socio/cultural and religious habits which reduce the bioavailabilty of certain essential elements. Through the widespread diseases that they cause, micronutrient deficiencies constitute a brake on socioeconomic development and are of considerable detriment to the world's already underprivileged groups (1).

It is interesting to note that the most recent reports (17) agree with the old ones (18) in considering the elements Se, Cu, Zn, Cr, and Mn to be beneficial for cardiovascular health whereas cadmium and lead seem to be associated with cardiovascular diseases. The significance of these associations in public health is uncertain but is consistent with the findings of beneficial health effects of these essential elements.

Of course, these observations cannot be construed to indicate a cause-effect relationship, but are consistent with the hypothesis that trace element deficiencies may exert harmful health effects on an endemic scale. Studies on the epidemiology of trace element deficiencies, after a period of interest several years ago, seem to have now lost priority. Perhaps the failure to identify consistent trends as compared to the relatively high research costs have discouraged investigators. A sort of "Micronutrient Renaissance" has recently started, as evidenced by increased interest in the role of trace elements in nutrition and in the elimination of malnutrition (18). At the recent congress of the International Society for Trace Element Research in Humans (ISTERH) many papers were presented on the role of trace elements in nutrition and in various pathologies. However, practically nothing new was said on the epidemiology of trace element deficiencies (19). These widespread deficiencies need to be addressed.

REFERENCES

1. Food and Agriculture Organization and World Health Organization. Major issue for nutrition strategies, Theme paper No. 6: Preventing specific micronutrient deficiencies. In: Report of the International Conference on Nutrition, Rome December 1992.
2. Food and Agriculture Organization. Human Nutrition in the Developing World. FAO, Rome 1997.
3. World Health Organization. Trace elements in human nutrition and health. World Health Organization, Geneva, 1996.
4. Chazot G, Abdulla M, Arnaud P. Eds. Current trends in trace element research. Smith-Gordon, London, 1989.
5. Ananda S. Prasad Ed. Essential and toxic trace elements in human health and disease. Alan R. Riss Inc. New York.1988.
6. Combs GF, Combs SB. The role of selenium in nutrition. Academic Press, Inc. New York, 1986.
7. Masironi R. Geochemistry, soils and cardiovascular diseases. Experientia 1987;531:68–74.
8. Shamberger RJ. Selenium in health and disease. In: Proceedings of a symposium on selenium and tellurium in the environment. Notre Dame Industrial Health Foundation, Pittsburgh,1976, pp.243–267.
9. Salonen JT. Association between cardiovascular death, myocardial infarction and serum selenium in a matched-pair longitudinal study. Lancet 1982;2:175–179.

10. Reis M.F. et al Eds. Trace elements in medicine, health and atherosclerosis. Smith-Gordon, London, 1995.
11. Klevay LM. ibid., chapters 2 and 25.
12. Mertz W. Ed. Trace elements in human and animal nutrition. Fifth edition, Vol. 1 and 2. Academic Press, Inc., New York,1986.
13. Masironi R. Trace elements and cardiovascular diseases. Bull World Hlth Organ 1969;40:302.
14. Masironi R, Shaper AG. Epidemiological studies of health effects of water from different sources. Ann Rev Nutr 1981;1:375–400.
15. Derry CW, Bourne DE, Sayed AR. The relationship between the hardness of treated water and cardio-vascular mortality in South African urban areas. S Afr Med J 1990;77(10):522–524.
16. Rylander R, Bonevik H, Rubenoowitz E. Magnesium and calcium in drinking water and cardiovascular mortality. Scand J Work Envir Hlth 1991;17(2):91–94.
17. Houtman JP. Trace elements and cardiovascular diseases. J Cardiovasc Risk 1996;3:18–25.
18. Underwood BA. Micronutrient malnutrition. Nutrition Today 1998;33:121–128.
19. International Society for Trace Element Research in Humans. New aspects of trace element research. Fifth International Conference, Lyon, France, 2–6 Sept, 1998.

7

Trace Element and Supplement Safety

John N. Hathcock, PhD

1. INTRODUCTION

Safety evaluation of the essential nutrients is undergoing rapid development and it may become standardized *(1–7)*. This progress occurs with a background knowledge that among the nutrients the trace elements pose particularly difficult challenges to find reasonable safety limits that will protect from toxicity but also allow the benefits of supplements. The difficulty with trace elements relates to both relatively narrow margins of safety and extensive interactions among them and with other substances.

The relative safety of the trace elements is described by the margins of safety between their minimum desirable intakes and the highest intakes that may be considered safe *(1)*. The upper level for safe intake for specific nutrients can be calculated through any of several published approaches: the Nutrient Safety Limit (NSL) *(1,2)*, the Reference Dose (RfD)(8), and the Upper Reference Intake Level (UL) *(7)*. The strengths and weaknesses of the NSL and RfD have been compared *(2,3)*. The NSL calculation uses the Recommended Dietary Allowance (RDA) or other recommended intake as a "floor" and either the No Observed Adverse Intake Level (NOAEL) or Lowest Observed Adverse Intake Level (LOAEL) as a "ceiling." The RfD does not directly account for nutritional benefits, but, in the case of zinc, the Uncertainty Factors (UF) were adjusted upward so that the RfD was not below the RDA for all age-gender groups *(9)*.

The Food and Nutrition Board has defined and set some UL values using a method that involves consideration of the nutritionally useful intake through expert judgment *(7)*. The UL method includes:

1. Identification of the critical adverse effect related to excessive intakes,
2. Dose-response assessment of the critical adverse effect to identify a NOAEL or LOAEL,
3. Uncertainty assessment and selection of a UF,
4. Calculation of the UL, and
5. Intake evaluation in relation to the RDA and UL.

Thus far, the National Academy of Science (NAS) has published UL values for only calcium, phosphorus, magnesium, and fluoride, as well as for a few vitamins. The Environmental Protection Agency (EPA) has set RfD values for boron, fluoride, manganese, selenium, and zinc *(10)*. The published RfD and UL values for trace elements, and the UF on which each is based, are shown in Table 1.

From: *Clinical Nutrition of the Essential Trace Elements and Minerals: The Guide for Health Professionals*
Edited by: J. D. Bogden and L. M. Klevay © Humana Press Inc., Totowa, NJ

Table 1
Reference Dose[a] (RfD) and/or Upper Reference Intake Level[b] (UL)

Value	B	Cr 3+	F	Mn	Se	Zn
NOAEL, amount/kg/d	8.8 mg[c]	1468 μg[c]	0.06 mg	0.14 mg	15 μg	None
LOAEL, mg/kg/d	29 mg[c]	None	0.12 mg	None	23 μg	1.0 mg
Composite SF (UF × MF)	100	1000	1	1	3	3
RfD, per kg	0.09 mg	1.0 mg	0.06 mg	0.14 mg	5 μg	0.3 mg
RfD, Daily Total (per 70 kg)	6.3 mg	70 mg	4.2 mg	9.8 mg	350 μg	21 mg[d]
UL, daily for adults	–	–	10.0 mg	–	–	–
RI = RDA or upper ESADDI for adult males	2.0	200 μg	3.8 mg	5.0	70 μg	15[d]
Ratio = RfD ÷ RI	3.15	350	2.1	1.96	5	1.4

[a] US Environmental Protection Agency (10).
[b] National Academy of Sciences (7).
[c] Data from animal studies.
[d] For adult men; the RfD equals the RDA for pregnant women; the RfD is less than the RDA for children.
SF = Safety Factor.
UF = Uncertainty Factor.
MF = Modifying Factor.
RDA = Recommended Dietary Allowance (18).
ESADDI = Estimated Safe and Adequate Daily Dietary Allowance (18).

All "safety limit" assessments are very dependent on identification of the critical effect, judgment of the data to identify the NOAEL or LOAEL, and evaluation of the associated uncertainty. The limit identified should be protective, feasible, and not preclude benefits that may occur at intakes above those officially sanctioned. Safety evaluations follow for the essential trace elements chromium, copper, fluoride, iodine, iron, manganese, molybdenum, selenium, and zinc, as well as the possbily essential trace element boron.

2. BORON

Boron has a low potential for causing obvious adverse effects in humans, as indicated by the widespread use of boric acid between 1870 and 1920 as a food preservative. This use of boric acid led to boron intakes of up to 500 mg per day without adverse effects other that nausea and loss of appetite (11). In pregnant rats, dietary boric acid can cause fetal development defects and growth deficits (12). In studies with dogs, high intakes of boric acid have caused testicular atrophy and decreased sperm production (13). Intakes of 500 mg boric acid (72 mg boron) per day for 50 days by adults have disturbed appetite and digestion (11).

In a study on dogs (13), adverse effects were found with an intake of 29 mg/kg/d over 38 wk of treatment, and this level became the LOAEL. The next lower dose of 8.8 mg/kg/d produced no adverse effects and therefore this intake became the NOAEL. The fetal development NOAEL in rats is higher than the NOAEL in male dogs. The EPA applied a 100-fold margin of safety to the NOAEL in dogs to calculate a "safe" intake (i.e., an RFD) of 0.09 mg/kg per day, or 6.3 mg per day in a 70 kg man (10).

For humans, the data are too scant and the effects too vague to identify a specific LOAEL value. Although more information is needed, the gastrointestinal effects associated with an intake of 500 mg of boric acid (72 mg boron) may be considered undesirable rather than harmful. Moreover, they should be self-limiting due to consumer awareness. Thus, no LOAEL value for boron intake by humans is identified.

The clinical trials with an upper intake of 3 mg per day produced no adverse effect but this intake may be too low to be a meaningful NOAEL for humans because few intake levels have been studied. The EPA RfD (equivalent to 6.3 mg/d in a 70 kg man), that was extrapolated from animals with a 100-fold safety factor, may be considered a safe level of human intake. This intake level could be suggested as a NOAEL, except that it would be a misnomer because it is based on calculation rather than observation. For boron intakes by adults, the RfD of 6.3 mg per day may be used as a well-substantiated human NOAEL; that is, it does not require application of any additional safety factor (equivalent to a safety factor of 1.0) to calculate a safe human intake.

3. CHROMIUM

No credible data or reports have shown adverse effects of chromium III (valence 3[+]) in humans, and animal data also suggest that orally administered chromium is extremely innocuous *(2,14,15)*. In addition, the Medline database lists no published cases of adverse reactions in humans.

In contrast, chromium VI (chromate, valence 6[+]) is clearly established as the work-related etiologic agent in lung disease, including lung cancer in chromate and stainless steel workers *(16)*. One report described chromosome breakage in vitro by high concentrations of chromium (III) picolinate added directly to cells *(17)*. These data showed that even at the high concentrations of chromium picolinate used in vitro, the only evidence for DNA damage resulted from picolinic acid, not chromium. Overall, such data do not provide appropriate evidence that chromium III in foods or dietary supplements carries any risk of causing DNA damage or cancer.

The EPA has reviewed all relevant data on chromium toxicity and calculated an RfD, a safety limit involving a margin of safety below the levels with evidence of adverse effects, for chromium III and also for chromium VI *(10)*. Application of a composite safety factor of 1,000 to the animal data gives an RfD of 1.47 mg/kg (15), which with rounding converts to 70 mg/d in the adult male. The RfD for chromium III (70,000 μg) is 350 times the upper value of the nutritional range (the Estimated Safe and Adequate Daily Dietary Intake) of 50–200 μg for adults *(18)*. Thus, chromium III has an extraordinarily wide margin of safety.

In contrast, hexavalent chromium (Cr^{6+}), a form not found in the diet, has significant toxic potential, and thus the RfD for chromium VI, calculated by the EPA for a 70 kg man, is only 335 μg/d *(15)*.

In summary, there is no evidence of toxicity in humans from orally ingested trivalent chromium (Cr^{3+}), and extrapolation from animal data indicates that it is extraordinarily safe. The benign character of chromium III should not be confused with the established toxicity of chromium VI.

There are no data on which to base a LOAEL for chromium III in humans. The highest intake reported for a group of people under good observation is 1,000 μg/d *(19)*, therefore this value is identified as the NOAEL. Because of the extremely high RfD calculated from animal data (70,000 μg/d) through application of a large safety factor (1,000), it is likely that the NOAEL is limited by experience with high intakes and not by any known potential for adverse effects.

4. COPPER

Copper is relatively nontoxic in most mammals, including humans *(20,21)*. Excess copper intakes that cause acute or chronic adverse effects are rare. Nevertheless, the adverse effects from acute intake of massive amounts of copper include epigastric pain, nausea, vomiting, and diarrhea *(22)*. These reactions tend to eliminate the large amounts of ingested copper that caused them, and thereby help reduce the risk of its more serious manifestations which can include coma, liver and kidney pathologies, and death.

Adverse effects related to longer-term ingestion of excess copper have been described in infants in India. These cases of "Indian childhood cirrhosis" resulted from heating milk formula in brass pots which leached large amounts of copper into the formula *(21)*. The intakes of copper associated with these cases are not known. Similar effects can be produced in animals by feeding them diets that contain very large amounts of copper (such as 2,000 mg per kilogram of feed).

There are no reports of adverse effects related to chronic intake of excess dietary copper by adults. The Food and Nutrition Board of the US National Academy of Sciences has set the nutritional range (the Estimated Safe and Adequate Daily Dietary Intake) at 1.5 to 3 mg, and the average diet in the United States supplies 1.0 to 1.5 mg/d *(18)* (*see* Chapter 4). A Food and Agriculture Organization/World Health Organization (FAO/ WHO) Expert Committee identified intakes of up to 0.5 mg/kg body weight as safe *(23)*, a level of intake equivalent to more than 25 mg/d for most adults. The Food and Nutrition Board concluded that occasional intakes of up to 10 mg are safe.

A LOAEL cannot be identified because of the absence of reports of adverse effects related to chronic intake, and the data on acute ingestion are not appropriate for identifying a chronic intake LOAEL.

The opinion of the FAO/WHO Expert Committee *(23)* might be interpreted as supporting a NOAEL of 25 mg/d or more, but the paucity of data on chronic high intakes warrants caution. A NOAEL of 10 mg/d is tentatively selected because it produces no known adverse effects and because of the substantial margin it provides below levels that may not be safe.

5. FLUORIDE

Fluoride toxicity is well-known and has been extensively reviewed *(7,10,24)*. The critical effects (i.e., those of significant adverse consequences and occurring at the lowest intakes) are dental fluorosis in children and skeletal fluorosis in adults. Excessive intakes in children before the permanent teeth are fully formed can result in dental fluorosis that manifests mainly as mottled brown discoloration and some increase in fragility. Dental fluorosis has been studied in relation to municipal drinking water fluoridation for the anticariogenic effect, and in relation to naturally occurring high-fluoride water supplies. The maximum safe fluoride intakes by children depend on age and body size. The NAS UL values are shown in Table 2. The critical effect, dose-response evaluation, and uncertainty assessment by the NAS are based on an extensive human database. The ready visibility of the critical adverse effect no doubt explains the extensive study it has received.

Excessive intakes of fluoride by adults do not result in dental fluorosis but instead result in skeletal fluorosis that results in increased risk of bone fracture. The NAS UL for adults is 10 mg per day, based on a NOAEL of 10 mg and a UF of 1.0, related to skeletal fluorosis. This evaluation, however, may somewhat underestimate the potency of fluoride

Table 2
Fluoride Upper Reference Intake Levels (UL) by Life–Stage Groups *(7)*

Life–Stage Group	Fluoride UL (mg/d)[a]
0 to 6 mo	0.7
6 to 12 mo	0.9
1 through 3 yr	1.3
4 through 8 yr	2.2
All other groups, including all male groups above 8 yr, and all female groups above 8 yr — including pregnant and lactating women.	10

[a]The marked increase in UL value after 8 yr of age reflects the lower fluoride intakes during tooth development that may cause dental mottling in children 1–8 yr-old. The fluoride intakes that can cause skeletal fluorosis are much higher.

to increase bone fracture risk *(25)*. Some epidemiological data suggest that an increased rate of bone fracture is associated with high drinking water fluoride concentrations (4 mg/L) and low drinking water calcium concentrations (15 mg/L) *(24)*. Assuming a daily intake of 1.5 L of drinking water, these data suggest that adverse effects of fluoride from this source might occur with intakes of 6 mg/d or more. If the fluoride intakes from foods and nonfluoridated water are 1 mg/d or less, and the intake from fluoridated toothpaste is approx 1 mg/d, the addition of these quantities to the 6 mg/d for high-fluoride water suggests that total intake of 8 mg/d increases the risk of bone fracture in persons who drink water with low calcium concentrations, and thus should be considered to be a LOAEL. This contrasts with the adult NOAEL of 10 mg/d identified by the NAS. Because of the conservative assumptions made, a UF of 1.3 may be adequate to calculate a UL from this 8 mg LOAEL. Thus, the calculated UL would be 6 mg. The UF of 1.3 for application to a conservative LOAEL of 8 mg seems reasonable in face of the NAS's identification of 10 mg as the NOAEL and their selection of a UF of 1.0 that leads to a calculated UL of 10 mg.

The epidemiological data do not present any clear pattern of association of fluoride intakes with cancer risk *(24)*. Animal studies are almost all negative for carcinogenicity of fluoride compounds found in water and food. The sole exception is the finding of "equivocal evidence" of carcinogenicity of sodium fluoride in the male Fisher 344/N rat. With the large number of studies performed, a single study that suggests possible significant effects is not surprising. No other data suggests an increased cancer risk related to fluoride consumption.

High intakes of fluoride can have adverse effects on the kidneys and the immune, gastrointestinal, genitourinary, and respiratory systems. All these effects occur at higher intakes than those that cause dental fluorosis in children and increased bone fracture risk in adults *(24)*. Thus, none of these effects is critical for evaluating the safety of fluoride for human consumption.

6. IODINE

Humans are remarkably tolerant to high intakes of iodine, except for rare instances of hypersensitivity to this element *(26)*. Although toxic effects are not observed in humans until daily intakes have exceeded 10,000 μg, intakes of 2,000 μg should be regarded as excessive and potentially harmful *(27)*. Residents of coastal regions in some areas of Japan have chronic daily intakes of iodine as high as 50,000 to 80,000 μg. Persons who have not been conditioned by iodine deficiency can maintain normal thyroid size and function when they are consuming several milligrams of dietary iodine per day, but previous deficiency can cause problems *(27)* *(see* Chapter 13   ).

For normal persons who have not been conditioned to iodine deficiency, no adverse effects have been identified at intakes of 1,000 μg/d in children or 2,000 μg/d in adults *(18)*. An intake of 1,000 μg/d is conservatively identified as the NOAEL for all except those previously deficient in iodine. Persons who were previously iodine deficient can respond with hyperthyroidism and iodine-induced thyroiditis when intakes exceed approx 200 to 300 μg/d. The data on adverse effects are so scattered and inconsistent that they are not useful in identifying a LOAEL.

7. IRON

For chronic, habitual intakes by persons who do not have a genetic defect that increases iron absorption and retention, iron has not been shown to have adverse effects at levels equal to several times the Recommended Dietary Allowance (RDA) of 10 mg for men and 15 mg for women *(18)*. Menstrual losses of iron account for the difference in RDA for men and women.

Chronic iron overload has resulted from several conditions or circumstances, including hereditary hemochromatosis, alcoholic liver disease, and excessive intake of dietary iron, especially from home-brewed alcoholic beverages *(28)*. Long-term daily ingestions of iron from some home-brewed alcoholic beverages may exceed 100 mg. This level of chronic iron intake, at least in combination with chronically high alcohol intakes, can lead to the liver disease "Bantu siderosis" that involves excessive storage of iron.

Hereditary hemochromatosis, a genetic disorder of iron uptake and storage, has a homozygous frequency of 3 to 4 per 1,000 in populations of European extraction *(see* Chapter 12) *(29)*. This condition may lead to excessive iron storage even at intake levels recommended for most of the population. There is no clear evidence that carriers for the gene (heterozygous condition) have any increased risk of excessive uptake and storage of iron, so the effect, if any, must be small compared with the effect in those who are homozygous.

The hypothesis and initial data *(30,31)* that high plasma ferritin levels or dietary iron causes an increased risk of heart disease have not been supported by subsequent evidence and evaluation *(32–37)*. The preponderance of evidence indicates that dietary iron does not increase the risk of heart disease.

For prolonged but not chronic use, such as in pregnancy, daily supplements of up to 60 mg are routinely and safely used. For other adults, the 95th percentile of intake has been reported to be 54 mg for men and 67 mg for women *(38)*. Many high-potency multivitamin and multimineral dietary supplements contain 27 mg of iron. Adverse effects have not been attributed to any of these intake levels.

Acute iron poisoning has occurred in children under three years of age who accidentally consumed massive amount of iron salts in the form of high-potency (usually 60 or 65 mg), single-nutrient iron supplements *(39)*. Such supplements are usually recommended for prenatal use. The quantities of iron involved in such cases are above 900 mg in a single ingestion. Such levels of iron override the intestinal regulatory mechanisms and lead to greatly increased plasma levels of iron. In contrast, no severe adverse effects other than mild gastrointestinal symptoms have been reported in association with acute ingestion of large numbers of children's multivitamins that contain iron. The adverse effects that may result from acute ingestion of large amounts of iron have no bearing on the safety of appropriately used iron supplements.

A large amount of experience supports a NOAEL value for longer-term iron supplementation of 18 to 65 mg per day (with little data on intermediate values). Data from chronic use of home-brewed alcoholic beverages brewed in iron pots supports a LOAEL of approx 100 mg/d, although the appropriate LOAEL may be higher for those who do not chronically consume large amounts of alcohol. Also, higher iron intakes for short periods are not known to cause harm.

8. MANGANESE

Manganese is often considered to be one of the least toxic of the trace elements for oral consumption (4,40,41). In animals, excess manganese may inhibit iron absorption and result in iron deficiency anemia. Additional adverse effects of manganese can include depressed growth, decreased appetite, and altered neurological functions. In contrast to the relatively low toxicity of oral manganese, environmental and workplace manganese exposures (mainly by inhalation) have led to a variety of severe neurological and brain effects, including ataxia, a pseudo Parkinson's disease, and behavioral changes (40). When administered to animals by injection, manganese is capable of producing central nervous system (CNS) toxicity (42).

Epidemiological reports from Greece suggest some evidence of adverse neurological effects in a high-manganese area, in comparison with lower manganese areas (10,43). The manganese content of well water averaged approx 2 mg/liter in the high-manganese area, suggesting an adult lifetime intake from water there to be approx 3 mg/d. Intake of manganese from food in the high-manganese area was initially estimated to be 10 to 15 mg/d, but this was later revised to 5 to 6 mg/d (10). These reports suggest that the total intake of manganese in the high area was either approx 8 to 9 mg or approx 13 to 18 mg, depending on which food intake data were used. These discrepancies have led others to conclude that the dietary data are not sufficient to permit reliable estimation of the total oral intake of manganese in these areas (44).

Several types of data show that oral manganese intakes up to 10 mg/d do not cause adverse effects in healthy adults (18,44–46). The epidemiological data from Greece are not inconsistent with this conclusion. Some epidemiological evidence indicates CNS toxicity of manganese in persons with liver disease, perhaps because of the prominent role of biliary excretion in manganese metabolism (see Chapter 17).

Several types of data show no adverse effects of manganese in adults with total oral intakes of 10 mg/d, and this value is identified as NOAEL. Due to uncertainties about the adverse effects and the total oral intakes of manganese in epidemiological studies, a LOAEL cannot be confidently estimated, although adverse effects are known.

9. MOLYBDENUM

Ruminant animals are susceptible to adverse effects of molybdenum under conditions of copper deficiency and marginal sulfur amino acid intakes (47). Men who consumed

10 to 15 mg of molybdenum per day for prolonged periods developed abnormally high serum uric acid levels and increased cellular xanthine oxidase activity *(48,49)*. Intakes as low as 0.54 mg (540 µg)/d have been associated with loss of copper in the urine *(18)*. It is not clear whether this effect has clinical consequences, but an increase in plasma uric acid levels observed with molybdenum intakes of 10 to 15 mg/d may result directly from excess activation of xanthine oxidase. No adverse effects were observed in an epidemiological study of men consuming molybdenum at a level of 5 µg/kg body weight in an area where the soil has a high molybdenum concentration and is deficient in copper *(50)*. The EPA has used this study as the basis for its regulatory assessment of molybdenum safety *(10)*.

The absence of adverse effects with molybdenum intakes of 5 µg/kg body weight is a sufficient basis to identify a NOAEL of 350 µg/d. Based on the increased plasma uric acid levels, a molybdenum LOAEL as high as 10 mg/d might be selected as the LOAEL. Although abnormal plasma uric acid levels are associated with that intake, there is little corroboration of the finding and the clinical impact is not clear. Thus, the data are not sufficiently clear to warrant identification of a specific LOAEL value.

10. SELENIUM

Excess selenium intake due to consumption of seleniferous plants by animals produces a wide range of adverse effects *(51)*. Chronic toxicity signs in livestock include cirrhosis, lameness, hoof malformations, hair loss, and emaciation. In laboratory animals, the signs most commonly include cirrhosis. The minimum dietary level of selenium recognized to produce adverse effects in farm animals is 4 to 5 µg/g dry weight of diet.

An episode of human poisoning by selenium involved a manufacturing error that resulted in a dietary supplement product which actually contained 182 times the amount of selenium declared on the label *(52,53)*. Adverse effects occurred within a few weeks and included effects on hair, nails, and liver. Human selenium poisoning in a high-selenium area of China also produced adverse effects on nails, hair, skin, the nervous system, and teeth *(54)*. The clinical signs included malformation and sloughing of nails, hair loss, dermatosis, nonspecific neuritis, and discoloration of the teeth. Because no specific biochemical or clinical indicators of selenosis are available, diagnosis involves the association of high intakes with characteristic adverse effects. Mild adverse effects have occurred in susceptible persons with intakes of 910 µg/d or more. No adverse effects have been associated with lower levels, but the ratio of plasma selenium to erythrocyte selenium has been found to increase with dietary intakes of 750 µg/d or more *(55)*. Human surveys in seleniferous areas of the US have failed to find any signs of selenium intoxication with intakes up to slightly more than 700 µg/d *(56)*. Because the chemical forms of selenium in foods grown in seleniferous areas are not known, the human data on adverse effects from chronically high intakes apply only to total dietary selenium and not to any specific form. No adverse effects were observed in the 8 to 10 yr clinical trial by Clark and coworkers *(57,58)* at daily supplemental intakes of 200 µg selenium in yeast.

With adverse effects established in a few individuals at chronic dietary intakes of 910 µg/d, this value may be identified as the LOAEL for skin, hair and nail effects and liver malfunction. The data of Yang and coworkers *(55)* did not find any overt adverse effects but found an increase in the ratio of plasma selenium to erythrocyte selenium at intakes 750 µg/d. Therefore, this intake level is not selected as a NOAEL. Although this change in ratio is not itself an adverse effect, it may indicate that the ability to eliminate excess selenium is nearly saturated. Application of regression methods to the data of Yang and coworkers (55,59) supports a NOAEL of 853 µg/d for the Chinese adult of 55 kg weight (60,61). The EPA has set the NOAEL at 0.015 mg/kg/d (10,60), a value that corresponds to a NOAEL of 1,050 µg for a 70 kg man, or 822 µg for a 55 kg adult. In the Chinese population with an average LOAEL of 910 µg selenium intake, the lower 95 percent confidence limit was 600 µg per day (62).

Considering these factors, a NOAEL is set at 200 µg supplemental selenium per day, based on the absence of adverse effects at this supplemental level in the clinical trial of Clark and coworkers (57,58), and on the substantial margin of safety it provides below the levels that are associated with adverse effects.

11. ZINC

Although certain folic acid-zinc interactions are well documented (63), the crucial issue is whether higher intakes of either zinc or folic acid have adverse consequences through disruption of the bioavailability or function of the other, and, if so, the levels associated with such effects. The reports of potential adverse effects through zinc-folic acid interactions describe the possibility that supplemental folic acid could adversely affect zinc nutriture (64–66), but more recent reports have not found any such interaction (67,68). There are no Medline reports of adverse effects of high zinc intakes through an antagonism of folic acid. The reports of anemia related to excess zinc intake all describe the microcytic, hypochromic anemia associated with copper deficiency, a condition that could also reflect interference with iron utilization (69–72). All anemia cases that have been associated with zinc involve intakes of more than 110 mg/d.

Supplements of 150 mg/d may also suppress lymphocyte stimulation response and might thereby compromise immune function (69,73). Supplements of 50 mg or more zinc per day decreased serum high-density lipoprotein (HDL) cholesterol levels (74). Total intakes of 60 to 64 mg/d decreased uptakes of copper (75) and iron (76), and decreased HDL cholesterol levels (75,77,78). The depressing effect of 60 mg of zinc intake on the copper-dependent form of the enzyme superoxide dismutase (E-SOD) (76) was most consistent and has been judged by the EPA as the most appropriate basis for the RfD for zinc (9,10).

There are no known adverse effects of zinc at chronic intakes of 30 mg/d and this level provides a substantial margin of safety below the levels associated with adverse effects. Therefore, 30 mg/d is identified as the NOAEL. Although there is no evidence of overt harm, a significant decrease in the copper-dependent SOD activity when longer-duration zinc intake is 60 mg is a reasonable basis for identifying this intake as the LOAEL. Much higher intakes for shorter periods have been taken without known adverse effects.

The changes in copper metabolism and nutriture that have been observed with zinc intakes in the range of 10 to 25 mg/d (79) are not known to lead to clinical consequences but that is a logical outcome if intake imbalances are chronic. Certainly, current assessments of zinc safety are based on changes in copper-dependent SOD, and thus are likely to reflect zinc antagonism of copper metabolism or function.

12. TRACE ELEMENT SUPPLEMENT SAFETY

The amounts of trace elements obtained from unfortified conventional foods vary widely with the types and amounts of specific foods in the diet, and these contents may be influenced by the composition of soil in the specific geographical locality, as well as the composition of the fertilizers used.

The only documented adverse effects related to trace element supplements have involved selenium and iron. In the early 1980s, a selenium supplement was misformulated to contain nearly 200-times the amount claimed on the label *(52,53)* and its consumption led to severe adverse effects on skin, hair, and nails within a few weeks. Accidental ingestions at one time of large numbers of high-potency (prenatal) iron tablets has caused severe adverse effects and some deaths in children under six years of age *(39)*.

There are no established adverse effects of properly manufactured trace element supplements that are used according to label recommendations. However, the margins of safety between dietary intakes and the levels that might cause adverse effects are narrower for most trace elements (with the notable exception of chromium) than for most vitamins. Thus, appropriate constraint in trace element supplement intake is advisable.

REFERENCES

1. Hathcock JN. Safety limits for nutrient intakes: Concepts and data requirements. Nutr Rev 1993;51:278–285.
2. Hathcock JN. Safety limits for nutrients. J Nutr 1996;126:2386S–2389S.
3. Hathcock JN. Vitamin and Mineral Safety. Council for Responsible Nutrition. Washington, DC, 1997.
4. Hathcock JN. Vitamins and minerals: efficacy and safety. Am J Clin Nutr 1997;66:427–437.
5. Mertz W, Abernathy CO, Olin SS, ed. Risk Assessment of Essential Elements. ILSI Press, Washington, DC,1994.
6. WHO Expert Committee on Trace Elements in Human Nutrition, Trace Elements in Human Nutrition and Health. World Health Organization, Geneva, Switzerland,1996.
7. Institute of Medicine, Standing Committee on the Scientific Evaluation of Dietary Reference Intakes, Dietary Reference Intakes for Calcium, Phosphorus, Magnesium, Vitamin D, and Fluoride. National Academy Press, Washington, DC, 1997.
8. Barnes DG, Dourson M. Reference dose (RfD): description and use in health risk assessments. Reg Toxicol Pharmacol 1988;8:471–486.
9. Cantilli R, Abernathy CO, Donohue JM. Derivation of the reference dose for zinc. In: Mertz W, Abernathy CO, Olin SS, ed. Risk Assessment of Essential Elements. ILSI Press, Washington, DC, 1994,pp: 113–126.
10. IRIS: Integrated Risk Information System Database IRIS-NCAR (non-carcinogenic). U.S. Environmental Protection Agency. Available from the U.S. National Library of Medicine through TOXLINE; 1997.
11. Nielsen FH. Other trace elements. In: Ziegler EE ,Filer LJ, ed. Present Knowledge of Nutrition, 7th Edition. ILSI Press, Washington, DC, 1996,pp. 353–377.
12. Price CJ, Strong PL, Marr MC, Myers CB, Murray FJ. Developmental toxicity NOAEL and postnatal recovery in rats fed boric acid during gestation. Fundamental and Applied Toxicology 1996;32:179–193.
13. Weir RJ, Fisher RS. Toxicological studies on borax and boric acid. Toxicology and Applied Pharmacology 1972;23:351–364.
14. Nielsen FW. Chromium. In: Shils ME, Olson JA, Shike M, ed. Modern Nutrition in Health and Disease, 8th ed. Lea and Febiger, Philadelphia, PA, 1994,pp. 264–268.
15. Dourson ML. Methods for establishing oral reference doses. In: Mertz W, Abernathy CO, Olin SS, ed. Risk Assessment of Essential Elements. ILSI Press, Washington, DC, 1994,pp. 51–61.
16. Gad SC. Acute and chronic systemic chromium toxicity. Sci Total Environ 1989;86:149–157.
17. Stearns DM, Wise JP, Sr, Patierno SR, Wetterhahn KE. Chromium (III) picolinate produces chromosome damage in Chinese hamster ovary cells. FASEB J 1995;9:1643–1648.
18. Food and Nutrition Board, Subcommittee on the Tenth Edition of the RDAs, Commission on Life Sciences, National Research Council, ed. Recommended Daily Allowances, 10th ed., National Academy Press, Washington DC, 1989.
19. Anderson R, Cheng N, Bryden N, Polansky M, Cheng N, Chi J, Feng J. Elevated intakes of supplemental chromium improve glucose and insulin variables in individuals with type 2 diabetes. Diabetes 1996;46:1786–1791.
20. Scheinberg IH, Sternlieb I. Copper toxicity and Wilson's disease. In: Prasad AS, ed. Trace Elements in Human Health and Disease, vol 1. Academic Press, New York, 1976,pp. 415–438.

21. Linder MC. Copper. In: Ziegler EE, Filer LJ, edS. Present Knowledge of Nutrition, 7th ed. ILSI Press, Washington, DC, 1996,pp. 307–319.
22. Turnlund JR, Copper. In: Shils ME, Olson JA, Shike M, eds. Modern Nutrition in Health and Disease, 8th ed. Lea & Fibiger, Philadelphia, 1994,pp. 231–241.
23. FAO/WHO (Food and Agriculture Organization/World Health Organization). Evaluation of Food Additives. WHO Technical Report Series No. 462, World Health Organization, Geneva, 1971.
24. Public Health Service, Ad Hoc Subcommittee on Fluoride. Review of Fluoride Benefits and Risks. Department of Health and Human Services, Bethesda, MD,1991.
25. Hathcock JN. Letter on fluoride safety to Food and Nutrition Board. National Academy of Sciences, Washington, DC,1997.
26. Clugston GA, Hetzel BS. Iodine. In: Shils ME, Olson JA, Shike M, eds. Modern Nutrition in Health and Disease, 8th ed. Lea and Febiger, Philadelphia, 1994,pp. 252–263.
27. Stanbury JB. Iodine deficiency and iodine deficiency disorders. In: Ziegler EE, Filer LJ, eds. Present Knowledge of Nutrition, 7th ed. ILSI Press, Washington, DC, 1996,pp. 378–383.
28. Fairbanks VF. Iron in medicine and nutrition. In: Shils ME, Olson JA, Shike M, eds. Modern Nutrition, Health and Disease, 8th ed. Lea and Febiger, Philadelphia, 1994, pp 185–213.
29. Yip R, Dallman PR. Iron. In: Ziegler EE,Filer LJ, ed. Present Knowledge of Nutrition, 7th Edition. ILSI Press, Washington, DC, 1996,pp. 277–292.
30. Sullivan JL. Iron and sex difference in heart disease risk. Lancet 1981;1:1293–1294.
31. Salonen JT, Nyyssonen K, Korpela H, Tuomilehto J, Seppanen R, Salonen R. High stored iron levels are associated with excess risk of myocardial infarction in eastern Finnish men. Circulation 1992;86:803–811.
32. Sempos CT, Looker AC, Gillum RF. Iron and heart disease: the epidemiologic data. Nutr Rev 1996;54:73–84.
33. Liao Y, Cooper RS, McGee DL. Iron status and coronary heart disease, negative findings from the NHANES I epidemiological follow-up study. Am J Epidem 1994;139:704–712.
34. Aronow WS. Serum ferritin is not a risk factor for coronary artery disease in men and women aged ≥ 62 years. Am J Cardio 1993;72:347–378.
35. Moore M, Folson AR, Barnes RW, Eckfeldt JH. No association between serum ferritin and asymptomatic carotid atherosclerosis; The Atherosclerosis Risk in Communities (ARIC) Study. Am J Epid 1995;141:719–723.
36. Baer DM, Tekawa IS, Hurley LB. Iron stores are not associated with acute myocardial infarction. Circulation 1994;89:2915–2918.
37. Morrison HI, Semenciw RM, Mao Y, Wigle DT. Serum iron and risk of fatal acute myocardial infarction. Epidemiology 1994;5:243–246.
38. Stewart ML, McDonald JT, Levy AS, Schucker RE, Henderson DP. Vitamin/mineral supplement use: A telephone survey of adults in the United States. J Am Dietetic Assoc 1985;85:1585–1590.
39. Food and Drug Administration. Iron-Containing Supplements and Drugs: Label Warning Statements and Unit-Dose Packaging Requirements. Fed Register 1995;60:8989–8993.
40. Keen CL, Zidenberg-Cherr S, Lonnerdal B. Nutritional and toxicological aspects of manganese intake: an overview. In: Mertz W, Abernathy CO, Olin SS, ed. Risk Assessment of Essential Elements. ILSI Press, Washington, DC, 1994,pp. 221–236.
41. Keen CL, Zidenberg-Cherr S. Manganese. In: Ziegler EE,Filer LJ, ed. Present Knowledge of Nutrition, 7th ed. ILSI Press, Washington, DC, 1996,pp. 334–343.
42. Ingersoll RT, Montgomery EB, Aphoshian HV. Central nervous system toxicity of manganese. 1. Inhibition of spontaneous motor activity in rats after intrathecal administration of manganese chloride. Fund Appl Toxicol 1995;26:106–113.
43. Kondakis XG, Makris N, Leotsinidis M, et al. Possible health effects of high manganese concentration in drinking water. Arch of Environ Health 1989;44:175–178.
44. Velazquez SF, Du JT. Derivation of the reference dose for manganese. In: Mertz W, Abernathy CO, Olin SS, ed. Risk Assessment of Essential Elements. ILSI Press, Washington, DC, 1994,pp. 253–268.
45. World Health Organization. Trace elements in human nutrition: Manganese. In: Technical Report Service 532 WHO Report of a WHO Expert Committee. Geneva, Switzerland, 1973,pp. 34–36.
46. Freeland-Graves JH, Bales CW, Behmardi F. Manganese requirements of humans. In: Kies C, ed. Nutritional Bioavailability of Manganese. American Chemical Society, Washington, DC, 1987,pp. 90–104.
47. Underwood EJ. Trace elements in human and animal nutrition, 4th ed. Academic Press, New York, 1977, pp. 109–131.

48. Nielsen FH. Ultratrace minerals. In: Shils ME, Olson JA, Shike M, eds. Modern Nutrition in Health and Disease, 8th ed. Lea and Febiger, Philadelphia, 1994,pp. 269–286.
49. Nielsen FH. Other trace elements. In: Ziegler EE, Filer LJ, eds. Present Knowledge of Nutrition, 7th ed. ILSI Press, Washington, DC, 1996, pp. 353–377.
50. Kovalskiy VV, Yarovaya GA, Shmavonyan DM. Changes of purine metabolism in man and animals under conditions of molybdenum biogeochemical provinces. Zh Obschch Biol 1961;22:179–191.
51. National Research Council, ed. Selenium in Nutrition, revised. National Academy Press, Washington, DC,1983.
52. Jensen R, Clossen W, Rothenberg R. Selenium intoxication — New York. Morbid Mortal Wkly Rep. 1984;33:157–158.
53. Helzlsouer K, Jacobs R, Morris S. Acute selenium intoxication in the United States. Federation Proceedings. 1985;44:1670.
54. Yang G, Wang S, Zhou R, Sun S. Endemic selenium intoxication of humans in China. Am J Clin Nutr 1983;37:872–881.
55. Yang G, Yin S, Zhou R, Gu L, Yan B, Liu Y, Liu Y. Studies of safe maximal daily dietary selenium intake in a seleniferous area in China, 2: relation between selenium intake and the manifestation of clinical signs and certain biochemical alterations in blood and urine. J Trace Elem Electrolytes Health Dis 1989;3:123–130.
56. Longnecker MP, Taylor PR, Levander OA, Howe M, Veillon C, McAdam PA, Patterson KY, Holden JM, Stampfer MJ, Morris JS, Willet WC. Selenium in diet, blood and toenails in relation to human health in a seleniferous area. Am J Clin Nutr 1991;53:1288–1294.
57. Clark LC, Combs GF, Turnbull BW, Slate EH et al. Effect of selenium supplementation for cancer prevention in patients with carcinoma of the skin. JAMA 1996;276:1957–1968.
58. Combs GF, Jr. Selenium and cancer prevention. In: HS Garewal ed. Antioxidants. Disease Prevention. CRC Press, Boca Raton, FL, 1997,pp:97–113.
59. Yang G, Zhou R, Yin S, Gu L, Yan B, Liu Y, Liu Y, Li X. Studies of safe maximal daily dietary selenium intake in a seleniferous area in China, 1: selenium intake and tissue levels of the inhabitants. J Trace Elem Electrolytes Health Dis 1989;3:77–87.
60. Poirier KA. Summary of the derivation of the reference dose for selenium. In: Mertz W, Abernathy CO, Olin SS, ed. Risk Assessment of Essential Elements. ILSI Press, Washington, DC, 1994,pp. 157–166.
61. Combs GF, Jr. Essentiality and toxicity of selenium: a critique of the recommended dietary allowance and the reference dose. In: Mertz W, Abernathy CO, Olin SS, ed. Risk Assessment of Essential Elements. ILSI Press, Washington, DC, 1994,pp. 167–183.
62. Yang G, Zhou R. Further observations on the human maximum safe dietary selenium intake in a seleniferous area of China. J Trace Elem Electrolytes Health Dis 1994;8:159–165.
63. Butterworth CE, Jr, Tamura T. Folic acid safety and toxicity: a brief review. Am J Clin Nutr 1989;50:353–358.
64. Mukherjee MD, Sandstead HH, Ratnaparkhl MV, Johnson LK, Milne DB, Stelling HP. Maternal zinc, iron folic acid and protein nutriture and outcome of human pregnancy. Am J Clin Nutr 1984;40:496–507.
65. Milne DB, Canfield WK, Mahalko JR, Sandstead HH. Effect of oral folic acid supplements on zinc, copper and iron absorption and excretion. Am J Clin Nutr 1984;39:535–359.
66. Simmer K, James C, Thompson RPH. Are iron-folate supplements harmful? Am J Clin Nutr 1987;45:122–125.
67. Tamura T, Goldenberg RL, Freeberg LE, Cliver SP, Cutter GR, Hoffman HJ. Maternal serum folate and zinc concentrations and their relationships to pregnancy outcome. Am J Clin Nutr 1992;56:365–370.
68. Kauwell GP, Bailey LB, Gregory JF, III Bowling DW, Cousins RJ. Zinc status is not adversely affected by folic acid supplementation and zinc intake does not impair folate utilization in human subjects. J Nutr 1995;125:66–72.
69. Greger JL. Zinc: overview from deficiency to toxicity. In: Mertz W, Abernathy CO, Olin SS, ed. Risk Assessment of Essential Elements. ILSI Press, Washington, DC, 1994, pp. 91–111.
70. Summerfield AL, Steinberg FU, Gonzalez JG. Morphologic findings in bone marrow precursor cells in zinc-induced copper deficiency anemia. Am J Clin Pathol 1992;97:665–658.
71. Gyorffy EJ,Chan H. Copper deficiency and microcytic anemia resulting from prolonged ingestion of over-the-counter zinc. Am J Gasterenterol 1992;87:1054–1055.
72. Frambach DA, Bendel RE. Zinc supplementation and anemia (letter). JAMA 1991;265:869.
73. Chandra RK. Excessive intake of zinc impairs immune responses. JAMA 1984;252:1443–1446.
74. Freeland-Graves JH, Friedman BJ, Han W, Shorey RL, Young R. Effect of zinc supplementation on plasma high-density lipoprotein and zinc. Am J Clin Nutr 1982; 35:988–992.

75. Fischer PWF Giroux A, L'Abbe AR. Effect of zinc supplementation on copper status in adult man. Am J Clin Nutr 1984;40:743–746.
76. Yadrick MK, Kenney MA, Winterfeldt EA. Iron copper and zinc status: response to supplementation with zinc or zinc and iron in adult females. Am J Clin Nutr 1989;49:145–150.
77. Hooper PL, Visconti L, Garry PJ, Johnson GE. Zinc lowers high-density lipoprotein-cholesterol levels. JAMA 1980;244:1960–1961.
78. Black MR, Medeiros DM, Brunett E, Welke R. Zinc supplementation and serum lipids in adult white males. Am J Clin Nutr 1988;47:970–975.
79. Sandstead HH. Requirements and toxicicity of essential trace elements illustrated by zinc and copper. Am J Clin Nutr 1995;61:621S–624S.

II TRACE ELEMENT AND MINERAL NUTRITION IN HEALTHY PEOPLE

8

Trace Element and Mineral Nutrition in Human Pregnancy

Theresa O. Scholl, PhD, MPH and
Thomas M. Reilly, PhD

1. INTRODUCTION

Minerals are nutrients that may function as enzymatic cofactors, as components of the skeletal system or as constituents of organic compounds. They are classed as macro- or micro-minerals (trace elements) depending upon the dietary requirement. Unlike animal studies that involve experimentally induced deficiencies of single nutrients, the link in humans between nutrient intake and the outcome of pregnancy is less secure. Except for rare occurrences, the inadequate intake of a single mineral is not an isolated event but occurs in conjunction with lifestyle factors and may be correlated with differences in education, occupation, ethnicity, and additional dietary inadequacies (energy, protein, and other minerals). This chapter will examine the documented influence of micro-minerals (iron, zinc, copper, selenium, iodine, chromium, fluoride, manganese, and molybdenum) and macro-minerals (calcium and magnesium) on the course and outcome of human pregnancy.

2. IRON AND PREGNANCY

Iron is essential for the formation of hemoglobin, which transports oxygen, and for the synthesis of enzymes that utilize oxygen to provide cellular energy *(1)*. For women in their reproductive years the need for iron is often greater than intake, due to factors such as iron loss with the onset of menstruation, and the increased requirements associated with pregnancy and lactation. In many women this may give rise to iron deficiency and eventually, iron deficiency anemia.

2.1. Anemia and Iron-Deficiency Anemia in Pregnancy

Iron deficiency is defined by three stages of increasing severity: depletion of iron stores (Stage 1), impaired hemoglobin production (Stage 2), and iron-deficiency anemia (IDA) (Stage 3). Anemia is an abnormally low concentration of hemoglobin (or hematocrit). Specific cut points have been formulated for its diagnosis by age, sex and, during pregnancy, by trimester (hemoglobin less than 110 g/L-first trimester, 105 g/L second trimester, and 110 g/L third trimester) *(1)*.

From: *Clinical Nutrition of the Essential Trace Elements and Minerals: The Guide for Health Professionals*
Edited by: J. D. Bogden and L. M. Klevay © Humana Press Inc., Totowa, NJ

Depending on the stage of gestation when anemia is assessed, it may be more or less difficult to separate truly anemic women from those whose anemia is attributable to hemodilution *(2)*. The increase in anemia during pregnancy is partly an artifact of maternal plasma volume expansion, a normal physiological response to pregnancy *(3)*. Although the maternal red blood cell mass also increases during gestation, its expansion and the expansion of the plasma volume occur at different times *(1,2)*. During the first and second trimesters hemoglobin concentration declines, reaching its lowest point early in the third trimester, and rising thereafter.

During pregnancy the diagnosis of iron deficiency anemia can be problematic. The choice of tests [serum ferritin, mean corpuscular volume (MCV), transferrin saturation, free erythrocyte protoporphyrin, hemoglobin response to a therapeutic trial with iron] depends on characteristics such as the underlying prevalence of iron deficiency and whether other factors (lead poisoning, infection, or thalassemia minor) are prevalent *(4)*. For example, physiologic alterations in maternal plasma volume and red cell mass with accompanying hemodilution mask the hemoglobin response to therapeutic iron trial in iron-deficient gravidas. MCV increases by about 5% in pregnancy and by itself is of limited diagnostic value *(5)*. Serum transferrin rises with the hormonal changes of pregnancy and there are subsequent decreases in transferrin saturation *(6)*. A combination of low hemoglobin and low serum ferritin (an indicator of iron stores) has been recommended to detect IDA *(1)*. Other causes of anemia during pregnancy, such as infection, are not characterized by low ferritin concentrations (<12 μg/L) *(1)*. However, since the concentration of ferritin may be reduced by hemodilution (increasing the false-positive rate) and increased by infection (increasing the false negative rate) *(5,6)* a new test based upon serum transferrin receptors may be used to improve detection *(7)*. Transferrin receptors reflect tissue iron and are said to be insensitive to inflammation and infection. They also appear stable over all periods of gestation, and thus may identify third trimester iron deficiency with increased precision *(7)*. Thus, in the future, a combination of tests (transferrin receptor concentration, serum ferritin, and hemoglobin) may be important to assess iron during pregnancy *(6)*.

Supplementation with iron is recommended during pregnancy to meet the demands of both the mother and rapidly growing fetus *(1)*. Anemia (low hemoglobin levels) and IDA sometimes also serve as indicators of overall poor maternal nutritional status during pregnancy. When overall dietary intake is inadequate, risk of anemia also is increased *(8–10)*.

2.2. Hemoglobin, Anemia, and Iron-Deficiency Anemia: Pregnancy Outcome

Evidence suggests that anemia and iron deficiencies are associated with an increased risk of infant low birth weight, preterm delivery, and perinatal mortality. The relationship between maternal hemoglobin and pregnancy outcome is U shaped with "low" hemoglobin probably reflecting the combination of true and physiologic anemia and "high" hemoglobin reflecting failure of the plasma volume to expand and/or possibly maternal infection.

Murphy et al. *(11)* studied 44,000 singleton pregnancies in women from Cardiff, Wales, who sought prenatal care by 24 wk gestation. The prevalence of anemia based upon "low" hemoglobin before week 24 (hemoglobin <104 g/L) among the women was 3.9%. Increased risk of preterm birth (<37 weeks) was associated with low hemoglobin when women entered care before week 13 or after week 20. For entrants between 20 and 24 wk, risk also was increased when hemoglobin was high. Risk of low birth weight (<2500 grams) was increased for women entering before 20 wk gestation. A high maternal hemoglobin concentration (>145 g/L) was also associated with hypertension and pregnancy-induced hypertension, both of which may reflect inadequate expansion of the maternal plasma volume.

Garn and colleagues *(12)* analyzed data from more than 50,000 consecutive pregnancies that were followed as part of the Collaborative Perinatal Project (CPP) using the lowest hematocrit any time during pregnancy, thus confounding the effects of true and physiologic anemia. Low (<0.29) and high (>0.39) hematocrit was associated with increased risks of fetal death, preterm delivery, and low birth weight. At the lowest hematocrit (<0.25), risks of preterm delivery, low birth weight, and fetal death were increased approximately two- to threefold for the white women. For black women, only the risk of fetal death was raised substantially (approximately two times higher). Overall, for both black and white gravidas, the risk of fetal death was increased appreciably when hematocrits were very high (>0.41).

Steer et al. *(13)* studied a multi-ethnic sample of women from the Northwest Thames region of London. For all ethnic groups, their data showed an increased risk of preterm delivery and infant low birth weight when the hemoglobin during the pregnancy was either low (<85 g/L) or high (>115 g/L).

Meis et al. *(14)* analyzed data from the Cardiff Birth survey, a population-based survey of data on the pregnancies of more than 25,000 Welsh women. Both low (<104 g/L) and high (>135 g/L) maternal hemoglobin at entry to care increased risk of preterm delivery. After controlling for other potential confounding variables, high hemoglobin remained a significant risk factor whereas low hemoglobin did not. However, early pregnancy bleeding, a factor which often gives rise to anemia and lowers hemoglobin concentration, was associated with nearly a twofold increase in risk of preterm birth.

Klebanoff and colleagues *(15)* examined the relationship of maternal anemia, estimated via hemoglobin or hematocrit during the second and third trimesters, to preterm birth. During the second trimester, anemia approximately doubled risk for preterm birth but during the third trimester, anemia was not a risk factor.

Higgins et al. *(16)* also found a strong inverse relationship between hemoglobin after 33 wk gestation and preterm birth; the effect of entry hemoglobin was weak and not statistically significant. The highest infant birth weights were associated with the lowest third-trimester maternal hemoglobin concentrations (<110 g/L). Birth weights were also related to the change in hemoglobin concentrations between entry and the third trimester; women with the greatest decreases gave birth to the largest infants.

Lu and colleagues *(17)* examined the relationship of maternal hematocrits to pregnancy. Before week 20 gestation, low hematocrits were weakly associated with an increased risk for preterm birth. After week 20, the relationship between maternal hematocrits and risk of preterm delivery reversed, although none of the adjusted odd ratios was statistically significant. Consistent with prior findings, high hematocrit before or after mid-pregnancy was associated with increased risk for preterm birth and for fetal growth restriction.

Lieberman et al. *(18)* examined the association of delivery hematocrit with spontaneous preterm birth in a sample of approx 8,000 Boston women. Each 5-point drop in hematocrit was associated with an approximately twofold increase in the risk of preterm delivery. In another publication from this cohort *(19)* the twofold difference in preterm delivery for blacks compared with whites, which had not been explained by known risk factors in earlier work *(20)*, was accounted for almost entirely by controlling for socioeconomic factors along with maternal anemia.

Klebanoff et al. *(2)* attempted to replicate the above results with data from the CPP. From prospective data they described changes in hemoglobin and hematocrit that were consequences of changes in plasma volume and red cell mass, which occur at different times during pregnancy. Because changes in red cell mass and plasma volume are asynchronous, lower hemoglobin concentrations typify the earlier stage of gestation when preterm births occur and higher hematocrits (and lower anemia risk) will characterize pregnancies that are delivered at a later stage of gestation. Consequently, when sampled at delivery, an increased risk of anemia and preterm delivery will be artifactually associated.

The above studies utilized hemoglobin alone as an indicator of maternal anemia. However, in Camden, N.J., Scholl and colleagues combined anemia per the Centers for Disease Control (CDC) criteria (CDC Reference) with low serum ferritin to index IDA *(1)*. Data from over 800 women in the Camden Study were utilized to examine total anemia, IDA, and anemia from causes other than iron deficiency at entry to prenatal care (16–17 wk of gestation) as risk factors for preterm delivery. At entry to care, the prevalence of anemia (using CDC standards *(40)* for hemoglobin) was high (27.9%), but the proportion with IDA (anemia with a serum ferritin of <12 µg/L) was lower than anticipated (3.5% of the cohort). Nevertheless, there was a better than twofold increased risk of preterm delivery with IDA. When vaginal bleeding was present at or before entry to care, risk of preterm delivery was increased fivefold for IDA and twofold for other anemia. When data from the cohort were examined at week 28 gestation, risk was not increased for women with iron deficiency anemia or anemia stemming from other causes *(21)*. Some, but not all, third trimester anemia is attributable to the expansion of the maternal plasma volume and at present this state is poorly differentiated from IDA late in pregnancy.

2.3. High Ferritin and Pregnancy Outcome

Recently the question has arisen whether a high concentration of serum ferritin, particularly during the third trimester of pregnancy, could be an acute phase reactant to subclinical maternal infection which would also serve as a marker for impending preterm delivery.

Ferritin is a sensitive indicator of iron storage except when the subject is in an inflammatory state; this is true for men and for women pregnant or not. In one of the first publications concerning ferritin and IDA during pregnancy, Puolakka et al. *(5)* commented that although women whose anemia was attributable to iron deficiency (absence of bone marrow iron) had low ferritin levels, those whose anemia was associated with infection (urinary tract infection) had levels that were increased approximately sixfold during the third trimester even when marrow iron could not be demonstrated. It is now well accepted that the ferritin, which can be synthesized by infiltrating macrophages, markedly increases when there is a physiologic stress. This effect is called an acute phase response *(22)*.

From their studies of Alabama women, both Tamura *(23)* and Goldenberg *(24)* found high levels of serum ferritin during the third trimester of pregnancy to be a marker for an increased risk for preterm delivery. Prospective data from Camden *(25)* indicate that high ferritin levels (90th percentile) during the third trimester which stem from the failure of ferritin to decline from entry (as expected with normal plasma volume expansion) increases risk of very preterm delivery eightfold and clinical chorioamnionitis more than twofold. Prospective data from Camden thus confirm the link between maternal ferritin during pregnancy, and very preterm delivery and extend them to markers for maternal infection. Data suggest, in addition, that IDA, and other markers for poor nutritional status (reduced concentrations of serum and red cell folate earlier in pregnancy) underlie the relationship of infection to preterm and very preterm delivery in Camden women.

Thus, maternal anemia, when diagnosed before mid-pregnancy, is associated with an increased risk of preterm birth. However, during the third trimester, anemia is a good prognostic sign, probably indicating the expansion of maternal plasma volume. While third trimester anemia usually is not associated with an increased risk of preterm birth, high levels of hemoglobin or hematocrit late in pregnancy are associated with increased preterm delivery. This increased risk may indicate failure of plasma-volume expansion but may as well be a marker for maternal infection.

3. CALCIUM AND PREGNANCY

The skeleton acts as the calcium reservoir of the body (99%) and when dietary calcium intake is low or poorly absorbed, calcium is withdrawn from bone to support serum calcium homeostasis (1) (see Chapter 14). During pregnancy, retention of an estimated 30 g of calcium is needed for mineralization of the fetal skeleton (1). In pregnant women, a calcium intake of 600 mg per day results in negative calcium balance (1). While the amount of dietary calcium intake and absorption required for optimal bone mineralization of the fetal and maternal skeleton is known (26), data suggest the opportunity for negative calcium balance when gravidas have calcium intakes less than 800 to 1,000 mg/d. One immediate consequence of this may be loss of maternal bone mass during pregnancy.

3.1. Pregnancy and Bone Mass

Several studies have examined longitudinally the change in bone mass with pregnancy (27–32) but, only two (27,28) have examined the influence of dietary calcium on bone mass as an independent variable. Lambke (27) evaluated 14 pregnant mature women in the second trimester and in the postpartum. He reported a significant decrease in trabecular bone and a small gain in cortical bone. Christiansen (28) studied serial changes in radial bone mass in 13 mature, white Danish women during pregnancy and found no change in radial bone mass. These women were, however, ingesting an average of 650 mg/d in calcium supplements, apart from their diet. Sowers et al. (29) has found no change in femoral bone mineral density in 32 women, aged 20–40 yr, with measurement prior to pregnancy and following delivery, compared to matched controls, but again the average calcium intake exceeded the RDA for both groups. Drinkwater et al. (30) studied changes in bone mineral density (pregravid and six weeks postpartum) in six women who experienced pregnancy and 25 controls; mean calcium intake was high (>1500 mg/day) in each group. Despite this, pregnancy was associated with significant decrements in bone at the femoral neck, and radial shaft; increased bone density was found for the tibia. Two uncontrolled studies (31–32) used single photon absorptiometry to assess bone and found no change over the course of pregnancy.

With the exception of one positive report (33), cross-sectional studies of bone mass and parity, generally confined to mature white women, have shown either an increased bone mass with parity or no effect of parity on bone mass (33–35). However, parity does not measure the effects of pregnancy but the cumulative effect of the reproductive experience, along with antecedents and consequences. For example, a positive correlation between parity and bone density may reflect greater antecedent hormonal integrity and possibly increased body weight of women who bear children compared to women who are infertile.

Calcium intake, particularly during growth, may be an important determinant of bone mineralization and thus bone density *(36)*. Higher calcium intakes during childhood and adolescence, are associated with higher bone mass at maturity *(37)*. Maternal growth and pregnancy often coincide and approximately half of all pregnant teenagers continue to grow while pregnant *(38)*. In case of pregnancy in a still-growing girl, calcium nutriture may be limited by maternal diet, but simultaneously driven by the need to retain enough calcium to mineralize two skeletons *(39)*. Presumably, continued maternal growth could affect the risk of osteoporosis and osteoporotic fractures in later life, particularly if the maternal diet was deficient in calcium during childhood and adolescence.

Sowers et al. *(39)*, in a cross-sectional study of two Iowa communities, reported that women with a first pregnancy before age 19 had, at maturity, a bone mass (measured at the mid-distal forearm) that was –0.52 standard deviation units (SDU) below other women. Calcium consumption was also related to bone density (-0.68 SDU for lower intakes), and the joint effect for early pregnancy and lower calcium intake, assuming additivity, exceeded –1 SDU in bone mass. A longitudinal study from a third community carried out 5 yr later also showed that bone mass was significantly reduced in those with a teenage birth *(40)*. Cross-sectional results by Fox and colleagues yielded similar results in perimenopausal women *(41)*.

Lower bone mineral density has been reported in parous minority women, compared to controls of the same ethnic group. Goldsmith *(42)* reported lower radial bone densities in 52 parous black women compared to black nulliparas. Among whites, parous women had a bone density 1% higher than nulliparous controls. Carter and Haynes *(43)* showed lower bone density was present in adult scoliotics. Parous black women were more likely to be scoliotic than nonparous blacks. There was no influence of parity among the white women who were examined. There is uncertainty about the extent to which small decrements in bone mass with parity among black women reflect an over-representation of women with adolescent childbearing.

3.2. Calcium, Hypertension and Preeclampsia

Another mechanism particularly active during pregnancy, is an increase in the tubular resorption of calcium, resulting in decreased urinary calcium excretion. Preeclampsia and gestational hypertension are common in nulliparous women and marked by hypocalciuria throughout pregnancy *(44–45)*. However, a significant proportion (about 66%) of women with low urinary calcium excretion levels never cross the line to develop frank gestational hypertension or preeclampsia *(45)*. Thus, preeclampsia may be a pathological manifestation of a calcium-conserving mechanism, which is associated with pregnancy and is more common in young, poor nulliparous women. On the other hand, hypocalciuria may be but a marker for preeclampsia, a response to an unknown and underlying metabolic perturbation.

Diets low in calcium, especially during pregnancy, have been associated with increased blood pressure levels through heightened smooth muscle reactivity. The pathogenesis of pregnancy induced hypertension (PIH) may or may not involve calcium in the maternal diet. Belizan and Villar *(46)* reported an inverse relationship between toxemia and dietary calcium from ecological-level data. More recently *(47)* gestational hypertension (but not preeclampsia) and maximum diastolic pressure were found to be weakly associated with low calcium intakes in primiparas. Several smaller scale clinical trials have confirmed that calcium supplementation is associated with decreased blood pressure (BP) during pregnancy *(48–49)*, findings which are consistent with reports of an inverse association between calcium and systolic blood pressure in nonpregnant subjects *(50–51)*.

A meta-analysis *(52)* of 14 randomized controlled trials of calcium supplementation involving more than 2,400 pregnant women showed statistically significant reductions in systolic and diastolic blood pressure with the administration of calcium salts (375–2,000 mg/d elemental calcium). Risk of preeclampsia was reduced more than twofold among women supplemented with calcium during these trials. Duration of treatment ranged from 10–22 wk, with most studies commencing calcium supplementation during the second trimester. While differences in risk of preeclampsia were significant in the aggregate, only two of nine of the studies examining this outcome obtained statistically significant findings.

A large randomized double-blind placebo controlled trial of 5,489 low-risk nulliparous women, however, showed no effect of calcium supplementation *(53)*. Pregnant women were enrolled at medical centers throughout the United States, prescreened for compliance with supplement use, and for conditions associated with abnormal calcium metabolism or increased risk of preeclampsia. Women were supplemented with 2 grams of elemental calcium (or placebo) beginning at 13–21 wk gestation until delivery. Calcium supplementation did not significantly reduce risk of preeclampsia, gestational hypertension without preeclampsia (either mild or severe), or pregnancy associated proteinuria without hypertension. Blood pressure was also unaffected. Between 20 and 40 wk gestation, systolic pressure was lower by 0.3 mm Hg and diastolic pressure was .03 mm Hg higher among the calcium supplemented; these small differences were not statistically significant. Likewise, risk did not differ when data were examined according to hypothesized moderating variables: quintile of dietary calcium intake at baseline, maternal age, urinary calcium excretion or gestation at entry to the study.

3.2.1. CALCIUM, PRETERM DELIVERY, AND INFANT LOW BIRTH WEIGHT

During pregnancy, an increased risk of PIH associated with lower calcium may result in an increased risk of preterm delivery; indicated preterm delivery is one method of reducing the maternal-fetal morbidity and mortality associated with preeclampsia and eclampsia *(54)*. Consequently, supplementation with calcium during pregnancy, if effective, may have a side effect of reduced preterm birth risk. Preeclampsia involves the failure to adequately perfuse many organs, including the placenta, and it is associated with fetal growth restriction and infant low birth weight (<2,500 grams).

Two calcium supplementation trials among high-risk women showed promising results. In Ecuador, among women with low calcium intake *(55,56)*, length of gestation was increased from 37.4 ± 2.3 wk for the placebo group (N=34) to 39.2 ± 1.2 wk (p<.01) for the calcium-supplemented group (N=22). Among teenagers from Baltimore *(48)*, the calcium-supplemented group had a lower incidence of preterm delivery (7.4%) compared with the placebo group (21.1%, p<.007). Further, life-table analysis demonstrated an overall shift to a higher gestational age in the calcium-supplemented group. A recent randomized controlled trial *(57)* of supplementation with 2,000 mg/d elemental calcium to 260 pregnant Ecuadorian teenagers (17.5 yr and under) increased gestation duration from 38.7 ± 0.3 wk (placebo) to 39.6 ± 0.4 wk (calcium supplement). Risk of PIH was reduced 80% in this trial with calcium supplementation. Baseline dietary calcium intake was low and amounted to less than 50% of the RDA for pregnancy.

On the other hand, a large calcium supplementation trial of over 1,000 adult women from Argentina showed a decrease in the incidence of PIH, but no effect on preterm delivery *(49)*. Buchler's meta-analysis *(52)*, cited previously, also showed no effect of calcium intake on preterm delivery or fetal growth restriction. Likewise, the clinical trial performed by Levine and colleagues *(53)*, discussed previously, also found no effect of calcium supplementation on obstetrical outcomes including preterm delivery and perinatal outcomes including birth weight, low birth weight, or fetal growth restriction. Thus, the ability of supplemental calcium to decrease the risk of preterm delivery, if genuine, may be confined to high-risk populations in which there is either a severe dietary restriction of calcium or a high demand for calcium as in adolescent pregnancy, where both the needs of the growing fetus and the mother must be met.

4. MAGNESIUM AND PREGNANCY

Magnesium is a divalent action essential for the release of parathyroid hormone during pregnancy. This hormone acts on the skeleton and also affects intestinal and kidney function *(1)*. When administered during pregnancy, magnesium sulfate reduces the risk of eclampsia in women with PIH *(58)* and the incidence of recurrent convulsions in eclamptic women *(58)*. Thus, the NIH Consensus Group recommended the administration of magnesium sulfate for control of preeclampsia and prevention of eclampsia during pregnancy *(59)*. These observations and recommendations support prior ecological studies suggesting an inverse relationship between the magnesium concentration in drinking water and risk of stillbirth *(60)* as well as older in vitro studies showing that the absence of magnesium in incubation medium potentiated vasoconstriction of isolated umbilical arteries and veins *(61)*. Thus, it was hypothesized that magnesium deficiency during pregnancy increased spasm of the maternal vessels, in the process increasing the likelihood of pregnancy-induced hypertension, preterm delivery, and infant low birth weight.

In the US, dietary magnesium intake is below the DRI (RDA) of 300–360 mg/d for nonpregnant and 350–400 mg/d for pregnant women, and on average magnesium balance is negative during pregnancy *(1)*. Low dietary intake, however, is offset by the fact that, when intake is low, absorption increases and more magnesium is retained by the kidneys *(1)*; consequently, magnesium deficiency is generally not observed among healthy free-living individuals. Failure to detect deficiency could be due to the lack of adequate laboratory tests to determine magnesium status *(see* Chapter 5).

Two randomized controlled studies have addressed use of magnesium supplements during pregnancy. Spalting and Spalting *(62)* administered magnesium or placebo to 568 pregnant women, allocated by odd or even date of birth. Magnesium supplementation was associated with fewer maternal hospitalizations, a reduced risk of preterm labor, and an increase in median gestation duration of about one day. When noncompliant patients were excluded, a procedure tantamount to converting a randomized trial to an observational study without control for confounding variables, some reduction in risk remained. These results were not replicated by Sibhai and colleagues *(63)* in their randomized and controlled study of 374 pregnant patients. Apart from higher levels of serum magnesium among supplemented women, there were no differences between the groups in risk of preeclampsia, preterm labor, fetal growth restriction, birth weight, or gestational age.

Three observational studies, which incorporated no control for confounding, have reported weak and inconsistent relationships between circulating magnesium and pregnancy outcome *(64–66)*. However, another well-done observational study of 965 Danish gravidas examined the influence of dietary and circulating magnesium and, in a smaller sample, tissue magnesium, on risk of pregnancy induced hypertension and pregnancy outcome *(67)* and found none. Magnesium intake, estimated from food, water and other nutritional supplements, was high and on average amounted to 446 mg/d. After control for important confounding variables, birth weight was inversely correlated with dietary magnesium intake (i.e., lower birth weight was associated with higher magnesium intake) but the effect was not statistically significant. Serum magnesium showed no effect on preeclampsia, or preterm labor. Likewise, the magnesium content of the rectus abdominis muscle (women with Caesarian Section) was found to be unrelated to pregnancy outcome or to risk of preeclampsia *(67)*.

5. ZINC AND PREGNANCY

Zinc is linked to DNA synthesis, facilitating cell division, and RNA synthesis, as required for protein synthesis *(1)*. These critical metabolic functions of zinc are uniquely essential for the promotion of both intrauterine growth and somatic growth of the offspring following birth.

5.1. Zinc Requirement during Pregnancy

The amount of absorbed zinc required to replace endogenous losses has been estimated to be 2.5 mg/d for nonpregnant women *(68)*. The average zinc content of the term fetus is approx 60 mg *(69)*. The total requirement for zinc during gestation is estimated to be 100 mg; approx 60% accumulates in the conceptus. An additional average need of 0.60 mg/d of zinc over nonpregnant needs has been estimated for the last 20 wk of gestation *(70)*, which appears to occur via an increase in intestinal zinc absorption *(71)*. A dietary zinc intake of 15 mg/day is recommended during pregnancy *(26)*.

5.2. Zinc and Congenital Malformations

The discovery of the first human clinical zinc deficiency syndrome in the Middle East in 1961 *(72)*, led Sever and Emanuel in 1973 to postulate that a relationship existed between poor maternal zinc status in humans and the high rate of central nervous system (CNS) anomalies *(73)*. Further support for the potential teratogenic effect of maternal zinc deficiency was documented by the poor reproductive performance of women with acrodermatitis enteropathica (AE), an autosomal recessive disorder causing inadequate zinc absorption *(74)*. Untreated AE is characterized by symptoms similar to zinc deficiency: hypozincemia, severe diarrhea, dermatitis, and alopecia. Case reports of adverse pregnancy outcome such as anencephaly and achondroplastic dwarfism in women with untreated AE suggested that the human fetus may be susceptible to the teratogenic effects of zinc deficiency *(74,75)*. Jameson *(76)*, Cavdar, et al. *(77)* and Soltan and Jenkins *(78)* reported associations between low maternal zinc concentrations and congenital malformations of the fetus. During routine screening for chromosomal abnormalities and fetal malformations, Baumah et al. *(79)* found that lower zinc concentrations in women with anencephalic fetuses, while Hinks et al. *(80)* documented a lower mean leukocyte zinc concentration in women diagnosed with fetuses having neural tube defects (NTDs). In one case-control study *(81)*, mean maternal serum zinc concentration at mid-pregnancy was determined to be higher in cases of NTDs when compared to control unaffected pregnancies. The authors concluded that this reflected a deficient maternal-fetal transfer of zinc in some women, which could influence critical events during fetal development.

One potential benefit of periconceptional zinc supplementation and reduced NTDs was reported by Cavdar et al. *(82)* who supplemented zinc sulfate to a woman with diagnosed zinc deficiency and prior history of recurrent anencephalic stillbirth. The outcome of her third pregnancy resulted in a healthy, well-developed 2,900 gram neonate. Cavdar, et al. *(82)* postulated that zinc therapy corrected her documented zinc deficiency.

In contrast to the above reports, stored serum samples from the 1991 Medical Research Council Vitamin Supplementation Trial for the prevention of NTDs were used by Hambidge et al. *(83)* to investigate the relationship of maternal zinc status in the causation of NTDs. No differences in serum zinc concentrations between cases of NTDs and controls were noted prior to conception, at study entry, or at 12 wk gestation. Mean serum zinc concentration was not significantly lower in women with NTD pregnancies when compared to unaffected pregnancies. These data weigh against the hypothesis that maternal zinc deficiency is a cause of NTDs. Thus, a proposed relationship between maternal zinc deficiency and congenital malformations awaits more definitive evidence from controlled studies.

5.3. Zinc, Fetal Growth, and Gestation

Due to the role of zinc as a cofactor for enzymes necessary to nucleic acid synthesis, it has been viewed as a potent modulator of intrauterine and postnatal growth. The possible relationship between maternal zinc status and birth weight has been intensely studied, but results have been inconsistent. Several studies have suggested that higher plasma or serum zinc concentrations may be a factor that facilitates fetal growth. In a study evaluating the effects of circulating nutrients on fetal growth, Crosby et al. *(84)* reported a positive correlation between plasma zinc concentrations at mid-gestation and gestational age-adjusted birth weight. Jameson *(76)* also reported a positive relationship between serum zinc concentrations measured at 14 wk gestation and birth weight. Women delivering preterm low birth weight infants (<2500 grams) had a lower mean serum zinc concentration when compared to women with normal weight term infants, although birth weights were not adjusted for gestational age in this study. Ghosh et al. *(85)* reported a positive correlation between birth weight and a mean serum zinc concentration at parturition in uncomplicated pregnancies. Singh et al. *(86)* also reported this relationship at parturition with a higher percentage of low birth weight infants born to the hypozincemic women when compared to normozincemic women. Neggers et al. *(87)* demonstrated a positive association between the mean maternal serum zinc concentration at 16 wk gestation and birth weight in a large lower socioeconomic status population. This association was observed for the entire sample, and separately for both ethnic groups studied. The serum zinc concentrations in the lowest quartile were associated with an 8 times greater frequency of low birth weight outcomes thus suggesting that a threshold for maternal serum zinc concentration may exist below which the incidence of low birth weight increased significantly. Kirksey et al. *(88)* examined the relationship of maternal zinc nutriture to birth weight and found that plasma zinc concentrations in the second trimester, along with pregnancy weight at 3 mo gestation, formed the best predictor model of birth weight from these pregnancies, accounting for 39% of the variance. Scholl and colleagues examined the relationship of dietary zinc intake in 818 Camden women *(9)* and reported increased risks of complications and adverse pregnancy outcomes in association with low intakes of dietary zinc (6 mg/d or less). These complications include increased inadequate gestational weight gain and IDA at entry to care. Poor outcomes involved increased risk of infant low birth weight (2 times higher), preterm, and very preterm delivery (2–3 fold greater). In the presence of IDA, the risk of very preterm delivery was increased greater than fivefold.

In contrast, other studies have reported an inverse relationship of maternal zinc status to birth weight. Metcoff et al. *(89)* examined adjusted birth weight in relation to maternal plasma zinc concentrations at 22 wk gestation. The mid-pregnancy plasma zinc concentrations were lower in women who delivered above-average birth weight infants suggesting that lower plasma zinc concentrations may reflect a more efficient placental transport of zinc to the fetus. McMichael et al. *(90)* also supported this relationship by reporting cases of intrauterine growth retardation (IUGR) in which the mean maternal serum concentration at 18 wk gestation was higher-than-average. These results suggested that elevated mid-pregnancy serum zinc concentrations may reflect defective fetal uptake of zinc, and that the normal maternal decline in circulating zinc concentrations may be an outcome rather than a cause of intrauterine growth retardation. Others *(91)* also demonstrated an inverse relationship between second trimester plasma zinc concentrations and birth weight suggesting this relationship may be partially explained by accelerated fetal uptake of zinc.

For a detailed discussion of appropriate zinc indices and laboratory tests useful for the assessment of zinc status in pregnancy *see* Chapter 5. Since serum or plasma zinc concentrations represent less than one percent of the total body zinc pool, much debate has focused on the possibility that these indices alone may not be reliable parameters for assessing zinc status. As a consequence, alternate zinc indices have been measured during gestation in relation to fetal growth. Pregnancy induces a state of polymorphonuclear leukocytosis and leukocytes have a high zinc content. Meadows et al. *(92)* demonstrated that the depletion of mean maternal leukocyte zinc concentration at parturition was associated with impaired fetal growth resulting in IUGR when compared to pregnancies with normal weight infants. No differences were noted between the mean leukocyte zinc concentration of women delivering preterm appropriate for gestational age (AGA) and normal weight infants. Meadows et al. *(93)* also demonstrated that the mean leukocyte zinc concentration in cord blood of infants with prolonged IUGR and infants with acute-onset IUGR were lower when compared to normal infants. In contrast, the mean leukocyte zinc concentration in cord blood for preterm infants was not depleted when compared to term infants. These results suggested that fetal zinc depletion was the result of maternal zinc depletion, and leukocytes may be useful for assessing zinc status in extrahepatic nucleated tissue.

Wells et al. *(94)* also supported an association between maternal leukocyte zinc depletion and identification of IUGR infants by demonstrating that the median maternal leukocyte zinc concentration during the third trimester rose progressively with birth weight percentiles. Maternal leukocyte zinc concentrations strongly predicted infant weight below the 10th percentile. This study documented an even distribution of the incidence of maternal smoking (29%) and complications of pregnancy (16%) which contributed to IUGR among all birth weight percentiles. Adenyi *(95)* reported hypozincemia at parturition in preeclamptic women with normal birth weight infants when compared to women delivering lower birth weight infants. When compared to the normal pregnant women, pre-eclamptic women delivering infants with lower birth weights displayed a lower mean leukocyte zinc concentration and a lower mean placental zinc concentration. Mean cord plasma zinc concentration was higher in normal birth weight infants when compared to lower birth weight infants of pre-eclamptic women. These data suggest that an enhanced provision of zinc to the fetus occurred in women resulting in higher birth weights and supports the work of others *(89–90,92,94)*.

Zinc concentrations are different in leukocyte sub-populations with polymorphonuclear (PMN) cells having less than half the zinc content of mononuclear (MN) cells. Simmer and Thompson *(96)* measured zinc concentrations in PMN and MN cells in women 24–48 h after parturition. Maternal zinc depletion was strongly associated with fetal growth retardation. When compared to mothers of appropriately grown infants, mothers delivering growth retarded infants had a lower mean zinc concentration in PMN cells and MN cells. In addition to a higher incidence of small for gestational age (SGA) infants, smoking women had a lower mean zinc concentration in PMN cells when compared to nonsmoking women. Simmer and Thompson *(96)* concluded that zinc depletion, partly due to an inadequate diet, was strongly associated with IUGR, and maternal smoking explained some of the reduction in cellular zinc possibly by decreasing zinc utilization.

Other studies have examined the potential influence of smoking on maternal zinc status and its relationship to birth weight. Kuhnert et al. *(97)* explored the influences of smoking on the relationship between maternal and fetal zinc status and birth weight. When compared to infants of nonsmoking women, infants of smokers had lower mean zinc concentrations in plasma and erythrocytes. The mean activity of plasma alkaline phosphatase, a zinc-dependent enzyme, was lower for infants of smoking women. A negative relationship between mean maternal plasma zinc and mean cord plasma zinc concentrations and birth weight was demonstrated in smoking women. These investigators concluded that infants of nonsmoking women appeared to maintain adequate zinc status by depleting maternal zinc stores, whereas infants of smokers appeared to become marginally zinc deficient due to a decreased availability of zinc.

Kynast and Saling *(98)* reported the effects of zinc supplementation of 20 mg/d on pregnancy outcome for women and controls between 12 and 34 wk gestation. Zinc treatment was associated with a lower incidence of SGA infants when compared to the placebo group. Zinc supplemented women had a lower incidence of preterm labor, placental abruption, vaginal bleeding, and fetal acidosis when compared to control subjects.

In a double-blind zinc supplementation trial, Cherry et al. *(99)* reported that a response to supplementation (30 mg/d zinc) was related to maternal pregravid weight and weight gain status for pregnant adolescents less than 25 wk gestation. Low serum zinc concentrations were more common in underweight and multiparous women. The frequency of preterm delivery was less in the zinc treated normal-weight women compared to the placebo group. Zinc treatment of underweight multiparous women was associated with increased gestational age by 2.8 wk at delivery. Zinc supplementation was also associated with a reduced need for assisted respiration in newborns of normal-weight women.

In a randomized double-blind placebo-controlled trial, Goldenberg et al. *(100)*, reported the effects of zinc supplementation of 25 mg/d on pregnancy outcome for African-American women. Women with plasma zinc concentrations below the median were randomized to zinc supplementation or placebo. Women were stratified after the fact by body mass index (BMI) into two groups (BMI ≥ 26 and BMI < 26) for pregnancy outcome analysis. This study documented an increased mean birth weight (126 grams) and head circumference (0.4 cm.) for infants of all women receiving zinc supplementation when compared to placebo group. Women with a BMI < 26 benefited most from zinc treatment with a 248 gram increase in infant birth weight and a 0.7 cm. larger infant head circumference. Although not associated with birth weight, plasma zinc concentrations were higher in the supplemented women. These investigators concluded that the improved birth weights and head circumferences for the zinc supplemented women with BMI < 26 was partly the result of increased fetal growth and increased gestational age of the offspring. In contrast, another double blind random-ized controlled trial conducted by Jonsson et al. *(101)* found no differences in maternal and fetal outcomes with zinc supplementation.

These studies have provided support for the possible relationship between maternal zinc status and compromised fetal development and fetal growth potential. Although these associations are by inference, studies do suggest that zinc may play a role in the many biological processes involved in the successful outcome of pregnancy.

6. COPPER AND PREGNANCY

Copper deficiency in animal models has been linked to infertility, abortion, stillbirths, skeletal defects, abnormal myelination, neonatal ataxia, anemia, decreased arterial elasticity, and impaired immune function. Copper deficiency has not been documented in human pregnancy *(1)*. However, several copper-dependent enzymes are essential for biological processes during gestation: cytochrome c oxidase (cellular respiration and energy production), superoxide dismutase (free radical defenses), lysyl oxidase (cross-linkage of elastin and collagen during connective tissue formation), ferroxidase I or ceruloplasmin (facilitation of iron transport and utilization), and dopamine B-hydroxy-lase (norepinephrine synthesis).

The concentration of copper in the human fetus increases substantially during gestation with 50% of the total deposited in hepatic stores. These reserves possibly protect the full-term infant against copper deficiency during the early postnatal months *(69)*. Low birth weight preterm neonates have low copper stores since two-thirds of fetal copper accretion occurs during the last 10 to 12 wk of pregnancy, especially the last 4 to 6 wk, at approx 0.28 mg/d *(69,102–104)*. Total copper retention during pregnancy is approx 30 mg, with 17–19 mg deposited in fetal tissue *(1,105)*. If a newborn was 3 kg, then 350 µg/d above an adult RDA could be adequate to meet the copper needs of a pregnant women *(105)*. This amount of copper may be difficult to achieve. Although RDA have not been formu-lated for copper during pregnancy, it has been suggested that the daily copper intake should be increased by 0.75 mg. above the 1.5 to 3.0 mg/d which has been recommended as safe and adequate for adults *(105)*. A selection of high copper-containing foods should be emphasized during pregnancy *(105)*.

The characteristics of Menkes' syndrome, an X-linked chromosomal disorder of copper metabolism and transport, suggest that human copper deficiency may contribute to CNS and connective tissue malformations (*see* Chapter 12). Although the exact mechanism has not been isolated, individuals with this syndrome display many similar abnormalities characteristic of copper-deficient newborn animals: in-utero growth failure from connec-tive tissue and skeletal disorders, and progressive degenerative CNS and blood vessel abnormalities. This genetic disorder provides evidence of the role of copper for normal fetal and neonatal development *(106–107)*. Copper excretion failure and resultant cirrhosis and CNS dysfunction characterize Wilson's disease, an autosomal recessive disorder of copper metabolism (*see* Chapter 12). Teratogenic effects during pregnancy have been associated with penicillamine therapy, a copper-chelating drug used for the treatment of Wilson's disease *(108–109)*. In contrast, other case reports have not supported the relationship of induced copper excretion and congenital anomalies with low dose penicillamine *(110)*. A further complication with the use of penicillamine, a nonspecific chelating agent, is the increased excretion of other transition metals in addition to copper, e.g., zinc.

Copper metabolism is markedly altered during pregnancy. In uncomplicated pregnancies, circulating copper and ceruloplasmin concentrations progressively increase during gestation to 2 to 3 times above nonpregnant values *(111–114)*. This increase is due to estrogen-stimulated synthesis of ceruloplasmin, which transports 90% of plasma copper and mobilizes hepatic copper stores. Maternal plasma copper concentration is 5–8 times higher than the cord plasma level at term *(106,115–116,129)*. Alterations in normal pregnancy-related changes in circulating copper are likely the result of problems associated with pregnancy rather than from inadequate copper intake *(1)*. In fact, circulating copper and ceruloplasmin concentrations have been commonly utilized for the assessment of adequate placental function and fetal well-being *(117–118)*. For a detailed description of appropriate copper indices and laboratory tests of copper status in pregnancy *see* Chapter 5.

Inconsistencies exist between studies describing the relationship of maternal copper status to pregnancy outcome. Diminished *(117–121)* and increased *(119,122–123)* circulating copper and ceruloplasmin concentrations have been documented in complicated pregnancies and pregnancies resulting in adverse outcomes when compared to normal pregnancies. However, other studies have reported no difference in maternal copper status with pregnancy complications *(124)*. Likewise, when compared to term pregnancies, hypocupremia was reported at parturition for women with preterm delivery *(125)*, while other reports documented higher circulating copper concentrations in mothers delivering preterm *(126)*. In contrast, no differences in maternal copper status at parturition were reported for women with preterm delivery by other investigators *(124)*.

The relationship between maternal copper status and fetal growth also remain inconclusive. No relationship was found between maternal plasma copper *(127–131)* or cord plasma copper status and neonatal birth weight *(128–129)*. However, other researchers reported weak positive associations between third trimester hair copper concentrations and birth weight *(114)*; and cord serum copper concentrations and birth length and head circumference *(132)*. Still other studies have documented negative associations between third trimester serum copper concentrations and newborn head circumference *(114)*; whereas other studies support an inverse relationship between maternal plasma copper concentrations at parturition and birth weight *(124,126,133)*, cord plasma copper concentrations and birth weight *(133)*, and head circumference and birth weight *(134)*. Much remains to be learned about the possible influence of maternal copper status on intrauterine growth and pregnancy outcome to enhance the present understanding of these relationships.

7. SELENIUM STATUS DURING PREGNANCY

Many studies have assessed the selenium status of populations with measurements of this mineral in whole blood, plasma, serum, erythrocytes, urine, and hair. Debate exists regarding the correlation between these static indices and true selenium status without the usage of a functional selenium measurement *(135)*. Considerable research has suggested the selenium-dependent enzyme glutathione peroxidase as a functional index. This selenoenzyme prevents lipid peroxidation of membranes by protecting against free radical damage *(136)*. Possible relationships between human selenium status and pregnancy outcome stem from well-established observations in animal models demonstrating the effects of selenium supplementation on improvements in growth and development. Fundamental processes of animal reproduction are compromised by selenium deficiency:

infertility due to fragility and dysmotility of sperm, embryonic loss before implantation, stillbirths, poor intrauterine growth, prematurity, placenta retention, and poor postnatal growth *(136–137)*.

In 1989 the RDA for selenium was established for the first time. The selenium allowance for nonpregnant 19 to 51+ yr old women is 55 µg/d *(26)*. Feeding high concentrations of selenium (150 µg/d) during metabolic balance studies resulted in retentions of 10 µg/d during 10 to 20 wk gestation, and 22 µg/d during 30 to 40 wk gestation *(138)*. However, metabolic balance studies have been reported to be misleading for determining selenium requirements since homeostasis changes over wide intakes of selenium *(1,137,139)*. By using the factorial method for establishing maternal selenium requirements, an average accretion of 6.5 µg/d would be necessary, and assuming an estimated 80% absorption efficiency *(139–140)*, the average increase in dietary selenium during pregnancy would be 10 µg/d. From these data, the 1989 RDA was determined to be 65 µg/d for pregnant women *(26)*.

During human pregnancy, approx 70% of fetal trace element reserves accumulate during the third trimester *(141)*. Factorial estimates of fetal selenium retention vary from an average of 1 µg/d to 14 µg/d during the third trimester *(1)*. When compared to full-term infants, preterm infants at birth have reduced plasma selenium concentrations *(142–143)*, and plasma glutathione peroxidase activity *(142)*. Total hepatic selenium content has also been reported to be lower in preterm than full-term infants *(144)*. These findings suggest that the preterm infant has limited selenium reserves, although normal for gestational age, and may be at-risk for selenium deficiency during the rapid postnatal growth period.

Changes in circulating maternal selenium concentrations have been documented in several studies. Some studies reported plasma selenium concentrations at parturition to be 60% lower *(145)*, and 90% *(146)* lower than nonpregnant controls. When compared to nonpregnant women, significantly lower maternal plasma selenium concentrations at parturition were also documented by other investigators *(126)*. Plasma selenium concentrations were significantly lower from 26 wk gestation through parturition when compared to nonpregnant levels *(147)*. This supports the work of others who have documented a decline in maternal serum selenium concentrations during the second and third trimesters of pregnancy *(148)*. Conversely, no significant differences in plasma selenium concentrations during early or late gestation when compared to nonpregnant women were reported by others *(138)*. Similarly, no significant differences were noted in longitudinal changes in maternal serum selenium concentrations, nor were these levels different than nonpregnant concentrations in another study *(113)*. Many studies have determined neonatal plasma selenium concentrations to be significantly lower than maternal concentrations during gestation *(126,132,145–146,149–150)*. No relationship between maternal plasma selenium concentrations and birth weight was reported by some investigators *(126,150)*; other investigators have documented a significant positive correlation between cord serum selenium concentrations and birth weight and head circumference *(132)*.

Studies have analyzed the selenium concentration in maternal erythrocytes since this index may reflect long-term selenium status, and have reported a gradual and significant decrease in erythrocyte selenium concentrations throughout pregnancy *(147,149)*. Other investigators found no significant changes during early and late gestation in erythrocyte selenium concentrations *(138)*.

Maternal plasma glutathione peroxidase activity at parturition has been shown to be significantly lower than enzyme activity in nonpregnant women *(138,150)*; especially after 26 wk gestation *(147)*. The activity of this enzyme declines more rapidly in plasma than in erythrocytes during pregnancy, especially following the 20th wk of gestation *(146–148)*. In contrast, other investigators have not found a progressive decline during pregnancy *(145,149)*.

The variations among study findings regarding circulating selenium concentrations and the activity of glutathione peroxidase during pregnancy are difficult to explain. They may reflect differences in the selenium content of soils or diets where study populations reside, dietary selenium intake, variations in laboratory analytical methodologies, or true differences in selenium status. Continued research is needed to determine the selenium needs during pregnancy and the influence of selenium status on the successful outcome of pregnancy.

8. IODINE STATUS IN PREGNANCY

The World Health Organization has estimated that developing countries have more than 1.5 billion people at risk for iodine deficiency disorders (IDDs) with 500 million suffering from goiter. Five million are affected by mental retardation as cretins, with 26 million suffering from lesser mental defects due to iodine deficiency *(151–152)*. Clearly, iodine deficiency is the most prevalent worldwide cause of preventable mental retardation *(152–153)*. Approximately 60 µg of iodine are required daily to maintain an adequate supply of thyroxine; hence iodine deficiency disrupts thyroid hormone production since it is an essential component of T4 and T3 (*see* Chapter 13). Intrauterine and postnatal somatic growth and neurologic development are severely compromised by iodine deficiency. Millions of children have been affected by cretinism, which involves severe mental and growth retardation, rigid spastic motor disorders, longstanding hypothyroidism, deaf mutism, and dwarfism, while milllions more suffer from milder forms of mental and physical dysfunction *(152,153)*.

During pregnancy, the fetus is vulnerable to iodine deprivation, especially when maternal thyroxine production is insufficient due to iodine deficiency *(152–154)*. Iodine deficiency has been associated with an increased incidence of fetal wastage and perinatal mortality and morbidity. Increased rates of spontaneous abortions, stillbirths, congenital anomalies, preterm deliveries, intrauterine growth retardation, low birth weight, and infant mortality have been reported *(152–154)*. These poor outcomes have been greatly reduced by prophylactic maternal iodine supplementation efforts *(155–158)*.

Maternal iodine deficiency increases risk of fetal hypothyroidism. When not corrected, the lack of thyroid hormone results in impaired brain development and cognitive function. The adverse influence of maternal iodine deficiency begins early in fetal life, since the fetal thyroid has the capacity to concentrate iodine and synthesize thyroxine by 10 to 12 wk of gestation. Fetal T4 secretion increases by mid-gestation and progressively rises until term *(154)*. The impact of maternal iodine deficiency becomes most apparent by the second trimester *(153)*. When iodine supplementation is implemented early in the second trimester, most of the fetal damage can be prevented. If the fetus is deprived of sufficient iodine until the third trimester, increased rates of perinatal mortality have been documented, and impaired growth, and neuromuscular and cognitive damage occur *(152–154)*. In endemic goiter areas, maternal iodine supplementation efforts prior to conception and during the first trimester of pregnancy have lowered rates of prematurity, still-births, and spontaneous abortions, as well as increased neonatal thyroxine concentrations, birth weights, and placental weights *(155)*. Endemic cretinism can be eliminated by iodine fortification programs *(158)*. To avoid compromised fetal and postnatal development maternal iodine deficiency must be corrected prior to conception *(159)*. Clearly, iodine supplementation efforts during pregnancy have become one of the most successful public health interventions aimed at preserving fetal neural development and postnatal cognitive attainment.

The suggested iodine allowance for pregnant women is an additional 25 μg/d over the nonpregnant women's need of 150 μg/d to meet the extra demands of the developing fetus *(26)*. The average iodine consumption in the US for 25 to 30-yr-old women has been estimated to be 170 μg/d, excluding iodine from iodized salt *(160)*. Iodine has been increasingly used in dough conditioners, in bread-making and as iodophors used for sanitizing equipment and dairy cows in the dairy industry *(139,153)*.

9. CHROMIUM, FLUORIDE, MANGANESE, AND MOLYBDENUM STATUS IN PREGNANCY

Chromium is markedly lower in the hair of parous women *(161,162)*. Chromium content of hair was found to decline between trimesters 1 and 3 among gravidas with gestational diabetes mellitus but not among nondiabetic controls *(163)*. Jovanovic-Petersen *(164)* randomly assigned 24 gestational diabetic women to receive chromium piccolinate (4 μg/d) or placebo. She found lower fasting glucose and insulin and lower peak plasma glucose and insulin following a 100 gram oral glucose load among gravidas given chromium. Severe glucose intolerance, however, was not improved by chromium supplementation. Since chromium facilitates the binding of insulin to its receptors, chromium deficiency during pregnancy has the potential to impair glucose tolerance and insulin resistance thus increasing risk of gestational diabetes; whether or not this actually occurs is uncertain *(1)*. Supplementation during pregnancy with chromium has not been recommended *(1)*.

At present, the role of fluoride in prenatal development is poorly understood. The degree of placental transport of fluoride to the fetus has been the subject of debate. Although the development of primary dentition begins as early as 10 to 12 wk gestation, and the formation of permanent molars and incisors occurs during the sixth and ninth months of pregnancy, no formal support for routine prenatal fluoride supplementation has been advocated by professional groups. Prenatal fluoride supplementation has not been endorsed by the American Dental Association *(1)*. Prospective studies have not provided sufficient evidence for the establishment of recommendations for fluoride supplementation as a means of protecting the teeth of offspring during human pregnancy.

Dietary manganese deficiency has not been observed in humans, although a few case studies have been reported. These are most commonly iatrogenic or occur as a complication of disease states *(165)*. There is a lack of adequate data on the accumulation of manganese in the conceptus during human pregnancy *(1)*, and maternal manganese deficiency in humans has not been documented. The Total Diet Study (1982 to 1986) documented the usual dietary manganese intake of 2 mg/d for 25 to 30-yr-old nonpregnant women *(160)*. Until more research provides evidence of problems with maternal manganese nutriture, manganese supplementation during pregnancy is not indicated.

Human molybdenum deficiency has not been described except when iatrogenic causes have been involved (i.e., molybdenum-deficient TPN solutions) *(1,165)*. No studies have been reported in humans suggesting that molybdenum deficiency exists during pregnancy. Molybdenum supplementation is not warranted at this time for pregnant women *(1)*.

10. SUMMARY AND CONCLUSIONS

The trace minerals have important functions that have the potential to influence the course and outcome of pregnancy. Iodine deficiency, for example, is a leading cause of cretinism and the associated mental retardation, which now are preventable through the iodinization of food. Iron deficiency is a leading cause of maternal anemia. Anemia and IDA are associated with increased risks of preterm delivery and infant low birth weight. However, for other trace minerals, many inconsistencies exist among studies describing the relationship of maternal status to pregnancy outcome and there is ongoing debate about risk that is attributable to deficiency. For example, calcium may be involved in the etiology of preeclampsia. However, the ability of supplemental calcium to decrease the risk of either preeclampsia and/or preterm delivery may be confined to high-risk populations in which there is either a severe dietary restriction of calcium or a high demand for calcium. Zinc deficiency is associated with poor pregnancy outcome but clinical trials have come to opposite conclusions about the efficacy of zinc supplementation. Since there is no agreed-upon indicator of zinc status, an underlying problem may be difficulty in the selection of individuals at risk, that is gravidas who are zinc deficient and thus may benefit from supplementation. Similar comments could be made about most of the other trace elements included in this chapter. Lack of sensitive and specific tests for trace element status limits detection of deficiencies and ultimately the recommendation to use supplements in the course of prenatal care.

REFERENCES

1. Institute of Medicine (US). Subcommittee on Nutritional Status and Weight Gain during Pregnancy. Nutrition During Pregnancy. National Academy Press, Washington, DC, 1990.
2. Klebanoff MA, Shiono PH, Berendes HW, Rhoads GG. Facts and artifacts about anemia and preterm delivery. JAMA 1989;262:511–515.
3. Whittaker PG, Macphail S, Lind T. Serial hematologic changes and pregnancy outcome. Obstet Gynecol 1996;88:33–39.
4. Dallman PR, Simmes MA, Stekel A. Iron deficiency in infancy and childhood. Am J Clin Nutr 1980;33:86–118.
5. Puolakka J, Janne 0, Pakarinen A, Jarvinen A, Vihko R. Serum ferritin as a measure of iron stores during and after normal pregnancy with and without iron supplements. Acta Obstet Gynecol Scand Suppil 1980;95:43–51.
6. Allen LH. Pregnancy and iron deficiency: unresolved issues. Nutr Rev 1997;55:91–101.
7. Carriaga MT, Skikne BS, Finley B, Cutler B, Cook JD. Serum transferrin receptor for the detection of iron deficiency in pregnancy. Am J Clin Nutr 1991;54:1077–1081.
8. Scholl TO, Hediger ML, Fischer RL, Shearer JW. Anemia and iron deficiency: increased risk of preterm delivery in a prospective study. Am J Clin Nutr 1992;55:985–988.
9. Scholl TO, Hediger ML, Schall JI, Fisher RL, Khoo CS. Low zinc intake during pregnancy: its association with preterm and very preterm delivery. Am J Epidemiol 1993;137:1115–1124.
10. Scholl TO. Hediger ML, Schall JI, Khoo CS, Fisher RL.1 Dietary and serum folate: their influence on the outcome of pregnancy. Am J Clin Nutr 1996;63:520–525.
11. Murphy JF, O'Riordan J, Newcombe RG, Coles EC, Pearson JF. Relation of haemoglobin levels in first and second trimesters to outcome of pregnancy. Lancet 1986;1:992–994.

12. Garn SM, Ridella SA, Petzold AS, Falkner F. Maternal hematologic levels and pregnancy outcomes. Sem Perinatol 1981;5:55–62.

13. Steer P, Alam MA, Wadsworth J, Welch A. Relation between maternal haemoglobin concentration and birth weight in different ethnic groups. BMJ 1995;310:489–491.

14. Meis PJ, Michielutte R, Peters TJ, Wells HB, Sands RE, Coles EC, Johns KA. Factors associated with preterm birth in Cardiff Wales. Am J Obstet Gynecol 1995;173:590–596.

15. Klebanoff MA, Shiono PH, Selby JV, Trachtenberg AL, Graubard BL. Anemia and spontaneous preterm birth. Am J Obstet Gynecol 1991;164:59–63.

16. Higgins AC, Pencharz PB, Strawbridge JE, Maughan GB, Moxiev JE. Maternal haemoglobin changes and their relationship to infant birth weight in mothers receiving a program of nutritional assessment and rehabilitation. Nutr Res 1982;2:641–649.

17. Lu ZM, Goldenberg RL, Cliver SP, Cutter G, Blankson M. The relationship between maternal hematocrit and pregnancy outcome. Obstet Gynecol 1991;77:190–194.

18. Lieberman E, Ryan KJ, Monson RR, Schoenbaum SC. Association of maternal hematocrit with preterm labor. Am J Obstet Gynecol 1988;159:107–114.

19. Lieberman E, Ryan KI, Monson RR, Schoenbaum SC. Risk factors accounting for racial differences in the rate of preterm birth. N Engl J Med 1987;317:743–748.

20. Shiono PH, Klebanoff MA, Graubard BI, Berendes ITW, Rhoads GG. Birth weight among women of different ethnic groups. JAMA 1986;255:48–52.

21. Scholl TO, Hediger ML. Anemia and iron–deficiency anemia: compilation of data on pregnancy outcome. Am J Clin Nutr 1994;59:492S–501S.

22. Beisel WR. Trace elements in the infectious processes. Med Clinics of North America 1978;60:831–849.

23. Tamura T, Goldenberg RL, Johnston KE, Cliver SP, Hickey CA. Serum ferritin: A predictor of early spontaneous preterm delivery. Obstet Gynecol 1996;87:360–365.

24. Goldenberg RL, Tamura T, DuBard M, Johnston KE, Copper RL, Neggers Y. Plasma ferritin and pregnancy outcome. Am J Obstet Gynecol 1996;175:1356–1359.

25. Scholl TO. High third trimester ferritin concentration: associations with very preterm delivery infection and maternal nutritional status. Obstet Gynecol 1998;92:161–165.

26. National Research Council (U.S.) Committee on Dietary Allowances. Recommended Dietary Allowances. 10th Edition. Washington, D.C. National Academy Press, 1989.

27. Lamke B, Brundin J, Moberg P. Changes of bone mineral content during pregnancy and lactation. Acta Obstet Gynecol Scand 1977;56:217–219.

28. Christiansen C, Rodbro P, Heinild B. Unchanged total body calcium in normal human pregnancy. Acta Obstet Gynecol Scand 1976;53:141–143.

29. Sowers MF, Crutchfield M, Jannausch M, et al. A prospective evaluation of bone mineral change in pregnancy. Obstet Gynecol 1991;77:841–845.

30. Drinkwater BL, Chestnut CH. Bone density changes during pregnancy and lactation in active women: a longitudinal study. Bone & Mineral 1991;14:153–160.

31. Kent GN, Price RI, Gutteridge DH, Allen JR, Rosman KJ, Smith M, Bhagat CI, Wilson SG, Retallack RW. Effect of pregnancy and lactation on maternal bone mass and calcium metabolism. Osteoporosis Int'l 1993;3 Supp: 44–47.

32. Cross NA, Hillman LS, Allen SH, Krause GF, Vieira NE. Calcium homeostasis and bone metabolism during pregnancy lactation and postweaning: a longitudinal study. Am J Clin Nutr 1995;61:514–523.

33. Nilsson BF. Parity and osteoporosis. Surg Gynecol Obstet 1969;129:27–28.

34. Aloia JF, Vaswani AN, Yeh JK, et al. Determinants of bone mass in postmenopausal women. Arch Int Med 1983;143:1700–1703.

35. Smith RW. Dietary and hormonal factors in bone loss. Fed Proc 1967;26:1737–1740.

36. Matkovic V, Kostial K, Simonovic I, et al. Bone status and fracture rates in two regions of Yugoslavia. Am J Clin Nutr 1979;32:540–549.

37. Sandler RB, Slemenda CW, LaPorte RE, et al. Postmenopausal bone density and milk consumption in childhood and adolescence. Am J Clin Nutr 1985;42:270–274.

38. Scholl TO, Hediger ML, Schall JI. Maternal growth and fetal growth: pregnancy course and outcome in the Camden Study. Ann NY Acad Sci 1997;817:281–291.

39. Sowers MF, Wallace RB, Lemke JH. Correlates of forearm bone mass among women during maximal bone mineralization. Prev Med 1985;14:585–596.

40. Sowers MF, Clark K, Wallace R, Jannausch M, Lemke J. Prospective study of radial bone mineral density in a geographically defined population of postmenopausal women. Caloif Tissue Int 1991;48:232–239.

41. Fox KM, Magaziner J, Sherwin R, Scott JC, Plato CC, Nevitt M, Cummings S. Reproductive correlates of bone mass in elderly women. Study of osteoporotic fractures research group. J Bone & Mineral Res 1993;8:901–908.
42. Goldsmith NF, Johnston JO. Bone mineral: effects of oral contraceptives pregnancy and lactation. J Bone Joint Surg 1975;57:A657–A668.
43. Carter OD, Haynes SG. Prevalence rates for scoliosis in U.S. adults: results from the first National Health and Nutrition Examination Survey. Int J Epidemiol 1987;16:537–544.
44. Sanchez-Ramos L, Sandroni S, Andres FJ, Kaunitz AM. Calcium excretion in preeclampsia. Obstet Gynecol 1991;77:510–513.
45. Sanchez-Ramos L, Jones DC, Cullen MT. Urinary calcium as an early marker for preeclampsia. Obstet Gynecol 1991;77:685–688.
46. Belizan JM, Villar J. The relationship between calcium intake and edema-proteinuria-and hypertension-gestosis: an hypothesis. Am J Clin Nutr 1980;33:2202–2210.
47. Marcoux S, Brisson J, Fabia J. Calcium intake from dairy products and supplements and the risks of preeclampsia and gestational hypertension. Am J Epidemiol 1991;133:1266–1272.
48. Repke JT, Villar J. Pregnancy-induced hypertension and low birth weight: the role of calcium. Am J Clin Nutr 1991;54:237–241S.
49. Belizan JM, Villar J, Gonzalez L, Campodonico L, Bergel E. Calcium supplementation to prevent hypertensive disorders of pregnancy. N Engl J Med 1991;325:1399–1405.
50. McCarron D, Morris CD, Roullet C, et al. Dietary calcium and blood pressure: modifying factors in specific populations. Am J Clin Nutr 1991;54:215–219S.
51. Bucher HC, Cook RJ, Guyatt GH, Lang LD, Cook DJ, Hatala R, Hunt DL. Effects of dietary calcium supplementation on blood pressure. JAMA 1996;275:1016–1022.
52. Bucher HC, Guyatt GH, Cook RJ, Hatala R, Cook DJ, Lang JD, Hunt D. Effect of calcium supplementation on pregnancy-induced hypertension and preeclampsia. JAMA 1996;275:1113–1117.
53. Levine RJ, Hauth JC, Curet LB, Sibai BM, Catalano PM, Morris CD, Der Simonian R, Esterlitz JR, Raymond EG, Bild DE, Clemens JD, Cutler JA. Trial of calcium to prevent pre-eclampsia. N Engl J Med 1997;337:69–76.
54. Lenfant C, Gifford RW, Zuspan FP. Consensus report: National high blood pressure education program working group report on high blood pressure in pregnancy. Am J Obstet Gynecol 1990;163:1689–1712.
55. Lopez-Jaramillo P, Narvaez M, Weigel RM, Yepez R. Calcium supplementation reduces the risk of pregnancy–induced hypertension in an Andes population. Br J Obstet Gynaecol 1989;96:648–655.
56. Lopez-Jaramillo P, Narvaez M, Felix C, Lopez A. Dietary calcium supplementation and prevention of pregnancy hypertension. Lancet 1990;335:293.
57. Lopez-Jaramillo P, Delgado F, Jacome P, Teran E, Ruano C, Rivera J. Calcium supplementation and the risk of preeclampsia in Ecuadorian pregnant teenagers. Obstet Gynecol 1997;90:162–167.
58. Lindheimer MD. Pre-eclampsia-eclampsia 1996: preventable? Have disputes on its treatment been resolved? Nephrology and Hypertension 1996;5:452–458.
59. The Eclampsia Collaborative Group: Which anticonvulsant for women with eclampsia? Evidence from the collaborative eclampsia trial. Lancet 1995;345:1455–1463.
60. Elwood JM. Anencephalus and drinking water composition. Am J Epidemiol 1977;105:460–468.
61. Altura BM, Altura BT, Carella A. Magnesium deficiency-induced spasms of umbilical vessels: relation to pre-eclampsia hypertension growth retardation. Science 1983;221:376–377.
62. Spatling L, Spatling G. Magnesium supplementation in pregnancy. A double-blind study. Brish J Obstet Gynaecol 1988;95:120–125.
63. Sibai BM, Villar L, MA, Bray E. Magnesium supplementation during pregnancy: A double-blind randomized controlled clinical trial. Am J Obstet Gynecol 1989;161:115–119.
64. Smolarczyk R, Wojcicka-Jagodzinska J, Romejko E, Pickarski P, Czajkowski K, Teliga J. Calcium-phosphorus-magnesium homeostasis in women with threatened preterm delivery. Int'l J Gynecol Obstet 1997;57:43–48.
65. Boston JL, Beauchene RE, Cruikshank DP. Erythrocyte and plasma magnesium during teenage pregnancy: relationship with blood pressure and pregnancy-induced hypertension. Obstet Gynecol 1989;73:169–174.
66. Standley CA, Whitty JE, Mason BA, Cotton DB. Serum ionized magnesium levels in normal and preeclampsia gestation. Obstet Gynecol 1997;89:24–27.
67. Skajaa K, Dorup I, Sandstrom BM. Magnesium intake and status and pregnancy outcome in a Danish population. Brish J Obstet Gynaecol 1991;98:919–928.

68. Hess F, King J, Margen S. Zinc excretion in young women on low zinc intake and oral contraceptive agents. J Nutr 1977;107:1610–1620.
69. Widdowson E, DaunceyJ, Shaw J. Trace elements in fetal and early postnatal development. Proc Nutr Soc 1974;33:275–284.
70. Swanson CA, King JC. Zinc and pregnancy outcome. Am J Clin Nutr 1987;46:763–771.
71. Fung E, Ritchie L, Woodhouse L, Roehl R, King. J. Zinc absorption in women during pregnancy and lactation: a longitudinal study. Am J Clin Nutr 1997;66:80–88.
72. Prasad AS. History of zinc in human nutrition In: AS. Prasad IE. Dreosti BS. Hetzel eds. Clinical Applications of Recent Advances in Zinc Metabolism. Alan R. Liss Inc, New York, 1982,pp. 1–17.
73. Sever LE, Emanuel I. Is there a connection between maternal zinc deficiency and congenital malformations of the central nervous system in man? Teratol 1973;7:117–118.
74. Hambidge KM, Neldner KH, Walravens PA. Zinc acrodermatitis enteropathica and congenital malformations. Lancet 1975;1:577–578.
75. Neldner KH, Hambidge KM. Zinc therapy of acrodermatitis enteropathica. N Engl J Med 1975; 292:879–888.
76. Jameson S. Variations in maternal serum zinc during pregnancy and correlation congenital malformations dysmaturity and abnormal parturition. Acta Med Scand 1976;59:321–337.
77. Cavdar AO, Arcasoy A, Baycu T, Himmetoglu O. Zinc deficiency and anencephaly in Turkey. Teratol 1980;22:141–149.
78. Soltan MH, Jenkins DM. Maternal and fetal plasma zinc concentration and fetal abnormality. Br J Obstet Gynaecol 1982;89:56–58.
79. Buamah PK, Russell M, Bates G, Ward AM, Skillen AW. Maternal zinc status: A determination of central nervous system malformation. Br J Obstet Gynaecol 1984;91:788–790.
80. Hinks LJ, Oglivy-Stuart A, Hambidge KM, Walker V. Maternal zinc and selenium status in pregnancies with a neural tube defect or elevated plasma alpha-fetoprotein. Br J Obstet Gynaecol 1989;98:61–66.
81. McMichael A, Dreosti I, Ryan P, Robertson E. Neural tube defects and maternal serum zinc and copper concentrations in mid-pregnancy: a case-control study. Med J Autralia 1994;161:478–482.
82. Cavdar AO, Bahceci M, Akar N, Erten J, Yavuz H. Effect of zinc supplementation in a Turkish woman with two previous anencephalic infants. Gynecol Obstet Invest 1991;32:123–125.
83. Hambidge M, Hackshaw A, Wald N. Nueral tube defects and serum zinc. Br J Obstet Gynaecol 1993;100:746–749.
84. Crosby WM, Metcoff J, Costiloe JP, Mameesh M, Sandstead HH, Jacob RA, McClain PE, Jacobson G, Reid W, Burns G. Fetal malnutrition: An appraisal of correlated factors. Am J Obstet Gynecol 1977;128:22 29.
85. Ghosh A, Fong LYY, Wan CW, Liang ST, Woo JSK, Wong V. Zinc deficiency is not a cause for abortion, congential abnormality and small-for-gestational age infant in Chinese women. Br J Obstet Gynaecol 1985;92:886–891.
86. Singh PP. Khushlani K, Veerwal PC, Gupta RC. Maternal hypozincemia and low birth weight infants. Clin Chem 1987;33:1950.
87. Neggers YH, Cutter GR, Acton RT, Alverez JO, Bonner JL, Goldenberg RL, Go RCP, Roseman JM. A positive association between maternal serum zinc concentration and birth weight. Am J Clin Nutr 1990;51:678–684.
88. Kirksey A, Wachs T, Yunis F, Srinath U, Rahmanifar A, McCabe G, Galal O, Harrison G, Jerome N. Relationship of maternal zinc nutriture to pregnancy outcome and infant development in an Egyptian village. Am J Clin Nutr 1994;60:782–792.
89. Metcoff J, Cottilo J, Crosby W, Bentle L, Sethachalam D, Sandstead H, Bodwell C, Weaver F, McClain P. Maternal nutrition and fetal outcome. Am J Clin Nutr 1981;34:708–721.
90. McMichael AJ, Dreosti IE, Gibson GT, Hartshorne JM, Buckely RA, Colley DP. A prospective study of serial maternal serum zinc levels and pregnancy outcome. Early Human Development 1982;7:59–69.
91. Mukherjee MD, Sandstead HH, Ratnaparkhi MV, Johnson LK, Milne DB, Stelling HP. Maternal zinc iron folic acid and protein nutriture and outcome of human pregnancy. Am J Clin Nutr 1984;40:496–507.
92. Meadows N, Ruse W, Smith MF, Day J, Keeling PWN, Scopes JW, Thompson RPH, Bloxam DL. Zinc and small babies. Lancet 1981;2:1135–1137.
93. Meadows N, Ruse W, Keeling PWN, Scopes JW, Thompson RPH. Peripheral blood leucocyte zinc depletion in babies with intrauterine growth retardation. Arch Dis Childhood 1983;58:807–809.
94. Wells JL, James DK, Luxton R, Pennock CA. Maternal leucocyte zinc deficiency at start of third trimester as a predictor of fetal growth retardation. Br Med J 1987;294:1054–1057.

95. Adeniyi FAA. The implications of hypozincemia in pregnancy. Acta Obstet Gynecol Scand 1987;66:579–582.
96. Simmer K, Thompson RPH. Maternal zinc and intrauterine growth retardation. Clin Sci 1985;68:395–399.
97. Kuhnert BR, Kuhnert PM, Lazebnik N, Erhard P. The effect of maternal smoking on the relationship between maternal and fetal zinc status and infant birth weight. J Am Coll Nutr 1988;7:309–316.
98. Kynast G, Saling E. Effect of oral zinc application during pregnancy. Gynecol Obstet Invest 1986;21:117–123.
99. Cherry FF, Sandstead HH, Rohas P, Johnson LK, Batson HK, Wang XB. Adolescent pregnancy: associations among body weight zinc nutriture and pregnancy outcome. Am J Clin Nutr 1989;50:945–954.
100. Goldenberg R, Tamura T, Neggers Y, Cooper R, Johnson K, DuBard M, Hauth J. The effects of zinc supplementation on pregnancy outcome. J Am Med Assoc 1995;274:463–468.
101. Jonsson B, Hauge B, Larsen MF, Hald F. Zinc supplementation during pregnancy: a double blind randomized trial. Acta Obstet Gynecol Scand 1996;75:725–729.
102. Wilson T, Lahey M. Failure to induce dietary deficiency of copper in premature infants. Peds 1960;25:40–45.
103. Campbell D. Trace elements needs in human pregnancy. Proc Nutr Soc 1988;47:45–53.
104. Shaw J. Trace elements in the fetus and young infant. II Copper, manganese, selenium, and chromium. Am J Dis Child 1980;134:74–81.
105. Klevay L, Medeiros D. Deliberations and evaluations of the approaches endpoints and paradigms for dietary recommendations about copper. J Nutr 1996;126:2419S–2426S.
106. Pleban P, Numerof B, Wirth F. Trace element metabolism in the fetus and neonate. Clin Endocrinol Metabol 1985;14:545–565.
107. Hurley L. Trace elements: iron copper iodine. In: Developmental Nutrition. Prentice Hall Englewood Cliffs NJ 1980, pp.183–198.
108. Solomon L, Abrams G, Dinner M, Berman L. Neonatal abnormalities associated with D-penicillamine treatment during pregnancy. N Engl J Med 1977;296:54–55.
109. Rosa F. Teratogen update: penicillamine. Teratol 1986;33:127–131.
110. Nunns D, Hawthorne B, Goulding P, Maresh M. Wilson's disease in pregnancy. Europe J Obstet Reprod Biol 1995;62:141–143.
111. Morriss F. Trace minerals. Seminars in Perinatology 1979;3:369–379.
112. Hambidge M, Droegemueller W. Changes in plasma and hair concentrations of zinc, copper, chromium, and manganese during pregnancy. Obstet Gynecol 1974;44:666–671.
113. Kundu N, Parke P, Petersen L, Palmer I, Olson O. Distribution of serum selenium, copper, and zinc in normal human pregnancy. Arch Environ Hlth 1985;40:268–273.
114. Vir S, Love A, Thompson W. Serum and hair concentrations of copper during pregnancy. Am J Clin Nutr 1981;34:2382–2388.
115. Heinken R, Marshall J, Meret S. Maternal fetal metabolism of copper and zinc at term. Am J Obstet Gynecol 1971;110:131–134.
116. Yamashita K, Ohno H, Doi R, Mure K, Ishikawa M, Shimizu T, Avai K, Taniquchi N. Distribution of zinc and copper in maternal and cord blood at delivery. Biol Neonate 1985;48:362–365.
117. Friedman S, Bahary C, Eckerling B, Gans B. Serum copper level as an index of placental function. Obstet Gynecol 1969;33:189–193.
118. O'Leary J. Serum copper levels as a measure of placental function. Am J Obstet Gynecol 1969;105:636–637.
119. Schenker J, Jiengreis E, Polishiek W. Serum copper levels in normal and pathological pregnancies. Am J Obstet Gynecol 1969;105:933–937.
120. Buamah P, Russell M, Milford-Ward A, Taylor P, Roberts D. Serum copper concentration significantly less in abnormal pregnancies. Clin Chem 1984;30:1676–1677.
121. Ozgunes H, Beksac M, Dura S, Kayakirilmaz K. Instant effect of induced abortion on serum ceruloplasmin activity copper and zinc levels. Arch Gynecol 1987;240:21–25.
122. Borella P, Szilagyi A, Than G, Csaba I, Giardino A, Facchinetti F. Maternal plasma concentrations of magnesium calcium zinc and copper in normal and pathological pregnancies. Sci Tot Environ 1990;99:67–76.
123. Fattah M, Ibrahim F, Ramadam M, Sammiur M. Ceruloplasmin and copper levels in maternal and cord blood and placenta in normal pregnancy and in pre-eclampsia. Acta Obstet Scand 1976;55:383–385.

124. Bro S, Berendtsen H, Norgaard J, Host A, Jorgensen P. Serum zinc and copper concentrations in maternal and umbilical cord blood. Relation to course and outcome of pregnancy. Scand J Clin Lab Invest 1988;48: 805–811.

125. Kiilholma P, Gionroos M, Erkkola R, Pakarinen P, Nanto V. The role of calcium, copper, iron, and zinc in preterm delivery and premature rupture of fetal membranes. Gynecol Obstet Invest 1984;17:194–201.

126. Wasowicz W, Wolkanin P, Bednarski M, Gromadzinska J, Sklodowska M, Grzybowski K. Plasma trace minerals (Se Zn Cu) concentrations in maternal and umbilical cord blood in Poland. Biol Trace Elem Res 1993;38:205–215.

127. Tuttle S, Aggett P, Campbell D, MacGillivray I. Zinc and copper nutrition in human pregnancy: a longitudinal study in normal primigravidae and in primigravidae at risk of delivering a growth retarded baby. Am J Clin Nutr 1985;41:1032–1041.

128. Bogden J, Thind I, Louvia D, Caterini H. Maternal and cord blood metal concentrations and low birth weight-a case control study. Am J Clin Nutr 1978;31:1181–1187.

129. Bogden J, Thind I, Kemp F, Caterini H. Plasma concentrations of calcium, chromium, copper, iron, magnesium, and zinc in maternal and cord blood and their relationship to low birthweight. J Lab Clin Med 1978;92:455–462.

130. Campbell-Brown M, Ward R, Haines A, North W, Abraham R, McFadyen I. Zinc and copper in Asian pregnancies - is there evidence for nutritional deficiency? Br J Obstet Gynecol 1985;92:875–885.

131. Okonofua F, Amoke F, Emofurieta W, Ugwu N. Zinc and copper concentration in plasma of pregnant women in Nigeria. Int J Gynecol Obstet 1989;29:19–23.

132. Arnaud J, Preziosi P, Mashako L, Galan P, Nsibu C, Favier A, Kapongo C, Hercberg S. Serum trace elements in Zairian mothers and their newborns. Eur J Clin Nutr 1993;48:341–348.

133. Okonofua A, Isinkaye V, Onwudiegwe F, Amole F, Emofurieta W, Ugwu N. Plasma zinc and copper in pregnant Nigerian women at term and their newborns. Int. J. Gynecol Obstet 1990;32:243–245.

134. Ghebremeskel K, Burns L, Burden T, Harbige L, Costeloe K, Powell J, Crawford M. Vitamin A and related essential nutrients in cord blood: relationships with anthropometric measurements at birth. Early Hum Devel 1994;39:177–188.

135. Diplock A. Indexes of selenium status in human populations. Am J Clin Nutr 1993;57:256S–258S

136. Bedwal R, Nair N, Sharma M, Mathur R. Selenium - Its biological perspectives. Med Hypotheses 1993;41:150–159.

137. Levander O. Selenium. In: W. Mertz ed. Trace Elements in Human and Animal Nutrition, Vol. 2, 5th Edition. Academic Press Inc, NY, 1986, pp. 209–279.

138. Swanson C, Reamer D, Veillon C, King J, Levander O. Quantitative and qualitative aspects of selenium utilization in pregnant and non-pregnant women: an application of stable isotope methodology. Am J Clin Nutr 1983;38:169–180.

139. Levander O, Whanger P. Deliberations and evaluations of the approaches, endpoints, and paradigms for selenium and iodine dietary recommendations. J Nutr 1996;126:2427S–2434S.

140. Levander O. Considerations in design of selenium bioavailability studies. Proceed FASEB 1983;42:1721–1725.

141. Morris F. Trace minerals. Sem Perinatol 1979;3:369–379.

142. Lochitch G, Jacobson B, Quigley G. Selenium deficiency in low birthweight neonates: an unrecognized problem. J Pediatr 1989;114:865–870.

143. Lombeck I. The evaluation of the selenium status of children. J Inherit Metab Dis 1983;6:83S–84S.

144. Bayliss P, Buchanan B, Hancock R, Zlotkin S. Tissue selenium accretion in premature and full term human infant and children. Biol Trace Elem Res 1985;7:55–61.

145. Perona G, Guidi G, Piga A, Cellerino R, Milani G, Colantti P, Moschini G, Stievano B. Neonatal erythrocyte glulathione peroxidase deficiency as a consequence of selenium imbalance during pregnancy. Br J Haematol 1979;42:567–574.

146. Rudolph N, Wong S. Selenium and glutathione peroxidase activity in maternal and cord plasma and red cells. Pediatr Res 1978;12:789–792.

147. Zachara B, Wardak C, Didkowski W, Maciag A., Marchaluk E. Changes in blood selenium and glutathione concentrations and glutathione peroxidase activity in human pregnancy. Gynecol Obstet Invest 1993;35:12–17.

148. McGlashan N, Cook S, Melrose W, Martin P, Chelkowska E, vonWitt R. Maternal selenium level and sudden infant death syndrome (SIDS). Aust NZ J Med 1996;26:677–682.

149. Butler J, Whanger P, Tripp M. Blood selenium and glutathione peroxidase activity in pregnant women: comparative assays in primates and other animals. Am J Clin Nutr 1982;36:15–23.
150. Zachara B, Wasowicz W, Giomadzinska J, Sklodowska M, Krasomski G. Glutathione peroxidase activity, selenium and lipid peroxide concentrations in blood from healthy Polish population in maternal and cord blood. Biol Trace Elem Res 1985;10:175–187.
151. World Health Organization Report to 43rd World Health Assembly, Geneva, Switzerland, 1990.
152. Howowell J, Hannon H. Teratogen update: iodine deficiency a community teratogen. Teratology 1997;55:389–405.
153. Stanbury J. Iodine deficiency and the iodine deficiency disorders. In: Ziegler E, Filer L, eds. Present Knowledge of Nutrition (7th ed.), International Life Science Institute Press, Washington, D.C., 1996, pp. 378–383.
154. Glinoer D. Maternal and fetal impact of chronic iodine deficiency. Clin Obstet Gynecol 1997,40:102–116.
155. Chaouki M, Benmiloud M. Prevention of iodine deficiency disorders by oral administration of lipiodol during pregnancy. Europ J Endocrinol 1994;130:547–551.
156. Glinoer D, DeNayer P, Delange F. A nonrandomized trial for treatment of mild iodine deficiency during pregnancy: maternal and fetal effects. J Clin Endocrinol Metab 1995;80:258–269.
157. Pedersen K, Laurberg P, Iverson E. Amelioration of some pregnancy associated variations in thyroid function by iodine supplementation. J Clin Endocrinol Metab 1993;77:1078–1083.
158. Pharoah P. Iodine supplementation trials. Am J Clin Nutr 1993;57:276S–279S.
159. Hertel B, Hary I. Thyroid function, iodine nutrition and fetal brain development. Clin Endocrinol 1979;11:445–460.
160. Pennington J, Young B, Wilson D. Nutritional elements in U.S. diets: the Total Diet Study, 1982 to 1986. J Am Diet Assoc 1989;89:659–664.
161. Hambidge KM, Rodgerson DO Comparison of hair chromium levels of nulliparous and parous women. Am J Obstet Gynecol 1969;103:320–321.
162. Mahalko JR, Bennion M. The effect of parity and time between pregnancies on maternal hair chromium concentration. Am J Clin Nutr 1976;29:1069–1072.
163. Aharoni A, Tesler B, Paltieli Y, Dori Z, Sharf M. Hair chromium content of women with gestational diabetes compared with non-diabetic pregnant women. Am J Clin Nutr 1992;55:104–107.
164. Jovanovic-Peterson L, Peterson CM. Vitamins and mineral deficiencies which may predispose to glucose intolerance of pregnancy. J Am Coll Nutr 1996;15:14–20.
165. Freeland-Graves J, Turnland J. Deliberations and evaluations of the approaches, endpoints and paradigms for manganese and molybdenum dietary recommendations. J Nutr 1996;126:2435S–2440S.

9 Trace Element and Mineral Nutrition During Lactation

Mary Frances Picciano, PhD

1. INTRODUCTION

Lactation is a vital aspect of the human reproductive process. Humans are among the over 4000 species of mammals who are distinguished from all other animals by the female possessing mammary glands capable of furnishing milk as the sole source of nutrition for their developing young immediately following birth *(1)*. Knowledge of human milk mineral contents and quantity transferred to the infant are essential to our understanding of maternal and infant nutritional requirements.

Human milk is a complex biological fluid that contains thousands of constituents in a variety of compartments. Minerals are present as ions, ion complexes in solution, ion complexes with proteins and as part of colloids. The mineral composition of human milk is not static and considerable changes occur over the course of lactation. Yet there is species-specificity for many minerals. Maternal nutritional factors can influence the mineral composition of human milk, notably several trace minerals, but generally milk mineral contents do not correlate well with either maternal dietary intake or circulating levels. Marked physiological changes occur during lactation that undoubtedly influence nutritional requirements. The most notable are the maintenance of elevated circulating prolactin and reduced estradiol. Nutritional adequacy during lactation is usually assessed from growth and biochemical indices of the nursing infant, and the volume of milk produced and its composition. Unfortunately, the impact of lactation on maternal nutrition status is seldom examined.

In this chapter, a brief discussion of the regulation of milk production is presented first to enable an assessment of total daily mineral secretion rates and infant intakes that are directly related to maternal and infant nutritional requirements. It is important to point out that mineral needs among lactating women and infants can vary widely, even when known influential factors are controlled for reasons that have not been adequately explored.

The major minerals in human milk that will be discussed are calcium, magnesium, phosphorus, sodium, potassium, and chloride. The first three of these minerals are present in milk as divalent cations; the others, as monovalent cations. Among the trace elements identified in human milk, iron, zinc, copper, manganese, chromium, selenium, molybdenum, nickel, iodine, aluminum, and fluorine will be discussed. For some of the trace minerals, information is fragmentary largely because of analytical difficulties.

From: *Clinical Nutrition of the Essential Trace Elements and Minerals: The Guide for Health Professionals*
Edited by: J. D. Bogden and L. M. Klevay © Humana Press Inc., Totowa, NJ

2. THE REGULATION OF HUMAN MILK SECRETION

The quantity of human milk secreted varies from 500 mL/d to over 1,000 mL/d *(2)*. Among diverse populations in the world, there is amazing consistency for measures of milk transferred to exclusively breast-fed infants. Mean values increase from 650 mL/d at 1 mo of lactation to approx 800 mL/d at 6 mo. Butte et al. *(3)* reported that milk volume was increased by 10–15% in women with low fat stores who secreted a milk low in fat so that total energy transfer was appropriately increased. There is substantial evidence that infant demand is the major regulatory factor for volume of milk secreted during lactation. Studies of early investigators *(4)* indicate that wet nurses could secrete greater than 3,000 mL/d and mothers of twins and triplets are reported to secrete 2,000 to 3,000 mL/d by nursing about 12–15 times per day *(5)*. Thus, the average quantity of milk secreted by lactating women for a normal single infant is far less than maternal capacity for milk production.

3. THE DIVALENT IONS: CALCIUM, MAGNESIUM, PHOSPHORUS

The amounts of calcium, magnesium, and phosphorus in human milk are in the millimolar range (Table1), far higher than the levels in maternal serum (Table 2). In humans, the concentrations of these minerals in milk are not affected by maternal intake. In contrast, Buck and Bales *(6)* found that, in lactating rats made magnesium-deficient, the concentration of magnesium in milk declined, lactation failure occurred, and the growth and development of the young were stunted.

Bovine milk contains about four times more calcium and four to five times more magnesium than human milk *(7,8)* and there are indications that these minerals are highly bioavailable from human milk. The differences in the binding patterns of these minerals in human and bovine milk may affect their bioavailability. About two-thirds of the calcium and a large fraction of the magnesium are bound to casein in bovine milk, while the casein in human milk binds only minor amounts of these minerals *(8)*. Newborns, whose digestive capacity is immature, may be unable to digest casein completely, and their ability to absorb casein-bound minerals may therefore likewise be limited.

Lactation places a high demand for calcium on women. Boass and Toverud *(9)* found that absorption of calcium increases in rats during lactation, apparently via increased nonactive transport. This increase may be due to the greater availability of glucose, stemming from increased food consumption; greater glucose availability leads to increased transport of water and, correspondingly, of calcium ions. Also, absorption may increase because calcium is removed more rapidly into circulation, leading to a diffusion gradient across the intestinal cell. A study of Gambian women, who traditionally consume a low-calcium diet, showed that calcium absorption was increased, apparently as an adaptation to low calcium intake. During lactation, the additional need for calcium seemed to be met by decreased calcium excretion rather than by a further increase in absorption *(10)*. Lactating women do experience a transient bone loss and calcium supplementation has little impact on lactation induced changes in calcium homeostasis *(11)*.

The concentrations of calcium, magnesium, and phosphorus in human milk initially increase with time postpartum. The level of calcium in human milk peaks after the first few weeks postpartum, then declines *(12–14)*; that of magnesium peaks between one and two months postpartum and subsequently levels off *(15)*. However, in a 6-mo study of

Table 1
Typical Concentrations of Selected Minerals in Human and Bovine Milks[1]

Mineral (unit)	Human Colostrum	Mature Milk	Bovine Milk
Calcium(mmol/L)	6.4 ± 1.7	6.5 ± 1.5	29.5
(mg/L)	255 ± 68	259 ± 59	1180
Magnesium (mmol/L)	1.5 ± 0.3	1.3 ± 0.3	4.9
(mg/L)	35.7 ± 6.4	31.4± 5.9	120
Phosphorus (mmol/L)	4.0 ± 0.8	4.8 ± 0.8	30.1
(mg/L)	124 ± 25	142 ± 25	930
Sodium (mmol/L)	17.9 ± 4.5	9.0 ± 4.1	25.2
(mg/L)	411 ± 4.0	207 ± 94	580
Potassium (mmol/L)	18.2 ± 2.1	13.9 ± 2.0	35
(mg/L)	712 ± 82	543 ± 78	1400
Chloride (mmol/L)	25.1 ± 1.6	12.8 ± 1.5	28.9
(mg/L)	888 ± 56	453 ± 53	1040
Iron (ug/mL)	0.97	0.4–0.76	0.2–0.6
Copper (ug/mL)	0.5–0.8	0.2–0.4	0.05–0.2
Zinc (ug/mL)	8–12	1–3	4
Manganese (ng/mL)	5–12	3–6	21
Selenium (ng/mL)[2]	32–41	15–20	10
Iodine (ng/mL)[3]		12–178	70–219
Molybdenum (ng/mL)	10–12	1–2	22
Chromium (ng/mL)		0.2–0.4	5–15
Nickel (ng/mL)		0.5–2	4–40
Aluminum (ng/mL)		4–14	27
Fluorine (ng/mL)		4–15	19

[1]Representative values are taken from: Jensen, R., ed. (1995) Handbook of Milk Composition. Academic Press, San Diego, CA

[2] Selenium content in human and bovine milk varies considerably. In selenium deficient areas of the word, representative values for human and bovine milks are 3–8 and 2–7 ng/mL, respectively. In China where selenium toxicity was evident, values for human milk were reported to be 283 ng/mL .

[3]Content of iodine in milks is highly dependent on intake.

breast-fed infants, Greer et al. (16) found that the serum calcium and magnesium levels of the infants increased over time. These findings were thought to be due to the fact that concentrations of serum calcium and magnesium are inversely related to the concentration of serum phosphorus. The concentration of phosphorus in milk peaks between 8 and 36 d postpartum, then begins to decline (17). The decrease in phosphorus intake of breast-fed infants over time may be responsible for the increase in serum levels of the calcium and magnesium.

Conversely, increased serum phosphorus leads to a decrease in serum calcium. This is one reason why infants are not fed unmodified cow's milk, which has about six times more phophorus than human milk (7). As infants have a limited ability to regulate serum calcium, hypocalcemia may result from excess phosphorus intake (17). The level of phosphorus in cow's milk-based formulas, however, is low enough that serum calcium should not be adversely affected.

Table 2
Comparison of Maternal Serum/Plasma Concentrations for Selected Minerals with
Corresponding Representative Values for Milk in Established Lactation

Mineral (unit)	Reference	Concentration in Serum/Plasma of Lactating Women[1]	Representative Milk Concentration
Calcium (mg/L)	Greer et al., 1982	91	259
Magnesium (mg/L)	Greer et al., 1982	22	331
Selenium (µg/L)	Mannan & Picciano, 1987	97	15–20
Zinc (µg/L)	Moser & Reynolds, 1983	790	1000–3000

[1] Values are for women during established lactation, greater than 1 month postpartum.
[2] Representative values for mature human milk are taken from: Jensen, R., ed. (1995) *Handbook of Milk Composition*. Academic Press, San Diego, CA.

4. THE MONOVALENT IONS: NA, K, CL

In general, the concentrations of sodium, potassium, and chloride in human milk do not vary to a great extent (Table 1). Under conditions such as mastitis, however, sodium and chloride may flow directly into milk through "leaky" junctions between mammary secretory cells, raising milk concentrations considerably *(12)*. Contents of sodium and chloride are higher in the milk of mothers who give birth to preterm infants than in those who deliver at term *(18)* indicating that tight junctions between mammary secretory cells are not yet well established.

Over the first 6 mo of lactation, the chloride content of human milk decreases by 10% or more; those of sodium and potassium decline by 25% or more *(12)*. Upon weaning, however, sodium and chloride concentrations in milk rise somewhat.

Cow's milk has considerably more chloride than human milk *(17)* and about two to three times the levels of sodium and potassium *(7,19)*. Human infants have an incomplete ability to excrete these minerals, which is one reason why unmodified cow's milk feeding of young infants is not recommended. Renal function of newborns is characterized by a low glomerular filtration rate and a low concentration capacity. The concentrations of these minerals in cow's milk-based formulas currently used in the United States are intermediate between those in human and cow's milk and do not furnish an excessive renal solute load to infants.

5. TRACE MINERALS

The trace minerals in human milk have been less well studied, and the variability in reported results is great. Although environmental factors may be responsible in part, methodological uncertainties are undoubtedly a source of conflicting results. In recent years, an awareness about trace mineral species in milk and resulting bioavailability has become apparent. Ratios and possible interactions of trace minerals in milk also are emerging as important nutritional considerations *(20)*. Gunshin et al. *(21)* found that the ratio of concentrations of molybdenum, cobalt, nickel, chromium, and manganese in human milk (100 : 6 : 15 : 27 : 40) was very close to the ratio in bovine milk (100 : 5 : 19 : 28 : 54). The similarity between these ratios may indicate that the balance between these trace minerals is regulated and has an effect on neonatal utilization.

5.1. Iron

Iron was the first trace mineral noted in milk and it remains the most extensively studied. There is a wide variation in the results reported. In humans, dietary intake of iron does not affect the iron concentration in milk. Iron deficiency is common among women and pregnant and lactating women often take iron supplements. Although iron supplementation has no effect on human milk iron content, it can replete maternal iron stores that are often diminished following pregnancy *(12)*. In a study of Nigerian women and infants, Murray et al. *(22)* found that iron in milk and status of breast-fed infants were similar, regardless of whether their mothers had low, average, or high iron status. In contrast, if lactating rats are given iron supplements or made iron-deficient, the level of iron in their milk changes dramatically *(12,23)*, an example of the fact that data from animal models is not always applicable to humans during lactation.

The concentration of iron is highest in colostrum. It declines significantly for about the first month of lactation, plateaus, then declines again in late lactation *(12,20,24)*. Some studies have indicated that prolonged exclusive breastfeeding can lead to inadequate iron intake and the development of iron deficiency in infants *(25,26)*.

Bovine milk contains slightly less iron than human milk *(27)*. Administration of unmodified bovine milk to infants can result in iron deficiency, as bovine milk, in addition to being a poor source of iron, increases intestinal blood loss and may inhibit iron absorption *(28)*. In contrast, although the iron content of human milk is also low, iron-deficiency anemia is rare in breast-fed infants in the first six months of life *(25)*. Iron bioavailability from human milk is reported to be greater than from bovine milk *(29,30)*. The greater bioavailability of iron from human milk as compared to bovine milk may be due in part to the very different binding patterns of iron in the two types of milk *(31)*. In bovine milk, 42% of iron is found in the lipid fraction, 24% bound to casein, 29% bound to whey proteins, and 32% to low-molecular-weight compounds. In human milk, between 16 and 46% of iron occurs in the lipid fraction, about 32% is bound to low-molecular-weight compounds, 9% to casein, and about 26% to whey proteins. Of the whey proteins, lactoferrin binds the majority of iron in human milk, whereas in bovine milk, the amount of lactoferrin is considerably less.

Lactoferrin, the major iron-binding protein in human milk, is thought to confer protection against bacterial infections in breastfed infants, who are known to have fewer gastrointestinal infections than formula-fed infants *(32)*. Earlier, it was thought that the mechanism of action was through sequestration of iron by lactoferrin, which prevented the growth of iron-dependent microorganisms. Recently, however, it was determined that lactoferrin also can bind to the surfaces of gram-negative bacteria, altering permeability and membrane function of the pathogens *(33)*.

It has also been postulated that lactoferrin may facilitate iron absorption. However, despite the much higher concentration of lactoferrin in human than in bovine milk, it is unlikely that lactoferrin alone accounts for the greater bioavailability of iron in human milk; its degree of saturation is too low: 6–9% *(31)*. Furthermore, heating of human milk denatures lactoferrin but does not affect the rate of iron absorption *(30)*. Other possible reasons for the high bioavailability of iron from human milk include the low concentrations of protein, calcium, and phosphorus, which inhibit iron absorption, and the high concentrations of lactose and ascorbate, which enhance iron absorption *(17)*. The small amount of iron in human milk may itself facilitate absorption, as small amounts of iron are more readily absorbed than large.

Not only the absolute amounts of iron in human milk, bovine milk, and formula are of interest, but also the relative amounts of iron and other minerals. In particular, it is known than high levels of either iron, copper, or zinc may influence the absorption of the other two elements, presumably due to competitive inhibition *(20,34)*. The Fe:Zn ratio of human milk is less than 1; in iron-fortified formula, it is greater than 2. Infants fed iron-fortified cow's milk-based formula often have lower plasma zinc levels than those given nonfortified formula, even though their zinc intakes are similar.

5.2. Zinc

There is great interindividual variation in the amount of zinc in human milk with typical amounts ranging from 1–3 µg/mL. The level of zinc in milk is always lower than that in the mother's serum, suggesting that the secretion of zinc into milk is tightly regulated (Table 2) *(35)*. Zinc is highest in colostrum and early milk, peaking about 2 d postpartum *(12,36)*. Milk zinc declines steeply for the first 3 mo postpartum, and then continues to decline gradually. By 7 or 8 mo of lactation, exclusive breastfeeding may not provide an infant with sufficient zinc, and there is some indication that growth-limiting zinc deficiency may be prevalent among otherwise healthy breast-fed infants *(37)*.

Dietary intake may affect the level of zinc in milk somewhat, although some authors have found no effect *(38)*. An increased zinc concentration in milk has been reported after maternal zinc supplementation *(12,36,39)*. Alternatively, mothers with very low zinc status may limit the zinc supply to their milk *(40)*.

The bioavailability of zinc in human milk is apparently high. Blakeborough et al. *(41)* found that plasma zinc of breast-fed infants was higher than that of formula-fed infants, even if infants were given zinc-fortified formula. Similarly, among adult women given 25 mg of zinc with either human milk, bovine milk, or formula, those who consumed the human milk showed the highest rise in plasma zinc, indicating that some component of human milk facilitates zinc absorption *(42)*.

There are several possible explanations for the high bioavailability of zinc from human milk. First, zinc binds to different macromolecules in human and cow's milk. In cow's milk, more than 95% of the zinc is bound to casein, whereas in human milk, the major protein component has been variously identified as lactoferrin or serum albumin *(41,43)*. It has been suggested that casein forms "a nonsoluble, poorly available complex with zinc" *(36)*, hindering zinc absorption. Second, about 29% of the zinc in human milk is bound to a low-molecular-weight ligand, which may facilitate zinc absorption *(44)*. Although the ligand was originally believed to be picolinic acid, it was later determined to be citrate. Bovine milk also contains a considerable amount of citrate, but the affinity of casein for zinc is higher than that of citrate, so that citrate does not bind zinc in bovine milk to a great extent. Cow's milk-based formulas are often made from milk that has been dialyzed and no longer contains citrate. Supplementation of formula with citrate may therefore facilitate zinc absorption *(45)*. Third, the high phosphorus level of bovine milk may impede zinc absorption, as there are reports that phosphate and phosphorus-containing compounds impair zinc bioavailability. Fourth, as with iron, the low concentration of zinc in human milk may lead to ready absorption *(17)*.

5.3. Copper

Human milk copper concentration is low with typical values ranging between 0.2 and 0.4 µg/mL (Table 1) . The amount of copper in milk is unaffected by maternal dietary intake *(26)*. Secretion of copper into milk, like that of zinc, is apparently actively controlled, as the copper level in milk is always less than maternal plasma copper concentration *(46)*.

The copper concentration in human milk is reported to peak around 1–8 d postpartum, decline for 3 mo, then plateau *(24,35,47)*. The decrease in human milk copper may be related to the decrease in total protein over time, as about 85% of the copper in milk is associated with the whey and casein fractions, most of which is protein-bound *(46)*.

5.4. Manganese

The concentration of manganese in human milk is very low: 3–6 ng/mL (Table 1) and may be influenced by dietary intake *(12)*. Manganese is highest in colostrum *(47)* and reported to decline between 1 and 4 mo postpartum then increase again *(46)*.

The level of manganese in bovine milk is about three- to four-fold higher than in human milk. The binding patterns also differ: the major manganese-binding compound in human milk is lactoferrin, whereas in bovine milk, the majority of manganese is bound to low-molecular-weight compounds *(48)*. All manganese in human milk is bound, although some occurs as free manganese in cow milk based formula. The effect of high-molecular-weight species on manganese absorption is unknown *(49)*.

Results from animal and human studies on the bioavailability of manganese are controversial. Chan et al. *(49)* found that far more manganese was transported into intestinal cells of rats fed bovine milk or formula than those fed human milk. These researchers hypothesized that the low-molecular-weight compounds binding manganese in bovine milk and formula are more easily taken up by intestinal cells, facilitating manganese absorption. On the other hand, Davidsson et al. *(50)* found that the percentage absorption of manganese by adult humans was higher from human milk than from cow's milk, cow's milk-based formula, or soy formula. These authors hypothesized that the binding of manganese to lactoferrin in human milk may aid absorption, and the high level of calcium in cow's milk may interfere with manganese absorption.

In humans, manganese deficiency is very rare. It has been reported in infants, however, and very low-birthweight infants may be at particular risk *(49)*. Manganese toxicity may also be of concern. Although a very large concentration of manganese is needed to produce toxicity in human adults, infants may be more vulnerable *(12)*. Young infants have an incomplete ability to excrete manganese. The high concentrations of manganese in some infant formulas are speculated to lead to a higher absolute retention of manganese than from human milk, even if the relative absorption is lower *(49)*. On average, feeding infants manganese-supplemented formulas is reported to result in a sixfold greater retention than when human milk is fed *(51)*. In the United States, formulas had been supplemented with manganese; however, that practice has been abandoned. Safe and adequate ranges of manganese intakes during infancy are not well defined.

5.5. *Chromium*

Human milk contains about 0.15–0.40 ng Cr/mL (Table1). Earlier studies reported much higher values for chromium in milk. Since the determination of chromium is very sensitive to contamination, the older values probably reflected analytical errors *(52,53)* (*see* Chapter 5).

The content of chromium in human milk is reported to be relatively constant throughout lactation *(54)*. Chromium intake does not appear to affect human milk chromium concentration, partly because as intake increases, absorption of chromium decreases, and chromium excretion in urine is enhanced.

It has been suggested that women are at risk for chromium depletion during lactation *(52)*. In general, the chromium intake in the United States is low, and lactating women lose 50% more chromium in their urine than nonpregnant women, in addition to losses due to milk secretion.

The level of chromium in bovine milk is about ten times higher than in human milk *(47)*; in formulas, it is 20–100 times higher *(55)*. Although chromium may be less available from formulas than from human milk, formula-fed infants are receiving exceedingly high amounts of chromium and potential consequences have not been evaluated.

5.6. *Selenium*

Human milk contains about 15–20 µg Se/L *(56)* although there is a wide range of reported values (Table 1). The selenium level of milk is highest in colostrum and declines with the progression of lactation in women unless they are receiving selenium supplements *(57)*. The initial selenium concentration of human milk also is strongly affected by maternal intake. Great geographical variation is seen: in areas where the selenium content of the soil is low, such as China and New Zealand, milk selenium concentrations as low as 3–5 µg/L are reported *(58)*, and selenium deficiency is common. Not only the amount but also the form of selenium consumed affects selenium levels in milk: selenium from vegetable sources is more bioavailable than that from animal sources *(59)*.

There is less selenium in bovine milk than in human milk. Little is known about the relative bioavailabilities of selenium from human and bovine milk, although 40–60% of the selenium in cow's milk is bound to casein, which may impede its absorption *(60)*. Most selenium in human milk is also protein-bound; Milner et al. *(61)* separated at least nine different selenoprotein-containing fractions in human milk. It is not known what effect, if any, this distribution pattern has on selenium bioavailability to infants.

McGuire et al. *(62)* reported that infants given selenium-supplemented formulas had a nearly 60% higher selenium intake than breast-fed infants but that both groups of infants had similar plasma selenium concentrations, indicating that utilization of selenium differs in infants fed human milk compared to selenium supplemented formula. Premature infants have baseline plasma selenium values that are lower than those of full-term infants and selenium status deteriorates rapidly unless they are fed human milk or selenium supplemented formula *(63,64)*. Recently, a high rate of respiratory morbidity was found to be directly related to selenium status of very low birth weight infants *(65)*.

5.7. *Molybdenum*

The molybdenum content of human milk has not been extensively examined. Analytical difficulties are largely responsible. Milk molybdenum concentration is reported to be high in colostrum (10–20 ng/mL), then to decline rapidly during the first 2 wk of lactation *(17)*. Approximately 40% of human milk molybdenum is associated with the fat fraction probably as part of the enzyme, xanthine oxidase, that is a major component of the milk fat globular membrane.

Little is known about the molybdenum requirements of infants, and molybdenum deficiency is rare. Bougle et al. *(66)* found that the milk of mothers of premature infants contains less molybdenum than that of mothers of full-term infants; however, although breast-fed premature infants may have low molybdenum intakes, there is little evidence that they are at risk of molybdenum deficiency.

Molybdenum toxicity is also of concern in some areas. Because molybdenum is metabolized as an anion, its gastrointestinal absorption is not restricted *(67)*. Thus, levels of molybdenum in body fluids likely reflect environmental levels much more than do levels of cationic elements. Infants (and adults) in areas with extremely high environmental levels of molybdenum, such as certain regions of India, are therefore at risk for molybdenum toxicity.

5.8. Nickel

Although nickel is considered to be a possibly essential trace element, very little is known about its metabolism during lactation. Human milk contains about 0.5–2.0 ng/mL *(67)* (*see* Chapter 2). Some researchers have reported much higher values, which may be due to contamination of milk samples by nickel from stainless steel equipment *(21)*. The concentration of nickel, like that of chromium, remains fairly steady throughout lactation.

5.9. Iodine

The concentration of iodine in human milk varies greatly, ranging from about 29 to 490 ng/mL *(68)*. The level of iodine varies with the time of day and the time postpartum. It does not vary significantly during a nursing. The variation in iodine concentration is primarily due to maternal intake. In North America, the average intake of iodine is quite high, due to consumption of iodized salt, and human milk on average contains far more iodine than infants need. In contrast, in some regions of the world, iodine intake is quite low, and iodine deficiency disorders are prevalent in both lactating women and their infants. Uptake of iodine by the mammary gland may compensate to a certain extent for low iodine intake. Vermiglio et al. *(69)* found evidence of enhanced iodine uptake in lactating women from an endemic goiter region in Sicily. Milk iodine content and urinary iodine excretion of breast-fed infants of subjects in the endemic goiter region and controls from an iodine sufficient region were found to be similar.

5.10. Aluminum

There is scant information on the aluminum content of human milk. Contents in blood and milk appear to reflect intake or environmental exposure. Human milk is reported to contain about 27 ng Al/mL., bovine milk, about 100 ng/mL, and formulas, anywhere from 14 to 1950 ng/ml *(70)*. Aluminum intake at high levels is neurotoxic to humans but because it is not very effectively absorbed, it is not viewed as an important toxicant in adults. However, the high levels of aluminum in some formulas could pose a risk to infants; cases of aluminum toxicity have been observed in formula-fed infants with renal failure who are unable to excrete excess aluminum *(70)*.

5.11. Fluorine

Human milk contains little fluorine, approx 4–15 ng/mL. The concentration of fluorine in milk is affected by dietary intake, but the effect is weak. Dirks et al. *(71)* reported that the milk from women who lived in towns where the water supply was fluoridated did not have significantly higher values for fluorine than milk from women in towns without fluoridated water.

In the past, fluoride supplementation was recommended for breastfed infants by the American Academy of Pediatrics *(72)* since human milk feeding provided so little fluoride. That policy was recently revised because of the growing incidence of dental fluorosis in the United States and other parts of the developed world *(73)*. No fluorine supplementation is currently recommended for the first 6 mo of life.

6. CONCLUSION

A complex interplay of homeostatic mechanisms influence the mineral composition of human milk and quantity transferred to the breastfed infant. With only few exceptions, maternal dietary deficiencies and excesses have little impact on milk mineral composition. Two notable exceptions are for the trace elements iodine and selenium, and the impact is observed only in extreme situations where deficient or toxic intakes have persisted for long periods of time. Our knowledge base is far from complete and information is sorely needed to provide meaningful dietary recommendations for the trace minerals to ensure nutritional adequacy for both the lactating woman and her nursing infant. In addition to infant performance indices, future research should include measures on the lactating woman, particularly in the second 6 mo postpartum. Human milk feeding is currently recommended for the entire first year of life *(74)* and few studies have extended the period of observation beyond 3 mo.

REFERENCES

1. Morris D. The Naked Ape. Corgi, London,1968.
2. Neville MC, Keller R, Seacat J, LutesV, Neifert M, Casey C, Allen JA Archer P. Studies in human lactation: Milk volumes in lactating women during the onset of lactation. Am J Clin Nutr 1988;48:1375–1386.
3. Butte NF, Villalp,o S, Wong WW, Flores-Huerta S, de Hernadez–Beltran M, O'Brian Smith E, Garza C. Human milk intake and growth faltering of rural Mesoameridian infant. Am J Clin Nutr 1992;55:1109–1116.
4. Macy IG, Huncher HA, Donelson E, Nemo B. Human milk flow. Am J Dis Child 1930;6:492–515.
5. Saint L, Smith M, Hartmann PE. The yield nutrient content of milk in eight women breast-feeding twins and one woman breast-feeding triplets. Br J Nutr 1986;56:49–58.
6. Buck, DR Bales J. Maternal dietary magnesium effects on lactation success and on milk yield composition in the rat. J Nutr 1983;113:2421–2431.
7. Blanc B. Biochemical aspects of human milk: Comparison with bovine milk. World Revof Nutr Dietetics 1981;36:1–89.
8. Fransson GB, Lonnerdal B. Distribution of trace elements and minerals in human cow's milk. Ped Res 1983;17:912–915.
9. Boass A, Toverud SU. Enhanced nonsaturable calcium transport in the jejunum of rats during lactation, but not during pregnancy. J Bone Miner Res 1997;12:1577–1583.
10. Fairweather-Tait S, Prentice A, Huemann KG, Jarjou LMA, Stirling DM, Wharf SG, Turnlund JR. Effect of calcium supplements and stage of lactation on the calcium absorption efficiency of lactating women accustomed to low calcium intakes. Amer J ClinNutr 1995;62:1188–1192.
11. Kalkwarf HJ, Specker BL, Ho M. Effects of calcium supplementation on calcium homeostasis and bone turnover in lactating women. J Clin Endocrinol Metab 1999;84:464–470.
12. Bates C, Prentice A. Vitamins, minerals, and essential trace elements. In: PN Bennett ed. Drugs in Human Lactation. Elsevier, Amsterdam, 1988,pp. 433–494.

13. Allen JC, Neville MC. Ionized calcium in human milk determined with a calcium-selective electrode. Clin Chem 1983;29:858–861.

14. Butte NF, Garza C, Smith EO, Wills C, Nichols BL. Macro- and trace-mineral intakes of exclusively breast-fed infants. The Amer J Clin Nutr 1987;45:42–48.

15. Dewey KG, Lonnerdal B. Milk nutrient intake of breast–fed infants from 1 to 6 months: Relation to growth fatness. J Pediatr Gastroenterol Nutr 1983;3:713–720.

16. Greer FR, Tsang RC, Levin RS, Searcy JE, Wu R, Steichen JJ. Increasing serum calcium and magnesium concentrations in breast-fed infants: Longitudinal studies of minerals in human milk and in sera of nursing mothers and their infants. J Ped 1982;100:59–64.

17. Flynn A. Minerals and trace elements in milk. Adv Food Nutr Res 1992;36:209–252.

18. Gross SJ, David RJ, Bauman L, Tomarelli RM. Nutritional composition of milk produced by mothers delevering preterm. J Pediatr 1980;96:641–644.

19. Allen JC, Keller RP, Archer P, Neville MC. Studies in human lactation: milk composition and daily secretion rates of macronutrients in the first year of lactation. Am J Clin Nutr 1991; 54:69–80.

20. Lonnerdal B. Effects of milk and milk components on calcium magnesium, and trace element absorption during infancy. Physiol Rev 1997;77:643–669.

21. Gunshin H, Yoshikawa M, Doudou T, Kato N. Trace elements in human milk, cow's milk, and infant formula. Agric Biol Chem 1985;49:21–26.

22. Murray MJ, Murray AB, Murray NJ, Murray MB. The effect of iron status of Nigerian mothers on that of their infants at birth and 6 months, and on the concentration of Fe in breast milk. Br J Nutr 1978;39:627–630.

23. Anaokar SG, Garry PJ. Effects of maternal iron nutrition during lactation on milk iron and rat neonatal iron status. Amer J Clin Nutr 1981;35:1505–1512.

24. Burguera M, Burguera JL Garaboto AM, Alarcon OM. Iron and copper content of human milk at early state of lactation in Venezuela women. Trace Elem Med 1988;5:60–63.

25. Haschke F, Vanura H, Male C, Owen G, Pietschnig B, Schuster E, Krobath E, Huemer C. Iron nutrition and growth of breast- and formula-fed infants during the first 9 months of life. J Pediatr Gastroenterol Nutr 1993;16:151–156.

26. Bates CJ, Prentice A. Breast milk as a source of vitamins, essential minerals, and trace elements. Pharmacol Ther 1994;62:193–220.

27. Anderson RR. Comparison of trace elements in milk of four species. J Dairy Sci 1992;75:3050–3055.

28. Ziegler EE, Fomon SJ, Nelson SE, Rebouche CJ, Edwards BB, Rogers RR, Lehman LJ. Cow milk feeding in infancy: further observations on blood loss from the gastrointestinal tract. J Pediatr 1990;116:11–18.

29. Saarinen UM, Siimes MA, Dallman PR. Iron absorption in infants: high bioavailability of breast milk iron as indicated by the extrinsic tag method of iron absorption and by the concentration of serum ferritin. J Pediatr 1979;91:36–39.

30. McMillan JA, Oski F, Lourie G, Romarelli RM, L,aw SA. Iron absorption from human milk, simulated human milk, and proprietary formulas. Pediatrics 1977;60:896–900.

31. Fransson GB, Lonnerdal B. Iron in human milk. J Ped 1980;96:380–384.

32. Villalpando S, Hamosh M. Early and late effects of breast-feeding: does breast-feeding really matter? Biol Neonate 1998;74:177–191.

33. Xanthou M. Immune protection of human milk. Biol Neonate 1998;74:121–133.

34. Craig WL, Balbach L, Harris S, Vyhmeister N. Plasma zinc and copper levels of infants fed different milk formulas. J Amer Col Nutr 1984;3:183 186.

35. Arnaud J, Favier A. Copper, iron, manganese and zinc contents in human colostrum and transitory milk of French women. Scien Total Environ 1995;159:9–15.

36. Bates CJ, Tsuchiya H. Zinc in breast milk during prolonged lactation: Comparison between the UK and Gambia. Eur J Clin Nutr 1990;44: 61–69.

37. Michaelson KF, Samuelson G, Granham TW, Lonnerdal B. Zinc intake, zinc status, and growth in a longitudinal study of healthy Danish infants. Acta Paediatrica 1994;83:1115–1121.

38. Vuori E, Makinen SM, Kara R, Duitunen P. The effects of the dietary intakes of copper, iron, manganese, and zinc on the trace element content of human milk. Amer J Clin Nutr 1980;33: 227–231.

39. Karra MV, Kirksey A, Galal O, Bassily NS, Harrison GG, Jerome NW. Zinc, calcium, and magnesium concentrations in milk from American and Egyptian women throughout the first 6 months of lactation. Amer J Clin Nutr 1988;47:642–648.

40. Bedwal RS, Bahuguna A. Zinc, copper and selenium in reproduction. Experientia 1994;50:626–640.

41. Blakeborough P, Salter DN, Gurr MI. Zinc binding in cow's milk and human milk. Biochem J 1983;209:505—512.

42. Casey CE, Walravens PA, Hambidge KM. Availability of zinc: Loading tests with human milk, cow's milk, and infant formulas. Pediatrics 1981;68:394–396.
43. Lonnerdal B, Hoffman B, Hurley LS. Zinc and copper binding proteins in human milk. Amer J Clin Nutr 1982;36:1170–1176.
44. Hurley LS, Lonnerdal B. Zinc binding in human milk: Citrate vs. picolinate. Nutr Rev 1982;40: 65–71.
45. Harzer G, Kauer H. Binding of zinc to casein. Amer J Clin Nutr 1982;35:981–987.
46. Casey CE, Neville MC, Hambidge KM. Studies in human lactation: Secretion of zinc, copper, and manganese in human milk. Amer J Clin Nutr 1989;112:642–651.
47. Casey CE, Hambidge KM, Neville MC. Studies in human lactation: Zinc, copper. manganese, and chromium in human milk in the first month of lactation. Amer J Clin Nutr 1985;41:1193–1200.
48. Lonnerdal B, Keen CL, Hurley LS. Manganese binding proteins in human and cow's milk. Amer J Clin Nutr 1985;41:550–559.
49. Chan WU, Bates JM, Rennert OM. Comparative studies of manganese binding in human breast milk, bovine milk and infant formula. J Nutr 1982;112:642–651.
50. Davidsson L, Cederblad A, Lonnerdal B, Sandstrom B. Manganese absorption from human milk, cow's milk, and infant formulas in humans. Amer J Clin Nutr 1989;43:823–827.
51. Dorner K, Dziadzka S, Hohn A, Sievers E, Odigs HD, Schulz-Lell G, Schaub J. Longitudinal manganese and copper balances in young infants and preterm infants fed on breast milk and adapted cow's milk formulas. Br J Nutr 1989;61:559–572.
52. Casey CE, Hambidge KM. Chromium in human milk from American mothers. Br J Nutr 1984;52:73–77.
53. Cocho JA, Cervilla JR, Rey-Goldar ML, Fdea-Lorenzo JR, Fraga JM. Chromium content in human milk, cow's milk, and infant formulas. Biol Trace Elem Res 1992;32:105–107.
54. Anderson RA, Bryden NA, Patterson KY, Veillon C, on MB, Moser-Veillon PB. Breast milk chromium and its association with chromium intake, chromium excretion, and serum chromium. Amer J Clin Nutr 1993;57:519–523.
55. Deelstra H, Van Schoor O, Robberecht H, Clara R, Eylenbosch W. Daily chromium intake by infants in Belgium. Acta Paediatrica 1988;77:402–407.
56. Smith AM, Picciano MF, Milner JA. Selenium intakes and status of human milk and formula-fed infants. Amer J Clin Nutr 1982;35:521–526.
57. McGuire MK, Burgert SL, Milner JA, Glass L, Kummer R, Deering R, Boucek R, Picciano MF. Selenium status of lactating women is affected by the form of selenium consumed. Amer J Clin Nutr 1993;58:649–652.
58. Levander OA, Moser PB, Morris VC. Dietary selenium intake and selenium concentrations of plasma, erythrocytes, and breast milk in pregnant and postpartum lactating and nonlactating women. Am J Clin Nutr 1987;46:694–698.
59. Debski B, Finley DA, Picciano MF, Lonnerdal B, Milner J. Selenium content and glutathione peroxidase activity of milk from vegetarian and nonvegetarian women. J Nutr 1989;119:215–220.
60. Debski B, Picciano MF, Milner JA. Selenium content distribution of human, cow and goat milk. J Nutr 1986;117:1091–1097.
61. Milner JA, Sherman L, Picciano MF. Distribution of selenium in human milk. Amer J Clin Nutr 1987;45:617–624.
62. McGuire MK, Burgert SL, Milner JA, Glass L, Kummer R, Deering R, Boucek R, Picciano MF. Selenium status of infants is influenced by supplementation of formula or maternal diets. Amer J Clin Nutr 1993;58:643–648.
63. Smith AM, Chan GM, Moyer-Mileur LJ, Johnson CE, Gardner BR. Selenium status of preterm infants fed human milk, preterm formula, or selenium-supplemented preterm formula. J Pediatr 1991;119:429–433.
64. Tyrala EE, Borschel MW, Jacobs JR. Selenate fortification of infant formulas improves the selenium status of preterm infants. Am J Clin Nutr 1996;64:860–865.
65. Darlow BA, Inder TE, Graham PJ, Slius KB, Malpos TJ Taylor BJ Winterbourn CC. The relationship of selenium status to respiratory outcome in the very low birth weight infant. Pediatrics 1995;96:314–319.
66. Bougle D, Bureau F, Foucault P, Dhuamel JF, Muller G, Drosdowsky M. Molybdenum content of term and preterm human milk during the first 2 months of lactation. Amer J Clin Nutr 1988;48:652–654.
67. Casey CE, Neville MC. Studies in human lactation 3: Molybdenum and nickel in human milk during the first month of lactation. Amer J Clin Nutr 1987;45:921–926.
68. Gunshin H, Yoshikawa M, Doudou T, Kato N. Trace elements in human milk, cow's milk, and infant formula. Agric Biol Chem 1985;49:21–26.

69. Vermiglio F, Lo Presti VP, Finocchiaro MD, Battiato S, Grasso L, Ardita FV, Mancuso A, Trimarchi F. Enhanced iodine concentrating capacity by the mammary gland, in iodine deficient lactating women of an endemic goiter region in Sicily. J Endocrinol Invest 1992;15:137–142.
70. De Curtis M, Napoitan E, Ciccimarra F, Mellone MC, Del Rio A. Aluminum content in human milk and in infant formulas (letter). EurJ Clin Nutr 1989;43:887.
71. Dirks OB, Jongeling-Eijndhoven JMPA, Flissebaalje TD, Gedalia I. Total and free ionic fluoride in human and cow's milk as determined by gas-liquid chromatography and the fluoride electrode. Caries Research 1974;8:181–186.
72. American Academy of Pediatrics/Committee on Nutrition. Fluoride supplementation for children: Interim policy recommendation. Pediatrics 1995;95:777.
73. Warren JJ, Kanellis MJ, Levy SM. Fluorosis of the primary dentition: what does it mean for permanent teeth? J Am Dent Assoc 1999;130:347–356.
74. American Academy of Pediatrics/Work Group on Breastfeeding. Breastfeeding and the use of human milk. Pediatrics 1997;100:1035–1039.

10 Trace Element and Mineral Nutrition in Adolescents

Velimir Matkovic, MD, Nancy E. Badenhop, and Jasminka Z. Ilich, PhD

1. INTRODUCTION

Adolescence is a critical and complex phase in human development characterized by major biological, psychological, and social changes. Puberty marks the beginning of accelerated physical growth, alterations in body composition, and sexual maturation. The growth spurt in female adolescents contributes about 16% to adult height, 54% to adult weight, 73% to adult body fat content, 40% to adult lean body mass, and about 37% to the whole body calcium (Fig. 1). Similar changes are present in males. All individuals during this period of life should be in a strong positive nitrogen balance and balance of minerals required for body building. Those changes influence teenagers' nutritional needs and status (Fig. 2). In addition, psychological changes involving the adolescent's search for independence and identity, desire for acceptance by peers, and preoccupation with physical appearance may affect eating habits, food choices, nutrient intake, and particularly status of certain minerals of which calcium (Ca), phosphorus (P), magnesium (Mg), iron (Fe), zinc (Zn), and selenium (Se) are the most important. During the last 20 years, the focus of nutrition research and recommendations for children has shifted from the prevention of nutritional deficiencies to the early establishment of recommended diets to prevent chronic diseases. These priorities may eventually lead to dietary guidelines for the prevention and treatment of those conditions by targeting predisposed individuals early in life *(3)*.

2. CALCIUM

As 99% of total body calcium (Ca) is found in bone, the need for calcium is largely determined by skeletal requirements (Fig. 3) (*see* Chapter 14). During adolescence the increase in total body calcium far outpaces the change in stature; 132% vs 19%, respectively (Fig. 4). Optimal calcium intake during growth refers to the level of consumption that is necessary for an individual to maximize peak adult bone mass. This was first indicated by an epidemiological study conducted in high and low calcium regions in Croatia *(4)*. In this study metacarpal cortical bone mass was measured in two

From: *Clinical Nutrition of the Essential Trace Elements and Minerals: The Guide for Health Professionals*
Edited by: J. D. Bogden and L. M. Klevay © Humana Press Inc., Totowa, NJ

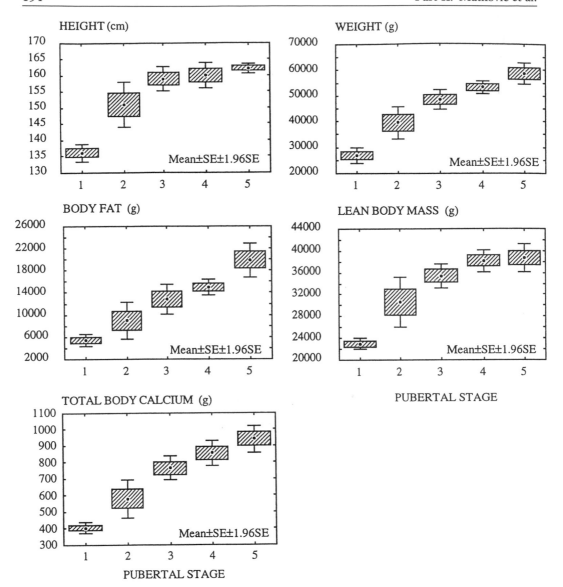

Fig. 1. Stature, body weight and composition in young females according to pubertal development (breast changes). Based on a cross-sectional study conducted in 80 healthy Caucasian females, age range 8–17 yr. Adapted from Matkovic et al. *(1)*.

rural populations who were accustomed to different lifetime calcium intakes primarily due to the variation in dairy product consumption. Both men and women from the high calcium region had higher bone mass than corresponding populations from the low calcium district, and this was true throughout the age range from 30 to 75+ yr. Both populations seemed to lose bone mass with age at the same rate. Thus, the men in the high calcium district had as much bone mass at 70 as did men from the low calcium region at the age of 30 yr. Although this was a cross-sectional study it suggested the importance of adequate nutrition during skeletal development. A similar discovery was made among various Chinese populations accustomed to different calcium intakes over a lifetime *(5)*.

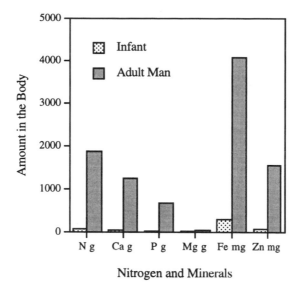

Fig. 2. Total body nitrogen and minerals in infants and young adults. The difference between these two phases of life represents the amount of mineral accumulated during childhood and adolescence. Adapted from Widdowson *(2)*.

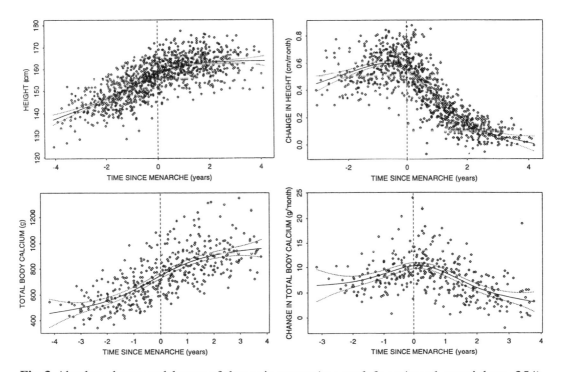

Fig. 3. Absolute change and the rate of change in stature (cm, top left; cm/month, top right; n=354) and total body calcium (g, bottom left; g/month, bottom right; n=90) with time since menarche (years) in a cohort of young females followed annually for 4 years. Total body calcium is considered a fraction (38%) of total body bone mineral content as measured by dual energy X-ray absorptiometry (DXA). Scatterplots shown with cubic splines and 95% confidence intervals. All participants were healthy Caucasian females from central Ohio.

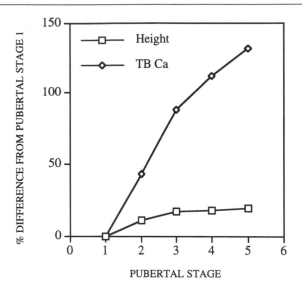

Fig. 4. Relative difference in the whole body calcium and stature between pubertal stage 1 and subsequent stages. Based on a cross-sectional study conducted in 80 healthy adolescent Caucasian females, ages 8–17 yr. Adapted from Matkovic et al. *(1)*.

In addition, several retrospective studies also showed that adult women who consumed more milk and dairy products during adolescence had higher bone mineral density at the forearm than those who did not *(6–9)*. Overall, it is likely that variations in calcium nutrition early in life may account for as much as a 5–10% difference in peak adult bone mass. Such a difference in peak adult bone mass, although small, may contribute to as much as a 50% reduction in hip fracture rate later in life *(4)*.

The results of balance studies suggest a threshold effect for calcium intake; body retention of calcium increases with increasing calcium intake up to a threshold, beyond which further calcium intake causes no additional increment in body retention of calcium (Table 1, Fig. 5) *(10)*. Below a certain threshold level of dietary calcium intake young individuals will not be able to reach genetically predetermined peak bone mass, while adults will be losing bone tissue at a faster rate than is necessary. Adequate calcium intake above a certain threshold level is therefore absolutely required for bone health during skeletal growth and consolidation. The key issue then in clinical nutrition during growth is not the calcium intake at zero balance, as it applies to adults for the maintenance of skeletal structure, but rather the level of positive calcium balance. According to calcium balance studies the threshold intake for adolescents is about 1500 mg/d *(10)*. The corresponding average calcium retention which saturates the skeletons of teenagers is about 400 mg/d. Recommendations for calcium nutrition should take into account that the calcium threshold is highly variable and depends on body size as well as stage of human development. When metacarpal cortical bone mass was separately examined in a segment of the population from the high and low calcium districts in Croatia, there was a larger discrepancy in the cortical bone mass per corresponding bone volume for persons of a larger body size than for the smaller individuals *(11)*. This indicates that calcium deficiency during growth could disproportionally affect individuals who are genetically predestined to reach a higher level in their peak bone mass, as they require more calcium.

Table 1
Calcium Intake Thresholds and Balances for Growing Individuals

Age group (years)	Threshold intake mg/day	Threshold balance mg/day
0–1	1090	+503
2–8	1390	+246
9–17	1480	+396
18–30	957	+114

The intake threshold for calcium is considered to be the level below which calcium retention in the body is a function of intake, and above which calcium retention is constant, irrespective of further increases in intake. This threshold intake should provide sufficient calcium to ensure maximal skeletal retention of calcium which will lead to peak bone mass formation. From Matkovic and Heaney (10).

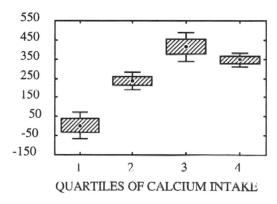

QUARTILES OF CALCIUM INTAKE

Fig. 5. Boxplots of calcium balances according to quartiles of calcium intake for adolescents. Mean ± SE ± 1.96SE. Calcium intake in quartile 4 >1500 mg/d. Adapted from Matkovic and Heaney (10).

The importance of a positive calcium balance during adolescent years is further emphasized by the need to meet not only the rapidly expanding skeletal compartment, but also losses of calcium through the skin (not measured in usual balance studies) which may amount to as much as 60 mg/d in adults (12). Young athletes could lose considerable calcium through sweat; this may be up to 60–80 mg/h of intensive training. Low calcium intake may lead to a negative calcium balance and bone loss, as reported for basketball players (13).

Adolescents, in general, absorb more calcium from their diet than either children or young adults. The concentration of serum calcitriol is the highest during peak growth; pubertal stages 3 and 4 (Fig. 6) (14–16). Urinary calcium increases during the period of adolescence and reaches its maximum by the age of 15–16 yr, or by the cessation of puberty (17). The mean urinary calcium output for young boys and girls aged 9 to 17 yr is about 130 mg/d (17,18). Mean urinary calcium excretion at an intake of about 500 mg/d is about 120 mg/d. Further increases in intake up to 1800 mg/d increase urinary calcium excretion only by 10–20 mg/d (19). This level of urinary calcium excretion of about 130 mg/d can, therefore, be considered as the mean obligatory urinary calcium loss for the age group 9–17 yr. The above indicate that urinary calcium excretion during adolescence is barely

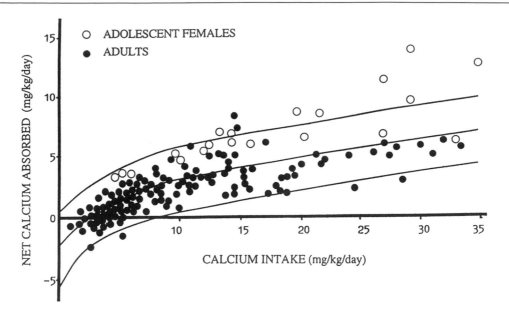

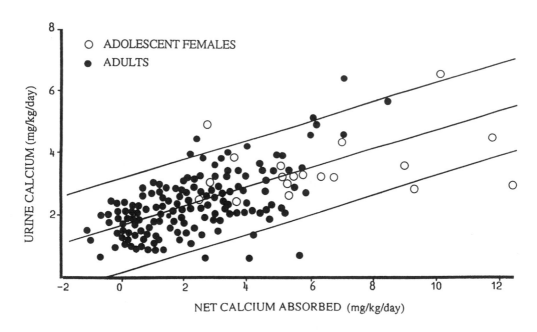

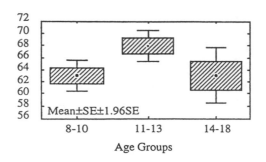

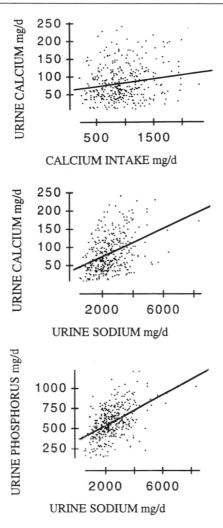

Fig. 7. The relationship between urinary calcium and calcium intake (top, R-squared=2.9%), urinary calcium and urinary sodium (middle, R-squared=17.4 %), and urinary phosphorus and urinary sodium (bottom, R-squared=25.3 %) in prepubertal females (n=370; ages 8–13 yr). Adapted in part from Matkovic et al. (22).

related to calcium intake (Fig. 7) (17–20). Body weight and age seem to be the principal determinants of urinary calcium excretion during this phase of life. More powerful relationships between urinary and dietary calcium definitely exist in adults (21). The explanation for the above is that adolescents retain the absorbed calcium in the skeleton rather than excreting it in the urine. Calcium in the urine is expected to rise, as a result of the increase in the filtered load of calcium, only after the skeletal compartment is being saturated with

---

Fig. 6. *(opposite page)* Net calcium absorption and calcium intake in adults and adolescents (bottom), and urinary calcium and net calcium absorption in adults and adolescents (middle). Adapted from Nordin and Marshall *(21)* and Matkovic et al. *(18)*. Note higher calcium absorption per mg/kg calcium intake in adolescents. Boxplots of serum calcitriol [1,25(OH)$_2$D$_3$] according to pubertal development. Adapted from Ilich et al. *(16)* (top).

calcium at intakes above the threshold level *(19)*. Renal excretion of calcium is believed to be regulated by parathyroid hormone and estrogens and is also influenced by dietary protein and sodium intake. High consumption of salt increases the obligatory calcium loss in the urine *(22)* (Fig. 7). A strong positive nitrogen balance is required for rapid pubertal development and growth and, therefore, the amounts of proteins commonly consumed by American teenagers have no influence on urinary calcium excretion *(22)*.

Several clinical trials showed that calcium intake (from milk or supplements) above the threshold standard was associated with an increase in bone mass in either children or adolescents *(18,23–28)*. Therefore, optimal calcium intake in childhood and adolescence is critical for achieving adult peak bone mass and also may contribute to the reduction in the incidence of bone fragility fractures during growth *(29,30)*. Nationwide surveys reveal that adolescents, especially females, consume inadequate amounts of calcium. In addition, psychological changes involving the adolescent's search for independence and identity, desire for acceptance by peers, and preoccupation with physical appearance may affect eating habits, food choices, nutrient intake, and ultimately nutritional status. As children reach their teen years they drink less milk and their calcium intake declines far below the current standard (1300 mg/d) and even more so in comparison to the calcium intake threshold of 1500 mg/d. Optimizing the calcium intake of young Americans is, therefore, of critical importance. Recent improvements in calcium intake have been reported for most age groups, however, young females showed a decrease in calcium intake as compared to a decade earlier *(31)*. The impact of suboptimal calcium intake on the health of Americans and the health care cost to the American public is of vital concern. It is thus appropriate that increasing calcium intake is a national health promotion and disease prevention objective in the Healthy People 2000 agenda *(32)*. Public health strategies to promote optimal calcium intake should have a broad outreach and should involve educators, health professionals, and the private and public sectors *(33)*.

To maintain adequate calcium intake, the NIH Consensus Conference Panel encourages adolescents to consume more calcium rich foods such as milk and other dairy products *(33)*. This approach of recommending the consumption of calcium-rich foods is consistent with current dietary guidelines (U.S. Department of Agriculture Food Guide Pyramid), which includes 2–3 servings per day of dairy products. This task to meet calcium requirements on a continuing daily basis presents a great challenge for some individuals *(33)*. Additional strategies include the consumption of calcium-fortified foods and calcium supplements. For many Americans, dairy products are the major contributors of dietary calcium because of their high calcium content and frequency of consumption. Other good food sources of calcium include some green vegetables (broccoli, kale, turnip greens), tofu processed with calcium salts, legumes, canned fish with bones, seeds, nuts, and certain fortified food products. Breads and cereals, although low in calcium, could contribute to calcium intake due to the frequency and amount of their consumption *(33)*.

As most of the dairy products contain fat there is a concern that this drive for extra calcium intake may perpetuate problems related to obesity *(3)*. A certain degree of body fatness (30% body fat and 12.2 ng/mL of serum leptin) is necessary to trigger puberty and the reproductive function in human females (Fig. 8). Obesity is of particular concern during adolescence; over the past 20 years, the prevalence of this condition has increased 39% among teenagers 12–17-yr-old *(34)*. It is important to realize that obesity during adolescence is a strong predictor of adult obesity. There is an assumption that nutrient density of calcium is different between teenagers who consume dairy products and those

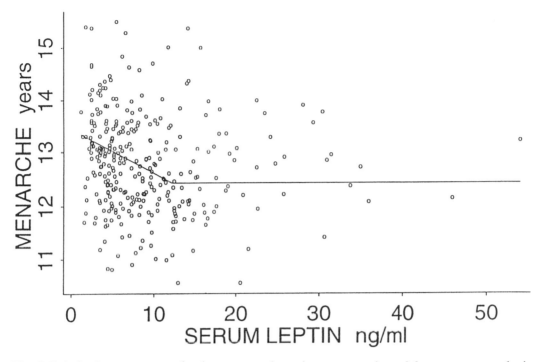

Fig. 8. Relation between serum leptin concentration prior to menarche and the age at menarche in 311 young females. The scatterplot shown is a linear-plateau least squares fit model. The 95% CI for the slope in the lower region, showing the inverse relation between menarche and leptin, is −0.12 to −0.05 (y). The 95% CI for the change point (serum leptin; ×*0) is 7.6–16.7 ng/mL. The scatterplot is shown with the 95% confidence curves and the regression line. Adapted from Matkovic et al. *(119).*

who take calcium supplements; higher density is expected among pill users, but this is unknown. Contrary to this, it can be assumed that children who take calcium supplements replace dairy products by inferior foods with regard to other nutrients, particularly fat and cholesterol content *(3).* A recent study which compared body composition and serum leptin levels in teenage females who were meeting their dietary calcium needs through dairy products as compared to calcium supplements, shows that consumption of dairy products does not lead to obesity as previously anticipated *(35,36)* . This applies to the goal of meeting new intake standards for calcium up to 1500 mg/d.

The World Health Organization recommendations for dietary calcium intakes for 11–15-yr-old adolescents are 600 to 700 mg/d and for 16–19-yr-old adolescents, 500 to 600 mg/d. Although those figures might satisfy some population groups characterized by small body frames, this is not enough for the vast majority of Western populations. It is apparent from these differences in recommended intakes that the amount of dietary calcium needed to sustain growth, as well as to provide maintenance, requires much more study particularly with regard to different populations. The standards for one ethnic group might not satisfy the requirements of another. Each country should develop its own standards specific for the people living in the region. Factors like ethnicity, stature and body frame, dietary habits, determinants of calcium economy in the body (sodium intake, sunlight exposure), and activity level all play a role. Ideally standards should be based on

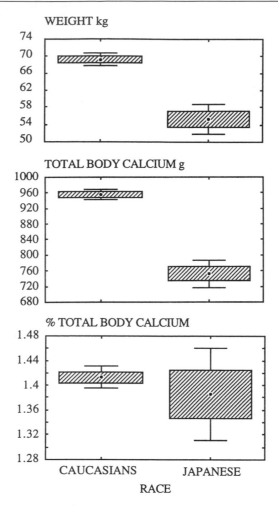

Fig. 9. Boxplots of body weight (top), total body calcium (middle), and percent total body calcium (bottom) in the group of young adult (18–50 yr) Caucasian (n=437) and Japanese (n=34) premenopausal women. Results presented as mean ± SE ± 1.96SE. Significant differences are present for body weight and total body calcium, but not for % total body calcium. Data for Japanese women kindly provided by Drs. Fujita and Tokita. The average total body calcium in the group of Japanese women is 752 ± 107 g while in Caucasians it is 956 ± 145 g. Subtracting 30 g of skeletal calcium at birth and assuming that most of the bone mass was accumulated by the age of 18 yr, the average Japanese and Caucasian women from the group were retaining 109 and 141 mg of calcium per day, respectively.

calcium intake thresholds obtained from balance studies and/or whole body bone mass measurements by DXA (38% of bone mineral content is calcium) at various calcium intakes. In the absence of metabolic wards or densitometry machines, simple but crude estimates could be based on body weight data. The whole body bone mineral content is about 3–4% of body weight irrespective of age, sex, or ethnicity. The best example is the comparison of the absolute and relative body calcium (derived from DXA) between two ethnic groups known for the significant differences in body frames: Caucasians vs Japanese (Fig. 9). Japanese have lower amounts of total body calcium but a comparable ratio of calcium to body weight.

3. PHOSPHORUS

Phosphorus is essential for normal bone and tooth formation and, therefore, plays a very important role during skeletal development. Out of about 700 g of phosphorus contained in the human body, approximately 85% is in the bone while the remaining part is in the soft tissues, where it plays an important role in energy storage and release systems. Phosphorus is a ubiquitous element present in almost all foods. Major dietary contributors of phosphorus are protein-rich foods and cereal grains; about half of the food phosphorus comes from milk and dairy products, as well as meat, poultry, and fish. Although phosphorus deficiency has been reported in adults taking large amounts of antacids, a widespread phosphorus deficiency syndrome in humans is practically unknown. This is to a large extent explained by the phosphorus homeostasis in the body. Most of the consumed phosphorus is excreted in the feces and in the urine. Phosphorus balance studies in adults showed that phosphorus output is equal to input at various intake levels from 700–1800 mg/d indicating excellent adaptation *(37)*. Due to the lack of balance studies at very low phosphorus intakes, Nordin concludes that it is almost impossible to calculate phosphorus requirements for adults *(37)*. There is presumably an intake below which adult humans go into negative balance; however, this figure is unknown. As phosphorus is an essential component of calcium hydroxyapatite crystal, growing individuals should be in a positive phosphorus balance. Phosphorus metabolism of adolescent females is presented in Fig. 10. As in adults phosphorus output (urinary and fecal excretion) is highly related to phosphorus input (dietary phosphorus), however, most of the young females were in a positive phosphorus balance of about 97±17 mg/d irrespective of their phosphorus intake. The regression line of phosphorus output on phosphorus intake for the particular intake range (800–2000 mg/d) has a slope of 0.96 and is almost parallel to the line of equality, with an intercept of –58. The difference between the lines is due to phosphorus retention in the body required primarily for skeletal development *(38)*. The data in Fig. 10 are for postpubertal girls (2 yr since menarche) who had a slower rate of growth and mineral accretion. A positive phosphorus balance of about 150–200 mg/d is expected during the pubertal growth spurt; age ~12. As sodium contributes to calcium excretion in the urine, it can also influence phosphorus excretion and affect phosphorus balance (Fig. 7).

Although phosphorus deficiency was never a real problem in human nutrition, a surplus of phosphorus in the diet was more of a concern and received considerable attention in the nutrition literature. Dr. Lenart Krook, a veterinarian from Sweden, first described a metabolic bone disease and secondary hyperparathyroidism in domestic animals who were consuming high amounts of phosphates in their diets with a Ca to P ratio of 1 : 5 *(39–41)*, although the calcium content of the diets was low. The above findings were attributed to calcium phosphate precipitation in the gut and decreased calcium absorption. Dr. Krook subsequently moved to Cornell University, New York, and jointly with Leo Lutwak proposed a hypothesis linking a periodontal bone disease (bone resorption around the tooth with the loss of lamina dura dentes) and osteoporosis in humans to the abnormal Ca/P ratio *(42)*. The assumption was that periodontal bone loss with concomitant development of periodontal disease preceeds the development of osteoporosis later on in life. Fuller Albright described periodontal bone loss in patients with primary hyperparathyroidism *(43)* and dental X-rays were part of the routine screening for the disease in the 1950s and 1960s, before the introduction of the radioimmunoassay for parathyroid hor-

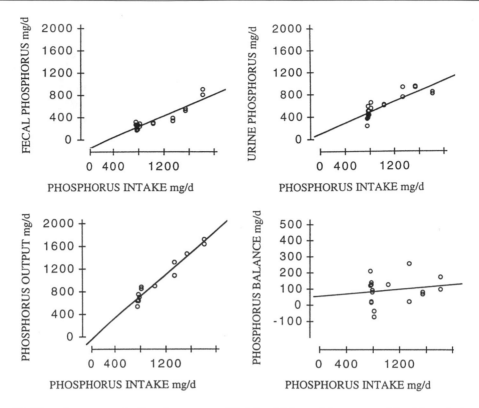

Fig. 10. Phosphorus metabolism in a group (N=20) of 14-yr-old teenage girls. The relationship between fecal phosphorus (Pf) and phosphorus intake (Pi) is best represented by the equation: Pf=0.48 Pi −153.8; R-squared 84.5%, p<0.0001. The relationship between urinary phosphorus (Pu) and phosphorus intake is represented by the equation: Pu=0.48Pi + 96; R-squared 73.8%, p<0.0001). Phosphorus output (Po) and phosphorus intake: Po=0.96Pi − 57.7; R-squared 95.7%, p<0.0001. There was no relationship between phosphorus balance and intake; the slope of the regression line was 0.037 and intercept 58. Phosphorus balances were conducted during the study of calcium metabolism, the data for which were previously presented *(18).*

mone. The premise of the Krook-Lutwak hypothesis was that the vast majority of young Americans consume too much phosphorus through the consumption of carbonated beverages containing phosphoric acid. Although this theory had several supporters among bone researchers *(44,45),* it was never accepted by the specialists in the field: periodontists and clinicians dealing with metabolic bone disease. The average Ca/P ratio in the diets of typical American teenagers is in range of 0.3–1.3 (Fig. 11). Within this range calcium intake is the main determinant of fecal calcium and not phosphorus intake (Fig. 12). A person needs to consume 25–80 cans (44 mg of phosphorus per can) of cola daily depending on the calcium intake, to drastically disturb the Ca/P ratio. In addition, subsequent balance studies with varying amounts of phosphorus in the diet did not find abnormalities in calcium metabolism in the form of decreased absorption and increased fecal excretion of calcium *(46–48).* In a more recent study phosphate supplementation (up to 2000 mg/ d) in a group of young men did not show any effect on calcium homeostasis or bone turnover markers *(49).* As milk and dairy products are the main source of calcium in the diet, they are also a good source of phosphorus with a Ca/P ratio of 1.3. The consumption

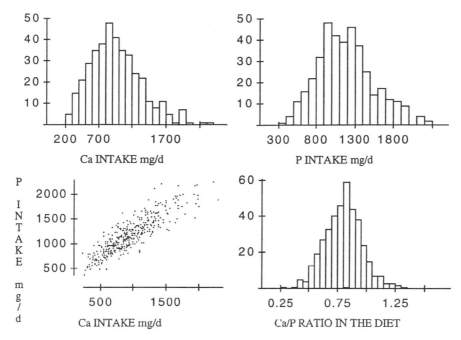

Fig. 11. Frequency histograms of calcium (Ca) intake (top left; mean intake 956±380 mg/d, range 220–2300 mg/d), phosphorus (P) intake (top right; mean intake 1180±360 mg/d, range 362–2251 mg/d), and calcium/phosphorus ratio in the diet (bottom right) in 392 prepubertal girls (ages 8–13 yr) from central Ohio; regression of phosphorus intake on dietary calcium intake for the same group of girls (R-squared 77%, p<0.0001) (bottom left). There is a normal distribution of Ca and P intakes in the population, as well as the Ca:P ratio (mean ratio 0.8±0.2, range 0.3 to 1.3). Results based on the 3-d food records analyzed by Nutritionist III software. Linear regression analysis indicates that diets rich in calcium also contain phosphate.

of milk should, therefore, be encouraged among adolescents because it contains both minerals important for skeletal mineralization in a favorable ratio.

4. MAGNESIUM

Most of the magnesium contained in the human body is in the skeleton (59%), 40% in the lean body mass, and 1% in the extracellular fluid. With regard to bone, magnesium concentrations are higher along the periosteal and the endosteal surfaces and equal between the two sexes (50). Magnesium concentrations in bone do not change with age in general, however, slightly higher concentrations were found among teenagers and lower concentrations among the very elderly (50). In teenagers as well as in adults, most of the magnesium consumed will be absorbed and excreted in the urine (Fig. 13). The data from a metabolic balance study conducted in teenage females shows that the relationship between magnesium intake and magnesium output is best explained by a linear equation with a slope of 1.04 (R-squared 68.8%). The regression line is almost parallel to the line of equality, however the intercept is –18.1 and not 0.0 as found in adults (37) (Fig. 13). This suggests that magnesium output is below magnesium intake due to the retention of magnesium in the body of growing individuals. When dietary magnesium is reduced, there is a concomitant decrease in urinary magnesium. Thus the adaptation to low

Ca FECES mg/d

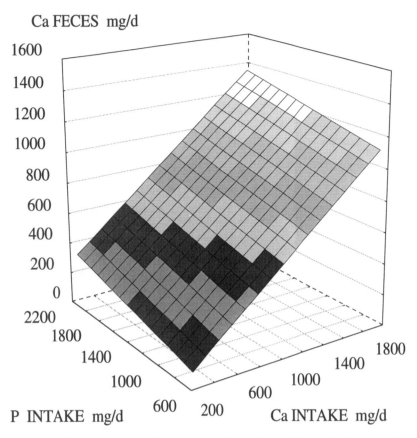

Fig 12. Three-dimensional representation (surface plot) of the relationship between fecal calcium (z), phosphorus intake (y), and calcium intake (x) in a group of adolescent females. Calcium intake was the main determinant of fecal calcium; phosphorus intake in range of 600 to 2200 mg/d had little influence on fecal calcium excretion.

magnesium intake by the fall in excretion is extremely efficient, not only in adults but also in growing individuals as well. Any diet providing enough nutrients to support life would also contain enough magnesium *(37)*. Dietary deficiency of magnesium is, therefore, unusual, but it can occur among teenagers after prolonged vomiting, diarrhea, or alcohol abuse. It has been suggested that magnesium intake may be a factor in lowering blood pressure in adults *(51)*. It is not known whether adequate magnesium intake during adolescence can protect against the future development of hypertension.

Total body magnesium increases from 1 g at birth to 23–27g in adults, with most of the gain occurring during adolescence. This equals an average magnesium retention rate of 3.0–4.0 mg/d, assuming that the majority of the adult total body magnesium pool is accumulated during the first two decades of life *(2)*. Greater retention rates would be expected during periods of accelerated growth, such as puberty, and lower rates would he expected during periods of slower growth. In either case, it seems likely that an adequate retention rate for magnesium during growth and development is quite low. The current dietary intake standard for magnesium for females aged 11–14-yr is 6.0 mg/kg body weight/d, which equals 280 mg at the mean body weight for this age group (52). Greger et al. reported slightly negative mean magnesium balances (~4 mg/d) in 14

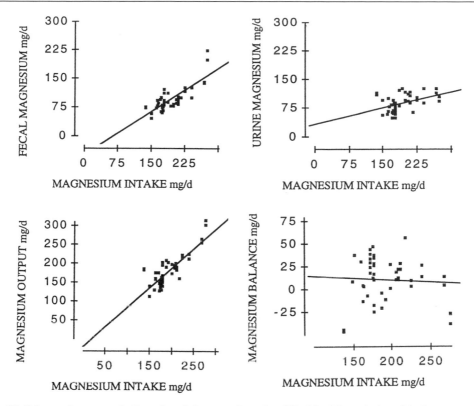

Fig. 13. Magnesium metabolism in adolescent females (N=46). The relationship between fecal magnesium (Mgf) and magnesium intake (Mgi) is best represented by the equation: Mgf=0.76 Mgi −50.8; R-squared 64.5%, p<0.0001. The relationship between urinary magnesium (Mgu) and magnesium intake is represented by the equation: Mgu=0.28Mgi + 32.6; R-squared 18.9%, p<0.0025). Magnesium output (Mgo) and magnesium intake: Mgo=1.037Mgi −18.1; R-squared 68.8%, p<0.0001. There was no significant relationship between magnesium balance and intake; the slope of the regression line was −0.038 and intercept 18.1; R-squared 0.3%, p=0.72. Magnesium balances are for twenty 14-yr-old teenage females [study conducted along with calcium balances previously presented *(18)*] that were combined with data accumulated by Andon et al. *(54)* for twenty-six young females (age 11.3 ± 0.5 yr).

adolescent girls consuming 3.3–5.6 mg/kg body weight/d *(53)*. In the study of Andon et al. a group of adolescent females ingested 176 mg/d (4.45 mg/ kg body weight/d) *(54)* which was well below the recommended dietary allowance and somewhat below the national average for magnesium consumption by 11-yr-old females of 217 mg. At this magnesium intake balance was positive and averaged 21 mg/d for all subjects. Four of 26 girls were in negative magnesium balance and three of these subjects consumed about 4.2 mg/kg body weight/day. Magnesium balance was strongly positive in all subjects with a magnesium intake > 5.0 mg/kg body weight/d. Although the importance of a positive magnesium balance during growth is not in question, a specific objective for magnesium retention has not been determined. This limitation notwithstanding, prediction intervals from the linear regression of magnesium balance on intake indicate that 95% of the girls would have a magnesium balance ~ 8.5 mg/d at the current recommended dietary allowance of 6.0 mg/kg body weight/d. Thus, the current recommended dietary allowance appears adequate for this age group relative to the anticipated expansion of the total body magnesium pool during growth. In addition, the values for these variables were very similar to those reported for adults, suggesting that magnesium utilization is similar in adolescent females and adults. Although magnesium intake in the study of Andon et al. (4.45 mg/kg body weight/d) was lower than the current recommended dietary allowance of 6.0 mg/kg body weight/d, it was sufficient to result in positive magnesium balance for the majority (85%) of subjects (54). Based on the 95% prediction interval from the regression of magnesium balance on intake, a magnesium intake of 6.0 mg/kg body weight/d would be sufficient to support magnesium retention consistent with the expansion of the total body magnesium pool during growth.

5. IRON

The body of a young adult contains only 3 to 5 g of iron. Most of this is found in the hemoglobin of red blood cells. Hemoglobin transports oxygen and carbon dioxide, respectively, to and from the cells of the body. Iron is also an essential element in the chain of enzyme-controlled reactions that releases energy. Iron may play an important role in bone formation acting as a cofactor with enzymes involved in collagen synthesis. In a recent study by Medeiros et al. it was found that the bone breaking strength was lower in iron deficient rats, suggesting that iron deficiency may play a role in bone fragility during growth (55), however, this remains to be confirmed in humans. Iron deficiency is still considered the most prevalent nutrient deficiency in the world, affecting about 10–20% of the population (56–58) (see Chapter 6), with teenage females being at the highest risk of developing anemia (59). Using serum ferritin as a determinant of iron deficiency and a cutoff value of 16 ng/mL, Hallberg et al. determined that the prevalence of iron deficiency among adolescent females in Sweden could be even higher, up to ~40% (59). Applying the same cutoff values for serum ferritin to young females from other countries, they estimated a similar prevalence of iron deficiency in adolescent females in Australia, Canada, and the United States of America (60). Although it is generally accepted that adolescent girls are particularly prone to develop iron deficiency anemia due to increased demands for growth, loss of iron with menstruation, and poor dietary habits, until recently there were no longitudinal studies conducted in this population showing that iron status is actually compromised upon the onset of menarche relative to the rate of growth and iron intake. The loss of iron with menstruation has been measured and reported numerous times, however studies showing the negative effect of the onset of menarche on iron status in adolescent females are rare (61,62). Bailey and coworkers showed in a cross-sectional study conducted among 67 young females aged 11–18 yr that postmenarcheal girls had lower ferritin levels than premenarcheal girls (63).

The estimated average amount of iron required for growth in teenage females is about 1.6 mg/d (64). This is primarily required for the expansion of the cellular compartments rich in iron like muscle tissue (myoglobin) and red blood cells (hemoglobin), both being represented in the lean body mass measurements by DXA (65). Most of the iron in a young adult woman of 65 kg is in the erythron (1700 mg), iron stores (300 mg), muscle tissue (120 mg), and transferrin (4 mg) (66). In a 4-yr longitudinal study conducted in teenage females we recently showed that pubertal growth spurt and menstrual status have adverse effects on iron stores of girls with low dietary iron intake (< 9 mg/d) (67). Approximately 45% of the total amount of iron of ~2.13 g will be incorporated into the lean body mass during the pubertal growth spurt (Fig. 14) (67). Depending on the rate of pubertal development, this requires a positive net tissue balance of 1–3 mg/d. The

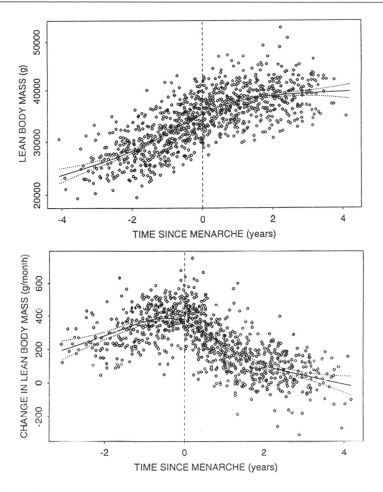

Fig. 14. Absolute (g) change (top) and the rate of change (g/month) (bottom) in lean body mass with time since menarche (years). Scatterplots shown with cubic spline and 95% confidence interval. Adapted from the study of Ilich et al. **(67)**.

recommended dietary allowance for iron of 15 mg/d, in spite of the relatively low absorption efficacy of 10–15%, should meet the demand of almost all female adolescents. One of the stated reasons in the literature for the compromised iron status in adolescent females, besides growth, is the loss of iron with menstruation. According to Hallberg et al. the average menstrual blood loss in 15-y-old girls is about 28 mL per period corresponding to a daily loss of about 0.4 mg iron *(62)*. Although the estimated menstrual losses in older women are usually higher, their requirements for iron are lower and thus, they might be able to better compensate for losses. Whether these losses actually cause a decrease in ferritin concentration with corresponding depletion of iron stores in young females is not clear and so far has not been appropriately evaluated. The negative association between the duration of the menstrual period and mean corpuscular volume, and hemoglobin, as found in the study of Ilich et al. *(67)*, confirms the above notations. When serum ferritin was studied in the lower and upper quartiles of cumulative iron intake in a group of teenage females (Fig. 15) *(67)*, there was an inverse relationship

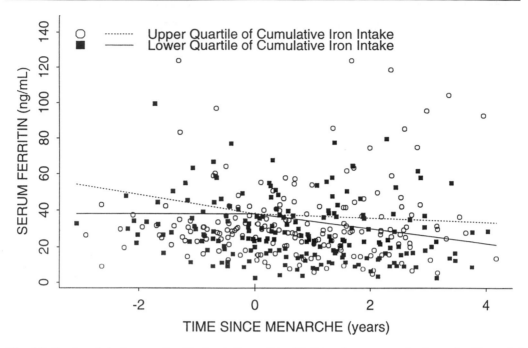

Fig. 15. Scatterplot of serum ferritin (ng/mL=μg/L) with time since menarche (years) with model fit representing upper (broken line) and lower (solid line) quartiles of cumulative iron intake (upper=open circles, lower=solid squares). The simultaneous effects of iron intake and the menstrual status on serum ferritin level, after being controlled for the gain in LBM, was evaluated among subjects in the upper and lower quartiles of cumulative iron intake. The indicator variable, upper, was created referring to the upper quartile of cumulative iron intake (I). This model was: serum ferritin μg/L = β_0 + β_1 * (Δ LBM g/year) + β_2 * I(t ≥ 0) * t + β_3 upper * t + β_4 * upper * I (t ≥ 0) * t + e. The fitted lines for this model for the upper quartile of cumulative iron intake before and after menarche were: y = 38.48 – 5.09 * t for t < 0 and y = 38.48 –1.36 * t for t ≥ 0, and the fitted lines for the lower quartile of cumulative iron intake before and after menarche were: y = 38.48 for t < 0 and y = 38.48 – 4.09 * t for t ≥ 0. The two fitted models representing ferritin levels of subjects with cumulative iron intake in the upper and the lower quartiles were significantly different from each other (p<0.018). The regression line representing ferritin level in menstruating (t > 0) females with cumulative iron intake above the 75th percentile has a less negative slope compared to the regression line fit to serum ferritin level of subjects with iron intake below the 25th percentile (p<0.08). Adapted from Ilich et al. *(67).*

between serum ferritin and the time since menarche but only in girls with low iron intake. The girls who were taking iron supplements or had higher habitual dietary iron intake were able to maintain their iron stores in spite of the loss of iron with menstruation. The difference in iron intake between the upper and the lower quartile groups of about 10 mg/ d, assuming 10–15% absorption efficacy, was high enough (0.8–1.2 mg/d retention) to match for the iron losses by menstruation, keeping the iron stores in balance *(67).*

The relationships between ferritin and mean corpuscular volume and hemoglobin among adolescents have been described by quadratic-plateau equations *(67).* Based on this analysis it was possible to estimate a threshold level below which hemoglobin and mean corpuscular volume were directly reflective of the serum ferritin concentration and above which they did not change regardless of the further increases of serum ferritin *(67).* This helps in understanding the development of anemia in teenage females. The serum ferritin threshold concentrations for adequate hemoglobin and mean corpuscular volume were 18.4 ± 0.59 ng/mL (95% CI, 17.8–19.0) and 37.6 ± 0.94 ng/mL (95% CI, 36.6–38.5), respectively, with corresponding values for hemoglobin and mean corpuscular volume of 13.4 g/dL and 88.1 μm^3. Although, not using the same mathematical model, Hallberg et al. found similar cutoff ferritin levels of 16–20 ng/mL and 30–40 ng/mL for hemoglobin and mean corpuscular volume, respectively in their population of 220 sixteen-year old girls. From the other selected dietary constituents only vitamin C showed a significant positive association with serum ferritin *(66)*. Hallberg and Solvell noted that ascorbic acid significantly increased (by an average of 20%) the absorption of nonheme iron, but did not effect the absorption of heme iron *(68)*. However, Hunt et al. found no influence of supplemental vitamin C on iron absorption in young adults aged 20–45 yr *(69)*.

A subgroup (7%) of teenage females in the study of Ilich et al. was iron deficient as judged by ferritin concentrations of ≤12 ng/dL as the internationally accepted cutoff value *(67)*. This percent becomes even higher (16%) when considering the cutoff of 16 ng/dL as proposed by Hallberg et al., as this was the level with no stainable iron in bone marrow smears *(59)*. In summary, data from the long term study of Ilich and coworkers *(67)* provide strong evidence that adequate dietary iron intake (>9 mg/d) precludes the negative effects of iron losses because of menstruation in the population of teenage females during their growth spurt.

6. ZINC

The adolescent population may be susceptible to a mild to moderate zinc deficiency as a result of poor eating habits and increased requirements for growth *(71)*. Teenagers who consume vegetarian diets, especially those that do not contain any animal products, are more likely to develop a deficiency. Numerous studies on nutrient intakes and zinc status indicate that adolescent females are consuming as low as one-half to two-thirds of the RDA for Zn *(72–75)*. Although severe zinc deficiency is rarely seen in the U.S., mild zinc deficiency has been reported in children and adolescents, leading to the low growth percentiles, diminished taste acuity, and low hair zinc levels *(71,76,77)*. The effect on growth may be mediated through insulin-like growth factor –1 (IGF-I); a direct link between zinc nutritional status and IGF-I was described in postmenopausal women *(78)*. In the study of McKenna et al. *(79)* adolescent females were consuming about 46% of the recommended dietary allowance (RDA) for zinc while in the metabolic ward, and about 67% of recommended dietary allowance in their self selected diet (RDA for adolescent females is 12 mg/d), which is in agreement with other nationwide surveys of Zn intake for this age group. The study did not show a relationship between zinc intake and zinc balance; five of the twenty-six subjects were in negative zinc balance irrespective of intake (whether the girls who were in negative zinc balance were zinc deficient could not be assessed from the study) *(79)*. A problem with assessing zinc nutriture is the lack of an adequate biochemical or laboratory marker of mild to moderate zinc deficiency (*see* Chapter 5). Nevertheless, a number of studies suggest that zinc deficiency may be a problem in the pregnant adolescent (*see* Chapter 8).

7. OTHER TRACE MINERALS

Fluoride (F) is an essential trace mineral found mostly in mineralized tissues. If fluoride is available during the development of teeth and bone, it is incorporated into their mineral structure; and makes teeth more resistant to decay. Studies showed that children raised in areas where there is one part per million of fluoride in the water have fewer cavities than children who do not drink fluoridated water. Caries experience per child is inversely related to the fluoride concentration of drinking water. There is no recommended dietary allowance for fluoride, but there is a suggested adequate intake which is shown to reduce the occurrence of dental caries to a maximum without causing unwanted side effects including dental fluorosis *(85)*. The estimated adequate intake for boys and girls ages 9 through 13-yr is 2.0 mg/d. For older boys and girls ages 14 to 18 yr the estimated adequate intake is 3.0 mg/d, *(85)*. In many areas of the country, fluoride is added to the drinking water at a level of one part per million as the WHO recommends *(80)*.

There is about 75–100 mg of copper (Cu) in the body, most of it being accumulated during rapid growth. A deficiency of copper among young individuals is very rare, although it has been found in severely malnourished children with disturbed growth and metabolism, along with deficiencies of other important nutrients. There is no recommended dietary allowance for copper; the suggested safe and adequate intake is 1.5 to 3.0 mg/d *(52)*. The average American diet provides about 2.0 mg of copper per day. In preadolescent and adolescent girls, fecal and urinary losses were at or near equilibrium with a dietary copper intake of 1–1.3 mg/d *(81–83)*.

Selenium (Se) is found in all body tissues, primarily in kidneys, liver, spleen, pancreas, and testicles. Selenium functions with vitamin E as an antioxidant, helping to prevent cell damage. Severe deficiency of selenium predisposes people to develop virus induced cardiomyopathy. This was described in children and women of childbearing age in China as well as in patients on total parenteral nutrition *(84)*. Some studies suggest that selenium may have anticancer activities; this remains to be confirmed. The selenium requirement increases during growth, however, recommendations for adolescents have been extrapolated from adult values. The National Research Council (1989) recommends an intake of 40–45 µg/d for teenage boys and girls 11–14 yr old and 50 µg/d for older adolescents *(52)*. Further research is necessary to precisely define selenium requirements during growth.

Chromium (Cr) helps regulating glucose metabolism in the body. Chromium is found in whole grains, meats, cheese, and eggs. The richest source of chromium is brewers yeast. Chromium-responsive impairment of glucose tolerance has been reported in malnourished children *(52)* suggesting that adolescents with type I diabetes mellitus may benefit from chromium supplements. The estimated safe and adequate intake of chromium for adolescents is between 50 and 200 µg/d.

Manganese (Mn) is important for reproductive function, skeletal development, cartilage formation, and for glucose metabolism. Manganese deficiency practically does not exist; it was only described in a human requiring a purified diet from which manganese was omitted. Whole grains and cereal products are the main dietary sources of manganese. The estimated adequate intake of manganese for teenagers is between 2.0 and 3.0 mg/d *(52)*.

Molybdenum (Mo) is a constituent of several enzymes including aldehyde oxidase, xanthine oxidase, and sulfite oxidase. Naturally occurring molybdenum deficiency has not been described either in animals or humans; it was produced artificially in goats by feeding them a low molybdenum diet. Deficient animals did not gain weight, had impaired reproduction, and shortened life expectancy. Most of the molybdenum consumed comes from milk, beans, breads, and cereals. Estimated safe and adequate intakes of molybdenum for adolescents are between 75 and 250 µg/d *(52)*.

Iodine (I) is incorporated into structure of the thyroid hormones (*see* Chapter 13). Of the 25 mg of iodine in the body approximately 50% is found in the thyroid gland. Thyroid hormones control energy metabolism and are important for reproduction and growth. Main sources of iodine are seafood and iodized salt. The recommended allowance for iodine for adolescents is the same as for adults and that is 150 µg/d. Pregnant teenage mothers require an extra 25 µg/d and lactating mothers require an extra 50 µg/d. Those increments are to cover the demands of the fetus and the infant *(52)*.

8. NUTRIENT INTERACTIONS

The National Academy of Sciences, Food and Nutrition Board, as well as the National Institutes of Health Consensus Panel on Optimal Calcium Intake recently increased calcium intake standards for teenagers to 1300 and 1500 mg/d, respectively *(33,85)*. However, there is a concern that high calcium intake may lead to decreased absorption of other important minerals.

There is evidence that high calcium intakes decrease gastrointestinal absorption and retention of magnesium in adults *(86,87)*. However, few data on this topic are available for the younger population. The study of Andon et al. conducted in healthy adolescent females shows that magnesium balance is not significantly affected by high calcium intake (1700 mg vs 700 mg Ca/d; supplementation with calcium citrate malate) *(54)*. The values reported for magnesium absorption and excretion were similar to those reported previously for adolescent females and adults. The amounts of calcium in the low- and high-calcium diets reflected current self-selected intakes among American adolescent females and the new recommendations to increase calcium intake. Approximately 40% of girls this age consume ~700 mg Ca/day in their self-selected diets, whereas several recent reports have recommended calcium intakes up to 1300–1500 mg/d to optimize peak bone mass acquisition during puberty. Participants in this study were selected from the placebo-controlled trial of calcium supplementation and bone mass acquisition. Thus, it was more likely that the observations reflected chronic magnesium utilization and not acute responses to increases in calcium intake. The period of intervention lasted six months. Previous studies in which a negative interaction between increased calcium intake and magnesium utilization were observed did not involve such a long experimental period. Magnesium absorption as assessed by an intestinal perfusion technique was shown to be significantly lower in the ileum of adult men who consumed a high- (1900 mg/d) compared with a low- (200 mg/d) calcium diet for 4 wk *(86)*. Based on literature accumulated before 1965, Seelig concluded that calcium intakes > 800 mg/d reduce magnesium balance *(87)*, however, more recent studies in adults showed that magnesium balance was not influenced by increasing calcium intakes from ~ 800 mg/d to 2400 mg/d *(88,89)*. Thus, it seems unlikely that a calcium intake somewhat greater than the one consumed (1700 mg/d) by young females in the study of Andon et al. *(54)* would have deleterious effects on magnesium balance. Greger et al. showed that fractional magnesium absorption in weanling rats was greater from a nonfat dry milk-based diet compared with diets containing different supplemental sources of calcium, including dibasic calcium phosphate, dolomite, oyster shell, chelated calcium from yeast, and calcium carbonate *(90)*. In contrast, Ilich et al. reported that a bolus infusion of calcium gluconate had no effect on endogenous magnesium absorption in chronically catheterized rats *(91)*. In adult humans, increasing calcium intake from 200 to 2000 mg/d with calcium gluconate had no significant effect on magnesium balance. Lewis et al. reported that magnesium balance in adults was not changed by supplementing a basal diet containing 700 mg Ca/d with an additional 900 mg Ca/d as either milk, calcium chloride, or calcium carbonate *(92)*. Thus, a range of calcium sources, including food sources (milk) and both soluble and insoluble calcium salts, have been evaluated in adults with no significant effect being noted on magnesium utilization. These data suggest that research findings of Andon et al. *(54)* with calcium citrate malate apply to other sources of calcium.

Adequate iron status is very important for menstruating adolescent girls and pregnant and lactating teenage females, as these groups are especially prone to develop iron deficiency anemia. These young women are also at risk of forming inadequate skeletal mass if calcium intake is below the threshold level (<1500 mg/d). For the majority of adolescent females in these groups, calcium supplementation is an important consideration, as most of them do not consume 1300–1500 mg/d of calcium from dairy products. It is, therefore, very important that well documented clinical studies examine the effects of calcium supplementation on iron status in these high risk individuals. It has been shown in several studies that calcium interferes with iron absorption and that the effect is dose-dependent *(68,93–98)*. Mixed results exist with regard to the effects when consumption of calcium occurs separately from the meals containing iron *(99–101)*. It also is not clear to what extent, if any, higher calcium intake (even when it interferes with iron absorption) might influence iron stores in the population. So far the longest study with calcium supplementation (1000 mg of calcium as calcium citrate malate) ever conducted did not show any interference of calcium with iron status of young females. The study was conducted in a large group of adolescent females who were followed for 4 yr from the premenarcheal to postmenarcheal period, representing the highest risk group for the development of iron deficiency anemia *(67)*. Both the dietary calcium and iron intakes among participants of this study were below the recommended intakes for these minerals; the recommended dietary allowance for iron is 15 mg/d. However, the calcium supplemented group reached total calcium intakes of about 1500 mg/d, raising the question of its influence on iron stores. The results of this study clearly show no effect of calcium supplementation taken at that level and in the form of calcium citrate malate on the iron status of young teenage females, assessed by serum ferritin and red blood cell indices (Table 2). Hemoglobin, hematocrit, and the corpuscular indices measured after 4 yr of intervention with calcium and placebo were not different between the groups, confirming the findings inferred from the ferritin study (Table 3).

According to some studies, calcium in food or as a supplement may decrease iron absorption by as much as 50% *(96,98)*. However, the inhibitory effect of calcium may be influenced by the compounds containing calcium and iron, the amount consumed, and whether the minerals are consumed separately or as part of a meal. In the study by Hallberg et al. different levels (40, 75, 165, 300, 600 mg/serving) of calcium as calcium chloride were added to wheat rolls or hamburger and caused a dose related inhibitory response up to 300 mg of calcium *(94)*. In addition, when milk and cheese containing 165 mg calcium were consumed with the control wheat rolls, iron absorption was reduced by 57% when milk was consumed and by 46% when cheese was consumed. In a similar study, Hallberg et al. demonstrated that 165 mg of calcium carbonate reduced heme iron absorption by 41% when consumed in a hamburger and by 48% when consumed in a wheat roll *(96)*. Cook et al. showed that calcium carbonate did not inhibit the absorption of ferrous sulphate when taken between meals at doses of 300 mg calcium and 37 mg Fe or 600 mg calcium and 18 mg Fe *(93)*. However, when 600 mg of calcium citrate or

Table 2
Calcium intake and serum ferritin levels for control and calcium supplemented
individuals from age 11 to age 15 yr. Data presented as a mean ± SD. p represents
the level of significance between the groups based on the two sample t-test. From
Ilich et al. *(67)*.

Age (y)	Calcium Intake (mg/d)			Serum Ferritin (ng/dL)		
	Control	Suppl	p-level	Control	Suppl	p-level
11	820±303	854±289	0.3104	29.3±17.9	29.1±16.9	0.8780
12	786±280	1589±353	0.0001	35.6±26.6	31.1±15.6	0.1174
13	826±326	1591±382	0.0001	32.3±15.5	31.1±16.8	0.5644
14	864±336	1551±441	0.0001	30.9±16.7	30.6±20.3	0.8787
15	799±397	1567±424	0.0001	29.5±17.0	29.6±19.1	0.9644

Table 3
Hematologic indices for the low (control) and high calcium (supplemented)
groups. Data presented as a mean ± SD. HGB=hemoglobin; HCT=hematocrit;
RBC=red blood cells; MCV=mean corpuscular volume; MCHC=mean
corpuscular hemoglobin concentration. From Ilich et al. *(67)*.

Variable	Control	Suppl	p-level
HGB (g/dL)	13.4±0.8	13.2±0.9	0.0971
HCT (%)	38.5±2.4	37.9±2.5	0.1814
RBC (M/µL)	4.4±0.3	4.4±0.3	0.3076
MCV (µm^3)	86.6±3.5	86.5±4.0	0.8065
MCHC (g/dL)	34.8±0.6	34.7±0.7	0.1147

calcium phosphate was consumed, the absorption of 18 mg ferrous sulfate was reduced
by 49% and 62%, respectively. In addition, all three calcium supplements had an inhibitory effect when consumed with a meal. Prather and Miller used a rat hemoglobin repletion assay to determine if the inhibitory effect of calcium was due to the calcium, the anion,
or a combination of the two. Low, medium, and high doses of either calcium carbonate,
calcium sulfate, sodium carbonate, or sodium sulfate were added to the repletion diet.
Calcium carbonate reduced iron bioavailability in a dose related manner. Calcium sulfate
and sodium carbonate also decreased iron bioavailability but only at the highest dose. Based
on these observations, it was concluded that both the cation and the anion together contribute to the inhibitory effect *(102)*. Dawson-Hughes et al. showed that iron retention was
significantly reduced by calcium carbonate or hydroxyapatite in postmenopausal women
when both were consumed in a test meal *(103)*. Similarly, Cook et al. found that iron
absorption was reduced when both minerals were taken together *(93)*.

Kalkwarf and Harrast *(104)* presented data on the effects of calcium carbonate on iron
status in a group of lactating (n=95) and nonlactating (n=92) women participating in a
double-blind placebo-controlled clinical trial. In a similar study, Minihane and
Fairweather-Tait *(105)* examined the effects of short-and long-term calcium carbonate
supplementation on iron status in a smaller group of young adult men and women. Both
studies investigated the effects of calcium intake with meals for six months with similar

doses of calcium (500 mg at two meals and 400 mg at three meals, respectively). In 1996 Lyn et al. *(106)* published data on the effect of long-term calcium supplementation given as calcium carbonate at a dose of 500 mg twice daily in-between meals on indices of iron status in a group (n=60) of malnourished lactating women from Gambia who were at risk of iron deficiency; baseline ferritin levels were low. Calcium supplements were given with supervision (100% compliance) and over a 12 mo period. Serum ferritin concentration was used as an index of iron status in each of the three studies mentioned above. The studies found no effect of long-term calcium supplementation in the form of calcium carbonate on iron status, regardles of the timing of the calcium supplementation. Minihane and Fairweather-Tait confirmed that calcium supplementation with a meal does significantly reduce iron absorption but does not affect long-term iron status. Hallberg *(107)* questioned the outcome of Minihane and Fairweather-Tait study *(105)* claiming that the period of 6 mo was not long enough to actually determine the effects of calcium supplementation on iron status especially when serum ferritin was the indicator. However, the study of Yan et al. *(106)* was 12 mo long, and did not show the adverse interaction between the minerals to support Hallberg's claim. Our study which lasted 48 mo and was conducted in menstruating adolescent females during peak growth did not show any effect of calcium supplementation on iron status *(67)*. It is possible that calcium-citrate malate (CCM), which was used in the study *(67)*, does not have an adverse effect on iron absorption as compared to other forms of calcium, however, this is highly unlikely as suggested by the results of the 6–12 mo studies with calcium carbonate *(104–106,108)*. The results of the study of Ilich et al. *(67)* are similar to those of Sokoll and Dawson-Hughes in which 107 premenopausal women (average age about 32 yr) were randomly assigned to receive either a placebo or 1000 mg/d of calcium as calcium carbonate for 12 wk *(108)*. Serum ferritin levels were not significantly different in the treatment and control groups at baseline and after 12 wk of supplementation. In a metabolic balance study by Snedeker et al. iron balance and serum ferritin were not significantly affected by intake of calcium up to 2382 mg/d *(100)*. Most recently, Reddy and Cook found no change in nonheme iron absorption, from a complete diet containing bread rolls tagged with extrinsically labeled radioiron, in the presence of varying amounts of calcium (from 280 to 1280 mg/d) *(109)*. This study was performed in healthy young women and men and was unique in that the effects were examined in the context of the complete and freely chosen diet instead of only in particular portions of food items or meals.

Several animal studies have shown that calcium interferes with the intestinal absorption of zinc resulting in lesions and parakeratosis *(110)* or retarded growth and decreased levels of zinc in tissues *(111–113)*. While some human studies have shown that increased calcium intake decreases zinc absorption *(114,115)*, others have been unable to confirm this *(100,116)*. However, in the study of McKenna et al. *(79)* we investigated if threshold intakes of approximately 1500 mg/d of calcium had any adverse effects on zinc metabolism, rather than determine at what level calcium intake influences zinc absorption. The study showed that long-term calcium supplementation with 1000 mg of calcium as CCM, in addition to dietary calcium, did not have detrimental effects on zinc balance of adolescent females consuming lower amounts of zinc (Fig. 16) *(79)*.

High calcium intake of about 1500 mg/d did not affect selenium balance and status in adolescent females. Selenium balances conducted in a group of teenage females (n=26) revealed relatively higher net selenium absorption (75%) comparable to adults, however, this was not affected by the amount of calcium in the diet *(117)*.

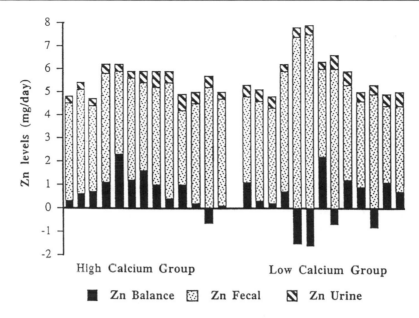

Fig. 16. Zinc balance study in young females at two levels of calcium intake. Each column represents average daily zinc balance per individual subject. Adapted from McKenna et al. *(79)*.

In summary, adolescence is the period of psychobiologic maturation during which the secondary physical growth spurt is completed and sexual maturity and the ability to reproduce are achieved. Healthy adolescents are in strong positive balance of nitrogen and the minerals required for body building. This is most obvious for major body minerals like calcium, phosphorus, magnesium, and iron. Teenagers do not suffer from a deficiency of phosphorus and magnesium and most of the trace elements (Cr, Cu, I, Mn, Mo, Se) due to the ubiquitous nature of these elements in the water and food supply, and/or due to a specific homeostatic control in the human body; however, there is a widespread belief that adolescents may be especially prone to develop calcium, iron, and zinc deficiencies. While calcium deficiency among teenagers may not be readily recognized due to its effect on peak bone mass and osteoporosis later in life, iron and zinc deficiency during pubertal growth could immediately lead to anemia and growth retardation. Zinc deficiency may influence bone accretion through its effect on IGF-I, however, this requires further confirmation. A recent study indicated that magnesium supplementation may suppress bone turnover in young adult males *(118)*, but whether this could be translated into a higher peak bone mass remains to be confirmed. Low fluoride concentrations in the drinking water may negatively influence the oral health of teenagers while its effect on peak bone mass may be negligible.

With regard to nutrient interactions, it can be concluded that high dietary calcium intake does not influence the nutritional status of some of the major minerals and trace elements (P, Mg, Fe, Zn, Se) in the body of adolescents. Therefore, public health measures to elevate calcium intakes among young Americans to the new standards (up to 1500 mg/d) are safe recommendations and should not trigger a concern for the possible induction of iron deficiency anemia, hypomagnesemia, zinc deficiency and growth retardation, or predispose young people to cardiomyopathy as the result of selenium deficiency.

REFERENCES

1. Matkovic V, Jelic T, Wardlaw GM, Ilich JZ, Goel PK, Wright JK, Andon MB, Smith KT, Heaney RP, Timing of peak bone mass in caucasian females and its implication for the prevention of osteoporosis. Inference from a cross-sectional model. J Clin Invest 1994;93:799–808.
2. Widdowson EM. Growth and body composition in childhood. In: Brunser O, Carrazza F, Gracey M, Nichols B, Senterre J, eds. Clinical nutrition of the young child. Raven Press, New York, 1985;1–21.
3. Miller GD, Jarvis JK, McBean LD. Handbook of dairy foods and nutrition. CRC Press, Boca Raton, 1995.
4. Matkovic V, Kostial K, Simonovic I, Buzina R, Brodarec A, Nordin, BEC. Bone status and fracture rates in two regions of Yugoslavia. Am J Clin Nutr 1979;32: 540–49.
5. Hu JF, Zhao XH, Jia JB, Parpia B, Campbell TC. Dietary calcium and bone density among middle-aged and elderly women in China. Am J Clin Nutr 1993;58:219–227.
6. Sandler RB, Slemenda C, LaPorte RE, Cauley JA, Schramm MM, Baresi M, Kriska AM. Postmenopausal bone density and milk consumption in childhood and adolescence. Am J Clin Nutr 1985;42:270–74.
7. Halioua L, Anderson JJB. Lifetime calcium intake and physical activity habits: independent and combined effects on the radial bone of healthy premenopausal Caucasian women. Am J Clin Nutr 1989;49:534–541.
8. Murphy S, Khaw KT, May H, Compston JE. Milk consumption and bone mineral density in middle aged and elderly women. BMJ 1994;308:939–941.
9. Soroko S, Holbrook TL, Edelstein S, Barrett-Connor E. Lifetime milk consumption and bone mineral density in older women. Am J Public Health 1994;84:1319–1322.
10. Matkovic V, Heaney RP. Calcium balance during human growth: evidence for threshold behavior. Am J Clin Nutr 1992;55:992–996.
11. Matkovic V, Ilich JZ. Calcium requirements during growth. Are the current standards adequate? Nutr Rev 1993;51:171–180.
12. Charles P, Taagehoj Jensen F, Mosekilde L, Hvid Hansen H. Calcium metabolism evaluated by 47Ca kinetics: estimation of dermal calcium loss. Clin Sci 1983;65:415–22.
13. Klesges RC, Ward KD, Shelton ML, Applegate WB, Cantler ED, Palmieri GMA, Harmon K, Davis J. Changes in bone mineral content in male athletes. Mechanisms of action and intervention effects. JAMA 1996;276:226–230.
14. Aksnes L, Aarskog D. Plasma concentrations of vitamin D metabolites in puberty: Effect of sexual maturation and implications for growth. J Clin Endocrinol Metab 1982;55:94–101.
15. Chesney RW, Rosen JF, Hamstra AH, DeLuca HF. Serum 1,25-dihydroxyvitamin D levels in normal children and in vitamin D disorders. Am J Dis Child 1980;134:135–139.
16. Ilich JZ, Badenhop NE, Jelic T, Clairmont AC, Nagode LA, Matkovic V. Calcitriol and bone mass accumulation in females during puberty. Calcif Tissue Int 1997;61:104–109.
17. Matkovic V. Calcium metabolism and calcium requirements during skeletal modeling and consolidation of bone mass. Am J Clin Nutr 1991;54:245S–260S.
18. Matkovic V, Fontana D, Tominac C, Goel P, Chesnut CH. Factors which influence peak bone mass formation: A study of calcium balance and the inheritance of bone mass in adolescent females. Am J Clin Nutr 1990;52:878–888.
19. Jackman LA, Millane SS, Martin BR, Wood OB, McCabe GP, Peacosk M, Weaver CM. Calcium retention in relation to calcium intake and postmenarcheal age in adolescent females. Am J Clin Nutr 1997;66:327–33.
20. Matkovic V, Ilich JZ, Skugor M. Calcium intake and skeletal formation. Challenges of modern medicine 1995;7:129–145.
21. Nordin BEC, Marshall DH. Dietary requirements for calcium. In: Nordin BEC, ed. Calcium in human biology. ILSI Human Nutrition Reviews. Berlin: Springer-Verlag 1988, pp. 447–471.
22. Matkovic V, Ilich JZ, Andon MB, Hsieh LC, Tzagournis MA, Lagger BJ, Goel PK. Urinary calcium, sodium, and bone mass of young females. Am J Clin Nutr 1995;62:417–425.
23. Johnston CC Jr, Miller JZ, Slemenda CW, Reister TK, Hui S, Christian JC, Peacock M. Calcium supplementation and increases in bone mineral density in children. N Eng J Med 1992;327:82–87.
24. Lloyd T, Andon MB, Rollings N, Martel JK, Landis RJ, Demers LM, Eggli DF, Kieselhorst K, Kulin HE. Calcium supplementation and bone mineral density in adolescent girls. JAMA 1993;270:841–844.
25. Chan GM, Hoffman K, McMurray M. Effect of dairy products on bone and body composition in pubertal girls. J Pediatrics 1995;126:551–556.

26. Bonjour JP, Carrie AL, Ferrarri S, Clavien H, Slosman D, Theintz G, Rizzoli R. Calcium-enriched foods and bone mass growth in prepubertal girls: a randomized, double-blind, placebo-controlled, trial. J Clin Invest 1997;99:1287–1294.

27. Cadogan J, Eastell R, Jones N, Barker ME. Milk intake and bone mineral acquisition in adolescent girls: randomised, controlled intervention trial. BMJ 1997;315:1255–60.

28. Lee WTK, Leung SSF, Wang SF, Xu YC, Zeng, WP, Lau J, Oppenheimer SJ Cheng JCY. Double-blind, controlled calcium supplementation and bone mineral accretion in children accustomed to a low-calcium diet. Am J Clin Nutr 1994;60:744–750.

29. Chan GM, Hess M, Hollis J, Book LS. Bone mineral status in childhood accidental fractures. Am J Dis Child 1984;139:569–70.

30. Goulding A, Cannan R, Williams SM, Gold EJ, Taylor RW, Lewis-Barned NJ. Bone mineral density in girls with forearm fractures. J Bone Miner Res 1998;13:143–148.

31. Fleming KH, Heimbach JT. Consumption of calcium in the U.S. :Food sources and intake levels. J Nutr 1994;124:1426S–1430S.

32. U.S. Department of Health and Human Services, Public Health Service. Healthy people 2000. National health promotion and disease prevention objectives. Jones and Bartlett Publ., Boston, 1992, pp. 1–153.

33. NIH Consensus Conference: Optimal calcium intake. JAMA 1994;272:1942–8.

34. Witschi J, Capper AL, Ellison RC. Sources of fat, fatty acids, and cholesterol in the diets of adolescents. J Am Diet Assoc 1990;90:1429–1431.

35. Badenhop NE, Ilich JZ, Skugor M, Landoll JD, Matkovic V. Changes in body composition and serum leptin in young females with high vs low dairy intake J Bone Min Res 1997;12:S487.

36. Badenhop NE, Ilich JZ, Matkovic V. Trends in food choices of calcium among teenage females over a 4-year period. J Bone Min Res 1998;13: S1.

37. Nordin BEC. Nutritional consideration. In : Nordin BEC, ed. Calcium, phosphate and magnesium metabolism. Churchill Livingstone, Edinburgh 1976, pp. 1–35.

38. Landoll JD, Mobley LS, Matkovic V. The relationship between phosphorus intake and output during growth. J Bone Min Res 1998;13:S1.

39. Krook L, Barrett RB. Simian bone disease - a secondary hyperparathyroidism. Cornell Vet 1962;52:459–492.

40. Krook L, Barrett RB, Usui K, Wolke RE. Nutritional secondary hyperparathyroidism in the cat. Cornell Vet 1963;53:224–240.

41. Krook L, Lowe JE. Nutritional secondary hyperparathyroidism in horse. Path Vet 1964,1:S1–S98.

42. Krook L, Whalen JP, Lesser GV, Lutwak L. Human periodontal disease and osteoporosis. Cornell Vet 1972;62: 371–391.

43. Albright F, Reifenstein EC. The parathyroid glands and metabolic bone disease. Williams & Wilkins Comp., Baltimore, 1948.

44. Jowsey J, Reiss E, Canterbury JM. Long term effects of high phosphate intake on parathyroid hormone levels and bone metabolism. Acta Othop Scand 1974;45:801–808.

45. Calvo MS, Kumar R, Heath H.III. Persistently elevated parathyroid hormone secretion and action in young women after four weeks of ingesting high phosphorus, low calcium diets. J Clin Endocrinol Metab 1990;70:133–134.

46. Spencer H, Menczel J, Lewin I, Samachson J. Effect of high phosphorus intake on calcium and phosphorus metabolism in men. J Nutr 1965;86:125–132.

47. Spencer H, Kramer L, Osais D, Norris C. Effect of phosphorus on the absorption of calcium and on calcium balance in men. J Nutr 1978;108:447–457.

48. Heaney RP, Recker RR. Effects of nitrogen, phosphorus, and caffeine on calcium balance in women. J Lab Clin Med 1982;99:46–55.

49. Whybro A, Jagger H, Barker M, Eastell R. Phosphate supplementation in young men: lack of effect on calcium homeostatis and bone turnover. Eur J Clin Nutr 1998;52:29–33.

50. Tsuboi S, Nakagaki H, Ishiguro K, Kondo K, Mukai M, Robinson C, Weatherell JA. Magnesium distribution in human bone. Calcif Tissue Int 1994;54:34–37.

51. Seelig MS. Interrelationship of magnesium and estrogen in cardiovascular and bone disorders, eclampsia, migraine and premenstrual syndrome. J Am Coll Nutr 1993;12:442–58.

52. Standing Committee on the Scientific Evaluation of Dietary Reference Intake, Food and Nutrition Board, Institute of Medicine, Dietary reference intake for calcium, phosphorus, magnesium, vitamin D, and fluoride. National Acadamy Press, Washington, DC, 1997.

53. Greger JL, Baligar P, Abernathy RP, Bennett GA, Peterson T. Calcium, magnesium, phosphorus, copper, and manganese balance in adolescent females. Am J Clin Nutr 1979;31:117–21.

54. Andon MB, Ilich JZ, Tzagournis MA, and Matkovic V. Magnesium balance in adolescent females consuming a low or high calcium diet. Am J Clin Nutr 1996;63:950–953.
55. Medeiros DM, Ilich JZ, Ireton J, Matkovic V, Shiry L, Wildman R. Femurs from rats fed diets deficient in copper or iron have decreased mechanical strength and altered mineral composition. J Trace Elem Exper Med 1997;10:197–203.
56. Cook JD, Finch CA, Smith NJ. Evaluation of the iron status of a population. Blood 1976;48:449–55.
57. Expert Scientific Working Group. Summary of a report on assessment of the iron nutritional status of the United States population. Am J Clin Nutr 1985;42:1318–1330.
58. Dallman PR. Biochemical basis for the manifestations of iron deficiency. Annu Rev Nutr 1986;6:13–40.
59. Hallberg L, Hulten L, Lindstedt G, Lundberg P-A, Mark A, Purens J, Svanberg B, Swolin B. Prevalence of iron deficiency in Swedish adolescents. Pediatr Res 1993;34:680–687.
60. Hallberg L, Bengtsson C, Lapidus L, Lundberg P-A, Hulten L. Screening for iron deficiency: an analysis based on bone-marrow examinations and serum ferritin determinations in a population sample of women. Br J Hematol 1993;85:787–98.
61. Bowering J, Sanchez AM, Irvin IM. A conspectus of research on iron requirement of man. J Nutr 1976;106:985–1074.
62. Hallberg L., Rossander-Hulten L. Iron requirements in menstruating women. Am J Clin Nutr 1991;54:1047–1058.
63. Bailey L, Ginsburg J, Wagner P, Noyes W, Christakis G, Dinning J. Serum ferritin as a measure of iron stores in adolescents. J Pediatr 1982;101:774–776.
64. Bothwell TH, Finch CA. Iron metabolism. Little, Brown and Co., Boston, 1962.
65. Pietrobelli A, Formica C, Wang Z, Heymsfield SB. Dual-energy X-ray absorptiometry body composition model: review of physical concepts. Am J Physiol 1996;271:E941–E951.
66. Hillman RS, Finch CA. Red Cell Manual. Ed 4. F.A. Davis Comp., Philadelphia, 1976, pp. 12–17.
67. Ilich-Ernst JZ, McKenna AA, Badenhop NE, Clairmont AC, Andon MB, Nahhas RW, Goel P, Matkovic V. Iron status, menarche, and calcium supplementation in adolescent girls. Am J Clin Nutr 1998;68:880–887.
68. Hallberg L, Solvell L. Absorption of hemoglobin iron in man. Acta Med Scand 1967;131:335–54.
69. Hunt JR, Gallagher SK, Johnson LK. Effect of ascorbic acid on apparent iron absorption by women with low iron stores. Am J Clin Nutr 1994;59:1381–1385.
70. Finch CA, Bellotti V, Sray S, Lipschitz DA, Cook JD, Pippard MJ, Huebers HA. Plasma ferritin determination as a diagnostic tool. West J Med 1986;145:657–63.
71. Donovan UM, Gibson RS. Iron and zinc status of young women aged 14 to 19 years consuming vegetarian and omnivorous diets. J Am Coll Nutr 1995;14:463–472.
72. Devine A, Rosen C, Mohan S, Baylink D, Prince RL. Effects of zinc and other nutritional factors on insulin-like growth factor 1 and insulin-like growth factor binding proteins in postmenopausal women. Am J Clin Nutr 1998;68:200–206.
73. Murphy S P, Calloway DH. Nutrient intakes of women in NHANES II, emphasizing trace minerals, fiber, and phytate. J Am Diet Assoc 1986;86:1366–1372.
74. Pilch SM, Senti FR. Analysis of zinc data from the second National Health and Nutrition Examination Survey (NHANES II). J Nutr 1985;115:1393–1397.
75. Greger JL, Higgins MM, Abernathy RP, Kirksey A, DeCorso MB, Baligar MS. Nutritional status of adolescent girls in regard to zinc, copper, and iron. Am J Clin Nutr 1978;31:269–275.
76. Sloane BA, Gibbons CC, Hegsted M. Evaluation of zinc and copper nutritional status and effects upon growth of southern adolescent females. Am J Clin Nutr 1985;42:235–241.
77. Butrimovitz GP, Purdy WC. Zinc nutrition and growth in a childhood population. Am J Clin Nutr 1978;31:1409–1412.
78. Hambidge MK, Hambidge C, Jacobs M, Baum DJ. Low levels of zinc in hair, anorexia, poor growth, and hypogeusia in children. Pediatr Res 1972;2:868–74.
79. McKenna AA, Ilich JZ, Andon MB, Wang C, Matkovic V. Zinc balance in adolescent females consuming a low- or high-calcium diet. Am J Clin Nutr 1997;65:1460–1464.
80. World Health Organisation, W.H.O. Expert Committee Report. W.H.O. Techn Rep Ser 146, 1958.
81. Engel RW, Price NO, Miller RF. Copper, manganese, cobalt, and molybdenum balance in pre-adolescent girls. J Nutr 1967;92:197–204.
82. Greger JL, Zaikis CS, Abernathy RP, Bennett OA, Huffman J. Zinc, nitrogen, copper, iron and manganese balance in adolescent females fed two levels of zinc. J Nutr 1978;108:1449–1456.
83. Price NO, Bunce GE. Effect of nitrogen and calcium on balance of copper, manganese, and zinc in preadolescent girls. Nutr Rep Int 1972;5:275–280.

84. Levander OA. A global view of selenium nutrition. Annu Rev Nutr 1987;7:227–250.
85. Dietary Reference Intakes. Food and Nutrition Board, Institute of Medicine, National Academy Press, Washington, DC, 1997.
86. Norman DA, Fordtran 35, Brinldey U. Ct al. Jejunal and ileal adaptation to alterations in dietary calcium. J Clin Invest 1981;67:1599–1603.
87. Seelig MS. The requirement of magnesium by the normal adult: summary and analysis of published data. Am J Clin Nutr 1964;14:342–90.
88. Spencer H, Norris C, Derler J, Osis D. Effect of oat bran muffins on calcium absorption and calcium, phosphorus, magnesium and zinc balance in men. J Nutr 1991;121:197–83.
89. Greger JL, Smith SA, Snedeker SM. Effect of dietary calcium and phosphorus levels on the utilization of calcium, phosphorus, magnesium, manganese, and selenium by adult males. Nutr Res 1981;1:315–25.
90. Greger JL, Krzykowski CE. Knazen RR, Krashoc CL. Mineral utilization by rats fed various commercially available calcium supplements or milk. J Nutr 1987;117:717–24.
91. Ilich JZ, Kimura RE, Smith AM. Duodenal magnesium infusions decrease intestinal calcium absorption in the chronically catheterized rat. J Optimal Nutr 1994;3:72–79.
92. Lewis NM, Marcus MSK, Behling AR. Greger IL. Calcium supplements and milk: effects on acid-base balance and on retention of calcium, magnesium, and phosphorus. Am J Clin Nutr 1989;49:527–33.
93. Cook JD, Dassenko SA, Whittaker P. Calcium supplementation: effect on iron absorption. Am J Clin Nutr 1991;53:106–11.
94. Hallberg L, Brune M, Eriandsson M, Sandberg A, Rossander-Hulten L. Calcium: effect of different amounts on nonheme- and heme-iron absorption in humans. Am J Clin Nutr 1991;53:112–19.
95. Hallberg L, Rossander–Hulten, L, Brune M, Gleerup A. Calcium and iron absorption: mechanism of action and nutritional importance. Euro J Clin Nutr 1992;46:317–327,.
96. Hallberg L, Rossander-Hulten, L, Brune M, Gleerup A. Inhibition of haem-iron absorption in man by calcium. Br J Nutr 1992;69:533–540.
97. Deehr MS, Dallal GE, Smith KT, Taulbee JD, Dawson-Hughes B. Effects of different calcium sources on iron absorption in postmenopausal women. Am J Clin Nutr 1990;51:95–9.
98. Monsen ER, Cook JD. Food iron absorption in human subjects IV. The effects of calcium and phosphate salts on the absorption of nonheme iron. Am J Clin Nutr 1976;29:1142–1148.
99. Rossander L, Hallberg L, Bjorn-Rasmussen E. Absorption of iron from breakfast meals. Am J Clin Nutr 1979;32:2484–2489.
100. Snedeker SM, Smith SA, Greger JL. Effect of dietary calcium and phosphorus levels on the utilization of iron, copper, and zinc by adult males. J Nutr 1982;112:136–43.
101. Turnlund JR, Smith RG, Kretsch MJ, Keyes WR, Shah AG. Milk's effect on the bioavailability of iron from cereal-based diets in young women by use of in vitro and in vivo methods. Am J Clin Nutr 1990;52:373–378.
102. Prather TA, Miller DD. Calcium carbonate depresses iron bioavailability in rats more than calcium sulfate or sodium carbonate. J Nutr 1992;122:327–332.
103. Dawson-Hughes B, Seligson FH, Hughes VA. Effects of calcium carbonate and hydroxyapatite on zinc and iron retention in postmenopausal women. Am J Clin Nutr 1986;44:83–88.
104. Kalkwarf HJ, Harrast SD. Effects of calcium supplementation and lactation on iron status. Am J Clin Nutr 1998;67:1244–1249.
105. Minihane AM, Fairweather-Tait SJ. Effect of calcium supplementation on daily nonheme-iron absorption and long-term iron status. Am J Clin Nutr 1998;68:96–102.
106. Yan L, Prentice A, Dibba B, Jarjou LMA, Stirling DM, Fairweather-Tait S. The effect of long-term calcium supplementation on indices of iron, zinc, and magnesium status in lactating Gambian women. Br J Nutr 1996;76:821–831.
107. Hallberg L. Does calcium interfere with iron absorption. Am J Clin Nutr 1998;68:3–4.
108. Sokoll LJ, Dawson-Hughes B. Calcium supplementation and plasma ferritin concentrations in premenopausal women. Am J Clin Nutr 1992;56:1045–1048.
109. Reddy MB, Cook JD. Effect of calcium intake on nonheme-iron absorption from a complete diet. Am J Clin Nutr 1997;65:1820–1825.
110. Forbes RM. Nutritional interactions of zinc and calcium. Fed Proc 1960;19:643–647.
111. Hoekstra WG, Lewis PK, Phillips PH, Grmmer RH. The relationship of parakeratosis, supplemental calcium and zinc to the content of certain body components of swine. J Anim Sci 1956;15:752–764.
112. Luecke RW, Hoeter JA, Brammell WS, Schmidt DA. Calcium and zinc in parakeratosis of swine. J Anim Sci 1957;16:3–11.

113. Dursun N, Aydogan S. Comparative effects of calcium deficiency and supplements on the intestinal absorption of zinc in rats. Jap J Physiol 1994;44:157–166.
114. Wood RJ, Hanssen DA. Effect of milk and lactose on zinc absorption in lactose-intolerant postmenopausal women. J Nutr 1988;118:982–986.
115. Argiratos V, Samman S. The effect of calcium carbonate and calcium citrate on the absorption of zinc in healthy female subjects. Eur J Clin Nutr 1994;45:198–204.
116. Wood RJ, Zheng JJ. Milk consumption and zinc retention in postmenopausal women. J Nutr 1990;120:398–403.
117. Holben D, Smith AM, Ha EJ, Ilich JZ, Matkovic V. Selenium (Se) absorption, balance, and status in adolescent females throughout puberty. Faseb J 1996;10:A532.
118. Dimai HP, Porta S, Wirnsberger G, Lindschinger M, Pamperl I, Dobnig H, Wilders–Trusching M, Lau KHW. Daily oral magnesium supplementation supresses bone turnover in young adult males. J Clin Endocrinol Metab 1998;83:2742–2748.
119. Matkovic V, Ilich JZ, Skugor M, Badenhop NE, Clairmont A, Goel P, Klisovic D, Nasseh RW, Landoll JD. Leptin is inversely related to age at menarche in human females. J Clin Endo Metab 1997.;82:3239–3245.

11

Trace Element Requirements in the Elderly

Ronni Chernoff, PhD, RD, FADA

1. INTRODUCTION

The nutritional requirements of older adults have attracted the interest of scientists and nutritionists in recent years. Until recently, the Recommended Dietary Allowances provided guidelines for adults over age 50 but without subdivision into more precise age ranges *(1)*. This leaves a broad gap in definitive recommendations for a large proportion of the population, particularly because life expectancy continues to increase; during the 20th century human life expectancy from birth has nearly doubled *(2)*. The risk for inadequate nutrition in older adults is related to a variety of physiologic, economic, and social factors.

As people age, there are changes in physiology that may contribute to alterations in trace mineral requirements. These changes include a decrease in total body protein, a reduction in total body water, a loss of bone density and a relative increase in body fat. The consequence of these changes is a decline in basal metabolic rate that requires reduced energy intake to avoid weight gain. A lower intake of calories will contribute to a lower intake of essential nutrients unless nutrition counseling is instituted before deficiencies occur. Nutrient dense foods are needed to overcome the potential decrease in nutrients due to a smaller volume of food.

These physiologic changes associated with advancing age may affect the efficiency with which the gastrointestinal tract functions. There may be changes in the proficiency of digestion and absorption of nutrients, including trace minerals. One syndrome that occurs more frequently in older adults is atrophic gastritis, a condition in which the production of hydrochloric acid is decreased leading to a relative hypochlorhydria which may impact the bioavailability or absorption of trace minerals. Absorptive surfaces of the small intestine may have senescent changes and the absorption of trace minerals may be, in some instances, impaired.

Health status may impair appetite or require dietary modifications which may contribute to inadequate consumption of all nutrients.

From: *Clinical Nutrition of the Essential Trace Elements and Minerals: The Guide for Health Professionals*
Edited by: J. D. Bogden and L. M. Klevay © Humana Press Inc., Totowa, NJ

2. IRON

Iron requirements remain fairly constant throughout adulthood for men; requirements decrease by about 50% for women after menopause compared to premenopausal requirements *(1)*. Tissue stores of iron are generally adequate in older adults and it appears that iron adequacy is related to dietary intake *(3)*. Epidemiologic studies have reported a relationship between high tissue iron stores and the risk of chronic disease. The absorption of dietary iron may be influenced by several dietary factors, including the intake of heme iron, supplemental iron, dietary ascorbic acid, and alcohol *(4)*.

2.1. Dietary Iron Deficiency

Dietary iron deficiency is frequently manifested as iron deficiency anemia. Iron deficiency that is severe enough to cause anemia may be associated with significant morbidity *(5)*. However, the data from the third National Health and Nutrition Examination Survey (NHANES III) indicate that the prevalence of iron deficiency anemia among American adults is presently very low; a low incidence of iron deficiency has also been reported in elderly Europeans *(6)*. Anemia is frequently seen in older adults who have chronic inflammatory diseases *(7)*. It is often difficult to differentiate between the anemia associated with chronic inflammatory processes and that associated with dietary iron deficiency. A diagnosis can be made using measures of serum ferritin, plasma transferrin receptors, and erythrocyte sedimentation rate *(8)*.

When there is a reduced incidence of iron deficiency, there is an increase in serum ferritin levels; this has been noted in men and postmenopausal women *(5)*. It has been postulated that an increase in tissue iron stores is a risk factor for ischemic heart disease *(9)*, although this has yet to be proven *(10,11)*. One study investigated the impact of stored iron in postmenopausal women *(12)*. After instituting a daily walking regimen in the subjects over a 24-wk period, the investigators noted a decrease in stored iron.

Relationships between dietary iron supplementation, an increase in serum ferritin, and the development of colorectal cancer have also been investigated with inconclusive results. *(13,14)* Nevertheless, iron supplementation in adults who are not iron deficient should be pursued with caution *(15)*.

2.2. Iron Deficiency Anemia

Although iron deficiency anemia is a relatively uncommon finding in the United States, anemia has been demonstrated to be a common finding in elderly people, with a higher incidence among hospitalized, institutionalized, and homebound older people *(16,17)*. Over the years, the etiology of this anemia has been questioned. Is it associated with advanced age or is there an underlying pathology that can be corrected? Is it associated with lifelong poor iron nutriture? Epidemiologic studies indicate that there is a higher prevalence of anemia among low socioeconomic status groups which had other indicators of poor nutritional status (i.e., low serum albumin, transferrin, and prealbumin). There does not appear to be a significant effect of age on the incidence of iron deficiency anemia.

There does seem to be a high incidence of nutrient deficiencies among elderly people which may contribute to the frequency of anemia. In particular, it may be related to inadequate intake of vitamins B_6, B_{12} *(18,19)*, folate *(19)*, and iron.

Iron is one of the nutrients that is often deficient in the diets of many older adults. Although the risk for iron deficiency is common throughout the world in premenopausal or pregnant women and in infants and young children, the risk changes because the physiologic need for iron changes with advancing age and with increased iron stores. For older males, iron stores average approximately 1200 mg. In women, average iron stores increase from about 300 mg to 800 mg in the decade after menopause; this occurs due to a cessation of blood loss from menstruation. Iron deficiency is not the most common anemia in elderly people although it may be more common among hospitalized older individuals (20). Perhaps the most common cause of iron deficiency anemia in elderly people is blood loss, usually from the gastrointestinal tract (21). There are, however, other anemias that are seen in elderly populations, often associated with chronic disease, inflammatory processes (22,23) or malnutrition.

In the elderly, iron deficiency sometimes manifests itself as a condition called restless leg syndrome. Iron supplementation can produce a significant reduction in symptoms (24).

If iron deficiency associated with poor dietary intake occurs, providing a diet rich in iron-containing foods should be the first option (3). If iron deficiency is associated with other causes, the most effective therapy is to first correct the underlying problem and then to restore iron status by administering oral iron salts, generally ferrous sulfate (20). To enhance absorption and decrease gastrointestinal side effects of iron salts, the daily dose should be divided and taken with meals. Older patients respond to this regimen as rapidly as do younger individuals, but it is very important to correct the underlying cause of iron deficiency.

There are individuals who have conditions that limit the use of oral iron supplements. For these patients, parenteral iron supplementation may be used for short-term therapy (25,26).

2.3. Hemochromatosis in the Elderly

Hemochromatosis is a metabolic disorder in which the intestinal mechanisms that regulate the absorption of iron are dysfunctional, thereby leading to an increase of tissue iron content (see also Chapter 12). This accumulation of iron with deposition in soft tissue leads to the functional failure of vital organs, including liver, heart, pancreas, and pituitary gland (27).

Although this condition is familial, symptoms may not appear until those afflicted are adults. The first manifestation is usually skin hyperpigmentation due to the deposition of excess iron in the basal layer of the skin and the associated increase in melanin production (27). Clinical outcomes due to the accumulation of iron include heart failure due to cardiomyopathy leading to cardiac fibrosis; diabetes with pancreatic involvement; hypogonadism; polyarthritis; and a high incidence of hepatic carcinoma (27–30).

In recent years, a genetic screening by measuring transferrin saturation and by measuring other iron status indicators have proved effective in identifying individuals who are homozygous for the genes associated with this disorder (31–34). Early diagnosis with appropriate treatment will increase longevity. Hemochromatosis can be expressed in any stage of life, even into the 7th or 8th decade (35). Treatment options may be phlebotomy or the use of parenteral and oral iron chelating agents (27).

3. ZINC

Zinc requirements for adults over age 51 were established at 15 mg for men and 12 mg for women (1). Although these recommended levels do not seem excessively high, there is evidence that they are not met in many older adults (36–38). In a summary of 10 studies, mean dietary intake of zinc was 50–67% of the recommended dietary intake *(1)*. An age-related decrease in zinc absorption is controversial with evidence that supports an alteration in absorption as well as data that support no changes with age *(39,40)*. Malabsorption syndromes may impair zinc nutriture since the absorption of zinc in the bowel appears to be a critical factor. Both prescription and over-the-counter medications may also interfere with zinc absorption or increase zinc losses, for example, diuretics, laxatives, and antacids *(41)*. Another aspect of the challenge in assessing zinc status is the ability to accurately measure it in elderly subjects; a lack of statistical correlation between serum zinc and dietary intake raises concerns about the utility of this measure *(42)*.

Recent reports indicate that, whether or not there is an age-related decrease in zinc absorption, there are nutrients that may inhibit or interfere with the absorption of zinc, for example, some dietary proteins *(43)*.

Zinc is an essential component of many biomembranes and in many physiologic processes, including DNA synthesis, protein synthesis, cell division, lymphocyte proliferation, and the production of other vital biologic elements such as helper T leukocytes and interleukin-2. Zinc deficiency is associated with skin changes, poor appetite, loss of taste acuity, delayed or impaired wound healing, neurosensory disorders, and cell-mediated immune disorders *(44,45)*.

Zinc inadequacy is widespread throughout the world so it is likely that many noninstitutionalized older people are at risk of deficiency because of their dietary intake or the possibility of poor absorption *(46,47)*. In a recent study, it was reported that dietary zinc intake was low in hospitalized elderly women, probably due to poor intake of energy and other nutrients. There is evidence that dietary zinc deficiency may exist in individuals who are hospitalized for a variety of reasons *(47)*, have rheumatoid arthritis *(48)*, and head and neck cancer *(49)*. In hypertensive patients, zinc status was affected by treatment with captopril which led to increased urinary zinc excretion *(50)*.

3.1. Zinc Supplementation

Zinc is a nutrient that is often supplemented in long-term care patients to enhance wound healing or to minimize skin breakdown. Prospectively, this therapy has not been demonstrated to be either efficacious or ineffective unless an individual is zinc deficient, however, in a percent of this population, anemia and copper deficiency may be exacerbated by zinc supplementation *(51)*. Zinc supplementation has been demonstrated to decrease plasma lipid peroxides in noninstitutionalized elderly people *(52)* and improve cell-mediated immune response *(53)*. In a study conducted in France, supplementation with 20 mg of zinc and 100 mcg of selenium proved adequate to correct deficiencies in these nutrients and to reduce the number of infectious episodes in institutionalized elderly *(54)*. There has also been some speculation that supplementation with zinc and other anti-oxidant nutrients may have a weak protective effect against age-related macular degeneration *(55)*. In other reports, the evidence that zinc has a great impact on different measures of immune function is less definite *(56,57)*, and there is evidence that declines in immune function in healthy, elderly individuals are not related to plasma zinc status *(57)*.

Zinc supplementation may interfere with the absorption of other like minerals; supplementation with other divalent minerals, such as calcium, may affect zinc absorption *(58)*. Future zinc recommendations may be based on the level of bioavailability of its source *(59,60)*.

4. IODINE

Iodine is an essential nutrient because it is necessary for the normal production and action of thyroxine and triiodothyronine, thyroid hormones (*see* Chapter 13). The recommended dietary allowance for iodine for adults is 150 μg/d *(1)*. Iodine deficiency is not common among adults although it has been reported in children. Iodine deficiency that may result in goiter, hypothyroidism, or cretinism is considered a public health problem in some communities *(61)*, particularly in developing countries *(62,63)*. Dietary intake of iodine in the United States, evaluated in the 1982–1991 Total Diet Studies, appears to be adequate *(37)* (*see* Chapter 4).

Iodine can easily and safely be supplemented by adding it to food products such as salt, bread, or dairy products *(64,65)*. Even in communities where dietary iodine insufficiency among elderly people has been demonstrated, it is difficult to evaluate due to great variability among those who use supplements *(66)*. In countries that have used iodized salt to successfully address an endemic iodine deficiency, iodine deficiency should theoretically not exist, however, among those who have reduced their dietary salt consumption, the assumption of adequate intake may prove to be erroneous *(67)*. Even where salt has been iodized because of low soil iodine concentrations, deficient intake in the population may emerge when assessed by urinary iodide excretion and measurement of thyroid hormones *(68)*.

In the United States, there does not appear to be a problem of iodine deficiency among older adults, however, high intake levels associated with iodine supplementation may lead to thyrotoxicosis *(41)*.

5. MAGNESIUM

Although not generally considered a trace mineral because of its requirement levels, magnesium is included here because of its importance in many metabolic reactions. The recommended dietary allowance for magnesium is 350 mg/d for men and 280 mg/d for women with no difference found for elderly adults *(1,69)*. The establishment of criteria for assessment of magnesium status is challenging due to the constancy of the serum magnesium concentration (between 0.7–1.1 mmol/L); there does not seem to be any age-related decrease in serum magnesium levels.

A working group on establishing new dietary allowances with updated recommendations has raised some interesting issues about new ways of determining dietary magnesium needs by using metabolic balance based on lean body mass or energy expenditure rather than on weight *(70)*. Additionally, the working group encourages further investigation into claims that magnesium may have a role in the prevention or treatment of heart disease or hypertension.

Using the present recommendations, it has been reported that intakes of magnesium in adults are marginal *(69)* thereby raising concern about the potential for deficiency in elderly people who have gastrointestinal disorders that impair the absorption of magnesium or renal conditions that affect its urinary excretion. In a study designed to evaluate the impact of achlorhydria, a gastrointestinal condition more common in older adults, there did not appear to be any significant malabsorption of magnesium *(71)*.

Hypomagnesemia may produce irritability and other mental changes as measured by electroencephalogram *(72)* although it may not be common, magnesium depletion should be considered when evaluating mental changes in older adults. Hypomagnesemia may also be a factor in depressed immune function; muscle atrophy; osteoporosis; hyperglycemia; hyperlipidemia; and other neuromuscular, cardiovascular, and renal symptomatologies that are associated with advancing age *(73)*. It may result from dietary insufficiency or from various chronic conditions associated with aging such as noninsulin dependent diabetes or the use of diuretics that enhance magnesium excretion. Hypermagnesemia is not seen very frequently but may be suspected in individuals who have renal insufficiency and are taking magnesium-containing antacids or laxatives *(69)*.

6. COPPER

Copper is one of the earliest identified essential trace minerals *(41)*. Copper is essential in the function of several enzymes and required in host defense mechanisms, bone strength, iron transport, cholesterol and glucose metabolism, myocardial contractility, and other functions *(74)*. Copper appears to be well-regulated by homeostatic mechanisms but these mechanisms are poorly understood; when copper intake and absorption are high, more copper is excreted and when copper intake is low, it is conserved, thus maintaining an appropriate body copper pool *(75,76)*. Approximately 30–40% of dietary copper is absorbed, probably through a carrier-mediated transport mechanism. Aging may decrease the efficiency of copper homeostasis which results in higher plasma copper concentrations in older people *(77)*.

There are no RDAs for copper, however, the Committee on Dietary Allowances has included copper in the Estimated Safe and Adequate Daily Dietary Intake (ESADDI) category and established the level at 1.5–3 mg/d for adults *(1)*. In a series of surveys *(78–80)*, it was demonstrated that many elderly individuals do not consume the ESADDI for copper, however when they consume diets that provide copper within the ESADDI range, they can maintain copper balance *(81)*.

Copper deficiency is difficult to diagnose. The manifestations of deficiency are anemia, neutropenia, and osteoporosis which are associated with many other etiologies, deficiencies, and conditions. Copper deficiency may also be related to hypercholesterolemia, hypertriglyceridemia, glucose intolerance, and hypertension, risk factors for cardiovascular disease *(41)*. Copper may have a role in the action of antioxidant therapy on arterial atherosclerosis and, therefore, on the development of coronary heart disease (82) *(see* Chapter 15).

It has been suggested that nontraditional evaluation methods (e.g., erythrocyte superoxide dismutase, platelet cytochrome-c oxidase) may be better indicators of copper status than plasma copper or ceruloplasmin concentrations *(83,84)* *(see* Chapter 5). Overt copper deficiency in healthy older people is not generally considered to be a major concern; however, acquired deficiency may occur in malabsorption syndromes and other conditions *(85)*. Copper deficiency may be induced by physiologically similar trace minerals. In particular, zinc competes for absorption sites with copper and with a high dietary intake ratio of zinc to copper, copper absorption will be impaired and may result in symptomatic copper deficiency including dyslipidemia *(86)*. In a study conducted on elderly institutionalized individuals, it was determined that aging does not seem to have an impact on copper status *(87)*.

When copper is ingested in excess amounts, copper toxicity is a potential problem, but there are mechanisms to protect against the development of this condition, including metal-binding proteins *(88)*. High serum copper has been associated with increased cardiovascular mortality from coronary heart disease in men dying from cardiovascular disease *(89)*.

Copper has an important role in immune functions. In copper deficiency, Interleukin-2 and T-cell proliferation are reduced; the number of neutrophils are reduced and their ability to generate superoxide anion and kill ingested microorganisms is also decreased *(90–92)*. Copper is a nutrient that receives too little attention in assessment of nutritional status in elderly people.

7. CHROMIUM

The essentiality of chromium was recognized when its role in glucose tolerance was identified *(93)*. Chromium has been demonstrated to improve the glucose/insulin interaction in subjects with known hypoglycemia, hyperglycemia, diabetes, and hyperlipemia with no detectable effects on normal controls. There appears to be improved insulin binding, number of insulin receptors, beta cell sensitivity, and insulin receptor enzymes when supplementation of 500 µg of chromium picolinate is given twice a day *(94)*. There is no Recommended Dietary Allowance for chromium but there is an ESADDI range of 50 to 200 µg *(1)*. There is some controversy about the adequacy of this range for elderly people. It has been reported that the intake of chromium is below the ESADDI range in the diets of elderly subjects *(95)*. However, there is more recent evidence that the ESADDI range may be too high based on crude evaluation methods that have since been refined *(96)*.

Although there are still many unanswered questions about the role of chromium in glucose metabolism, chromium deficiency is characterized by impaired glucose tolerance, altered plasma lipid profile, and peripheral neuropathy *(41)*. One of the challenges in the assessment of chromium status is the lack of a definitive method for measuring it; most investigators are assessing chromium nutriture by inference: adding chromium to the diet and looking for an improvement of symptoms *(97,98)*. Chromium supplementation should be approached with some caution. However, trivalent chromium (CrIII) has been shown to have a large safety range and is well-tolerated at levels up to 1 mg/d *(99,100)* (*see* Chapter 7). The use of chromium supplements, usually as chromium picolinate, for extended periods or at high dosages, may lead to an accumulation of chromium (III) which may lead to DNA damage *(101)*.

8. SELENIUM

Selenium requirements in the United States have been established as 70 µg/d for males and 55 µg/d for females *(1)* however, the World Health Organization requirements are lower at 40 µg/d for males and 30 µg/d for females. Selenium is known to be an essential nutrient for humans *(102)* and its deficiency causes Keshan Disease (cardiomyopathy) and is related to the development of Kashin-Beck Disease (an osteoarthropathy), both of which were identified in China in areas where soil selenium is very low *(41)*. Selenium deficiency has also been linked to cancer *(103)*, muscular dystrophy, and cardiovascular disease *(104,105)*.

The problem of low soil selenium has been identified in locales other than China *(106,107)* and has been addressed in other countries in various ways; in Finland, for example, selenium has been added to fertilizers with a measurable increase in serum selenium among its citizens *(108)*. Selenium supplementation has been reported to restore selenium levels in many studies, but there are also reports that indicate there may be additional factors aside from selenium, including viral infection *(109)*, that contribute to the development of Keshan Disease *(110)*.

In elderly, institutionalized individuals, infection is a serious problem and trace mineral nutriture may have a role. In one study, supplementation with antioxidant minerals, including selenium, reduced the incidence of infection significantly although antioxidant vitamin supplementation did not have a similar effect *(111)*. In another study, decreased selenium and its relationship to senile cataracts was explored; the investigators conclusions attributed the development of the cataracts to defective antioxidant systems including selenium deficiency *(112)*. Aging is associated with a decline in immune function regardless of living situation. In another study, immune function in healthy, elderly people was maintained with supplementation of trace minerals and other micronutrients *(113)*. Others have shown that immune status in elderly subjects can be restored with moderate supplementation of antioxidant vitamins and minerals *(114)*.

Selenium status in elderly individuals seems to be related more to diet and to lifestyle than it is to their age or to institutionalization *(115)* although there does appear to be a negative correlation in some institutionalized populations for some nutrients, including selenium *(116)*. Other conditions in which supplementation with selenium may be appropriate are for individuals who are dependent on enteral or parenteral feedings for extended periods of time, particularly patients who are losing intestinal secretions *(117)* (*see* Chapter 20).

For patients who are suspected of being selenium deficient, selenium supplementation is a reasonable therapy. In one prospective, randomized, double-blind study, selenium supplementation in parenterally fed patients did not appear to have a major impact on cardiac function or on skeletal myopathy *(118)*. However, in another investigation conducted on patients who were sustained on enteral feeding for an extended period, selenium supplementation led to an improved serum profile and an alleviation of their symptoms which included muscle pain and weakness, gait disturbance, palpitation, and shortness of breath *(119)*.

Assuring adequate intake of selenium is important in the elderly, however, large doses may lead to toxicity. Selenium toxicity symptoms include nausea, vomiting, hair loss, nail changes, irritability, fatigue, and peripheral neuropathy *(120)*. Selenium nutriture can be assessed by monitoring serum or erythrocyte levels of selenium or selenium-dependent glutathione peroxidase concentrations *(121,122)*.

9. ALUMINUM

Aluminum has not been identified as an essential nutrient and seems to have no specific requirement in any metabolic process, however, it does deserve some mention due to its controversial association with the development of senile dementia of the Alzheimer's type and other toxic reactions *(41,123)*. Exposure to aluminum may occur when aluminum-containing over-the-counter remedies are used indiscriminately, or there is excessive use of aluminum cookware, utensils, and foil wraps with high acid foods such as tomato. However, the exposure to aluminum in cooking does not add aluminum to food in any significant amounts *(124)*. Ingestion of large amounts of aluminum may occur through the use of antacids, buffered analgesics, some anti-ulcer products, anti-diarrheal remedies, and other medications *(125)*. This exposure may become a problem if there is a preexisting medical condition, such as renal disease (*see* Chapter 16). Patients who are dialyzed with aluminum-containing dialysates or treated with parenteral fluids that include aluminum may be at risk for toxicity. Clinical signs of toxicity include osteodystrophy, encephalopathy, and anemia *(126)*.

Aluminum is not absorbed in large amounts under normal circumstances, however, it has been suggested that with genetic predisposition, advanced age, or mucosal damage, aluminum may be absorbed in greater quantities. This may allow greater central nervous system exposure to aluminum, which may, in turn, contribute to its deposition in the brain *(127)*. Some investigators believe that these factors contribute to the development of Alzheimer's disease. Others have reported that the aluminum depositions are located in structural sites that are not necessarily associated with this disease *(128)*. During the 1980s there were many reports that supported this theory *(129–132)* but other hypotheses suggest other etiologies *(133,134)*. What belies the aluminum exposure theory is that the first case of Alzheimer's disease with aluminum-containing neurofibrillary plaques in the brain was first described in 1907, long before aluminum use in cookware, dialysis fluids, or over-the-counter drugs *(135)*.

10. OTHER TRACE MINERALS

There is very little evidence that there are significant differences for trace element requirements in older adults than for the remainder of the population. Manganese deficiency is extremely difficult to define or identify. Although there are some reports that other dietary components interfere with manganese absorption *(136–140)*, it has been postulated that marginal manganese deficiency is not easily recognized *(41)*.

Boron is a micromineral that is often considered as an adjunct to calcium metabolism with a positive effect on bone mineralization *(141)*. There may be a relationship between boron and magnesium, with the net effect being excretion of calcium. In individuals who were put on low magnesium diets, boron supplementation increased urinary calcium excretion. In this study, supplementation with boron did not change plasma boron concentrations and fecal excretion accounted for nearly all the extra boron. There seems to be a homeostasic mechanism that functions to maintain plasma levels *(142)*. The establishment of recommended dietary allowances for an essential trace mineral requires clear evidence of essentiality despite less clear information regarding deficiencies. Thus far, criteria for boron requirements are still unclear *(143)*.

The essentiality of lead is unclear although there does seem to be a link with iron metabolism *(144)*. Human requirements are unknown and lead has gotten more attention when lead toxicity occurs. Although more commonly recognized in children living in poverty, lead poisoning from ingesting lead-based paint has been reported in elderly institutionalized individuals *(145)*.

What may be clinically significant about elevated lead levels is a link to elevated blood pressure. It has been reported that blood lead is a significant predictor of increased diastolic and systolic blood pressure *(146)*. Low level exposure to lead has also been linked to impaired renal function in older adults *(147)*.

11. CONCLUSIONS

For some trace elements, there is a great deal of information regarding requirements for older adults as well as associations with the development or exacerbation of medical conditions. For other minerals, there is very little data available on either requirements or age-related alterations in metabolism. Clearly some of these elements have roles in the maintenance of health (e.g., immune function integrity *[148]*) but there is a compelling need for research in the physiologic requirements for the essential trace elements and minerals in elderly individuals.

REFERENCES

1. Food and Nutrition Board, National Research Council. Recommended Dietary Allowances, 10th edition, National Academy Press, Washington, DC, 1989.
2. Chernoff R. Demographics of aging. In: Chernoff R. ed. Geriatric Nutrition: A Health Professional's Handbook, 2nd edition, Aspen Publishers, Gaithersburg, MD. 1999.
3. Roebothan BV, Chandra RK. The contribution of dietary iron to iron status in a group of elderly subjects. Int J Vitam Nutr Res 1996;66:66–70.
4. Fleming DJ, Jacques PF, Dallal GE, et al. Dietary determinants of iron stores in a free-living elderly population: The Framingham Heart Study. Am J Clin Nutr 1998;67:722–733.
5. Lynch SR, Baynes RD. Deliberations and evaluations of the approaches, endpoints and paradigms for iron dietary recommendations. J Nutr 1996;126(9 Suppl): 2404S–2409S.
6. Lesourd B, Decarli B, Dirren H. Longitudinal changes in iron and protein status of elderly Europeans. SENECA Investigators. Eur J Clin Nutr 1996;50(Suppl 2): S16–S24.
7. Chiari MM, Bagnoli R, DeLuca PD, et al. Influence of acute inflammation on iron and nutritional status indexes in older inpatients. J Am Geriatr Soc 1995;43:767–771.
8. Ahluwalia N, Lammi-Keefe CJ, Bendel RB, et al. Iron deficiency and anemia of chronic disease in elderly women: a discriminant-analysis approach for differentiation. Am J Clin Nutr 1995; 61:590–596.
9. Tzonou A, Lagiou P, Trichopoulou A, et al. Dietary iron and coronary heart disease risk: a study from Greece. Am J Epidemiol 1998;147:161–166.
10. Reunanen A, Takkunen H, Knekt P, et al. Body iron stores, dietary iron intake and coronary heart disease. J Inter Med 1995;238:223–230.
11. Sempos CT, Looker AC, Gillum RF. Iron and heart disease: the epidemiologic data. Nutri Rev 1996;54:73–84.
12. Naimark BJ, Ready AE, Sawatzky JA, et al. Serum ferritin and heart disease: the effect of moderate exercise on stored iron levels in postmenopausal women. Canadian J Cardiol 1996;12:1253–1257.
13. Tseng M, Sandler RS, Greenberg ER, et al. Dietary iron and recurrence of colorectal adenomas. Cancer Epidemiology, Biomarkers & Prevention 1997;6:1029–1032.
14. Ullen H, Augustsson K, Gustavsson C, et al. Supplementary iron intake and risk of cancer: reversed causality? Cancer Lett 1997;114(1–2):215–216.
15. Johnson MA, Fischer JG, Bowman BA, et al. Iron nutriture in elderly individuals. FASEB J 1994;8:609–621.
16. Beard JL, Richards RE, Smiciklas-Wright H, et al. Iron nutrition in rural homebound elderly persons. J Nutr Elderly 1996;15:3–19.
17. Smieja MJ, Cook DJ, Hunt DL, et al. Recognizing and investigating iron-deficiency anemia in hospitalized elderly people. Canadian Med Assoc J 1996;155:691–696.
18. Hash RB, Sargent MA, Katner H. Anemia secondary to combined deficiencies of iron and cobalamin. Arch Fam Med 1996;5:585–588.
19. Charlton KE, Kruger M, Labadarios D, et al. Iron, folate and vitamin B_{12} status of an elderly South African population. Eur J Clin Nutr 1997;51:424–430.
20. Kohli M, Lipschitz DA, Chatta GS. Impact of nutrition on declines in hematopoiesis. In: Chernoff R. ed. Geriatric Nutrition: A Health Professional's Handbook, 2nd edition, Aspen Publishers, Gaithersburg, MD, 1999.
21. Moses PL, Smith RE. Endoscopic evaluation of iron deficiency anemia. A guide to diagnostic strategy in older patients. Postgraduate Med 1995;98:213–216, 222–224.
22. Walter T, Olivares M, Pizarro F et al. Iron, anemia, and infection. Nutr Rev 1997;55:111–124.
23. Chiari MM, Bagnoli R, De Luca PD, et al. Influence of acute inflammation on iron and nutritional status indexes in older inpatients. J Am Geriatr Soc 1995;43:767–771.
24. O'Keeffe ST, Gavin K, Lavan JN. Iron status and restless legs syndrome in the elderly. Age & Ageing 1994;23:200–203.
25. Kumpf VJ. Parenteral iron supplementation. Nutr Clin Practice 1996;11:139–146.
26. Burns DL, Mascioli EA, Bistrian BR. Effect of iron-supplemented total parenteral nutrition in patients with iron deficiency anemia. Nutrition 1996;12:411–415.
27. Weintraub LR. The many faces of hemochromatosis. Hospital Practice 1991;26:49–59.
28. Niederau C, Fischer R, Purschel A, et al. Long–term survival in patients with hereditary hemochromatosis. Gastroenterology 1996;110:1107–1119.
29. Adams PC, Kertesz AE, Valberg LS. Clinical presentation of hemochromatosis: a changing scene. Amer J Med 1991;90:445–449.

30. Montgomery KD, Williams JR, Sculco TP, et al. Clinical and pathologic findings in hemochromatosis hip arthropathy. Clin Ortho Related Res 1998;347:179–187.
31. Phatak PD, Sham RL, Raubertas RF, et al. Prevalence of hereditary hemochromatosis in 16031 primary care patients. Ann Int Med 1998;129:954–961.
32. Powell LW, Summers KM, Board PG, et al. Expression of hemochromatosis in homozygous subjects. Implications for early diagnosis and prevention. Gastroenterology 1990;98:1625–1632.
33. Balan V, Baldus W, Fairbanks V, et al. Screening for hemochromatosis: a cost-effectiveness study based on 12,258 patients. Gastroenterology 1994;107:453–459.
34. Adams PC, Gregor JC, Kertesz AE, et al. Screening blood donors for hereditary hemochromatosis: decision analysis model based on a 30-year database. Gastroenterology 1995;109:177–188.
35. Crosby WH. Old age and hemochromatosis. J Amer Med Assoc 1992;268:802.
36. Fosmire G, Manuel P, Smiciklas-Wright H. 1984; Dietary intakes and zinc status of an elderly rural population. J Nutr Elderly 1992;4:19–30.
37. Pennington J. Intakes of minerals from diets and foods: Is there a need for concern? J Nutr 1996;126:2304S–2308S.
38. Solomons N. Trace elements in nutrition of the elderly 1:established RDAs for iron, zinc, and iodine. Postgraduate Med 1986;79:231–242.
39. Bales C, Steinman L, Freeland-Graves J, et al. The effect of age on plasma zinc, uptake, and taste acuity. Am J Clin Nutr 1986;44:664–669.
40. Couzy F, Kastenmayer P, Mansourian R, et al. Zinc absorption in healthy elderly humans and the effect of diet. Am J Clin Nutr 1993;58:609–694.
41. Fosmire G. Trace metal requirements. In: Chernoff R. ed. Geriatric Nutrition: A Health Professional's Handbook, 2nd edition, Aspen Publishers, Gaithersburg, MD,1999.
42. Artacho R, Ruiz–Lopez MD, Gamez C, et al. Serum concentration and dietary intake of Zn in healthy institutionalized elderly subjects. Sci Total Environ 1997;205:159–165
43. Davidson L, Almgren A, Sandstrom B, et al. Zinc absorption in adult humans: the effect of protein sources added to liquid test meals. Br J Nutr 1996;75:607–613.
44. Prasad AS. Zinc: an overview. Nutrition 1995;11(1Suppl):93–99.
45. Weiffenbach JM, Baum BJ, Burghauser R. Taste thresholds: quality specific variation with human aging. J Gerontology 1982;37:372–377.
46. Mares-Perlman JA, Subar AF, Block G, et al. Zinc intake and sources in the US adult population: 1976–1980. J Amer Coll Nutr 1995;14:349–357.
47. Schmuck A, Roussel AM, Arnaud J, et al. Analyzed dietary intakes, plasma concentrations of zinc, copper, and selenium, and related antioxidant enzyme activities in hospitalized elderly women. J Amer Coll Nutr 1996;15:462–468.
48. Kremer JM, Bigaouette J. Nutrient intake of patients with rheumatoid arthritis is deficient in pyridoxine, zinc, copper, and magnesium. J Rheumatology 1996;23:990–994.
49. Doerr TD, Prasad AS, Marks SC, et al. Zinc deficiency in head and neck cancer patients. J Amer Coll Nutr 1997;16:418–422.
50. Golik A, Zaidenstein R, Dishi V, et al. Effects of captopril and enalapril on zinc metabolism in hypertensive patients. J Amer Coll Nutr 1998;17:75–78.
51. Eleazer GP, Bird L, Egbert J, et al. Appropriate protocol for zinc therapy in long term care facilities. J Nutr Elderly 1995;14:31–38.
52. Fortes C, Agabiti N, Fano V, et al. Zinc supplementation and plasma lipid peroxides in an elderly population. Eur J Clin Nutr 1997;51:97–101.
53. Fortes C, Forastiere F, Agabiti N, et al. The effect of zinc and vitamin A supplementation on immune response in an older population. J Amer Geriatr Soc 1998;46:19–26.
54. Girodon F, Lombard M, Galan P, et al. Effect of micronutrient supplementation on infection in institutionalized elderly subjects: a controlled trial. Ann Nut Metab 1997;41:98–107.
55. Mares-Perlman JA, Klein R, Klein BE, et al. Association of zinc and antioxidant nutrients with age–related maculopathy. Arch Ophthalmology 1996;114:991–997.
56. Gardner EM, Bernstein ED, Dorfman M, et al. The age-associated decline in immune function of healthy individuals is not related to changes in plasma concentrations of beta-carotene, retinol, alpha-tocopherol or zinc. Mech Age Dev 1997;94:55–69.
57. Weksler ME. Immune senescence: deficiency or dysregulation. Nutr Rev 1995;53:S3–S7.
58. Wood RJ, Zheng JJ. High dietary calcium intakes reduce zinc absorption and balance in humans. Am J Clin Nutr 1997;65:1803–1809.

59. Sandstead HH, Smith JC, Jr. Deliberations and evaluations of approaches, endpoints and paradigms for determining zinc dietary recommendations. J Nutr 126(9 Suppl):2410S–2418S.

60. Hunt JR. Bioavailability algorithms in setting Recommended Dietary Allowances: lessons from iron, applications to zinc. J Nutr 126(9 Suppl):2345S–2353S.

61. Dunn JT. Seven deadly sins in confronting endemic iodine deficiency, and how to avoid them. J Clin Endocrinol Metab 1996;81:1332–1335.

62. Ali O. Iodine deficiency disorders: a public health challenge in developing countries. Nutrition 1995;11(5 Suppl):517–520.

63. Hou X, Chai C, Qian Q, et al. The study of iodine in Chinese total diets. Sci Total Environment 1997;193:161–167.

64. Brussaard JH, Hulshof KF, Lowik MR. Calculated iodine intake before and after simulated iodization Dutch Nutrition Surveillance System;. Annals Nutr Metab 1995;39:85–94.

65. Ranganathan S, Reddy V. Human requirements of iodine & safe use of iodised salt. Indian J Med Res 1995;102:227–232.

66. Pedersen KM, Iversen E, Laurberg P. Urinary iodine excretion and individual iodine supplementation among elderly subjects: a cross-sectional investigation in the commune of Randers, Denmark. Eur J Endocrinol 1995;132:171–174.

67. Als C, Lauber K, Brander L, et al. The instability of dietary iodine supply over time in an affluent society. Experientia 1995;51:623–633.

68. Thomson CD, Colls AJ, Conaglen JV, et al. Iodine status of New Zealand residents as assessed by urinary iodide excretion and thyroid hormones. Br J Nutr 1997;78:901–912.

69. Lindeman RD. Mineral requirements. In: Chernoff R. ed. Geriatric Nutrition: A Health Professional's Handbook, 2nd edition, Aspen Publishers, Gaithersburg, MD,1999.

70. Shils ME, Rude RK. Deliberations and evaluations of the approaches, endpoints and paradigms for magnesium dietary recommendations. J Nutr 1996;126(9 Suppl):2398S–2403S.

71. Serfaty-Lacrosniere C, Wood RJ, Voytko D, et al. Hypochlorhydria from short-term omeprazole treatment does not inhibit intestinal absorption of calcium, phosphorus, magnesium or zinc from food in humans. J Amer Coll Nutr 1995;14:364–368.

72. Penland JG. Quantitative analysis of EEG effects following experimental marginal magnesium and boron deprivation. Magnesium Res 1995;8:341–358.

73. Durlach J, Durlach V, Bac P, et al. Magnesium and ageing. II. Clinical data: aetological mechanisms and pathophysiological consequences of magnesium deficit in the elderly. Magnesium Res 1993;6:379–394.

74. Olivares M, Uauy R. Copper as an essential nutrient. Am J Clin Nutr 1996;63:791S–796S.

75. Turnlund J. Human whole-body copper metabolism. Am J Clin Nutr 1998;67(5 Suppl):960S–964S.

76. Aggett PJ, Fairweather-Tait S. Adaptation to high and low copper intakes: its relevance to estimated safe and adequate daily dietary intakes. Am J Clin Nutr 1998;67(5 Suppl):1061S–1063S.

77. Wapnir RA. Copper absorption and bioavailability. Am J Clin Nutr 67(5 Suppl):1054S–1060S.

78. Schmuck A, Roussel A-M, Arnaud J, et al. Analyzed dietary intakes, plasma concentrations of zinc, copper, selenium, and related antioxidant enzyme activities in hospitalized elderly women. J Amer Coll Nutr 1996;15:462–468.

79. Pennington J, Young B, Wilson D. Nutritional elements in US diets: results from the total diet study, 1982 to 1986. J Amer Diet Assoc 1989;89:659–664.

80. Gibson R, Anderson B, Sabry J. The trace metal status of a group of post-menopausal vegetarians. J Amer Dietetic Assoc 1983;82:246–250.

81. Solomons N. Trace elements in nutrition of the elderly, 2: E SADDIs for copper, manganese, selenium, chromium, molybdenum, and flouride. Postgrad Med 1986;79:251–263.

82. O'Leary VJ, Tilling L, Fleetwood G, et al. The resistance of low density lipoprotein to oxidation promoted by copper and its use as an index of antioxidant therapy. Atherosclerosis 1996;119:169–179.

83. Milne DB. Copper intake and assessment of copper status. Am J Clin Nutr 1998;67(5 Suppl):1041S–1045S.

84. Milne DB, Nielsen FH. Effects of a diet low in copper on copper-status indicators in postmenopausal women. Am J Clin Nutr 1996;63:358–364.

85. Sandstead HH. Requirements and toxicity of essential trace elements, illustrated by zinc and copper. Am J Clin Nutr 1995;61(3 Suppl):621S–624S.

86. Beshgetoor D, Hambidge M. Clinical conditions altering copper metabolism in humans. Am J Clin Nutr 1998;67(5 Suppl):1017S–1021S.

87. Gamez C, Artacho R, Luiz-Lopez MD, et al. Serum copper in institutionalized elderly subjects: relations with dietary intake of energy, specific nutrients and haematological parameters. Sci Total Environ 1997;201:31–38.

88. Dameron CT, Harrison MD. 1998; Mechanisms for protection against copper toxicity. Am J Clin Nut 675 Suppl;, 1091S–1097S.

89. Reunanen A, Knekt P, Marniemi J, et al. Serum calcium, magnesium, copper and zinc and risk of cardiovascular death. Eur J Clin Nutr 1996;50:431–437.

90. Percival SS. Copper and immunity. Am J Clin Nutr 1998;67(5 Suppl):1064S–1068S.

91. Kelley DS, Daudu PA, Taylor PC, et al. Effects of low-copper diets on human immune response. Am J Clin Nutr 1995;62:412–416.

92. Percival SS. Neutropenia caused by copper deficiency: possible mechanisms of action. Nutr Rev 1995;53:59–66.

93. Schwarz K, Mertz W. Chromium (III) and the glucose tolerance factor. Arch Biochem Biophys 1959;85: 292–295.

94. Anderson A. Nutritional factors influencing the glucose/insulin system: chromium. J Amer Coll Nutr 1997;16:404–410.

95. Offenbacher E. Chromium in the elderly. Biol Trace Elem Res 1992;32:123–131.

96. Stocker B. 1996; Chromium in Ziegler E, Filer L Jr Eds; Present Knowldge in Nutrition 7th edition, Washington DC:ILSI Press.

97. Urberg M, Zemel M. Evidence for synergism between chromium and nicotinic acid in the control of glucose tolerance in elderly humans. Metabolism 1987;36:896–899.

98. Martinez O, MacDonald A, Gibson R, et al. Dietary chromium and effect of chromium supplementation on glucose tolerance of elderly Canadian women. Nutr Res 1985;5:609–620.

99. Anderson RA. Chromium as an essential nutrient for humans. Regul Toxicol & Pharmacol 1997;26(1 Pt2):S35–41.

100. McCarty MF. Subtoxic intracellular trivalent chromium is not mutagenic: implications for safety of chromium supplementation. Med Hypoth 1997;49:263–269.

101. Stearns DM, Belbruno JJ, Wetterhahn KE A prediction of chromium (III) accumulation in humans from chromium dietary supplements. FASEB J 1995;9:1650–1657

102. Foster LH, Sumar S. Selenium in health and disease: a review Crit Rev Food Sci Nutr 1997;37:211–228.

103. Anonymous. Dietary selenium repletion may reduce cancer incidences in people at high risk who live in areas with low soil selenium. Nutr Rev 1997;55:277–279.

104. Hughes K, Ong CN. Vitamins, selenium, iron, and coronary heart disease risk in Indians, Malays, and Chinese in Singapore. J Epidemiol Commun Health 1998;52:181–185.

105. Levander OA. Selenium requirements as discussed in the 1996 joint FAO/IAEA/WHO expert consultation on trace elements in human nutrition. Biomed Environ Sci 1997;10(2–3):214–219.

106. Maksimovic ZJ, Djujic I. Selenium deficiency in Serbia and possible effects on health. Biomed Environ Sci 10(2–3):300–306.

107. Kadrabova J, Mad'aric A, Ginter E. Determination of the daily selenium intake in Slovakia. Biol Trace Element Res 1998;61:277–286.

108. Aro A, Alfthan G, Varo P. Effects of supplementation of fertilizers on human selenium status in Finland. Analyst 1995;120:841–843.

109. Bogden JD, Bendich A, Kemp FW, et al. Daily micronutrient supplements enhance delayed-hypersensitivity skin test responses in older people. Am J Clin Nutr 1994;60:437–447.

110. Xu GL, Wang SC, Gu BQ, et al. Further investigation on the role of selenium deficiency in the aetiology and pathogenesis of Keshan Disease. Biomed Environ Sci 1997;10:316–326.

111. Johnson MA, Porter MH. Micronutrient supplementation and infection in institutionalized elderly. Nutr Rev 1997;55(11 Pt1):400–404.

112. Karakucuk S, Ertugrul Mirza G, Faruk Ekinciler O, et al. Selenium concentrations in serum, lens and aqueous humor of patients with senile cataract. Acta Opthalmologica Scandinavica 1995;73(4):329–332.

113. Pike J, Chandra RK. Effect of vitamin and trace element supplementation on immune function indices in healthy elderly. Int J Vit Nutr Res 1995;65(2):117–121.

114. Monget AL, Richard MJ, Cournot MP, et al. Effect of 6 month supplementation with different combinations of an association of antioxidant nutrients on biochemical parameters and markers of the antioxidant defence system in the elderly. Eur J Clin Nutr 1996;50(7):443–449.

115. Ducros V, Faure P, Ferry M. et al. The sizes of the exchangeable pool of selenium in elderly women and their relation to institutionalization. Br J Nutr 1997;78(3):379–396.
116. Monget AL, Galan P, Preziosi P, et al. Micronutrient status in elderly people. Int J Vit Miner Res 1996;66(1):71–76.
117. Gramm HJ, Kopf A, Bratter P. The necessity of selenium substitution in total parenteral nutrition and artificial alimentation. J Trace Elements Med Biol 1995;9(1):1–12.
118. Rannem T, Ladefoged K, Hylander E, et al. The effect of selenium supplementation on skeletal and cardiac muscle in selenium-depleted patients. J Parenteral Enteral Nutr 1995;19(5):351–355.
119. Yagi M, Tani T, Hashimoto T, et al. Four cases of selenium deficiency in postoperative long-term enteral nutrition. Nutrition 1996;12:40–43.
120. Levander OA, Burk R. Selenium. In: Ziegler E, Filer L, Jr. eds. Present Knowledge in Nutrition, 7th edition. ILSI Press,Washington, DC, 1996.
121. Neve J. Human selenium supplementation as assessed by changes in blood selenium concentration and glutathione peroxidase activity. J Trace Elements Med Biol 1995;9:65–73.
122. Longnecker MP, Stram DO, Taylor PR, et al. Use of selenium concentration in whole blood, serum, toenails, or urine as a surrogate measure of selenium intake. Epidemiology 1996;7:384–390.
123. Shin RW. Interaction of aluminum with paired helical filament tau in involved in neurofibrillary pathology of Alzheimer's disease. Gerontology 1997;43(Suppl 1):16–23.
124. Pennington J. Aluminum content of foods and diets. Food Addit Contam 1988;5:161–232.
125. Lione A. Aluminum intake from non–prescription drugs and sucrafalate. Gen Pharmacol 1985;16:223–228.
126. Wills M, Savory J. Aluminum toxicity and chronic renal failure. In: Sigel H, ed. Metal Ions in Biological Systems. Marcel Dekker,New York, 1988.
127. Perl D. Aluminum and Alzheimer's disease, methodological approaches. In: Sigel H ed. Metal Ions in Biological Systems. Marcel Dekker, New York,1988;.
128. Kasa P, Szerdahelyi P, Wisniewski HM. Lack of topographical relationships between sites of aluminum deposition and senile plaques in the Alzheimer's disease brain. Acta Neuropathologica 1995;90:526–531.
129. McDermott J, Smith I, Iqbal K, et al. Brain aluminum in aging and Alzheimer's disease. Neurology 1979;29:809–814.
130. McLachlan DRC, Kruck TPA, VanBerkum MFA. Aluminum and neurodegenerative disease: therapeutic implications. Am J Kidney Dis 1985;5:322–329.
131. McLachlan DRC. Aluminum and Alzheimer's disease. Neurobiology Aging 1986;7:525–532.
132. Markesbery WR, Ehmann WD, Hossain TIM, et al. Instrumental neuron activation analysis of brain aluminum in Alzheimer's disease and aging. Annals Neurology 1981;10:511–516.
133. Bertholf RL. Aluminum and Alzheimer's disease: perspectives for a cytoskeletal mechanism. CRC Criti Rev Clin Lab Sci 1987;25:195–210.
134. Eichorn GL. Is there any relationship between aluminum and Alzheimer's disease? Experimental Gerontology 1993;28(4–5):493–498.
135. Alzheimer A. Über eine eigenartige erkrangkung der hirnrinde. All Z Psychiatr 1907;64:146–148.
136. Hallfrisch J, Powel A, Carafelli C, et al. Mineral balances of men and women consuming high fiber diets with complex or simple carbohydrates. J Nutr 1987;118:760–773.
137. Schwartz R, Apgar B, Wien E. Apparent absorption and retention of Ca, Cu, Mg, Mn, and Zn from a diet containing bran. Am J Clin Nutr 1986;43:444–455.
138. Lin P-H, Freeland-Graves J. Effects of simultaneous ingestion of calcium and manganese in humans. In: Bales C, ed. Mineral Homeostasis in the Elderly. Alan R Liss, Inc., New York, 1989.
139. Freeland-Graves J, Bales C, Behmardi F. Manganese requirements in humans. In: Kies C, ed. Nutritional Bioavailability of Manganese. American Chemical Society,Washington, 1987.
140. Dougherty V, Freeland-Graves J, Behmardi F, et al. Interactions of iron (Fe) and manganese in males fed varying levels of dietary manganese. Fed Proc 1987;46:914.
141. Meacham SL, Taper LJ, Volpe SL. Effect of boron supplementation on blood and urinary calcium, magnesium, and phosphorus, and urinary boron in athletic and sedentary women. Am J Clin Nutr 1995;61(2):341–345.
142. Hunt CD, Herbel JL, Nielsen FH. Metabolic responses of postmenopausal women to supplemental dietary boron and aluminum during usual and low magnesium intake: boron, calcium, and magnesium absorption and retention and blood mineral concentrations. Am J Clin Nutr 1997;65(3):803–813.
143. Hunt CD, Stoecker BJ. Deliberations and evaluations of the approaches, endpoints and paradigms for boron, chromium and fluoride dietary recommendations. J Nutr 1996;126(9 Suppl):2441S–2451S.

144. Nielsen FH. Ultratrace elements. In: Shils ME, Olson JA, Shike M, eds. Modern Nutrition in Health and Disease, 8th edition, Lea & Febiger, Philadelphia, 1994,pp.269–286.
145. Roberge RJ, Martin TG, Dean BS, et al. Ceramic lead glaze ingestions in nursing home residents with dementia. Am J Emerg Med 1994;12(1):77–81.
146. Menditto A, Morisi G, Spagnola A, et al. Association of blood lead to blood pressure in men aged 55 to 75 years: effect of selected social and biochemical cofounders. NFR Study Group. Environmental Health Perspectives 1994;102 (Suppl 9):107–111.
147. Kim R, Rotnitsky A, Sparrow D, et al. A longitudinal study of low-level lead exposure and impairment of renal function. The Normative Aging Study. JAMA 1996;275(15):1177–1181.
148. Bogden JD. Studies on micronutrient supplements and immunity in older people. Nutr Rev 1995;53:S59–S65.

III   TRACE ELEMENT AND MINERAL NUTRITION IN DISEASE

Genetic Disorders of Trace Element Metabolism

Gregory J. Anderson, MD and
Gordon D. McLaren, MD

1. INTRODUCTION

The spectrum of diseases which are passed on from parent to offspring i.e., the inherited or genetic diseases, encompasses most aspects of metabolism. The field of mineral metabolism is no exception and there exist a number of significant genetic abnormalities in humans affecting iron, copper, and zinc homeostasis. These diseases can lead to a deficiency of the metal in the tissues (e.g., Menkes disease — copper, acrodermatitis enteropathica — zinc) or an excess (e.g., hemochromatosis — iron, Wilson disease — copper) and thus can mimic the situations found in nutritional deficiency of the metal or those associated with excess exposure and toxicity. Although by their nature genetic disorders are often very rare, some are found in populations at sufficiently high frequencies that they represent a major health issue and can influence nutritional policies for the adequacy and safety of dietary trace element intake. The best example of this is the iron overload disease hemochromatosis, the most common of all autosomally inherited genetic diseases with an incidence in some populations as high as 1 in 250–300 *(1,2)*. In populations where hemochromatosis is prevalent there have been active campaigns to prevent the fortification of dietary staples with iron since this will accelerate iron accumulation in susceptible members of the population.

In addition to their obvious clinical implications for affected individuals, the analysis of genetic disorders of metal metabolism at both the phenotypic and genotypic level has contributed enormously to our understanding of normal trace element metabolism. In recent years this has been most apparent in the area of copper metabolism where the application of contemporary genetic and molecular technologies led first to the identification of the Menkes disease gene, a plasma membrane copper transporter, and then the Wilson disease gene. These discoveries have in turn spawned an extensive series of studies that have begun to link cellular and whole body phenotypes to their underlying molecular mechanisms. A similar revolution has begun in the area of iron homeostasis. The analysis of human genes has been supported and extended substantially by studies

From: *Clinical Nutrition of the Essential Trace Elements and Minerals: The Guide for Health Professionals*
Edited by: J. D. Bogden and L. M. Klevay © Humana Press Inc., Totowa, NJ

of their homologs in experimentally more tractable organisms such as yeast and mice. Indeed the analysis of human trace element metabolism has always drawn heavily on experimental animal models.

In this chapter we will describe briefly the major genetic diseases associated with abnormalities in iron, copper, and zinc metabolism. These include relatively well-known diseases such as hemochromatosis, Wilson disease and Menkes disease, as well as some less well studied clinical entities. Features of some of these are summarized in Fig. 1. The genes affected in a number of these diseases have now been identified, so the current state of knowledge of the molecular mechanisms underlying each disorder will be summarized. Wherever appropriate, some information will be provided on the contributions model organisms have made to the understanding of the molecular basis of trace element metabolism. Genetic disorders involving the other six essential trace elements (Cr,F,I,Mn,Mo,Se) have not been described and thus are not discussed in this chapter.

2. DISORDERS OF IRON METABOLISM

Hereditary disorders of iron metabolism in humans for the most part comprise conditions associated with an increased body storage iron level, or iron overload. Whereas body storage iron normally amounts to about 1 g or less, patients with the inherited disorder known as hemochromatosis may have iron stores that range anywhere from 4– 5 g to as high as 20–40 g or more in advanced cases *(3)*. Several other types of iron overload with a genetic component are also described. In some of these disorders (e.g., thalassemia major), the iron overload is secondary to another, primary, metabolic defect, yet affected individuals may accumulate amounts of iron comparable to the levels seen in patients with hereditary hemochromatosis *(4)*. From a clinical standpoint, severe iron overload causes damage to vital organs and, if untreated, may be fatal. In contrast, another inherited disorder of iron metabolism called the hyperferritinemia/cataract syndrome shows disease manifestations that are not associated with systemic iron overload *per se.*

2.1. Hemochromatosis

In patients with hereditary hemochromatosis (HHC) the normal mechanism by which the body maintains iron balance is disrupted, permitting continued iron absorption in excess of needs and progressive accretion of body iron stores. The increased absorption eventually leads to accumulation of iron to toxic levels, resulting in tissue damage involving the liver, heart, pancreas, joints, and other organs *(3)*. HHC is inherited in an autosomal recessive manner. The affected gene has long been known to be located on the short arm of chromosome 6 *(5)*, and, in 1996, Feder et al. *(6)* described a strong candidate gene telomeric to the major histocompatibility complex. The gene, which has been designated HFE, encodes an MHC class I - like protein of unknown function. Most patients with hemochromatosis are homozygous for a mutation producing a single amino acid substitution of tyrosine for cysteine at position 282 (abbreviated as C282Y). A second mutation, resulting in the substitution of histidine for asparagine at position 63 (abbreviated as H63D) has also been described. The relevance of the H63D mutation is controversial, but some patients with clinical manifestations of hemochromatosis are compound heterozygotes for the C282Y and H63D mutations. How the defective gene alters the body's ability to limit iron absorption in patients with hemochromatosis is unknown.

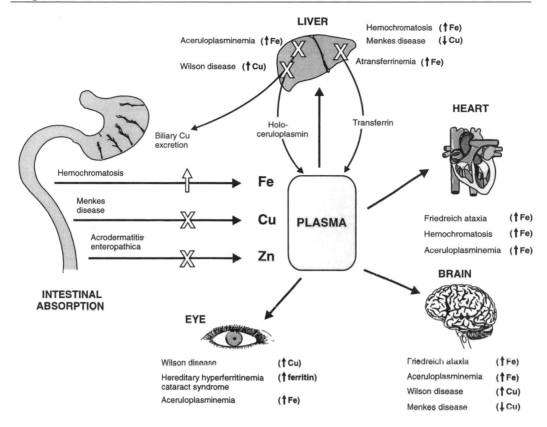

Fig. 1. Sites of basic defects and major organ involvement in some inherited disorders of iron, copper, and zinc metabolism. For each organ depicted a list of diseases which manifest pathology in that organ is given. After each disease the metal-related phenotype is given with upward pointing arrows indicating metal (or ferritin) deposition and downward pointing arrows metal depletion. Open crosses indicate known sites of defects where the normal function is diminished, whereas the open arrow indicates enhanced iron absorption in hemochromatosis.

Patients with HHC have increased iron absorption from birth. It is usually not until the fourth or fifth decade of life, however, that tissue iron concentrations reach toxic levels, although some individuals may develop symptoms at an early age *(7)*. In addition, patients with markers of an ancestral haplotype in the region of the HFE gene tend to have more severe disease expression even though they have the same HFE mutation as other, less severely-affected homozygotes *(8)*. Other factors that can influence expression of the disease include blood loss, the amount of iron in the diet, ingestion of medicinal iron compounds, and alcohol consumption, which may enhance intestinal iron absorption. Female homozygotes of childbearing age generally accumulate iron more slowly than male homozygotes. In general, approximately two-thirds of male homozygotes and one-half of female homozygotes develop full disease expression. The reason for the lack of disease expression in some homozygotes is unknown. Heterozygotes generally do not develop clinically significant degrees of iron overload. Some heterozygous individuals have a moderately elevated serum iron concentration and increased transferrin saturation, but complications attributable to iron overload alone in heterozygotes are extremely rare *(9)*. Occasionally, heterozygosity for hemochromatosis in combination with another condition that predisposes to increased iron absorption (such as porphyria cutanea tarda, β-thalassemia minor, or hereditary spherocytosis) can produce iron overload *(10)*.

The clinical manifestations of hemochromatosis are attributable to tissue damage resulting from accumulation of markedly increased amounts of iron in excess of the ability of cells to sequester the element in relatively nontoxic storage forms as ferritin and hemosiderin. An elevated level of intracellular iron catalyzes production of toxic free radicals such as the hydroxyl radical *(11)* causing lipid peroxidation and cell damage *(12–14)*. One of the main target organs is the liver and patients with advanced iron overload develop hepatic fibrosis that eventually progresses to frank cirrhosis *(15)*. A role for alcohol abuse has been advocated in the pathogenesis of the liver damage, but patients with hemochromatosis who have never consumed alcoholic beverages have developed cirrhosis *(16)*, indicating that iron overload alone is sufficient to produce the lesion. Cardiac manifestations include restrictive cardiomyopathy and arrhythmias. Glucose intolerance resulting from damage to pancreatic islet cells is common. Other endocrinological manifestations of the disease include gonadal dysfunction — impotence in men and amenorrhea in women — as a consequence of accumulation of toxic iron levels in the anterior pituitary, and hypothyroidism. Neurological symptoms include increased susceptibility to fatigue and memory difficulties. Hyperpigmentation, with a bronze or slate-gray cast, is the result of increased melanin production rather than cutaneous iron deposition per se. Patients with iron overload appear to have an increased risk of infection, often with opportunistic organisms such as *Listeria* monocytogenes, *Yersinia enterocolitica*, or *Candida* species, and primary septicemia with Vibrio vulnificus after consumption of shellfish has been reported *(10)*. In recent reports, it has been shown that in many cases the first symptom related to iron overload in HHC is arthritis (for a review see *[1]*).

Patients having any of these manifestations should be tested for iron overload with a screening serum transferrin saturation test, as almost all homozygous affected individuals with HHC have elevated serum iron and transferrin saturation levels *(17)*. A sustained elevation of transferrin saturation coupled with an increased serum ferritin concentration in the absence of some other explanation (e.g., liver disease, history of multiple blood transfusions) is presumptive evidence of iron overload consistent with HHC *(18)*. The diagnosis may be confirmed by performing a percutaneous liver biopsy, which should be examined with hematoxylin and eosin, iron, and connective tissue stains. A quantitative chemical determination of the liver iron concentration should also be performed if possible, as this is more accurate than histological assessment *(15)*. Genetic testing for mutations in the HFE gene can be used to confirm the diagnosis, but failure to find an HFE-associated mutation does not rule out the diagnosis. Approximately 90% of patients with hemochromatosis are homozygous for C282Y *(6)*, although this varies from one geographical area to another. Patients with typical clinical features of hemochromatosis who do not carry this mutation may suffer from a mutation in some other gene controlling iron metabolism. For this reason, and because not all C282Y homozygotes have phenotypic expression of the disease, genetic testing is not recommended for population screening at this time *(19)*. Therefore, the current recommendation is to test for iron overload using transferrin saturation as the initial screen, and this approach is being evaluated in a number of primary care settings *(20)*. The diagnosis of hemochromatosis in an individual patient indicates the need for family studies to identify relatives who also have the disease, and this is one situation where genetic testing may be a useful adjunct to transferrin saturation and serum ferritin for screening. For example, if the proband in a given family is homozygous for C282Y, then affected siblings will also be C282Y homozygotes.

Treatment consists of iron-removal therapy by repeated phlebotomy. Blood is removed in amounts of 450–500 mL weekly until a state of iron depletion is reached (21). Some patients tolerate phlebotomy more often, up to two or three times a week. Iron depletion is indicated by the onset of anemia with failure of the hematocrit or hemoglobin to return to baseline for two weeks after the last phlebotomy and is confirmed by a decreased serum ferritin level. The patient's pretreatment total body iron stores can be calculated retrospectively from the volume of blood removed and the hematocrit at the time of each phlebotomy (22). Removal of a total of at least 4 g iron is considered to be consistent with a diagnosis of HHC. Subsequently, the patient must continue with maintenance phlebotomy therapy (generally 3–4 times a year) for life in order to prevent reaccumulation of excess iron. Serum ferritin should be checked at least annually, to insure that the desired level (preferably in the low-normal range i.e., 20–50 ng/mL) is being maintained. Phlebotomy treatment appears to prevent further progression of many disease manifestations with the notable exception of the risk of primary hepatocellular carcinoma, which occurs in approximately one-third of patients who already have cirrhosis at the time of diagnosis (3). In some cases, reversal of hepatic fibrosis has been observed. Congestive heart failure and arrhythmias in particular may be ameliorated by phlebotomy, but diabetes and joint damage generally are not reversible. This emphasizes the importance of early diagnosis and prompt iron removal therapy. Indeed, patients with HHC who are identified in precirrhotic stages of the disease and treated with effective phlebotomy therapy have a normal life expectancy (23). Moreover, all disease manifestations can be prevented completely by phlebotomy therapy in patients diagnosed before the onset of any organ damage.

The mechanism by which a mutation in the HFE gene leads to increased intestinal iron absorption in hemochromatosis is unknown. The mucosal phase of iron absorption comprises three steps: uptake of dietary iron from the intestinal lumen, retention of some of this dietary iron in the mucosal epithelial cell, and transfer of iron from the mucosa to circulating transferrin in the plasma (24). In vitro studies of mucosal biopsies and in vivo studies of iron absorption in patients with hemochromatosis have indicated both increased iron uptake by the intestinal mucosa and increased transfer of mucosal iron to the systemic circulation (25–27). However, compartmental analysis of mucosal iron kinetics in patients with HHC has indicated that the rate of transfer of mucosal iron to the plasma is inappropriately high for the level of body iron stores, and this abnormality accounts for almost 90% of the increased iron absorption observed in hemochromatosis (28,29). In trying to understand the basic pathogenic mechanisms underlying hemochromatosis, an important observation has been that the mucosal epithelium in this disorder contains remarkably little ferritin in comparison with patients having other forms of iron overload, despite comparable degrees of systemic iron loading (30–32). This relative paucity of ferritin appears to be attributable to a low intracellular iron level rather than a defect in ferritin synthesis, as iron regulatory protein (IRP) activity levels in mucosal biopsies of HHC patients are appropriate for the mucosal ferritin concentration (31). The presence of an iron deficient mucosa is consistent with the observed elevated rate of iron absorption, but indicates that there is a defect in the way the body informs the mucosal epithelium of body iron requirements.

There is a deficiency of iron in bone marrow macrophages in hereditary hemochromatosis, and iron deposition in hepatic parenchymal cells generally is much more prominent than in Kupffer cells (3). This is in sharp contrast to certain other types of iron overload (e.g., that due to multiple blood transfusions) where iron is deposited initially in Kupffer cells and accretion in hepatocytes tends to be a late event. Consistent with these observations, increased efflux of iron from the reticuloendothelial system has been demonstrated in hemochromatosis patients (33), suggesting the possibility of a defect in the control of reticuloendothelial processing or release. Taken together, these observations, and other studies indicating an increased rate of transfer of mucosal iron to the plasma (28,29), are consistent with a systemic defect involving accelerated release of iron not only from the reticuloendothelial system but also from other tissues, including the intestinal mucosa.

Recent studies have shown that the HFE gene product is associated with both β_2-microglobulin and the transferrin receptor on the plasma membrane and thus may play some role in regulating the entry of iron into cells (34). This capability is lost as a result of the C282Y mutation in HHC (35), and it is tempting to speculate that the defective HFE protein in patients with hemochromatosis interferes in some way with the ability of the enterocyte to take up iron from plasma transferrin. This would explain the paucity of intracellular iron in the small intestinal mucosal epithelium in patients with hemochromatosis, despite increased intestinal iron absorption and body iron overload. In turn, a lack of iron in the mucosal intracellular pool in patients with hemochromatosis could result in changes in the rate of iron transport from the intestinal lumen to the systemic circulation. Interestingly, β_2-microglobulin knockout mice also lack the ability to limit transfer of iron from the intestinal mucosa to the plasma, and these mice develop iron overload with a predominance of iron accumulation in hepatocytes but relatively little iron in Kupffer cells (36). Reconstitution with normal hematopoietic cells after lethal irradiation in these mice led to redistribution of hepatic iron from parenchymal to Kupffer cells but did not correct the mucosal defect. If HFE is also expressed in the reticuloendothial system, it is possible that the same defect responsible for increased iron absorption in HHC could promote rapid egress of iron from monocytes and macrophages, leading to the characteristic tissue iron distribution, with a relative paucity of reticuloendothial iron despite increased parenchymal cell iron deposition in the liver and other organs.

2.2. African Iron Overload

Iron overload occurs commonly among indigenous peoples of sub-Saharan Africa who consume home-brewed beer that is fermented in steel drums. This traditional beverage contains a high concentration of iron in a highly bioavailable form (10). The hepatic iron levels in affected individuals tend to be higher than in alcoholic liver disease, and the histological changes associated with alcohol are rarely seen. Serum transferrin saturation levels typically are elevated to the same extent as in hereditary hemochromatosis. However, unlike HHC, in which hepatocellular iron deposition predominates, African iron overload is characterized by prominent iron deposition both in hepatocytes and in Kupffer cells. In some areas of southern Africa, necropsy studies have indicated that the prevalence of iron overload of a degree sufficient to cause cirrhosis is in excess of 10% (10). African iron overload has been considered until recently to be solely a consequence of increased dietary iron intake, but only a minority of individuals who regularly consume traditional beer have iron overload and new data suggest that beer drinkers with iron overload also have an inherited tendency to absorb excessive amounts of iron from dietary sources *(37)*. Unlike the gene for HHC in Caucasians, the putative gene involved in African iron overload appears not to be HLA-linked. It is reasonable to expect that this problem also may exist among African-Americans, and there have been occasional reports of iron overload in this population *(38,39)*. In addition, the possible presence of an iron-loading gene in the African-American population is suggested by an analysis of results from the second U.S. National Health and Nutrition Examination Survey (NHANES II). Mixture distribution analysis of transferrin saturation data among Caucasians demonstrated the presence of two distributions: a major population (possibly representing normal individuals) with a lower mean transferrin saturation and a minor population (possibly representing hemochromatosis heterozygotes) with a higher mean saturation *(40)*. A similar bimodal distribution of transferrin saturation values was observed among African-Americans in the same survey *(41)*. These results are consistent with the existence of a non-HLA-linked iron loading gene in this population. Further studies are needed to determine whether such an iron loading gene may represent a public health concern among African-Americans.

2.3. Autosomal Dominant Iron Overload

There has been one report of a large Melanesian kindred with a hereditary form of iron overload occurring in about one-third of family members. This disorder appears to be inherited as an autosomal dominant trait *(42)*. The pattern of iron deposition in the liver in affected individuals reportedly resembles that of hereditary (HLA-linked) hemochromatosis in Caucasians. Unlike the latter, however, no evidence of linkage to HLA was found in the Melanesian family. Thus, the affected individuals in this family may have a mutation in a gene involved in the control of iron metabolism that is distinct from the HFE gene that is mutated in most patients with HHC.

2.4. Hypotransferrinemia

Hypotransferrinemia or atransferrinemia is a very rare recessively inherited disorder characterized, as its name suggests, by very low or undetectable plasma transferrin levels. Affected individuals have a severe hypochromic, microcytic anemia which does not respond to iron therapy, but, paradoxically, there is massive iron loading in the tissues. Hepatic iron deposition has been observed within both hepatocytes and Kupffer cells *(43)*. Summaries of the described cases are provided by Hamill et al. *(43)* and Hayashi et al. *(44)*. The disorder has been treated effectively by infusions of apotransferrin or fresh-frozen plasma, sometimes in conjunction with iron chelators *(43–45)*. The molecular defect underlying hypotransferrinemia in humans has not been identified, but in a rodent model for this disorder, the hypotransferrinemic mouse, a splicing defect in the transferrin gene interferes with transferrin synthesis and is responsible for the very low levels of the protein *(46)*.

Transferrin is the major plasma iron transport protein and it plays an essential role in moving iron from sites of absorption (the small intestine) and storage (particularly the liver) to tissues in the body where it is required for metabolic functions *(47)*. The most important of these is the erythroid marrow where iron is needed for hemoglobin production. It might be expected that individuals lacking transferrin would have difficulty in absorbing iron and delivering it to tissues, but for most tissues this is not the case. Hypotransferrinemic individuals absorb iron very efficiently from the diet and deposit this iron in the liver and to a lesser extent in other body tissues *(44,45,48)*. The accumulation of iron to toxic levels within cells provides the pathological basis of this disease *(48,49)*. Many studies have now shown that nontransferrin bound iron can be taken up by cells much more efficiently than transferrin-bound iron *(50)*. Thus transferrin is not required for iron delivery to tissues per se, but it is required to regulate the delivery of iron to cells. In contrast to most tissues, the erythroid marrow has an absolute requirement for transferrin-bound iron and this explains the anemia which develops in hypotransferrinemia.

2.5. Hereditary Hyperferritinemia Cataract Syndrome

Hereditary hyperferritinemia cataract syndrome (HHCS) is a rare disorder in the regulation of the synthesis of the iron storage protein ferritin. It is inherited as an autosomal dominant trait. Clinically the condition is characterized by early onset bilateral cataracts and an elevated serum ferritin level in the absence of iron overload *(51,52)*. Venesection therapy leads to the rapid appearance of microcytic anemia without a significant decline in serum ferritin levels *(51,53)*, suggesting that iron overload is not the cause of the elevated ferritin concentration.

Molecular investigations have demonstrated that mutations in the ferritin gene underlie HHCS. Iron regulates the expression of the H and L subunits of ferritin at the translational level via cytosolic iron-dependent RNA-binding proteins known as iron regulatory proteins (or IRPs) that interact with a stem-loop structure in the 5' end of the ferritin mRNA called an iron responsive element (IRE). It is point mutations or deletions in the IRE of the L-ferritin gene which are responsible for the high ferritin synthesis in HHCS *(54–56)*. The binding of IRPs to the ferritin IRE normally blocks ferritin translation, but if there are mutations in the IRE then the IRP will no longer bind effectively and ferritin synthesis will proceed unchecked. How a defect in the regulation of ferritin can lead to cataracts remains to be elucidated, but the limited phenotype-genotype correlations which have been carried out indicate a direct relationship between the serum ferritin level and cataract severity *(57)*. Significantly, one study has shown a high concentration of L-ferritin in the lens of a patient with HHCS *(58)*, suggesting that a direct role of lens ferritin deposits rather than an indirect role of the high serum ferritin level is responsible for lens damage. Mechanisms proposed for how ferritin might potentiate this pathology include a role for the protein in promoting oxidative damage within the lens *(54,55)* or a disruption of the equilibrium between water soluble lens proteins as a result of the high local concentration of ferritin *(58)*.

2.6. Friedreich Ataxia

Friedreich ataxia (FRDA) is an autosomal recessive neurodegenerative disorder which usually appears before adulthood although the age of onset is variable *(59,60)*. The disorder is characterized by a variety of nervous system defects including progressive gait and limb ataxia. However, there are also nonneurological manifestations of the disease including cardiomyopathy and diabetes mellitus. The neurological defects in FRDA result from the degeneration of specific sets of neurons in the central and peripheral nervous system. The cardiac defects and diabetes are thought to result from the same underlying cellular defect that leads to neuronal damage. The tissues affected in FRDA are those showing a high dependence on oxidative metabolism and, as a consequence, the disease has been considered to be a mitochondrial disorder.

The gene affected in FRDA was recently identified by positional cloning and is known as frataxin *(61)*. In most FRDA patients, the defect in the frataxin gene is an expansion of an intronic trinucleotide repeat although point mutations have been found in a small percentage of affected individuals. These gene defects lead to severely reduced levels or absence of frataxin mRNA. The frataxin gene encodes a 210 amino acid protein with significant homology to proteins of unknown function in the worm Caenorhabditis elegans and the yeast Saccharomyces cerevisiae. The sequences of frataxin and its homologs indicated a putative mitochondrial targeting motif and this has now been confirmed experimentally *(62–64)*. Frataxin is widely expressed in body tissues *(62)*.

The link between FRDA and iron homeostasis was made from the observation that the deletion of the yeast homolog of frataxin (YFH1) leads to mitochondrial iron overload *(65,66)*. It is suspected that the elevated iron concentration within the mitochondrion leads to oxidative damage of various proteins such as iron sulfur proteins which in turn leads to mitochondrial dysfunction. How disruption of YFH1 leads to iron accumulation in the mitochondrion has yet to be elucidated. However, these data would suggest that YFH1 and, by inference, frataxin, play critical roles in iron traffic into or out of mitochondria. Evidence of iron accumulation in the cells of FRDA patients is very limited at present, but one study did find the accumulation of iron in cardiac myocytes *(67)*, one of the tissues affected in the disease. In addition, Rotig et al. *(68)* have presented direct evidence for free radical-mediated damage to mitochondrial enzymes in FRDA tissues. Much remains to be learned about frataxin and the role it plays in the pathogenesis of FRDA but these studies promise to greatly increase our knowledge of mitochondrial iron homeostasis in mammals, a critical area of iron metabolism very poorly understood at present.

2.7. Aceruloplasminemia

Aceruloplasminemia is a rare disorder characterized by neurological abnormalities, retinal degeneration, diabetes and, as its name suggests, a complete deficiency of circulating ceruloplasmin *(69)*. It is inherited in an autosomal recessive manner. Although ceruloplasmin is a copper-containing protein, it is now clear that aceruloplasminemia is a disorder of iron metabolism rather than of copper metabolism, and indeed copper homeostasis is not impaired in aceruloplasminemic patients. Affected individuals show iron deposition in the liver (both hepatocytes and Kupffer cells), brain (basal ganglia, thalamus), retina, pancreas, heart, kidney, spleen, and thyroid *(70–73)*. Consistent with tissue iron deposition is an elevated serum ferritin concentration, but, paradoxically, the serum iron concentration is low and patients often have a mild anemia *(70,74)*. While aceruloplasminemia usually proves fatal, the demonstration that tissue iron deposition is the likely cause of the pathology underlying the disease has led to the investigation of the therapeutic effects of the iron chelator desferrioxamine (DFO) *(75)*. DFO was able to reduce iron stores and prevent progression of the neurological symptoms of the disease indicating that the chelator has some therapeutic utility. Molecular analysis of the ceruloplasmin gene in several aceruloplasminemic patients has revealed a number of defects leading to premature truncation of the protein at the carboxy terminus *(69)*. These studies imply that ceruloplasmin plays an important function in body iron homeostasis.

An explanation for the role of ceruloplasmin in iron metabolism can be found in studies of the biochemistry and physiology of the protein. While 95% of the plasma copper in vertebrates is found in ceruloplasmin *(76)*, this copper is bound during biosynthesis and it is unlikely that ceruloplasmin has a primary function as a copper transport protein.

However, the copper in ceruloplasmin plays an essential role in enabling the protein to oxidize a number of substrates via the reduction of oxygen *(77)*. In vivo, the most relevant of these activities appears to be the oxidation of Fe(II) to Fe(III), i.e., ceruloplasmin has a ferroxidase activity *(76)*. Aceruloplasminemic patients lack serum ferroxidase activity consistent with the loss of critical copper binding residues in the C-terminal region of the protein *(69)*. Various physiological studies have shown that the ferroxidase activity of ceruloplasmin is necessary for the mobilization of iron from tissues and its subsequent incorporation as ferric iron into circulating apotransferrin *(78,79)*. Since ceruloplasmin is important for the normal trafficking of iron out of tissues, when synthesis of the protein is disrupted, such as in aceruloplasminemia, iron will accumulate in tissues and exert toxic effects. While the liver is responsible for most ceruloplasmin synthesis, small amounts are also synthesized in the CNS since the protein does not cross the blood-brain barrier *(80)*. The absence of CNS ceruloplasmin synthesis in aceruloplasminemia is likely to underlie the CNS iron deposition observed in this disease. The role of ceruloplasmin in tissue iron release explains why affected individuals have elevated serum ferritin concentrations (since the ferritin level will reflect iron stores) but reduced serum iron levels (since tissue iron release is impaired).

Current understanding of aceruloplasminemia has provided considerable insight into the role of copper in iron homeostasis but many significant questions remain and recent developments in the field suggest more complex interactions between the physiology of copper and iron. For example, a recent study *(81)* has indicated that ceruloplasmin gene expression is induced under iron deficient conditions. This could be an adaptive response to ensure adequate mobilization of storage iron in times of increased demand by the erythropoietic tissues, but this issue must be explored further. Other recent data have indicated that a membrane-bound ceruloplasmin homolog (known as hephaestin) is highly expressed in the small intestine and plays a role in intestinal iron absorption by participating in the release of iron at the basolateral membranes *(82)*. This study raises the possibility that while plasma ceruloplasmin may be the major mediator of iron release from parenchymal cells, there may be further ceruloplasmin homologs which play more specialized roles in iron trafficking in specific tissues and cell types.

2.8. Inherited Iron Deficiency Syndromes

Each of the seven disorders of iron metabolism described above is characterized by iron overload of one form or another. Inherited disorders of iron deficiency are rarely observed and there are only occasional reports of refractory anemias which may fall within this category. Buchanan et al. *(83)* described such an anemia in three siblings and a similar situation involving two siblings was described by Hartman and Barker *(84)*. In each of these families the anemia responded partially, but not completely, to parenteral iron treatment, indicating that the anemia was not due solely to an intestinal iron absorption defect but also involved tissue iron utilization. The reason for the relative paucity of inherited iron deficiency disorders is not clear. It may indicate that the liabilities of iron excess are more severe than the liabilities of iron depletion, or simply that the deleterious effects of iron deficiency are more insidious and difficult to recognize clinically. The human body is well adapted to mount an effective response to iron depletion by increases in intestinal iron absorption and iron uptake by body cells, but it is ill-adapted to disposing of excess iron. These differences in physiological response may contribute to the relative frequency of iron overload disorders.

2.9. Increased Iron Absorption Associated with Other Inherited Disorders

Several disorders of hemoglobin production are associated with increased intestinal iron absorption, including homozygous β-thalassemia (thalassemia major and thalassemia intermedia), double heterozygosity for β-thalassemia and hemoglobin E, and hemoglobin H disease *(10)*. These inherited anemias are common in parts of the world where malaria is endemic and can produce iron overload of an extent comparable to that in hereditary hemochromatosis. The mechanism of increased iron absorption in these disorders is unclear but is thought to be related in some way to a high degree of ineffective erythropoiesis which may cause the demand for iron to exceed the rate at which the element can be recycled from the reticuloendothelial system. Patients with β-thalassemia major generally are dependent on transfusions of red blood cells to maintain an adequate blood hemoglobin level and since humans lack an effective mechanism for actively increasing iron excretion *(85)*, blood transfusion therapy is also a major factor in the development of iron overload in this disease. In advanced cases, the pattern of iron deposition can be difficult to distinguish from HHC, and patients suffer most of the same kinds of toxicity, including cirrhosis of the liver, diabetes, and congestive heart failure. Excess iron can be reduced by using infusions of the iron chelating drug desferrioxamine. Transfusion therapy also reduces the erythropoietic stimulus, and iron absorption may decrease to normal levels and no longer represent a major contribution to the development of iron overload. The combination of blood transfusion therapy and iron removal with desferrioxamine currently appears to offer the best hope for most thalassemic patients, although bone marrow transplantation is under active investigation as a treatment for patients with a suitable donor. For patients with milder thalassemic syndromes, who develop iron overload solely as the result of increased intestinal iron absorption, the optimal form of management is yet to be determined.

Other inherited disorders of red blood cell production that are associated with ineffective erythropoiesis and increased intestinal iron absorption include a number of anemias with impaired incorporation of iron into hemoglobin. These conditions, called sideroblastic anemias, occur in both congenital (hereditary) and acquired forms and are characterized by the presence of increased numbers of so-called ringed sideroblasts, iron-laden red blood cell precursors containing abnormal mitochondrial iron deposits often forming a ring around the nucleus. A major degree of iron overload may occur in these conditions, even in the absence of severe anemia. As with the thalassemia syndromes, increased iron absorption in patients with sideroblastic anemia is thought to be attributable to the markedly increased ineffective erythropoiesis, but the mechanism remains unknown. Iron absorption is also increased in patients with hereditary pyruvate kinase deficiency, and severe iron overload in the absence of a history of multiple blood transfusions develops in some cases. Affected individuals may have a severe hemolytic anemia and often benefit from splenectomy, which may reduce the rate of hemolysis and result in a higher blood hemoglobin level *(10)*.

2.10. Inherited Rodent Disorders of Iron Metabolism

Although laboratory animal strains with inherited defects of iron metabolism have arisen with less frequency than those with defects in copper metabolism (see below), there are several inherited rodent anemias which have shown great promise in helping us to understand fundamental aspects of mammalian iron homeostasis. These include microcytic anemia (mk), sex-linked anemia (sla) and hemoglobin deficit (hbd) in the mouse, and the Belgrade rat *(86)*. None of these strains appears to have a well-defined human counterpart, although some refractory anemias in humans could be due to mutations in the homologous human genes.

The phenotypes of mk mice and Belgrade rats are similar *(86,87)*. Both strains develop a moderate to severe iron deficiency in which most body tissues appear to be affected. The animals show defective intestinal iron absorption, which certainly contributes to their anemia, but bypassing the small intestine by the parenteral administration of iron only leads to a partial correction of their condition indicating that iron delivery to other body tissues is impaired *(88,89)*. Supporting this is the demonstration in Belgrade rats that the delivery of transferrin-bound iron is defective in several cell types isolated from these animals *(90)*. The gene affected in mk mice has recently been identified as a transmembrane divalent metal transporter known as DMT1 (formerly Nramp2 or DCT1)*(91)*, and subsequent studies have confirmed that the basic defect in the Belgrade rat results from a mutation in the same gene *(92)*. A detailed analysis of the role of the *DMT1* protein in body iron homeostasis has yet to be carried out, but current evidence suggests that it performs two major functions: (1) to transport iron across the endosomal membrane of most body cells, and (2) to transport dietary iron into intestinal epithelial cells (either across the brush border membrane or across the membrane of a subcellular vesicle). The endosomal location is likely to explain why transferrin-bound iron delivery is disrupted in mk and Belgrade cells *(92)*. A third rodent anemia, hbd, has a phenotype superficially similar to the mk/Belgrade phenotype, but the locus maps to a different chromosome so DMT1 is clearly not the affected gene. The limited data available for hbd mice suggests that these animals are unable to effectively deliver transferrin-bound iron to developing erythroid cells *(93)*.

Mice carrying the sla mutation develop an iron-deficiency anemia as a result of a defect in intestinal iron absorption, or more specifically, in the release of newly absorbed iron from the cells of the intestinal epithelium into the body *(87)*. The sla gene has recently been mapped *(94)* and was identified using a positional candidate approach *(82)*. The gene has been named hephaestin and it encodes a membrane-bound homolog of ceruloplasmin. The importance of ceruloplasmin ferroxidase in iron release from cells has been detailed in Subheading 2.7. and it has been postulated that hephaestin also acts as a ferroxidase. However, in this case the protein plays a more specialized role in mediating the release of iron from enterocytes. The high expression of hephaestin in the intestinal epithelium is consistent with this, but some expression is observed in other tissues such as the kidney, heart, and brain so the protein may perform some more generalized function in tissue iron export.

The application of genetics to the isolation of the genes affected in rodent anemias has enabled two proteins with critical roles in mammalian iron metabolism to be identified. The fact that no corresponding human disorders have been identified may indicate that dysfunction of these molecules is lethal in humans. These advances serve to highlight the value of experimental animal models in the elucidation of physiological pathways involved in the handling of trace elements that may help clarify the mechanism of related disorders. For example, dysregulation of iron absorption in the human disease hemochromatosis is attributable to a mutation in HFE *(6)* resulting in elevated release of iron from enterocytes *(28,29)*. Although the target of HFE regulation is not known, control of the activity of hephaestin could provide the means to regulate iron export from the intestine. The human homologs of DMT1 and hephaestin have been cloned *(82,95)* and their roles in various diseases of iron metabolism are currently under investigation.

3. DISORDERS OF COPPER METABOLISM

An adequate dietary intake of copper is essential for normal metabolic functions and the normal adult human contains 70–100 mg of the metal. Although a far less abundant metal than iron, copper shares with iron the characteristic of two stable oxidation states, a property which makes it invaluable in electron transfer reactions. Consequently copper is a critical co-factor in a number of important enzymes such as cytochrome c oxidase, lysyl oxidase, superoxide dismutase, and dopamine β-hydroxylase. Normal copper homeostasis will be discussed here only in relation to genetic defects of copper metabolism.

3.1. Menkes Disease and Occipital Horn Syndrome

Menkes disease (MD) and occipital horn syndrome (OHS)(also known as X-linked cutis laxa) are disorders of copper homeostasis which show X-linked recessive inheritance (96). Molecular studies have shown that both disorders result from mutations in the same gene, a membrane copper transporter known as ATP7A (97,98). The major clinical problems in MD are progressive neurodegenerative disease and a variety of connective tissue abnormalities, but other disturbances associated with the disease include hypopigmentation, hypothermia, thrombosis, skeletal problems, and hyperbilirubinemia. The life expectancy of MD patients is very low and most die in early childhood. Patients with OHS show much milder disease and usually manifest only connective tissue defects and mild neurological problems. Consequently their prognosis is generally good with a high life expectancy (96,99). Several individuals with phenotypes which lie between those of MD and OHS have been reported (96). The basis of the pathogenesis of these diseases lies in a deficiency of critical copper-dependent enzymes (96,98). The connective tissue defects result from the decreased activity of the enzyme lysyl oxidase which is required for the cross linking of collagen and elastin. The neurological defects appear to result from an inadequate supply of copper across the blood-brain barrier at a time in development when the brain is particularly sensitive to copper deficiency. Deficiencies in the activity of cytochrome c oxidase and other essential copper-dependent brain enzymes are the likely causes of abnormal brain metabolism. In view of this apparent copper deficiency, the main form of treatment for MD patients has been the administration of copper in various forms (summarized in [96] and [98]). While some chelated forms of copper have not proved effective, copper-histidine administration has been shown to lead to some clinical improvement (100).

Individuals with MD have a profound abnormality in copper transport in most body cells. There is a significant decrease in the intestinal absorption of copper and, consequently, affected individuals have low levels of copper and ceruloplasmin in the plasma (96). Although, superficially, decreased intestinal absorption would appear to account for the decreased activity of copper-dependent enzymes in the body, the situation is somewhat more complex. While histological examination reveals a severe deficiency of copper in the liver and brain, other tissues, notably the intestine and kidney, show copper accumulation (96,98,101). These data, combined with similar studies in the mottled mouse (a valuable animal model for MD - see Subheading 3.3.), indicate that most tissues in patients with MD accumulate copper if it is available. The major exception is the liver (102,103). The tissue accumulation of copper results from a defect in cellular copper efflux. Indeed this efflux defect has been demonstrated using fibroblasts cultured from MD patients which readily accumulate copper (104,105). The copper which accumulates within the cells becomes bound to metallothionein and is not transported into the cellular compartment(s) where copper-containing enzymes are synthesized. In the small intestine, the failure of the epithelial cells to export copper to the body makes a major contribution to the apparent copper deficiency in MD.

The MD gene, known as MNK or ATP7A, was isolated by positional cloning and found to encode a membrane copper transporter belonging to the P-type ATPase family *(106–108)*. The 1500 amino acid protein contains 8 membrane spanning domains, an N terminal metal binding motif consisting of regularly spaced cysteine residues, an ATP binding cassette, phosphorylation and phosphatase domains, and a transmembrane cation channel. The ATP7A gene is expressed in all tissues studied except the liver, an expression pattern consistent with the clinical manifestations of the disease *(96,106)*. A large number of mutations in ATP7A have been described in patients with MD *(109–111)*. These include partial deletions of the gene in many patients with severe disease. In OHS, several splicing mutations have been identified and in these individuals both normal and shortened transcripts have been detected *(112,113)*. The presence of some normal message no doubt allows the synthesis of some functional copper transporter.

Since the cloning of the MNK gene several groups have begun to investigate the role the copper transporter plays in cellular copper efflux. A valuable tool for these studies has come from Camakaris et al. *(114)* who showed that cell lines which had been selected for their resistance to very high levels of copper in the culture medium were not defective in the ability to take up copper but rather were able to excrete it very effectively. They subsequently showed that the ATP7A gene was amplified in these cells *(114)* and have used them to investigate the subcellular localization of ATP7A *(115)*. When cells are grown in a basal medium containing a very low level of copper, ATP7A is located predominantly in the Golgi apparatus. However, when the copper concentration of the medium is elevated, there is a translocation of the ATPase from the Golgi to the plasma membrane. Further experiments suggested that there was a continual, vesicle-mediated recycling of ATP7A between the Golgi and the plasma membrane. This novel mechanism for ligand-mediated translocation of ATP7A to the plasma membrane helps to explain the role of the transporter in cellular copper homeostasis. In times of copper excess, the MNK protein located on the plasma membrane plays an important role in copper efflux to prevent copper from accumulating to toxic levels within the cell. However, in times of copper depletion the predominant localization of MNK in the Golgi complex may play an important role in copper delivery to essential copper-dependent enzymes within the cell. Several other groups have now confirmed the localization of ATP7A to the trans-Golgi network *(116,117)*.

3.2. Wilson Disease

While Menkes disease is a disorder of copper deficiency, Wilson disease (WD) is an autosomal recessive disorder characterized by copper overload with progressive deposition of copper in the liver, brain, kidneys, and the cornea *(96,118,119)*. Copper is an essential metal, but, like iron and other trace metals, it is toxic when present in excess and copper that cannot be adequately sequestered within the cell is able to catalyze reactions leading to the production of cytotoxic oxygen radicals *(see* Chapter 1). These in turn can lead to significant tissue damage. Consequently, individuals with Wilson disease develop chronic liver disease (which can lead to fibrosis and cirrhosis and ultimately liver failure), neurological symptoms such as behavior and movement disorders, renal tubular dysfunction, and pigmented rings in the cornea (Kayser-Fleischer rings) *(96,120,121)*. Kayser-Fleischer rings are a particularly consistent feature of the disease and are found in essentially all patients with neurological disease and 95% of all patients *(96)*, but the presentation can be quite variable *(122)*. Wilson disease should be considered in the differential diagnosis of all patients with chronic liver disease and in individuals over 12 yr of age with neurological symptoms. Since the pathology seen in Wilson disease is a consequence of copper accumulation in certain tissues, treatment strategies have been based on the use of copper chelators such as penicillamine and trientine and in most cases gradual but significant clinical improvement is observed *(121)*. The earlier treatment is commenced the better the prognosis and if therapy begins before severe tissue damage has occurred then life expectancy is normal. In cases of severe liver damage due to Wilson disease, orthotopic liver transplantation has proved very effective *(123)*.

Biochemically WD is characterized by low plasma ceruloplasmin and copper concentrations, increased urinary copper excretion, and a greatly increased hepatic copper level *(96)*. The deficiency in ceruloplasmin is not related to a defect in the synthesis of the protein per se, but to impaired incorporation of copper into the protein. There is also a major impairment of biliary copper excretion in WD *(124)*. Under normal physiological conditions, most of the copper in excess of body requirements is excreted into the bile but in Wilson disease this pathway is defective. The failure of Wilson patients to incorporate copper into ceruloplasmin and into the biliary excretion pathway suggests a defect in the trafficking of copper into one or more intracellular compartments. The sequence of events in the progression of Wilson disease has been summarized by DiDonato and Sarkar *(98)*. First there is an accumulation of copper in the hepatic cytosol as a result of the inability of these cells to divest themselves of excess metal. With increasing copper deposition, lysosomes containing copper, probably as copper metallothionein, appear and ultimately the high copper concentrations lead to hepatocellular damage with the consequent release of large quantities of nonceruloplasmin bound copper into the circulation. This copper can cause erythrocyte damage leading to hemolytic anemia and becomes deposited in other tissues such the brain, kidney, and cornea.

The Wilson disease gene (WND) was identified by a combination of positional cloning and its hypothesized homology to the MNK gene *(125–127)*. This hypothesis proved to be correct and despite the differences in the pathogenesis of Menkes and Wilson disease, the WND and MNK genes are very closely related. The two genes are 57% identical and, like MNK, WND encodes a copper transporting P-type ATPase (which has been designated ATP7B) *(98,128)*. Structurally, ATP7B, like ATP7A, has 8 transmembrane domains, an N-terminal metal binding domain, an ATP-binding domain, phosphorylation and phosphatase domains and a transmembrane cation channel. An analysis of the molecular defects found in ATP7B in patients with Wilson disease has revealed greater than 50 mutations, mainly point mutations and small deletions, spread throughout the gene *(129,130)*. There tends to be some clustering of the mutations in the regions required for ATPase activity and relatively few mutations have been identified in the metal binding region. A significant proportion of WD patients do not have mutations in the ATP7B coding region suggesting that the mutations occur in regulatory regions of the gene. This wide spectrum of mutations helps to explain the considerable variation in the clinical expression of Wilson disease and the variability in the age of onset *(130)*.

The distribution of expression of the ATP7B gene is restricted to tissues which show pathology in Wilson disease viz., the liver, brain, and kidney as well as the placenta *(125–127)*. At the subcellular level, most interest has centered on the hepatic localization of ATP7B since reduced biliary copper excretion and reduced incorporation of copper into ceruloplasmin (which mainly occurs in the liver) are major pathological features of the disorder. The disturbance of both ceruloplasmin synthesis and biliary copper export made it unlikely that ATP7B was restricted to the canalicular membrane, and it was proposed that the protein was more likely to reside in an intracellular compartment (such as the Golgi apparatus) which would affect both processes *(119,131)*. Subsequently ATP7B has been shown to reside in the trans-Golgi network (TGN) *(132,133)*. Interestingly, in the presence of increased intracellular copper the protein has been shown to translocate from the TGN to a population of cytoplasmic vesicles *(132)*, a behavior strikingly similar to that of the Menkes disease protein ATP7A *(115)*. Further studies using both mammalian and yeast cells have provided direct evidence that ATP7B is indeed a copper transporter and have demonstrated that the effect of one of the major ATP7B mutations in Wilson disease patients (H1069Q) is to destabilize the protein and lead to its premature degradation *(134,135)*.

3.3. Rodent Models for Studying Copper Homeostasis

Our understanding of disorders of copper metabolism has been enhanced considerably by the ongoing analysis of a series of rodent mutants with abnormalities in the homologs of the Menkes or Wilson disease genes *(96,136)*. The murine locus mottled has long been considered to encode the mouse homolog of MNK and this has now been proven at the molecular level. The corresponding murine gene has been designated Atp7a *(137–140)*. For Wilson disease there are both mouse (toxic milk or Tx) and rat (Long-Evans Cinnamon or LEC) mutants, and the relevant gene in each species has been designated Atp7b *(141,142)*. Recent studies on the distribution of the Atp7a and Atp7b genes during development have suggested that Atp7a plays a critical role in cellular copper homeostasis while Atp7b may play a more specific role in the synthesis of particular copper-containing proteins in various tissues *(143)*.

A large number (approximately 20) of mottled mutants are known, and these span the spectrum from very mild disease showing only connective tissue abnormalities to very severe disease with pronounced neurological manifestations *(140,144)*. In several alleles death occurs in utero. This range of disease symptoms spans and even extends the range of symptoms seen in the human disorders from occipital horn syndrome to full Menkes disease. The availability of such an extensive resource of mutant mice has proved extremely useful in investigating phenotype-genotype correlations and molecular defects in a number of the mottled alleles have now been identified *(138–140)*. Cell lines isolated from several of the mottled mutants have been used to study cellular copper homeostasis in relation to genotype *(145)*. The disorders in the Tx mouse and the LEC rat, like Wilson disease, are inherited in an autosomal recessive manner and lead to impaired biliary excretion of copper, a reduced incorporation of copper into ceruloplasmin and extensive hepatic deposition of copper. However, the phenotype of the Tx mouse (and possibly the LEC rat) differs from Wilson disease patients in that it produces copper-deficient milk leading to copper deficiency in the pup *(146)*. It is now clear that both the human and mouse defects result from the disruption of homologous genes, so the difference in phenotype may relate to the specific mutation found in Tx mice. Despite this phenotypic difference, the availability of these animal strains has proved an important resource in helping to understand the pathogenesis of Wilson disease *(147)* and for assessing various therapeutic approaches *(148)*.

4. DISORDERS OF ZINC METABOLISM

Zinc is an essential trace element and the normal adult human contains 1.5–2.5 grams of the metal. It is incorporated as a co-factor into a large number of proteins where it plays a major role in protein structure, but it also has a catalytic role in some enzymes. There are very few inherited disorders of zinc metabolism and, in contrast to iron and copper, genetic disorders of zinc overload are unknown. This presumably relates to the fact that zinc is far less toxic than either of the other two metals. Zinc deficiency can occur occasionally as a result of dietary insufficiency or due to the inherited condition acrodermatitis enteropathica which will be considered in Subheading 4.1.

4.1. Acrodermatitis Enteropathica

There are several inherited zinc deficiency syndromes in mammals but the only human disorder of this type is the autosomal recessive condition acrodermatitis enteropathica (AE). Affected individuals present with severe zinc deficiency during infancy and major symptoms include extensive dermatitis, alopecia, and diarrhea *(149,150)*. Growth defects, some neurological symptoms (particularly mental depression), impaired immunologic function and decreased resistance to infections may also occur. In untreated patients the overall mortality rate is approximately 20% *(150)* but therapy using oral zinc supplementation is highly effective and has been found to ameliorate or cure all symptoms of AE. Biochemically, reduced zinc levels are found in the plasma, urine, and hair, as well as in various tissues, but there is considerable overlap between the values in AE patients and those of normal individuals and these measures should be interpreted with caution *(150)*. The pathological consequences of AE relate to the critical role zinc plays in cellular metabolism since the metal is present in a large number of enzymes and other proteins in both catalytic and structural roles *(151)*.

The molecular basis of AE has yet to be defined and the defective gene has not been identified nor even mapped. However, a major manifestation of the disease is decreased intestinal absorption of zinc *(152,153)*. There are some data to suggest that there is a zinc binding substance in breast milk which facilitates zinc absorption and that once the child is weaned onto cow's milk the symptoms of zinc deficiency are exacerbated *(150)*, but despite this a clear defect in intestinal absorption is present. Sandstrom et al. *(154)* suggested that the decreased intestinal zinc absorption seen in AE individuals may be secondary to changes in intestinal morphology which are induced as part of a more generalized cellular defect of zinc homeostasis. Support for this comes from studies which demonstrate that fibroblasts from AE patients take up zinc more slowly than fibroblasts from normal individuals *(155,156)*. Decreased zinc accumulation and 5' nucleotidase (a zinc-dependent enzyme) activity were also lower in AE fibroblasts but the effect was only transient in culture *(155,157)*. Using these same cells, Grider and Mouat *(158)* used two-dimensional gel electrophoresis to identify two novel proteins which were present in normal fibroblasts but absent from AE fibroblasts. The function of these proteins is not known, nor is it known whether their deficiency in AE cells is a primary or secondary consequence of the AE mutation. The elucidation of the basic molecular defect underlying AE promises to be an important step in our understanding of the transport pathways underlying body zinc homeostasis.

4.2. Inherited Zinc Deficiency in Animals

Inherited zinc deficiency also occurs in mice and cattle *(159)*. The bovine disorder known as Adema disease (or lethal trait A 46) is an inherited zinc deficiency which affects Friesian cattle and appears to be phenotypically very similar to AE *(160)*. It is inherited in an autosomal recessive manner and affected animals develop diarrhea, skin lesions, and neurological abnormalities and, if left untreated, calves will die within several months *(160,161)*. In affected, pregnant cows there is an increased frequency of abortion. These features are all characteristic of zinc deficiency and plasma zinc levels are indeed decreased. Adema disease, like AE, can be treated very effectively by oral zinc therapy and all the clinical and biochemical abnormalities of afflicted calves are reversed by this treatment *(161)*.

In the mouse strain known as lethal milk (lm), there is a defect in the transfer of zinc from the maternal blood to the milk and pups suckled on homozygous affected mothers become zinc deficient *(162,163)*. Mortality amongst the pups is high but those which survive develop the characteristic symptoms of zinc deficiency including dermatitis, stunted growth, and alopecia *(164)*. As with other zinc deficiencies, zinc administration, either to the dams or to the pups themselves, is an effective therapy. Lethal milk is inherited in an autosomal recessive manner and maps to chromosome 2. The affected gene has recently been isolated serendipitously and has been designated Znt4 *(165)*. Znt4 is a member of a family of genes encoding membrane zinc transporters. It is expressed in a number of tissues but at particularly high levels in mammary epithelial cells and the brain. Preliminary functional studies suggest that Znt4 is a zinc export protein and this is consistent with the demonstrated defect in the transfer of zinc into the milk. Whether the lethal milk mutant is the mouse equivalent of AE remains to be determined, but the identification of the Znt4 gene will enable this issue to be addressed.

5. CONCLUSION

Inherited disorders of trace element metabolism are generally very rare and many remain clinical oddities, but some, and most notably hemochromatosis, are sufficiently common to be of significance for population health. The major features of some of these disorders are summarized in Figure 1 and Table 1. Over the last decade the application of modern molecular genetics has enabled the genes affected in many of these diseases to be identified. The availability of genetic testing which follows from these discoveries can be of considerable value to the clinician in diagnosis, but as yet these advances have had relatively little impact on therapy. The treatment of these disorders has traditionally been on an empirical basis, and the tried and proven treatment modalities are likely to remain the mainstay of therapy in the near future. In time, however, methodological advances may enable gene therapy approaches to be used for at least some of these diseases. An additional benefit of the analysis of inherited disorders of metal metabolism in both humans and animals has been the knowledge we have gleaned on normal metal homeostasis. Proteins which have proved difficult to isolate by traditional biochemical approaches have succumbed to contemporary molecular methods using inherited disorders as a source material. The identification of these new molecules has enabled us to place metabolic pathways involving metals on a more precise mechanistic basis, and this has important implications for understanding trace element nutrition.

Table 1
Summary of Some Genetic Diseases of Trace Metal Metabolism

Disease	Metal-related Phenotype	Chromosomal Location	Gene Affected	Population Frequency[a]	Main Clinical Features
Hemochromatosis	Iron overload	6	HFE	1:250	Liver disease
African iron overload	Iron overload	Unknown	Unknown	Common?[b]	Liver disease
Atransferrinemia	Iron overload	3	Transferrin	Rare[c]	Liver disease, heart disease
Aceruloplasminemia	Iron overload	3	Ceruloplasmin	Rare[c]	Neurological disease
Hereditary hyperferritinemia cataract syndrome	Lenticular ferritin deposition	19	L-ferritin	Rare[d]	Bilateral cataracts
Friedreich Ataxia	Iron overload (mitochondria)	9	Frataxin	1:50,000	Neurological disease, heart disease
Wilson Disease	Copper overload	13	ATP7B	1:30,000	Liver disease, neurological disease
Menkes Disease	Copper deficiency	X	ATP7A	1:100,000–1:250,000	Neurological disease, connective tissue disorders
Acrodermatitis enteropathica	Zinc deficiency	Unknown	Unknown	1:500,000	Dermatitis, alopecia, diarrhea

[a] The incidences reported are generally for populations in which the disease is most prevalent. Some disorders may be relatively "common" in some populations but absent in others.

[b] While iron overload in subsaharan Africa is relatively common, the proportion due to inherited factors has yet to be determined.

[c] These disorders are extremely rare and only a small number of cases of each has been described.

[d] There is insufficient experience with this disorder for an accurate incidence to be given, but individuals with unexplained elevated ferritin levels are not uncommon (1:200–300) and one of the possible causes for this elevation in some people may be HHCS.

ACKNOWLEDGMENTS

Portions of the authors' work reported in this chapter were supported by grants from the National Health and Medical Research Council of Australia (GJA) and the U.S. Department of Veterans Affairs (GDM). The authors thank Kym Doyle for commenting on a draft of this chapter.

REFERENCES

1. Edwards CQ, Griffen LM, Goldgar D, Drummond C, Skolnick MH, Kushner JP. Prevalence of hemochromatosis among 11,065 presumably healthy blood donors. N Engl J Med 1988;318:1355–1362.
2. Leggett BA, Halliday JW, Brown NN, Bryant S, Powell LW. Prevalence of haemochromatosis amongst asymptomatic Australians. Br J Haematol 1990;74:525–530.
3. Powell LW, Jazwinska EC, Halliday JW. Primary iron overload. In: Brock JH, Halliday JW, Pippard MJ, Powell LW, eds. Iron Metabolism in Health and Disease. WB Saunders Company, London, 1994, pp. 227–270.
4. Pippard MJ. Secondary iron overload. In: Brock JH, Halliday JW, Pippard MJ, Powell LW, eds. Iron Metabolism in Health and Disease. WB Saunders Company, London, 1994, pp. 271–309.
5. Simon M, Bourel M, Genetet B, Fauchet R. Idiopathic hemochromatosis: demonstration of recessive transmission and early detection by family HLA typing. N Engl J Med 1977;297:1017–1021.
6. Feder JN, Gnirke A, Thomas W, Tsuchihashi Z, Ruddy DA, Basava A, Dormishian F, Domingo R, Ellis MC, Fullan A, Hinton LM, Jones NL, Kimmel BE, Kronmal GS, Lauer P, Lee VK, Loeb DB, Mapa FA, McClelland E, Meyer GA, Mintier GA, Moeller N, Moore T, Morikang E, Prass CE, Quintana L, Starnes SM, Schatzman RC, Brunke KJ, Drayna DT, Risch NJ, Bacon BR, Wolff RK. A novel MHC class I-like gene is mutated in patients with hereditary haemochromatosis. Nat Genet 1996;13:399–408.
7. Muir WA, McLaren GD, Braun W, Askari A. Evidence for heterogeneity in hereditary hemochromatosis: evaluation of 174 individuals in nine families. Am J Med 1984;76:806–814.
8. Crawford DHG, Powell LW, Leggett BA, Francis JS, Fletcher LM, Webb SI, Halliday JW, Jazwinska EC. Evidence that the ancestral haplotype in Australian hemochromatosis patients may be associated with a common mutation in the gene. Am J Hum Genet 1995;57:362–367.
9. Bulaj ZJ, Griffen LM, Jorde LB, Edwards CQ, Kushner JP. Clinical and biochemical abnormalities in people heterozygous for hemochromatosis. N Engl J Med 1996;335:1837–1839.
10. Gordeuk VR, McLaren GD, Samowitz W. Etiologies, consequences and treatment of iron overload. Crit Rev Clin Lab Sci 1994;31:89–123.
11. Halliwell B, Gutteridge JMC, Cross CE. Free radicals, antioxidants, and human disease: Where are we now? J Lab Clin Med 1992;119:598–620.
12. Bacon BR, Tavill AS, Brittenham GM, Park CH, Recknagel RO. Hepatic lipid peroxidation in vivo in rats with chronic iron overload. J Clin Invest 1983;71:429–439.
13. Britton RS, O'Neill R, Bacon BR. Chronic dietary iron overload in rats results in impaired calcium sequestration by hepatic mitochondria and microsomes. Gastroenterology 1991;101:806–811.
14. Sharma BK, Bacon BR, Britton RS, Park CH, Magiera CJ, O'Neill R, Dalton N, Smanik P, Speroff T. Prevention of hepatocyte injury and lipid peroxidation by iron chelators and alpha-tocopherol in isolated iron-loaded rat hepatocytes. Hepatology 1990;12:31–39.
15. Bassett ML, Halliday JW, Powell LW. Value of hepatic iron measurements in early hemochromatosis and determination of the critical iron level associated with fibrosis. Hepatology 1986;6:24–29.
16. Powell LW, Kerr JFR. The pathology of the liver in hemochromatosis. Pathobiol Annual 1975;5:317–337.
17. McLaren CE, McLachlan GJ, Halliday JW, Webb SI, Leggett BA, Jazwinska EC, Crawford DHG, Gordeuk VR, McLaren GD, Powell LW. Distribution of transferrin saturation in an Australian population: relevance to the early diagnosis of hemochromatosis. Gastroenterology 1998;114:543–549.
18. Powell LW, George DK, McDonnell SM, Kowdley KV. Diagnosis of hemochromatosis. Ann Intern Med 1998;129:925–931.
19. Burke W, Thomson E, Khoury MJ, McDonnell SM, Press N, Adams PC, Barton JC, Beutler E, Brittenham G, Buchanan A, Clayton EW, Cogswell ME, Meslin EM, Motulsky AG, Powell LW, Sigal

E, Wilfond BS, Collins, FS. Hereditary hemochromatosis Gene discovery and its implications for population-based screening. JAMA 1998;280:173–178.

20. McDonnell SM, Phatak PD, Felitti V, Hover A, McLaren GD. Screening for hemochromatosis in primary care settings. Ann Intern Med 1998;129:962–970.

21. Barton JC, McDonnell SM, Adams PC, Brissot P, Powell LW, Edwards CQ, Cook JD, Kowdley KV. Management of hemochromatosis. Ann Intern Med 1998;129:932–939.

22. McLaren GD. Iron overload disorders. In: Mazza JJ, ed. Manual of Clinical Hematology. Little Brown and Company, Boston, 1995, pp. 115–145.

23. Niederau C, Fisher R, Sonnenberg A, Stremmel W, Trammpisch HJ, Strohmeyer G. Survival and causes of death in cirrhotic and non-cirrhotic patients with primary hemochromatosis. N Engl J Med 1985;313:1256–1262.

24. McLaren GD, Nathanson MH, Saidel GM.1995; Compartmental analysis of intestinal iron absorption and mucosal iron kinetics. In: Siva Subramanian KN, Wastney ME, eds. Kinetic Models of Trace Element and Mineral Metabolism During Development. CRC Press, Boca Raton, pp. 187–204.

25. Cox TM, Peters TJ. Uptake of iron by duodenal biopsy specimens from patients with iron deficiency anaemia and primary haemochromatosis. Lancet 1978;i:123–124.

26. Marx JJ. Mucosal uptake, mucosal transfer and retention of iron, measured by whole-body counting. Scand J Haematol 1979;23:293–302.

27. Powell LW, Campbell CB, Wilson E. Intestinal mucosal uptake of iron and iron retention in idiopathic haemochromatosis as eveidence for a mucosal abnormality. Gut 1970;11:727–731.

28. McLaren GD, Nathanson MH, Jacobs A, Trevett D, Thomson W. Control of iron absorption in hemochromatosis. Mucosal iron kinetics in vivo. Ann NY Acad Sci 1988;526:185–198.

29. McLaren GD, Nathanson MH, Jacobs A, Trevett D, Thomson W. Regulation of intestinal iron absorption and mucosal iron kinetics in hereditary hemochromatosis. J Lab Clin Med 1991;117:390–401.

30. Francanzani AL, Fargion S, Romano R, Piperno A, Arosio P, Ruggeri G, Ronchi G, Fiorelli G. Immunohistochemical evidence for a lack of ferritin in duodenal absorptive epithelial cells in idiopathic hemochromatosis. Gastroenterology 1989;96:1071–1078.

31. Pietrangelo A, Casalgrandi G, Quaglino D, Gualdi R, Conte D, Milani S, Montosi G, Cesarini I., Ventura E, Cairo G. Duodenal ferritin synthesis in genetic hemochromatosis. Gastroenterology 1995;108:208–217.

32. Whittaker P, Skikne BS, Covell AM, Flowers C, Cooke A, Lynch SR, Cook JD. Duodenal iron proteins in idiopathic hemochromatosis. J Clin Invest 1989;83:261–267.

33. Fillet G, Beguin Y, Baldelli L. Model of reticuloendothelial iron metabolism in humans: abnormal behavior in idiopathic hemochromatosis and in inflammation. Blood 1989;74:844–851.

34. Parkkila S, Waheed A, Britton RS, Bacon BR, Zhou XY, Tomatsu S, Fleming RE, Sly WS. Association of the transferrin receptor in human placenta with HFE, the protein defective in hereditary hemochromatosis. Proc Natl Acad Sci USA 1997;94:13198–13202.

35. Waheed A, Parkkila S, Zhou XY, Tomatsu S, Tsuchihashi Z, Feder JN, Schatzman RC, Britton RS, Bacon BR, Sly WS. Hereditary hemochromatosis: effects of C282Y and H63D mutations on association with β_2-microglobulin, intracellular processing, and cell surface expression of the HFE protein in COS-7 cells. Proc Natl Acad Sci USA 1997;94:12384–12389.

36. Santos M, Schilham MW, Rademakers LH, Marx JJ, de Sousa M, Clevers H. Defective iron homeostasis in β_2-microglobulin knockout mice recapitulates hereditary hemochromatosis in man. J Exp Med 1996;184:1975–1985.

37. Gordeuk V, Mukiibi J, Hasstedt SJ, Samowitz W, Edwards CQ, West G, Ndambire S, Emmanual J, Nkanza N, Chapanduka Z, et al. Iron overload in Africa. Interaction between a gene and dietary iron content. N Engl J Med 1992;326:95–100.

38. Barton JC, Edwards CQ, Bertoli LF, Shroyer TW, Hudson SL. Iron overload in African Americans. Am J Med 1995;99:616–623.

39. Wuropa RP, Gordeuk VR, Brittenham GM, Khiyami A, Schechter GP, Edwards CQ. Primary iron overload in African Americans. Am J Med 1996;101:9–18.

40. McLaren CE, Gordeuk VR, Looker AC, Hasselblad V, Edwards CQ, Griffen LM, Kushner JP, Brittenham GM. Prevalence of heterozygotes for hemochromatosis in the white population of the United States. Blood 1995;86:2021–2027.

41. Gordeuk VR, McLaren CE, Looker AC, Hasselblad V, Brittenham GM. Distribution of transferrin staurations in the African-American population. Blood 1998;91:2175–2179.

42. Eason RJ, Adams PC, Aston CE, Searle J. Familial iron overload with possible autosomal dominant inheritance. Aust N Z J Med 1990;20:226–230.
43. Hamill RL, Woods JC, Cook BA. Congenital atransferrinemia. A case report and review of the literature. Am J Clin Pathol 1991;96:215–218.
44. Hayashi A, Wada Y, Suzuki T, Shimizu A. Studies on familial hypotransferrinemia: unique clinical course and molecular pathology. Am J Hum Genet 1993;53:201–213.
45. Goya N, Miyazaki S, Kodate S, Ushio B. A family of congenital atransferrinemia. Blood 1972;40:239–245.
46. Huggenvik JI, Craven CM, Idzerda RL, Bernstein S, Kaplan J, McKnight GS. A splicing defect in the mouse transferrin gene leads to congenital atransferrinemia. Blood 1989;74:482-486.
47. Baker E, Morgan EH. Iron transport. In: Brock JH, Halliday JW, Pippard MJ, Powell LW, eds. Iron Metabolism in Health and Disease. WB Saunders Company, London, 1994, pp. 63–95.
48. Bernstein SE. Hereditary hypotransferrinemia with hemosiderosis; a murine disorder resembling human atransferrinemia. J Lab Clin Med 1987;110:690–705.
49. Simpson RJ, Konijn AM, Lombard M, Raja KB, Salisbury JR, Peters TJ. Tissue iron loading and histopathological changes in hypotransferrinaemic mice. J Pathol 1993;171:237–244.
50. Craven CM, Alexander J, Eldridge M, Kushner JP, Bernstein S, Kaplan J. Tissue distribution and clearance kinetics of non-transferrin-bound iron in the hypotransferrinemic mouse: a rodent model for hemochromatosis. Proc Natl Acad Sci USA 1987;84:3457–3461.
51. Girelli D, Olivieri O, De Franceschi L, Corrocher R, Bergamaschi G, Cazzola M. A linkage between hereditary hyperferritinaemia not related to iron overload and autosomal dominant congenital cataract. Br J Haematol 1995;90:931–934.
52. Bonneau D, Winter Fuseau I, Loiseau MN, Amati P, Berthier M, Oriot D, Beaumont C. Bilateral cataract and high serum ferritin: a new dominant genetic disorder? J Med Genet 1995;32:778–779.
53. Martin ME, Fargion S, Brissot P, Pellat B, Beaumont C. A point mutation in the bulge of the iron-responsive element of the L ferritin gene in two families with the hereditary hyperferritinemia-cataract syndrome. Blood 1998;91:319–323.
54. Girelli D, Corrocher R, Bisceglia L, Olivieri O, De Franceschi L, Zelante L, Gasparini P. Molecular basis for the recently described hereditary hyperferritinemia-cataract syndrome: a mutation in the iron-responsive element of ferritin L-subunit gene (the "Verona mutation") Blood 1995;86:4050–4053.
55. Beaumont C, Leneuve P, Devaux I, Scoazec JY, Berthier M, Loiseau MN, Grandchamp B, Bonneau D. Mutation in the iron responsive element of the L ferritin mRNA in a family with dominant hyperferritinaemia and cataract. Nat Genet 1995;11:444–446.
56. Girelli D, Corrocher R, Bisceglia L, Olivieri O, Zelante L, Panozzo G, Gasparini P. Hereditary hyperferritinemia-cataract syndrome caused by a 29-base pair deletion in the iron responsive element of ferritin L-subunit gene. Blood 1997;90:2084–2088.
57. Cazzola M, Bergamaschi G, Tonon L, Arbustini E, Grasso M, Vercesi E, Barosi G, Bianchi PE, Cairo G, Arosio P. Hereditary hyperferritinemia-cataract syndrome: relationship between phenotypes and specific mutations in the iron-responsive element of ferritin light-chain mRNA. Blood 1997;90:814–821.
58. Levi S, Girelli D, Perrone F, Pasti M, Beaumont C, Corrocher R, Albertini A, Arosio P. Analysis of ferritins in lymphoblastoid cell lines and in the lens of subjects with hereditary hyperferritinemia-cataract syndrome. Blood 1998;91:4180–4187.
59. Koenig M, Mandel JL. Deciphering the cause of Friedrich ataxia. Curr Opin Neurobiol 1997;7:689–694.
60. Gray JV, Johnson KJ. Waiting for frataxin. Nat Genet 1997;16:323–325.
61. Campuzano V, Montermini L, Molto MD, Pianese L, Cossee M, Cavalcanti F, Monros E, Rodius F, Duclos F, Monticelli A, Zara F, Canizares J, Koutnikova H, Bidichandani SI, Gellera C, Brice A, Trouillas P, De Michelle G, Filla A, De Frutos R, Palau F, Patel PI, Di Donato S, Mandel J-L, Cocozza S, Koenig M, Pandolfo M. Friedreich's ataxia: autosomal recessive disease caused by an intronic GAA triplet repeat expansion. Science 1996;271:1423–1427.
62. Koutnikova H, Campuzano V, Foury F, Dolle P, Cazzalini O, Koenig M. Studies of human mouse and yeast homologues indicate a mitochondrial function for frataxin. Nat Genet 1997;16:345–351.
63. Wilson RB, Roof DM. Respiratory deficiency due to loss of mitochondrial DNA in yeast lacking the frataxin homologue. Nat Genet 1997;16:352–357.
64. Campuzano V, Montermini L, Lutz Y, Cova L, Hindelang C, Jiralerspong S, Trottier Y, Kish SJ, Faucheux B, Trouillas P, Authier FJ, Durr A, Mandel JL, Vescovi A, Pandolfo M, Koenig M. Frataxin is reduced in Friedreich ataxia patients and is associated with mitochondrial membranes. Hum Mol Genet 1997;6:1771–1780.

65. Babcock M, de Silva D, Oaks R, Davis-Kaplan S, Jiralerspong S, Montermini L, Pandolfo M, Kaplan J. Regulation of mitochondrial iron accumulation by Yfh1p, a putative homolog of frataxin. Science 1997;276:1709–1712.

66. Foury F, Cazzalini O. Deletion of the yeast homologue of the human gene associated with Friedreich's ataxia elicits iron accumulation in mitochondria. FEBS Lett 1997;411:373–377.

67. Lamarche JB, Shapcott D, Cote M, Lemieux B. Cardiac iron deposits in Friedreich's ataxia. In: Lechtenberg R, ed. Handbook of Cerebellar Diseases. Marcel Dekker, New York, 1993,pp. 373–377.

68. Rotig A, de Lonlay P, Chretien D, Foury F, Koenig M, Sidi D, Munnich A, Rustin P. Aconitase and mitochondrial iron-sulphur protein deficiency in Friedreich ataxia. Nat Genet 1997;17:215–217.

69. Gitlin JD. Aceruloplasminemia. Pediatr Res 1998;44:271–276.

70. Miyajima H, Nishimura Y, Mizoguchi K, Sakamoto M, Shimizu T, Honda N. Familial apoceruloplasmin deficiency associated with blepharospasm and retinal degeneration. Neurology 1987;37:761–767.

71. Logan JI, Harveyson KB, Wisdom GB, Hughes AE, Archbold GP. Hereditary ceruloplasmin deficiency dementia and diabetes. Quarter J Med 1994;87:663–670.

72. Morita H, Ikeda S, Yamamoto K, Morita S, Yoshida K, Nomoto S, Kato M, Yanagisawa N. Hereditary ceruloplasmin deficiency with hemosiderosis: a clinicopathological study of a Japanese family. Ann Neurol 1995; 37:646–656.

73. Yoshida K, Furihata K, Takeda S, Nakamura A, Yamamoto K, Morita H, Hiyamuta S, Ikeda S, Shimizu N, Yanagisawa N. A mutation in the ceruloplasmin gene is associated with systemic hemosiderosis in humans. Nat Genet 1995;9:267–272.

74. Okamoto N, Wada S, Oga T, Kawahata Y, Baba Y, Habu D, Takeda Z, Wada Y. Hereditary ceruloplasmin deficiency with hemosiderosis. Hum Genet 1996;97:755–758.

75. Miyajima H, Takahashi Y, Kamata T, Shimizu H, Sakai N, Gitlin JD. Use of desferrioxamine in the treatment of aceruloplasminemia. Ann Neurol 1997;41:404–407.

76. Harris ZL, Klomp LWJ, Gitlin JD. Aceruloplasminemia: an inherited neurodegenerative disease with impairment of iron homeostasis. Am J Clin Nutr 1998;67(suppl), 972S–977S.

77. Calabrese L, Carbonaro M, Musci G. Presence of coupled trinuclear copper cluster in mammalian ceruloplasmin is essential for efficient electron transfer to oxygen. J Biol Chem 1993;264:6183–6187.

78. Roeser HP, Lee GR, Nacht S, Cartwright GE. The role of ceruloplasmin in iron metabolism. J Clin Invest 1970;49:2408–2417.

79. Osaki S, Johnson DA, Frieden E. The mobilization of iron from the perfused mammalian liver by a serum copper enzyme ferroxiase I. J Biol Chem 1971;246:3018–3023.

80. Klomp LWJ, Gitlin JD. Expression of the ceruloplasmin gene in the human retina and brain: implications for a pathogenic model in aceruloplasminemia. Hum Mol Genet 1996,5.1989–1996.

81. Mukhopadhyay CK, Attieth ZK, Fox PL. Role of ceruloplasmin in cellular iron uptake. Science 1998;279:714–717.

82. Vulpe CD, Kuo Y-M, Murphy TL, Cowley L, Askwith C, Libina N, Gitschier J, Anderson GJ. Hephaestin: a ceruloplasmin homologue implicated in intestinal iron transport and its defect in the sla mouse. Nat Genet 1999;21:195–199.

83. Buchanan GR, Sheehan RG. Malabsorption and defective utilization of iron in three siblings. J Pediatr 1981;98:723–728.

84. Hartman KR, Barker JA. Microcytic anemia with iron malabsorption: an inherited disorder of iron metabolism. Am J Hematol 1996;51:269–275.

85. McCance RA, Widdowson EM. Absorption and excretion of iron. Lancet 1937;ii:680–684.

86. Bannerman RM, Edwards JA, Pinkerton PH. Hereditary disorders of the red cell in animals. Prog Hematol 1973;8:131–179.

87. Russell ES. Hereditary anemias of the mouse: a review for geneticists. Adv Genet 1979;20:357–459.

88. Bannerman RM, Edwards JA, Kreimer Birnbaum M, McFarland E, Russell ES. Hereditary microcytic anaemia in the mouse; studies in iron distribution and metabolism. Br J Haematol 1972;23:235–245.

89. Garrick M, Scott D, Walpole S, Finkelstein E, Whitbred J, Chopra S, Trivikram L, Mayes D, Rhodes D, Cabbagestalk K, Oklu R, Sadiq A, Mascia B, Hoke J, Garrick L. Iron supplementation moderates but does not cure the Belgrade anemia. Biometals 1997;10:65–76.

90. Farcich EA, Morgan EH. Diminished iron acquisition by cells and tissues of Belgrade laboratory rats. Am J Physiol 1992;262:R220–R224.

91. Fleming MD, Trenor CC, Su MA, Foernzler D, Beier DR, Dietrich WF, Andrews NC. Microcytic anaemia mice have a mutation in Nramp2, a candidate iron transport gene. Nat Genet 1997;16:383–386.

92. Fleming MD, Romano MA, Su MA, Garrick LM, Garrick MD, Andrews NC. Nramp2 is mutated in the anemic Belgrade (b) rat: evidence for a role for Nramp2 in endosomal iron transport. Proc Natl Acad Sci USA 1998;95:1148–1153.
93. Garrick LM, Edwards JA, Hoke JE, Bannerman RM. Diminished acquisition of iron by reticulocytes from mice with hemoglobin deficit. Exp Hematol 1987;15:671–675.
94. Anderson GJ, Murphy TL, Cowley L, Evans BA, Halliday JW, McLaren GD. Mapping the gene for murine sex-linked anemia: an inherited defect of intestinal iron absorption in the mouse. Genomics 1998;48:34–39.
95. Kishi F, Tabuchi M. Human natural resistance-associated macrophage protein 2: gene cloning and identification. Biochem Biophys Res Commun 1998;251:775–783.
96. Danks DM. Disorders of copper transport. In: Scriver CR, Beaudet AI, Sly WS, Valle D, eds. The Metabolic Basis of Inherited Disease. McGraw-Hill, New York, 1995, pp. 2211–2235.
97. Vulpe CD, Packman S. Cellular copper transport. Annu Rev Nutr 1995;15:293–322.
98. DiDonato M, Sarkar B. Copper transport and its alterations in Menkes and Wilson diseases. Biochim Biophys Acta 1997;1360:3–16.
99. Tumer Z , Horn N. Menkes disease: recent advances and new aspects. J Med Genet 1997;34:265–274.
100. Kaler SG. Diagnosis and therapy of Menkes syndrome, a genetic form of copper deficiency. Am J Clin Nutr 1998;67(suppl):1029S–1034S.
101. Lucky AW, Hsia YE. Distribution of ingested and injected radiocopper in two patients with Menkes' kinky-hair disease. Pediatr Res 1980;13:1280–1284.
102. Camakaris J, Mann JR, Danks DM. Copper metabolism in mottled mouse mutants: copper concentrations in tissues during development. Biochem J 1979;180:597–604.
103. Darwish HM, Hoke JE, Ettinger MJ. Kinetics of Cu(II) transport and accumulation by hepatocytes from copper-deficient mice and the brindled mouse model of Menkes disease. J Biol Chem 1983;258:13621–13626.
104. Goka TJ, Stevenson RE, Hefferan PM, Howell RR. Menkes' disease: a biochemical abnormality in cultured human fibroblasts. Proc Natl Acad Sci USA 1976;73:604–606.
105. Camakaris J, Danks DM, Ackland L, Cartwright E, Borger P, Cotton RGH. Altered copper metabolism in cultered cells from Menkes' syndrome and mottled mouse mutants. Biochem Genet 1980;18:117–131.
106. Vulpe C, Levinson B, Whitney S, Packman S, Gitschier J. Isolation of a candidate gene for Menkes disease and evidence that it encodes a copper-transporting ATPase. Nat Genet 1993;3:7–13.
107. Chelly J, Tumer Z, Tonnesen T, Petterson A, Ishikawa Brush Y, Tommerup N, Horn N, Monaco AP. Isolation of a candidate gene for Menkes disease that encodes a potential heavy metal binding protein. Nat Genet 1993;3:14–19.
108. Mercer JF, Livingston J, Hall B, Paynter JA, Begy C, Chandrasekharappa S, Lockhart P, Grimes A, Bhave M, Siemieniak D, et al. Isolation of a partial candidate gene for Menkes disease by positional cloning. Nat Genet 1993;3:20–25.
109. Das S, Levinson B, Whitney S, Vulpe C, Packman S , Gitschier J. Diverse mutations in patients with Menkes disease often lead to exon skipping. Am J Hum Genet 1994;55:883–889.
110. Tumer Z, Tonnesen T, Horn N. Detection of genetic defects in Menkes disease by direct mutation analysis and its implications in carrier diagnosis. J Inherit Metab Dis 1994;17:267–270.
111. Tumer Z, Lund C, Tolshave J, Vural B, Tonnesen T, Horn N. Identification of point mutations in 41 unrelated patients affected with Menkes disease. Am J Hum Genet 1997;60:63–71.
112. Das S, Levinson B, Vulpe C, Whitney S, Gitschier J, Packman S. Similar splicing mutations of the Menkes/mottled copper-transporting ATPase gene in occipital horn syndrome and the blotchy mouse. Am J Hum Genet 1995;56:570–576.
113. Kaler SG, Gallo LK, Proud VK, Percy AK, Mark Y, Segal NA, Goldstein DS, Holmes CS, Gahl WA. Occipital horn syndrome and a mild Menkes phenotype associated with splice site mutations at the MNK locus. Nat Genet 1994;8:195–202.
114. Camakaris J, Petris MJ, Bailey L, Shen P, Lockhart P, Glover TW, Barcroft C, Patton J, Mercer JF. Gene amplification of the Menkes (MNK; ATP7A) P-type ATPase gene of CHO cells is associated with copper resistance and enhanced copper efflux. Hum Mol Genet 1995;4:2117–2123.
115. Petris MJ, Mercer JF, Culvenor JG, Lockhart P, Gleeson PA, Camakaris J. Ligand-regulated transport of the Menkes copper P-type ATPase efflux pump from the Golgi apparatus to the plasma membrane: a novel mechanism of regulated trafficking. EMBO J 1996;15:6084–6095.

116. Dierick HA, Adam AN, Escara Wilke JF, Glover TW. Immunocytochemical localization of the Menkes copper transport protein (ATP7A) to the trans-Golgi network. Hum Mol Genet 1997;6:409–416.

117. Yamaguchi Y, Heiny ME, Suzuki M, Gitlin JD. Biochemical characterization and intracellular localization of the Menkes disease protein. Proc Natl Acad Sci USA 1996;93:14030–14035.

118. Roberts EA, Cox DW. Wilson disease. Baillieres Clin Gastroenterol 1998;12:237–256.

119. Bingham MJ, Ong TJ, Summer KH, Middleton RB, McArdle HJ. Physiologic function of the Wilson disease gene product, ATP7B. Am J Clin Nutr 1998;67(suppl) 982S–987S.

120. Dobyns WB, Goldstein NP, Gordon H. Clinical spectrum of Wilson's disease. Mayo Clin Proc 1979;54:35–42.

121. Sternlieb I. Perspectives on Wilson's disease. Hepatology 1990;12:1234–1239.

122. Schilsky ML, Sternlieb I. Overcoming obstacles to the diagnosis of Wilson's disease. Gastroenterology 1997;113:350–353.

123. Polson RJ, Rolles K, Calne RY, Williams R, Marsden D. Reversal of severe neurological manifestations of Wilson's disease following orthotopic liver transplantation. Quarter J Med 1987;244:685–691.

124. Gibbs K, Walshe JM. Biliary excretion of copper in Wilson's disease. Lancet 1980;ii:538–539.

125. Bull PC, Thomas GR, Rommens JM, Forbes JR, Cox DW. The Wilson disease gene is a putative copper transporting P-type ATPase similar to the Menkes gene. Nat Genet 1993;5:327–337.

126. Yamaguchi Y, Heiny ME, Gitlin JD. Isolation and characterization of a human liver cDNA as a candidate gene for Wilson disease. Biochem Biophys Res Commun 1993;197:271–277.

127. Tanzi RE, Petrukhin K, Chernov I, Pellequer JL, Wasco W, Ross B, Romano DM, Parano E, Pavone L, Brzustowicz LM, et al. The Wilson disease gene is a copper transporting ATPase with homology to the Menkes disease gene. Nat Genet 1993;5:344–350.

128. Bull PC, Cox DW. Wilson disease and Menkes disease: new handles on heavy-metal transport. Trends Genet 1994;10:246–252.

129. Shah AB, Chernov I, Zhang HT, Ross BM, Das K, Lutsenko S, Parano E, Pavone L, Evgrafov O, Ivanova Smolenskaya IA, Anneren G, Westermark K, Urrutia FH, Penchaszadeh GK, Sternlieb I, Scheinberg IH, Gilliam TC, Petrukhin K. Identification and analysis of mutations in the Wilson disease gene (ATP7B): population frequencies genotype-phenotype correlation and functional analyses. Am J Hum Genet 1997;61:317–328.

130. Thomas GR, Forbes JR, Roberts EA, Walshe JM, Cox DW. The Wilson disease gene: spectrum of mutations and their consequences. Nat Genet 1995;9:210–217.

131. Bingham MJ, Ong TJ, Ingledew WJ, McArdle HJ. ATP-dependent copper transporter in the Golgi apparatus of rat hepatocytes transports Cu(II) not Cu(I). Am J Physiol 1996;271:G741–G746.

132. Hung III, Suzuki M, Yamaguchi Y, Yuan DS, Klausner RD, Gitlin JD. Biochemical characterization of the Wilson disease protein and functional expression in the yeast Saccharomyces cerevisiae. J Biol Chem 1997;272:21461–21466.

133. Yang XL, Miura N, Kawarada Y, Terada K, Petrukhin K, Gilliam T, Sugiyama T. Two forms of Wilson disease protein produced by alternative splicing are localized in distinct cellular compartments. Biochem J 1997;326:897–902.

134. Payne AS, Kelly EJ, Gitlin JD. Functional expression of the Wilson disease protein reveals mislocalization and impaired copper-dependent trafficking of the common H1069Q mutation. Proc Natl Acad Sci USA 1998;95:10854–10859.

135. Yuan DS, Stearman R, Dancis A, Dunn T, Beeler T, Klausner RD. The Menkes/Wilson disease gene homologue in yeast provides copper to a ceruloplasmin-like oxidase required for iron uptake. Proc Natl Acad Sci USA 1995;92:2632–2636.

136. Camakaris J, Phillips M, Danks DM, Brown R, Stevenson T. Mutations in humans and animals which affect copper metabolism. J Inherit Metab Dis 1983;6(Suppl 1):44–50.

137. Levinson B, Vulpe C, Elder B, Martin C, Verley F, Packman S, Gitschier J. The mottled gene is the mouse homologue of the Menkes disease gene. Nat Genet 1994;6:369–373.

138. Reed V, Boyd Y. Mutation analysis provides additional proof that mottled is the mouse homologue of Menkes' disease. Hum Mol Genet 1997;6:417–423.

139. Cecchi C, Biasotto M, Tosi M, Avner P. The mottled mouse as a model for human Menkes disease: identification of mutations in the Atp7a gene. Hum Mol Genet 1997;6:425–433.

140. Grimes A, Hearn CJ, Lockhart P, Newgreen DF, Mercer JF. Molecular basis of the brindled mouse mutant (Mo(br)): a murine model of Menkes disease. Hum Mol Genet 1997;6:1037–1042.

141. Theophilos MB, Cox DW, Mercer JF. The toxic milk mouse is a murine model of Wilson disease. Hum Mol Genet 1996;5:1619–1624.

142. Wu J, Forbes JR, Chen HS, Cox DW. The LEC rat has a deletion in the copper transporting ATPase gene homologous to the Wilson disease gene. Nat Genet 1994;7:541–545.
143. Kuo YM, Gitschier J, Packman S. Developmental expression of the mouse mottled and toxic milk genes suggests distinct functions for the Menkes and Wilson disease copper transporters. Hum Mol Genet 1997;6:1043–1049.
144. Mercer JF. Menkes syndrome and animal models. Am J Clin Nutr 1998;67(suppl):1022S–1028S.
145. Masson W, Hughes H, Papworth D, Boyd Y, Horn N. Abnormalities of copper accumulation in cell lines established from nine different alleles of mottled are the same as those found in Menkes disease. J Med Genet 1997;34:729–732.
146. Biempica L, Rauch H, Quintana N, Sternlieb I. Morphological and chemical studies on a murine mutation (toxic milk) resulting in hepatic copper toxicosis. Lab Invest 1988;59:500–508.
147. Nagano K, Nakamura K, Urakami K-I, Umeyama K, Uchiyama H, Koiwai K, Hattori S, Yamamoto T, Matsuda I, Endo F. Intracellular distribution of the Wilson's disease gene product (ATPase7B) after in vitro and in vivo exogenous expression in hepatocytes from the LEC rat an animal model of Wilson's disease. Hepatology 1998;27:799–807.
148. Yoshida K, Tokusashi Y, Lee G-H, Ogawa K. Intrahepatic transplantation of normal hepatocytes prevents Wilson's disease in Long-Evans Cinnamon rats. Gastroenterology 1996;111:1654–1660.
149. Aggett PJ. Acrodermatitis enteropathica. J Inherit Metab Dis 1983;6(Suppl 1):39–43.
150. Van Wouwe JP. Clinical and laboratory diagnosis of acrodermatitis enteropathica. Eur J Pediatr 1989;149:2–8.
151. Vallee BL, Falchuk KH. The biochemical basis of zinc physiology. Physiological reviews 1993;73:79–118.
152. Atherton DJ, Muller DPR, Aggett PJ, Harries JT. A defect in zinc uptake by jejunal biopsies in acrodermatitis enteropathica. Clin Sci 1979;56:505–507.
153. Weissman K, Hoe S, Knudson L, Sorensen SS. ^{65}Zinc absorption in patients suffering from acrodermatitis enteropathica and in normal adults assessed by whole-body counting technique. Br J Dermatol 1979;101:573–579.
154. Sandstrom B, Cederblad A, Lindblad BS, Lonnerdal B. Acrodermatitis enteropathica: zinc metabolism, copper status and immune function. Arch Pediatr Adolesc Med 1994;148:980–985.
155. Grider A, Young EM. The acrodermatitis enteropathica mutation transiently affects zinc metabolism in human fibroblasts. J Nutr 1996;126:219–224.
156. Vazquez F, Grider A. The effect of the acrodermatitis enteropathica mutation on zinc uptake in human fibroblasts. Biol Trace Elem Res 1995;50:109–117.
157. Grider A, Lin YF, Muga SJ. Differences in the cellular zinc content and 5'-nucleotidase activity of normal and acrodermatitis enteropathica (AE) fibroblasts. Biol Trace Elem Res 1998;61:1–8.
158. Grider A, Mouat MF. The acrodermatitis enteropathica mutation affects protein expression in human fibroblasts: analysis by two-dimensional gel electrophoresis. J Nutr 1998;128:1311–1314.
159. Chesters JK. Zinc metabolism in animals: pathology, immunology, and genetics. J Inherit Metab Dis 1983;6 (Suppl 1):34–38.
160. Weismann K, Flagstad T. Hereditary zinc deficiency (Adema disease) in cattle, and animal parallel to acrodermatitis enteropathica. Acta Derm Venereol 1976;56:151–154.
161. Machen M, Montgomery T, Holland R, Braselton E, Dunstan R, Brewer G, Yuzbasiyan-Gurkan V. Bovine hereditary zinc deficiency: lethal trait A 46. J Vet Diagn Invest 1996;8:219–227.
162. AcklandML and MercerJF.1992; The murine mutation, lethal milk, results in production of zinc-deficient milk J Nutr 122 1214-1218.
163. Lee DY, Shay NF, Cousins RJ. Altered zinc metabolism occurs in murine lethal milk syndrome. J Nutr 1992;122:2233–2238.
164. Piletz JE, Ganschow RE. Lethal milk mutation results in dietary zinc deficiency in nursing mice. Am J Clin Nutr 1978;31:560–562.
165. Huang L, Gitschier J. A novel gene involved in zinc transport is deficient in the lethal milk mouse. Nat Genet 1998;17:292–297.

13 Trace Element and Mineral Nutrition in Endocrine Diseases

John T. Dunn, MD

1. INTRODUCTION

The endocrine system is classically subdivided into six secretory organs — the pituitary/hypothalamus, thyroid, adrenal, parathyroid, pancreas, and gonads. Most of these produce more than one hormone. Singly and in combination, they modulate many systems and processes in the body. Other tissues also produce hormones and could appropriately be considered as part of the endocrine system, e.g., gut and kidney. The thyroid's dependence on iodine is the most important interaction between trace metals and endocrine disease and receives the most extensive coverage in this chapter. The parathyroids are essential to calcium homeostasis and their role is also discussed in detail. Most of the remaining endocrine systems have a relatively minor relationship with trace elements and minerals.

2. THYROID

2.1. The Thyroid's Need for Iodine

Iodine is an essential component of the thyroid hormones, thyroxine (T_4) and 3,5,3'-triiodothyronine (T_3), constituting respectively, 64% and 59% of their molecular weights. Several international groups including the International Council for Control of Iodine Deficiency Disorders, the World Health Organization, and the Food and Nutrition Board of the US National Academy of Sciences, recommend 150 µg iodine as the minimum daily adult ration (1). The urinary iodine concentration is a convenient marker for iodine nutrition, with optimal levels in the 100–300 µg/L range.

Iodine can be ingested through food and water in a variety of chemical forms. Most is released as iodide (I^-) in the stomach and then transported across the gastric mucosa to the circulatory system. The thyroid gland actively extracts iodide from the circulating blood via its sodium/iodide symporter. Once in the thyroid cell, iodide reaches the apical region where it is oxidized by thyroid peroxidase and attaches to thyroglobulin (2). The latter is a 660,000 kDa glycoprotein consisting of two identical chains, each of 2750 residues including 67 tyrosyls (for human thyroglobulin). The initial reaction is the iodination of selected tyrosyls to form monoiodotyrosine or diiodotyrosine within the

From: *Clinical Nutrition of the Essential Trace Elements and Minerals: The Guide for Health Professionals*
Edited by: J. D. Bogden and L. M. Klevay © Humana Press Inc., Totowa, NJ

polypeptide chain. Further action of the peroxidase couples two diiodotyrosyl residues to produce T_4 at the acceptor site, still within thyroglobulin's polypeptide chains, and leaving dehydroalanine at the donor site. Human thyroglobulin has four major hormonogenic sites. The most important, site A, is very close to the N-terminus, at residue 5, and depending on the animal species, accounts for about 40% of thyroglobulin's T_4. The second most important site, site B, is about 200 residues from the C-terminus. The third site, site C, is two residues from the C-terminus, and is particularly associated with T_3 formation in some species. The fourth major site, site D, is in the midportion of the molecule and is especially sensitive to TSH stimulation in some species.

Hormone-containing thyroglobulin is stored in the lumen of the thyroid follicle, where it constitutes the so-called colloid. For hormone release, thyroglobulin is degraded, first in endosomes and then lysosomes *(3)*. Three lysosomal endopeptidases, cathepsins L, B, and D, are important to thyroglobulin's degradation. Each has characteristic cleavage sites, and the activity of cathepsins B and L is regulated by TSH. Lysosomal exopeptidases, particularly dipeptidyl peptidase I, provide further breakdown. Free thyroid hormone is then carried to the thyroid's basal membrane, and released into the circulation. There it attaches to thyroid binding proteins, principally thyroxine binding globulin and transthyretin. They carry hormone to selected tissues, particularly liver, muscle, heart, kidney, and developing brain. At each target, thyroxine is deiodinated intracellularly to triiodothyronine, the active hormone form. Within tissues, thyroid hormones exert specific effects on cellular metabolism, mostly by influencing the synthesis and action of proteins, particularly enzymes. TSH acts at many steps in thyroidal iodine metabolism, increasing iodide uptake, thyroglobulin iodination, formation of both T_3 and T_4, and thyroglobulin proteolysis to release free hormone.

2. 2. Iodine Deficiency

Insufficient iodine lowers production and availability of thyroid hormone, so the major effect of iodine deficiency is hypothyroidism. The extent of the clinical manifestations depends on the severity of the iodine deficiency and the individual's success in adapting to it *(4)*. The major defense against inadequate circulating hormone is the pituitary, which responds by increasing TSH secretion. All of TSH's many effects on thyroid metabolism are aimed at increasing the efficient production and release of thyroid hormone.

The first clinical manifestation of iodine deficiency is thyroid enlargement or goiter (the term means simply an enlarged thyroid) (Fig. 1). Like a muscle asked to work harder, the thyroid's response to the increased demand for hormone is hyperplasia. Often this adaptation of the thyroid is sufficient to maintain the euthyroid state. For instance, in much of western Europe, with moderate iodine deficiency, the average thyroid size is considerably greater than in the iodine-sufficient United States, but serious features of hypothyroidism are probably not more frequent. Goiter is frequently and erroneously dismissed as a cosmetic inconvenience and an insignificant competitor for health care spending, particularly in developing countries, but it is important in its own right. A large goiter can cause significant compression on the trachea and esophagus. Longstanding-hyperplasia eventually leads to nodularity, including autonomous nodules, that may later, somewhat paradoxically, produce excessive thyroid hormones and make the subject hyperthyroid (toxic nodular goiter) *(5)*. The annual health-related costs incurred by iodine-deficient Germany for goiter alone have been estimated at about 1 billion dollars *(6)*.

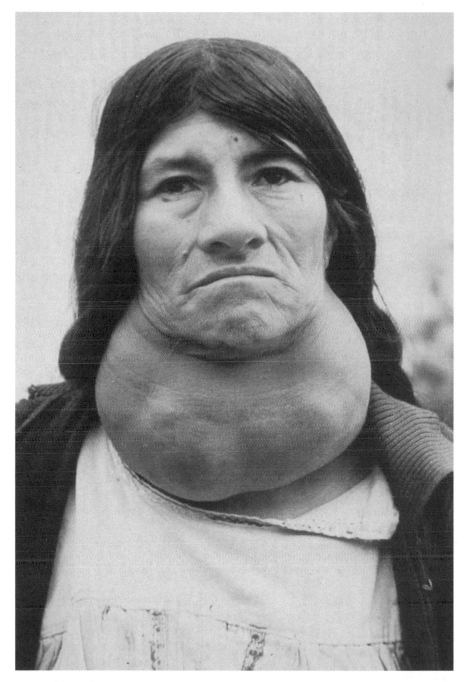

Fig. 1. Large multinodular goiter from iodine deficient area of Latin America (courtesy, Dr. A. Pardo).

If the adaptive mechanisms are inadequate to meet the challenge of iodine deficiency, insufficient thyroid hormone is produced and the subject becomes clinically hypothyroid. The manifestations vary with the individual, but typically include fatigue, somnolence, cold intolerance, constipation, menorrhagia, and dry skin. Prolonged hypothyroidism promotes atherosclerosis and hypertension, and these may not be completely reversible when euthyroidism is restored.

Hypothyroidism, from iodine deficiency or any other cause, is a much more serious condition for the fetus and young infant than for the adult, because adequate thyroid hormone is essential for proper maturation of the central nervous system, particularly its myelination. A large clinical and experimental literature has cataloged the consequences of hypothyroidism in early development *(7)*. The principal effects are mental and physical retardation. The problem is further complicated in iodine deficient regions because the mother is also iodine deficient, and the fetus depends on maternal thyroid hormone during the first trimester. The United States and other iodine-sufficient western countries routinely employ neonatal screening to detect and provide early treatment for the one in 4000 infants who have congenital hypothyroidism, usually from thyroid aplasia. With prompt recognition and treatment, only minimal permanent defects occur. In iodine deficient countries, including much of Europe, neonatal screening demonstrates an increased incidence of transient neonatal hypothyroidism, manifested by increased blood spot TSH determination *(8)*. While most of these infants appear to improve spontaneously, they may retain mild degrees of permanent impairment, but the extent of this consequence is uncertain.

Severe iodine deficiency during early human development can produce cretinism (Fig. 2). The cardinal feature, severe mental retardation, may be accompanied by varying degrees of growth stunting, deaf mutism, and delayed neuromuscular development. The literature occasionally makes a distinction between "neurological" and "myxedematous" forms of cretinism *(7)*. In addition to mental retardation, the latter usually show hypothyroidism and markedly short stature, whereas the former may have only the mental retardation with varying degrees of deaf mutism and gait disturbances. Many cretins are otherwise healthy, with good eyesight, intact hand coordination, and strong bodies.

Iodine deficiency also causes reproductive loss and decreased infant survival. Spontaneous abortions are frequent. Studies from a number of developing countries have shown that correction of iodine deficiency, in the absence of other apparent change, dramatically decreases neonatal and early infant mortality *(9,10)*.

Iodine deficiency has similar adverse effects on other animals. Examples are hairless pig malady, increased abortions in cattle, stunted growth in piglets, and decreased egg laying in chickens. All these effects are preventable with adequate iodine, and addition of iodine to feeds has been a standard practice in modern agriculture for almost a century. The consequences of iodine deficiency on both the animals and people in affected regions result in socioeconomic backwardness that further complicates human existence in these areas.

In principal, iodine deficiency is easy to correct *(11)*. Fortification of salt with potassium iodate or potassium iodide is the favored approach, because salt is a universal dietary requirement, its sources are usually limited and susceptible to control and the technology is simple and inexpensive. Great strides have been made in the last 10 yr in promoting universal salt iodization in developing countries. For countries that import all their salt, control is fairly simple but it may be much more difficult in others with widespread remote salt sources. Other measures are periodic (yearly) administration of capsules of iodized vegetable oil (200–400 mg iodine in a single dose), tablets of potassium iodide or Lugol's iodine solution, administered every several weeks or months, or iodized water. For the latter, at the simplest level, potassium iodide or iodate is added to standing drinking water in schools or homes. Simple devices can add iodine (I_2) to running water and achieve both correction of iodine deficiency and water purification. Occasionally other vehicles, such as candy, sugar, and bread, are used for iodization and may be appropriate under special circumstances, but salt is usually more practical.

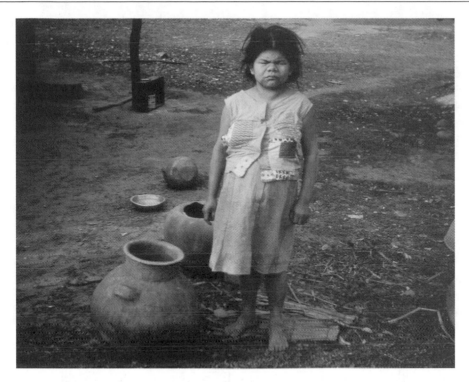

Fig. 2. Severe adult endemic cretin, with short stature, mental retardation, and deaf mutism, from area of severe iodine deficiency.

The magnitude of iodine deficiency as a public health problem deserves emphasis (*see* Chapter 6). Most countries of the world, including highly industrialized ones, such as western Europe, have at least some degree of iodine deficiency. The World Health Organization estimated that 29% of the world's population lives in areas of iodine deficiency and risks its consequences *(12)*. In some developing countries, the goiter prevalence, an indicator for iodine deficiency, is over 50%. A meta-analysis estimated that iodine deficiency caused an average loss of 13 IQ points per person in affected areas, making it the leading cause of preventable mental retardation in the world *(13)*. Numerous studies have shown the benefits of correction of iodine deficiency, not only for people but for animals and the economy. The World Summit for Children of 1990 pledged the virtual elimination of iodine deficiency by the year 2000. In 1997, we estimated that of the world's 150 most populous nations, 41 (27%) had achieved sustainable elimination of iodine deficiency, 32 (21%) were rapidly approaching elimination, 59 (39%) continued with mild or moderate deficiency, 2 (2%) had severe iodine deficiency, and the situation was unknown in 16 (11%) *(14)*. These figures represent considerable improvement within the decade of the 1990s, but completing the task and sustaining the achievement require continued effort *(15)*.

2.3. Iodine Excess

Acute iodine excess is rare. Iodine (I_2) taken in concentrated doses irritates oral and intestinal mucosa. Occasionally patients have reactions to iodine-containing radiocontrast dyes, manifested by a rash and other allergic features. Most iodine-sufficient people can ingest huge amounts of iodine, several hundred mg daily, without significant effect. An exception occurs in areas of iodine deficiency, where many people, particularly the older ones, have autonomous nodules as the result of their longstanding iodine deficiency (5). The synthesis of thyroid hormone in such nodules is unchecked, and when provided with large amounts of iodine, they overproduce hormone and cause hyperthyroidism. An example of this so-called iodine-induced hyperthyroidism is an older individual with nodular goiter who undergoes a procedure using iodine-containing radiocontrast medium, such as cardiac catheterization, or is treated with amiodarone (containing about 75 mg iodine in a daily dose) and develops clinical hyperthyroidism.

Iodine-induced hyperthyroidism also occurs in a more chronic form (5). Many, perhaps most, successful iodine prophylactic programs provoke an increase in hyperthyroidism, particularly in older subjects with nodular goiters. Usually this effect is transient in the population, and the hyperthyroidism can be treated satisfactorily. Occasionally, this complication can be serious and even fatal in situations with inadequate medical care. Awareness of this possibility leads to early diagnosis and prompt treatment. While iodine-induced hyperthyroidism is an unfortunate consequence of successful iodine prophylaxis, its significance to the community is dwarfed by the importance of eliminating iodine deficiency for the proper development of the young (1).

High levels of iodine are associated with an increased incidence of autoimmune thyroid disease. Several clinical subtypes are recognized, all having autoantibodies directed to the thyroid. In Graves' disease, antibodies to the TSH receptor stimulate the thyroid to over-produce thyroid hormone, leading to clinical hyperthyroidism. In chronic thyroiditis or Hashimoto's disease, the autoantibodies are destructive, leading to hypothyroidism and occasionally goiter. Subjects with Graves' disease usually also have the destructive antibodies and so eventually become hypothyroid as well. Many patients with Graves' disease, and some with Hashimoto's, have associated eye abnormalities, characterized by protrusion, irritation, muscle swelling, and an increase in retrobulbar fat. This ophthalmopathy is also immunologically mediated but details of its relationship to the thyroid disease are unclear.

Several lines of evidence point to a role for iodine in the pathogenesis of autoimmune thyroid diseases. The incidence of autoimmune thyroid diseases is generally correlated epidemiologically with levels of dietary iodine intake. Long-term observations in several countries that have increased their dietary iodine document an increased prevalence of autoimmune thyroid disease (16). Several experimental models show induction of chronic thyroiditis with increasing iodine administration (17). Iodination of thyroglobulin increases its antigenicity, and monoclonal antibodies developed to human thyroglobulin recognize several iodinated epitopes (18).

Epidemiologic studies also show an increase in papillary thyroid cancer with increasing iodine ingestion (19). Many of these cancers are found incidentally at autopsy, and appear biologically unimportant. A rough correlation exists between dietary iodine levels in a population and the incidence of papillary cancer. Longitudinal studies in some areas have correlated increasing dietary iodine with the incidence of papillary cancer. The mechanism is not known.

2.4. Selenium

The last decade has witnessed a growing awareness of a role for selenium in thyroid action and disease. As described above, T_4 is converted to T_3, the active form of the hormone, by deiodinases. The type I 5'-deiodinase is found in the thyroid, kidney, and the liver, while type II is localized principally in the central nervous system. Selenium deficiency markedly impairs type I activity in liver and kidney, and decreases T_4 deiodination. In the thyroid, selenium is an integral component of glutathione peroxidase, which acts in reducing hydrogen peroxide. Selenium deficiency lowers the metabolism of hydrogen peroxide. Contempre and colleagues *(20)* have proposed that myxedematous cretinism develops from the combined deficiencies of selenium and iodine. In studies with rats they found necrotic and fibrotic thyroids typical of myxedematous cretinism. Mitchell et al. *(21)* noted that the increased demand for peroxidase activity in iodine deficiency would increase the requirement for selenium. Epidemiologic support for this pathogenesis comes from Congo, where myxedematous cretins are most common and the combined severe deficiencies of iodine and selenium coexist. Corvilain *(22)* also hypothesized that selenium deficiency, by decreasing thyroxine deiodination and enhancing thyroxine synthesis, might save thyroxine for the fetal brain and protect it from neurological cretinism.

2.5. Calcitonin

The major product of the thyroid gland is the thyroid hormones made by the follicular cells. In addition, the parafollicular cells of the thyroid make and secrete calcitonin, a 32 amino acid peptide of uncertain physiologic role. Experimentally, calcitonin increases renal excretion of calcium and inhibits osteoclastic bone resorption. It has clinical importance as a pharmacologic agent for reducing serum calcium, and also as a highly specific marker for medullary carcinoma of the thyroid.

3. PARATHYROID

The parathyroid glands, usually two on each side, are located immediately behind, or occasionally within, the two thyroid lobes. They make parathormone (PTH) an 84 residue polypeptide that regulates the metabolism of calcium and phosphate, by mobilizing calcium and phosphate from bone, decreasing renal excretion of calcium, and increasing renal retention of phosphate and vitamin D. The parathyroids respond to circulating levels of calcium by raising or lowering PTH secretion, to keep the subject eucalcemic.

Hyperparathyroidism ensues when excess secretion occurs. The most common cause is a hypersecretory parathyroid tumor. Most are benign single adenomas, but they may occasionally be multiple or malignant. Clinical manifestations are kidney stones, hypertension, osteoporosis, and poorly characterized musculoskeletal discomfort. Today most cases are asymptomatic and discovered incidentally by routine laboratory screens that include a serum calcium. In addition to hypercalcemia, other laboratory features include a low serum phosphate, normal albumin, and high serum chloride. The diagnosis is confirmed with a serum PTH measurement that is inappropriately high for the serum calcium. Neck ultrasound or sestimibi imaging may help in localizing an adenoma. A 24-h urinary calcium excretion should be obtained to exclude familial hypercalcemic hypocalciuria, an uncommon benign condition. With widespread use of routine screening blood chemistry, detection in the asymptomatic stage is the rule. More advanced disease produces higher serum calcium levels and additional symptoms of somnolence, cardiac arrhythmias, and bone fractures.

Another cause of hyperparathyroidism is hyperplasia. This typically involves all the parathyroid glands. In multiple endocrine neoplasia type IIA, medullary carcinoma of the thyroid, pheochromocytoma, and hyperparathyroidism coexist. This syndrome occurs as an autosomal dominant and is linked to one of several specific mutations in the ret proto-oncogene. Kidney failure also causes hyperparathyroidism. Renal loss of calcium leads to parathyroid hyperplasia, initially with low or normal calcemia (secondary hyperparathyroidism), but later autonomy may develop, leading to hypercalcemia (tertiary hyperparathyroidism).

The most common treatment for hyperparathyroidism is surgery. The clinical setting frequently helps in predicting whether an adenoma or hyperplasia is more likely. At operation, the surgeon can usually diagnose an adenoma by its size. The other parathyroids should be identified, because adenomas are occasionally multiple or a suspected case of adenoma may turn out to be hyperplasia. If a single adenoma is found, it alone is removed. With hyperplasia, most parathyroid tissue is removed, usually leaving approximately one-half of one gland. Some surgeons transplant remaining parathyroid tissue to the forearm so that if hyperplasia recurs, the gland can be easily reached for resection. Many decisions on approach must be made at the time of operation and it is essential to involve a surgeon with extensive experience.

Following successful surgery, many patients become transiently hypocalcemic with the sudden removal of excess PTH stimulation on the bones ("hungry bone syndrome"). The previously suppressed normal parathyroids may take some time to resume function, and during this interval the patient needs treatment with calcium and synthetic vitamin D. In most instances, this reactive hypoparathyroidism is transient, but sometimes it is permanent, particularly after extensive neck surgery. This consequence occurs more commonly with operations for other purposes, such as for thyroidectomy or for neck cancer. With proper balancing of synthetic vitamin D and oral calcium, the serum calcium can be kept in the normal range. Patients with hypoparathyroidism need to be followed regularly to avoid over-treatment that can lead to hypercalcemia and consequent renal damage from hypercalciuria. However, in most instances this regulation is straightforward, and after initial adjustment, maintenance is of minimal inconvenience to the patient.

Spontaneous hypoparathyroidism is rare. In the adult, the usual cause is atrophy, probably autoimmune in nature. A much more common cause for hypoparathyroidism is neck surgery, described previously, in which the parathyroids are damaged or removed. In either spontaneous or postsurgical hypoparathyroidism, the clinical features are those of hypocalcemia, particularly paresthesias circumorally and peripherally. When the hypocalcemia is severe, tetany and cardiac arrhythmia may ensue. The treatment is vitamin D and calcium, as outlined above.

4. PANCREAS

The major hormones of the pancreas are insulin and glucagon. The basic action of insulin is to regulate glucose utilization. It increases glucose transport, decreases gluconeogenesis, increases fatty acid transport and triglyceride synthesis and promotes protein synthesis. Glucagon is a counter-regulatory hormone that balances effects of insulin. Insulin deficiency produces diabetes mellitus, an extremely common disorder that contributes heavily to chronic cardiovascular and renal disease. Two types are recognized. Type I typically occurs early in life, with almost complete destruction of beta cells. Its pathogenesis involves environmental insults and autoimmune destruction. Type II typically occurs later in life in association with obesity and insulin resistance.

A number of studies have looked at trace elements in diabetes, especially zinc. The available literature generally agrees that urinary zinc excretion is increased in diabetes, but serum zinc levels have usually been in the normal range. Zinc in leukocytes has been normal, but erythrocytes have either lower levels or have less capacity to respond to exogenous zinc. Various studies have suggested that zinc absorption may be lower in diabetics and that growth in diabetic children may be negatively correlated with zinc excretion (23). These considerations have led to recommendations for zinc supplementation in diabetics, but in one study (24) zinc treatment increased the blood hemoglobin A1C, a marker for hyperglycemia, and the authors suggested large doses of zinc supplementation might have adverse affects.

Measurements of other trace elements in the urine of diabetics have reported lower amounts of copper and chromium, and higher amounts of manganese and magnesium. Copper deficiency in rats increased serum cholesterol, glucose, and glycated hemoglobin (25,26). In two healthy human volunteers, experimentally induced copper deficiency appeared to impair glucose tolerance that returned to normal after repletion of copper (27). Other studies suggested a correlation between urinary copper excretion and the diabetic complications of increased infections and neuropathy (28), and associated retinopathy, hypertension, and microvascular disease with higher concentrations of copper in the plasma (29).

A relationship between chromium and carbohydrate metabolism has been recognized for years (30). Chromium appears to potentiate the action of insulin at the receptor level. Treatment of subjects with apparently inadequate chromium improves the glucose tolerance in diabetes or malnutrition. Supplementation of chromium is also reported to ameliorate hypoglycemia, a postulated effect of improved insulin deficiency (30). Chromium levels decrease with age and have been suggested as a factor in increased risk for developing impaired glucose metabolism and diabetes (31). Studies supplementing diabetics with chromium have been effective in lowering triglycerides, but it has been more difficult to show effects on glycemia (32). Manganese deficiency is associated with decreased insulin production in experimental animals, suggesting either a role for manganese in insulin biosynthesis or a depletion of pancreatic beta cells with the deficiency.

5. ADRENAL

The adrenal gland has two anatomically and functionally distinct components, the cortex and medulla. The cortex produces cortisol (a glucocorticoid) and aldosterone (a mineralocorticoid), and the medulla produces catecholamines, principally epinephrine. Cortisol has many effects on metabolism. It promotes gluconeogenesis and amino acid degradation in the liver, particularly during fasting, stimulates fat breakdown and affects tissue growth, especially in fetal tissues. Glucocorticoids are widely used pharmacologically, particularly for their antiinflammatory properties. Well-defined clinical syndromes of excess or inadequate glucocorticoids exist but neither hormone has a direct or specific relationship to trace metals as far as is known. Aldosterone acts on the kidney to promote sodium reabsorption and potassium excretion. Copper deficiency in rats diminished the response to excess NaCl as shown by lowered plasma levels of aldosterone, angiotensin converting enzyme, and renin, relative to controls (33).

Epinephrine is the main catecholamine of the adrenal. Clinically it increases the rate and output of the heart, alters blood flow in smooth muscles, and inhibits insulin secretion, thus increasing circulating glucose. Pheochromocytomas are tumors (usually but not invariably found in the adrenal medulla), that secrete epinephrine or norepinephrine to produce hypertension, flushing, and tachycardia.

Copper deficiency is the principal connection between trace metals and the catecholamines. Most data are limited to experimental animals. Copper-deficient mice develop cardiac hypertrophy, and in one study had increased norepinephrine and dopamine levels in the urine, without change in epinephrine *(34)*. Clinical correlation in humans of these limited studies is not available.

6. PITUITARY AND HYPOTHALAMUS

The major hormones of the pituitary are thyrotropin (TSH), adrenocorticotropin (ACTH), follicle stimulating hormone (FSH), luteinizing hormone (LH), growth hormone, and prolactin. The first four of these act as stimulating hormones, respectively, to the thyroid, adrenal cortex, and gonads, to direct the secretion of their hormones. As its name implies, growth hormone promotes metabolism and growth in many tissues. Prolactin stimulates the breast to secrete milk. The pituitary hormones regulate peripheral secretion of target organs through a feedback system, whereby pituitary secretion responds reciprocally to circulating levels of the peripheral hormone. For example, pituitary secretion of TSH is governed by circulating T_4 concentrations; low circulating T_4 increases TSH secretion, and high T_4 suppresses it. The hypothalamus secretes releasing hormones for each of these pituitary hormones: thyroid releasing hormone (TRH) for TSH and prolactin, corticotropin releasing hormone (CRH) for ACTH, gonadotropin releasing hormone (GnRH) for LH and FSH, and growth hormone releasing factor (GRF) for growth hormone. These releasing hormones act in coordination with the pituitary and peripheral hormones to maintain homeostasis. The posterior pituitary secretes antidiuretic hormone or vasopressin. It regulates water balance through actions on the kidney.

Most clinical disorders of the pituitary and hypothalamus relate to hypersecretory tumors, mass effects from nonsecretory tumors, or deficiencies from a variety of causes. The literature contains very little reliable or recent information on the influence of trace metals and minerals on pituitary and hypothalamic function.

7. REPRODUCTION

The important gonadal hormones are estrogen in the female and testosterone in the male, made respectively in the ovary and testis. They act at tissue-sensitive receptors to promote development of sexual characteristics. The reproductive system is complex, requiring balance and feedback among the relevant hypothalamic, pituitary, and gonadal hormones. Performance of the system is influenced generally by nutrition and proper function of other endocrine systems, including the thyroid, adrenal, pancreas, and pituitary. The clinical disorders relate to dysfunction or imbalance among any members of this complex system. The literature shows little recent or reliable data on a relationship between the human reproductive system and trace metals and minerals in clinical disease. One study reported a reversible decreased sperm count in four of five middle-aged men with experimentally restricted zinc intake *(35)*. More data exist for experimental and agricultural animals. For example, reproduction in cattle is adversely affected by deficiencies of calcium, phosphorus, and selenium *(36)*. Zinc deficiency is associated with fetal mortality and malformation in rats *(37)*. The extensive effects of iodine deficiency were cited previously. To avoid these effects, modern agricultural practice routinely incorporates trace elements and minerals in animal feeds.

8. SUMMARY

Iodine deficiency is the most important interaction between the endocrine system and trace elements and minerals. Iodine is an essential component of the thyroid hormones, and its deficiency produces mental retardation, goiter, hypothyroidism, reproductive impairment, and increased child mortality. Most countries harbor some areas with iodine deficiency and risk its consequences, with about 29% of the world's population at risk as of 1993. Major national and international efforts have greatly reduced this number, through a vigorous program of iodized salt. Selenium is a component of the deiodinases that convert thyroxine into the active form, triiodothyronine, and its deficiency also contributes to inadequate thyroid hormone action. The parathyroid glands regulate calcium and phosphate metabolism in bone and kidney. Hyperparathyroidism from adenomas is a common clinical condition, producing hypercalcemia, osteoporosis, and renal impairment, but can be treated effectively with surgery. Zinc excretion increases in diabetes mellitus, but its clinical importance is unclear. Deficiencies of copper, chromium, and manganese may impair glucose metabolism but the extent and clinical importance is not established. Copper deficiency may affect plasma levels of aldosterone and affect urinary excretion of catecholamines. Scattered reports show adverse affects on reproductive outcome from deficiencies in calcium, phosphorus, selenium, and zinc, as well as iodine. Little information exists on the effects of trace elements on pituitary function. In summary, the most important trace elements and minerals that impinge on the endocrine system are iodine and calcium with probable but less well established roles for sélenium, zinc, and copper.

REFERENCES

1. Dunn JT, Semigran J, Delange F. The prevention and management of iodine-induced hyperthyroidism and its cardiac features. Thyroid 1998;8:101–106.
2. Dunn JT. Thyroglobulin: chemistry and biosynthesis. In: Braverman LE, Utiger RD, eds. Werner and Ingbar's The Thyroid. A Fundamental and Clinical Text. Lippincott-Raven, Philadelphia, PA, 1996, pp. 85–95.
3. Dunn AD. Thyroglobulin retrieval and the endocytic pathway. In: Braverman LE, Utiger RD, eds. Werner and Ingbar's The Thyroid. A Fundamental and Clinical Text. Lippincott-Raven, Philadelphia, PA, 1996, pp. 81–84.
4. Delange F. The disorders induced by iodine deficiency. Thyroid 1994;4:107–128.
5. Stanbury JB, Ermans AE, Bourdoux P, Todd C, Oken E, Tonglet R, Vidor G, Braverman LE, Medeiros-Neto G. Iodine-induced hyperthyroidism: occurrence and epidemiology. Thyroid 1998;8:83–100.
6. Pfannenstiel P. The cost of continuing iodine deficiency in Germany and the potential cost benefit of iodine prophylaxis. IDD Newsletter 1998;14(1):11–12.
7. Stanbury JB, ed. The Damaged Brain of Iodine Deficiency. Cognizant Communication Corp, New York, 1994.
8. Delange F, Heidemann P, Bourdoux P, et al. Regional variations of iodine nutrition and thyroid function during the neonatal period in Europe. Biol Neonate 1986;49:322–330.
9. Thilly C, Lagasse R, Roger G, Bourdoux P, Ermans AM. Impaired fetal and postnatal development and high perinatal death-rate in a severe iodine deficient area. In: Thyroid Research VIII. Proceedings of the Eighth International Thyroid Congress. Australian Academy of Science, Canberra 1980, pp. 20–23.
10. DeLong GR, Leslie PW, Wang S-H, Jiang X-M, Zhang M-L, Rakeman MA, Jiang J-Y, Ma T, Cao X-Y. Effect on infant mortality of iodination of irrigation water in a severely iodine-deficient area of China. Lancet 1997;350:771–773.
11. Dunn JT, van der Haar F. A Practical Guide to the Correction of Iodine Deficiency. International Council for Control of Iodine Deficiency Disorders. The Netherlands, 1990.
12. WHO/UNICEF/ICCIDD: Global prevalence of iodine deficiency disorders. MDIS Working Paper #1. Micronutrient Deficiency Information System, World Health Organization, Geneva, 1993.

13. Bleichrodt N, Born MP. A metaanalysis of research on iodine and its relationship to cognitive development. In: Stanbury J.B, ed. The Damaged Brain of Iodine Deficiency. Cognizant Communication Corporation, New York, 1994, pp. 195–200.

14. Dunn JT. The epidemiology and prophylaxis of iodine deficiency worldwide. In: Reiners C, Weinheimer B, eds. Schilddruse 1997, Walter de Gruyter & Company, Berlin, 1998, pp. 3–7.

15. Dunn JT. Seven deadly sins in confronting endemic iodine deficiency, and how to avoid them. J Clin Endocrinol Metab 1996;81:1332–1335.

16. Roti E, Vagenakis AG. Effect of excess iodide: clinical aspects. In: Braverman LE, Utiger RD, eds. Werner and Ingbar's The Thyroid. A Fundamental and Clinical Text. Lippincott-Raven, Philadelphia, PA, 1996, pp. 316–327.

17. Hutchings PR, Cooke A, Dawe K, Champion BR, Geysen M, Valerio R, Roitt M. A thyroxine-containing peptide can induce murine experimental autoimmune thyroiditis. J Exp Med 1992;175:869–872.

18. Kurata A, Ohta K, Mine M, Fukuda T, Ikari N, Kanazawa H, Matsunaga M, Izumi M, Nagataki S. Monoclonal antihuman thyroglobulin antibodies. J Clin Endocrinol Metab 1984;59:573–579.

19. Harach HR, Williams ED. Thyroid cancer and thyroiditis in the goitrous region of Salta, Argentina, before and after iodine prophylaxis. Clin Endocrinol 1995;43:701–706.

20. Contempre B, Dumont JE, Denef JF, Many MC. Effects of selenium deficiency on thyroid necrosis, fibrosis and proliferation: a possible role in myxoedematous cretinism. Eur J Endocrinol 1995;133:99–109.

21. Mitchell JH, Nicol F, Beckett GJ, Arthur JR. Selenoenzyme expression in thyroid and liver of second generation selenium- and iodine-deficient rats. J Mol Endocrinol 1996;16:259–267.

22. Corvilain B, Contempre B, Longombe AO, Goyens P, Gervy-Decoster C, Lamy F, Vanderpas JB, Dumont JE. Selenium and the thyroid: how the relationship was established. Am J Clin Nutr 1995;57(2 Suppl):244S–248S.

23. Nakamura T, Higashi A, Nishiyama S, Fujimoto S, Matsuda I. Kinetics of zinc status in children with IDDM. Diabetes Care 1991;14:553–557.

24. Cunningham JJ, Fu A, Mearkle PL, Brown RG. Hyperzincuria in individuals with insulin-dependent diabetes mellitus: concurrent zinc status and the effect of high-dose zinc supplementation. Metabolism: Clinical and Experimental 1994;43:1558–1562.

25. Klevay LM. An increase in glycosylated hemoglobin in rats deficient in copper. Nutr Rep Int 1982;26:329–334.

26. Saari JT, Bode AM, Dahlen GM. Defects of copper deficiency in rats are modified by dietary treatments that affect glycation. J Nutr 1995;125:2925–2934.

27. Klevay LM, Canfield WK, Gallagher SK, Henriksen LK, Lukaski HC, Bolonchuk W, Johnson LK, Milne DB, Sandstead HH. Decreased glucose tolerance in two men during experimental copper depletion. Nut Rep Int 1986;33:371–382.

28. el-Yazigi A, Hannan N, Raines DA. Urinary excretion of chromium, copper, and manganese in diabetes mellitus and associated disorders. Diabetes Research 1991;18:129–134.

29. Walter RM. Jr, Uriu-Hare JY, Olin KL, Oster MH, Anawalt BD, Critchfield JW, Keen CL. Copper, zinc, manganese, and magnesium status and complications of diabetes mellitus. Diabetes Care 1991;14:1050–1056.

30. Anderson RA. Recent advances in the clinical and biochemical effects of chromium deficiency. In: Prasad AS, ed. Essential and Toxic Trace Elements in Human Health and Disease: An Update. Wiley-Liss, New York, 1993; pp. 221–234.

31. Davies S, McLaren Howard J, Hunnisett A, Howard M. Age-related decreases in chromium levels in 51,665 hair, sweat, and serum samples from 40,872 patients - implications for the prevention of cardiovascular disease and type II diabetes mellitus. Metabolism: Clinical & Experimental 1997;46:469–473.

32. Lee NA, Reasner CA. Beneficial effect of chromium supplementation on serum triglyceride levels in NIDDM. Diabetes Care 1994;17:1449–1452.

33. Moore RJ, Hall CB, Carlson EC, Lukaski HC, Klevay LM. Acute renal failure and fluid retention and kidney damage in copper-deficient rats fed a high-NaCl diet. J Lab Clin Med 1989;113:516–524.

34. Gross AM, Prohaska JR. Copper-deficient mice have higher cardiac norepinephrine turnover. J Nutr 1990;120:88–96.

35. Abbasi AA, Prasad AS, Rabbani P, DuMouchelle E. Experimental zinc deficiency in man. Effect on testicular function. J Lab Clin Med 1980;96:544–550.

36. Hurley WL, Doane RM. Recent developments in the roles of vitamins and minerals in reproduction. J Diary Sci 1989;72:784–804.

37. Rogers JM, Keen CL, Hurley LS. Zinc deficiency in pregnant Long-Evans hooded rats: teratogenicity and tissue trace elements. Teratology 1985;31:89–100.

14 Trace Element and Mineral Nutrition in Skeletal Health and Disease

Robert P. Heaney, MD, FACP, FAIN

1. INTRODUCTION

Bone is a largely extracellular tissue: cells make up only ~5% of bone volume. The bulk of bone, the intercellular material, is a dense, virtually anhydrous structure, with half of its volume made up of organic fibrillar molecules, mainly collagen, and the other half made up of a mineral (i.e., calcium phosphate, best characterized as an imperfect carbonate-apatite with variable stoichiometry). Thus two minerals, calcium and phosphate, have a unique nutritional relationship to bone, inasmuch as they are its bulk constituents. The mechanical properties of the skeleton are direct functions of its mineral mass, other things being equal. The nutritional relationship of these minerals to bone is, thus, straightforward, involving bulk transfer from food sources to bone.

The skeleton evolved in marine vertebrates as a reservoir of phosphate, present in sea water in only negligible concentrations. When vertebrates emerged onto dry land, the skeleton became mechanically important as well. But it retained its primitive homeostatic functions, helping to maintain extracellular fluid (ECF) ionized calcium and inorganic phosphate (P_i) concentrations. The former function had, in a marine habitat, been served by the control of calcium ion flux across the gill membranes.

Bone tissue is laid down by cells; its integrity is monitored by cells; and its structure is continuously revised by cells. For these activities the cells of bone are as dependent upon micro-nutrients as are all other cells and tissues of the body. Thus, distinction needs to be made between bulk (or macro-) minerals and trace (or micro-) minerals. In the former category I will discuss briefly calcium and phosphorus and in the latter, copper, zinc, manganese, and fluoride. Magnesium occupies an intermediate position — functioning for bone mainly as a micro-nutrient, but present in the diet and in bone itself in quantities approaching the levels of the macro-minerals.

2. NUTRITION AND SKELETAL STRENGTH

Because the principal function of the skeleton in humans is mechanical, the principal consequence of nutritional problems relating to the skeleton is structural weakness, i.e., fragility. Thus, the discussion of the role of minerals in skeletal health will be mainly in terms of their impact on bone strength.

From: *Clinical Nutrition of the Essential Trace Elements and Minerals: The Guide for Health Professionals*
Edited by: J. D. Bogden and L. M. Klevay © Humana Press Inc., Totowa, NJ

Bone is very much a living tissue, with its cells responding both to systemic influences and to strain patterns within the bony structure. Nevertheless, the mechanical properties of bone reside exclusively in the intercellular, nonliving, two-phase composite of fibrous protein and mineral. The inherent mechanical properties of this material are largely (though not entirely) determined at the time a unit of bone is formed. Since the total skeleton is turned over at a rate of only 8–10% per year, and only currently forming bone will be affected by current metabolic conditions, classical nutritional stresses have predictably small effects on current bone strength. The bulk of bone is, in effect, isolated from the systemic and environmental influences that can rapidly produce outspoken effects in soft tissues. This is not to say that there are no effects on bone. Bone cells, damaged by current nutritional problems, may die or otherwise fail in one or another of their monitoring functions. But the effects of that failure may not become evident until many years later, and they are, accordingly, extremely difficult to study in intact organisms.

3. MACRO-MINERALS

3.1. Calcium

Calcium is the fifth most abundant element in the earth's crust and is found in high concentrations in the plant foods which constitute the diet of the high primates today, and which presumably constituted the diet of the evolving hominids, as well. Hunter-gatherer peoples in East Africa today have diets with calcium densities greater than 70 mg/100 kCal (1), 3–4× the calcium density of diets in the industrialized nations. This change in the calcium density of technologically advanced humans was due to the agricultural revolution, with its shift to a predominantly cereal-based diet. This change occurred for various populations from 2,000–10,000 years ago (see Chapter 3). Human physiology is the result of millennia of adaptation to environmental conditions, and the agricultural revolution is, by comparison, a very recent event. In brief, our physiologies are paleolithic, while our diets are modern. Given calcium abundance in the available foods, the human (and primate) calcium economies are optimized to prevent toxicity rather than to deal with scarcity. Net intestinal absorption of calcium is poor (typically between 10% and 20% in adults), dermal losses unregulated, and renal conservation weak. As a result, the dietary requirement for calcium is relatively high. (With sodium, a trace mineral in the hominid diet, our physiology exhibits the opposite behavior.)

The skeleton constitutes the body's nutrient reserve for calcium. The bony reservoir for calcium and phosphate functions not by adding or withdrawing mineral as such, but by adding or removing bone. Thus, the calcium and phosphate concentrations in bone remain constant, at about 270 mg/g and 375 mg/g bony material, respectively (2). When the body needs calcium that it cannot get from food, it tears down bone and scavenges the calcium released in the process. In this way, unbalanced withdrawals from the skeletal reserves inevitably decrease bone strength.

Unlike most nutrient reserves, calcium is not stored as such, and the size of the reserve cannot grow without limit (as is the case, for example, for reserves of energy or the fat soluble vitamins, both of which can increase to the point of producing morbidity). Bone mass is limited first by the genetic program, and then by prevailing levels of mechanical utilization. In this latter respect, bone mass density is regulated (the supply of available nutrients permitting) so as to produce bending in any direction on the order of 0.1 percent during the loading experienced in routine activities. Absorbed calcium in excess of what is needed to produce this degree of stiffness is simply excreted. Thus, while high calcium diets will not produce more bone than is currently needed, low calcium diets either limit the achieving of the genetic potential or result in one-sided withdrawals that, over the years, express themselves as age-related bone loss.

Although there has been confusion about the precise importance of dietary calcium in ensuring skeletal integrity through most of the 20th century, there is now a fairly general scientific consensus that high calcium intakes are important throughout life *(3,4)*. An abundance of studies clearly shows that high calcium intakes [i.e., substantially above the 1989 RDAs *(5)*] augment bone acquisition during growth, slow bone loss in the aged, and reduce fractures at all ages, but especially in the elderly, when fragility fractures predominate. Various consensus panels and nutritional policy summaries agree that calcium intake during adolescence and old age needs to be about 1500 mg/d, and at all other ages after infancy, at least 1000 mg/d *(4,6)*. The background and rationale for these recommendations have been described extensively elsewhere *(6–8)*, and will not be discussed further here.

3.2. Phosphorus

Phosphorus, as phosphate, is a bulk mineral not only for bone, but in a sense for all cellular tissues as well, since it is a major structural component of all nucleic acids, as well as of the energy machinery of the cell. Unlike calcium, which is present in abundance both in most soils and in fresh and marine waters, available phosphate is a trace element in nature. Its abundance limits biomass, and most of the available phosphate in the biosphere will be found as protoplasm — both plant and animal. But animals at the top of the food chain, whether eating plant or animal tissues, necessarily consume their phosphate as well. Because there is relatively little difference in phosphate densities among various soft tissues and organisms, a diet adequate in other nutrients is almost always adequate in phosphate as well. Thus, true dietary phosphorus deficiency is rare. For this reason, many nations have not bothered even to promulgate a phosphorus requirement.

But skeletal phosphate deficiency does occur, although mainly for metabolic, rather than for dietary reasons. The skeletal requirement for phosphorus is mediated by the extracellular fluid inorganic phosphorus (ECF P_i) concentration *(6)*. Disorders of this mediation include mainly the various hypophosphatemic syndromes due to renal tubular defects, and vitamin D deficiency (in which release of phosphate from skeletal reserves is impeded, and in which the evoked increase in parathyroid hormone lowers the renal phosphate threshold and drives serum P_i down below levels needed for mineralization of newly forming bone). The lower limit for normal ECF P_i is a function of age (and hence of relative osteogenesis), being highest in infancy (~1.8 mmol/L) when bone deposition per unit body mass is at its lifetime peak, and falling by the adult years to ~0.9 mmol/L *(6)*. Levels appreciably below these values both limit mineral addition to bone and lead to osteoblastic cellular dysfunction. The osteoblast is particularly vulnerable to low P_i concentrations because mineralization further depletes the periosteoblastic ECF of its P_i. When severe, this osteoblast dysfunction is expressed histologically and clinically as rickets and osteomalacia.

4. MICRO-MINERALS

The cellular apparatus of bone responsible for forming, monitoring, and revising skeletal structures is as dependent upon the full array of micro-nutrients as is any other tissue. However, for reasons already discussed, many micro-nutrient deficiencies, even if they have profound effects on bone cell function, will not express themselves immediately as changes in bone strength. Thus there are relatively few unique skeletal manifestations of micro-nutrient effects in adults whose skeletons are fully formed before developing a nutrient deficiency. However, for three of the micro-nutrients, there is a reasonably firm evidential base for a clear role in skeletal development and maintenance, and these will be reviewed briefly here. The three are copper, zinc, and manganese. A fourth, fluoride, has effects both on the mineral of bone itself and on osteoblast function.

4.1. Copper

Copper has been recognized as an essential nutrient for nearly 70 years. The principal sources of copper in the diet are shellfish, nuts, legumes, whole grain cereals, and organ meats. True dietary copper deficiency is considered to be rare and to be confined to special circumstances, such as with total parenteral nutrition or infants recovering from malnutrition. Recognized manifestations have usually centered on disorders of hemopoiesis, mainly as an iron-refractory, hypochromic anemia, and leukopenia. Osteoporosis or fragility fractures have not been generally considered to be a part of the syndrome. However, copper-deficient premature infants have underdeveloped, weak bones that fracture easily and respond to copper supplementation (9); copper deficiency in sheep and dogs results in a skeletal syndrome similar to human osteoporosis (10–13); and in one human with copper deficiency due to a copper transport defect, the patient's morbidity included osteoporosis (14).

In addition to its many other functions in the body, copper plays a unique role in connective tissue formation. Copper is the co-factor for lysyl oxidase, the enzyme responsible for posttranslational formation of covalent cross-links between collagen fibrils (15). These cross-links are important for connective tissue strength, both in tension and in compression, as they prevent the fibrils from sliding along one another's length.

Whether significant copper deficiency develops in adult humans is uncertain, and whether such deficiency would play a role in human osteoporosis is still unknown. Howard et al. (16) found significantly lower bone density in ostensibly healthy postmenopausal women with low serum copper levels, and the difference became larger after adjusting for differences in calcium intake. Since vertebral trabecular bone turns over relatively rapidly, an effective copper deficiency lasting for as little as a year or two could substantially alter material properties of this portion of the skeleton. Oxlund and his colleagues have found a reduction in collagen cross-links in the vertebral trabecular bone of patients dying with osteoporosis (17), compatible with what might be expected in copper deficiency. More to the point, bone strength was proportional to the extent of cross linkage (18), just as theory predicts (15), and copper-deficient animals have bone with impaired mechanical properties (19).

4.2. Zinc

Zinc has been recognized as essential for growth and health for nearly half a century. It is a known constituent of about 300 enzymes, including alkaline phosphatase, and plays a role in other proteins, such as the estrogen receptor molecule. Its principal sources in the human diet are red meat, whole grain cereals, shellfish, and legumes.

A 70 kg adult body contains 2–3 g zinc, about half in bone. Most of this bony zinc is located on the surfaces of the calcium phosphate crystals and probably has no metabolic significance. Many cations present in the mineralizing environment adsorb to the oxygen-rich phosphate groups on crystal surfaces and get stuck there as free water is displaced by new mineral deposition. A fortuitous consequence of this situation is that urine zinc reflects bone resorption. Thus Herzberg et al. *(20)* have shown that urine zinc rises with age, is higher in patients with osteoporosis, and is reduced when postmenopausal women are given estrogen *(21)*. While some etiologic connection between zinc and osteoporosis cannot be ruled out, these observations are most easily explained as reflections of the enhanced bone resorption found in many patients with osteoporosis, the elevated resorption of the estrogen-deprived, postmenopausal state, and the well-known antiresorptive effect of estrogen. Urinary zinc excretion probably functions as a marker for bone resorption, rather than as a reflection of the underlying disease mechanisms.

On the other hand, of known nutrients, zinc is the one most strongly related to serum IGF-1 *(22)*, a growth factor known to be osteotrophic even in adults. In this connection, Bonjour et al. *(23)* have shown the importance of IGF-1 in recovery from hip fracture. In an observational study from Sweden, fracture risk was higher in individuals with low zinc intakes *(24)*, and, after adjusting for other nutrients, the risk gradient showed the expected dose-response relationship. New et al. *(25)* in a dietary survey of nearly 1,000 British premenopausal women found high zinc intakes to be associated with higher bone density values at both spine and hip.

Suggestive paleolithic evidence connecting zinc intake with bone status is provided by ancient skeletons discovered in Canary Island cave burials (where contamination by, or leeching of minerals into, ground water is considered not to have occurred). Bones with normal zinc content per unit ash, concentrated in one region of the Islands, tended to be robust, while those with low zinc contents, on another island, were found to be osteoporotic *(26)*. Zinc content of bone, as suggested above, is determined by the circulating zinc levels when bone is mineralizing, and thus low bone zinc probably reflects low zinc intake throughout life. Whether this exposure played an etiologic role in the low bone mass of these skeletal remains is conjectural.

4.3. Manganese

Whereas manganese is recognized as an essential nutrient, its precise role in nutrition is much less well characterized than that of copper and zinc. Although manganese deficiency is well recognized in both laboratory and farm animals, there is no generally recognized manganese deficiency syndrome in humans. Manganese is widely distributed in foods and is especially rich in tea.

Bone manganese content is, like that of copper and zinc, a reflection mainly of serum levels prevailing at the time bone is formed, and thus a reflection of dietary manganese. Bone manganese probably has no other metabolic significance, *per se*. Manganese is capable of activating many enzymes, but for most the effect is nonspecific. Manganese is, however, believed to be the preferred metal ion for certain glycosylations and related reactions involved in mucopolysaccharide synthesis. In this connection, manganese deficiency could interfere with both cartilage and bone matrix formation.

Animals reared on manganese-deficient diets exhibit general growth retardation, but careful measurements indicate that long bone growth is disproportionately affected *(10)*, possibly reflecting a specific problem with endochondral bone formation. There is also indication of delayed skeletal maturation, suggesting a role of manganese in chondrogenesis. Strause et al. *(27)* showed this quite nicely in a rat model in which demineralized bone powder is implanted subcutaneously. In control animals cartilage forms around the powder implant, then osteogenesis occurs. In manganese-deficient animals neither development took place. In further work, Strause et al. *(28)* showed that manganese-deficient rats had both disordered regulation of calcium homeostasis and decreased bone mineral density. Because histology was not performed, it is not possible to say whether this represented impaired mineralization or osteoporosis. Finally, Reginster et al. *(29)* found low serum manganese in a group of 10 women with osteoporosis. What significance any of these findings may have for human osteoporosis is uncertain.

4.4. Fluoride

Fluorine, the most electro-negative of all the elements, is not an essential nutrient in the usual sense, but it acts in the body at four intake levels that are, respectively, beneficial, cosmetic, therapeutic, and toxic. At intakes in the range of 0.5–2.0 mg/d, fluoride confers caries resistance on tooth enamel in children so long as the intake occurs at the time of enamel formation. At intakes in the range of 2–8 mg/d, fluoride produces tooth mottling, judged a cosmetic rather than a health problem. At intakes in the range of 20–80 mg/d, fluoride is an osteoblast mitogen and stimulates new bone formation, especially in the cancellous bone of the central skeleton. With treatments lasting 2–5 yr, this effect has been used to advantage in the treatment of osteoporosis. However, long continued exposure at this intake level leads to osteosclerosis, and in some populations, exuberant osteophyte formation and calcification of ligaments around joints, with consequent crippling arthritis. This effect is the basis for both endemic and industrial fluorosis. At intake levels above 80 mg/d, fluoride becomes increasingly toxic, leading to osteomalacia, mucosal burns, neuromuscular conduction defects, and ultimately death.

The pharmacology of fluoride is poorly worked out, but it is commonly believed that the therapeutic range for osteoblastic new bone formation involves blood levels between 95 and 190 ng/mL *(30)*, and that toxicity ensues at blood levels above 190. By contrast, blood levels of individuals living in communities with fluoridated water supplies are typically ~60 ng/mL.

Fluoride fits neatly into the apatite crystal lattice of bone mineral and tooth enamel, replacing the hydroxyl group, and thereby converting hydroxyapatite to fluorapatite. Bone fluoride concentration tends to rise throughout life, but even in cases of fluorosis never reaches anything approaching full replacement of hydroxyl ions by fluoride in bone mineral. At peak bone strength (see below) about 4–6% of the hydroxyl sites in bone mineral are substituted by fluoride ions, and in skeletal fluorosis the degree of replacement ranges from 10–30% of the theoretical maximum.

Because of the symmetry of the fluoride ion, the fluorapatite crystal is a more stable structure than hydroxyapatite and thus more resistant to acid dissolution. This is the basis of caries resistance. Presumably the same effect would render bone mineral more resistant to osteoclastic resorption, particularly on exposure long enough to incorporate fluoride uniformly throughout the skeleton. However, the antiosteoclastic action of therapeutic fluoride is very rapid in onset and cannot be explained by the greater resistance to dissolution of bone mineral. Instead it is probably due to a direct effect on the resorbing cell itself.

Because the physical properties of the mineral phase of bone change with progressive substitution of fluoride into hydroxyapatite, there has been uncertainty as to whether bone produced under therapeutic loads of fluoride might be mechanically weaker than normal. Turner et al. *(31)* showed, in rats fed controlled fluoride intakes from weaning, that bone strength peaked at a bone fluoride concentration of ~1200 ppm, with a significant positive correlation between bone strength and bone fluoride at all lower bone content values. Rich and Feist had earlier shown very similar behavior, with a peak bone strength in rats at a bone fluoride level closer to 3000 ppm *(32)*. (The bone fluoride level at these peak strength values is approximately equivalent to that which would be achieved by an intake in humans in the range of 1–3 mg/d.) In both studies higher intakes resulted in bone which was mechanically weaker than normal. At the same time it must be noted that fragility is not a recognized part of fluorosis, in which bone fluoride levels are much higher than this optimum value. This is probably because the extra bone of the syndrome compensates for the small decline in intrinsic bone strength.

Taken together, these data predict greater bone mass and bone strength in human populations ingesting optimally fluoridated water. However, the observational data on this point are decidedly mixed, with greater bone mass and fewer fractures reported in some studies *(33,34)*, no difference in others *(35)*, and even more fractures in some *(36)*. Perhaps the best of the available studies comes from a random sample of the population around Kuopio, Finland, in which, after adjusting for other variables, individuals ingesting water fluoridated at a level of 1–1.2 mg/L had 3% greater spine bone mass and 1% greater density at the femoral neck than individuals with water fluoride levels under 0.3 mg/L *(37)*. The two groups, both still relatively young, reported no difference in fracture rates.

Thus, given the promotion of caries resistance, the likely — if small — improvement in bone mass associated with intakes in the range of 1–2 mg/d, and the therapeutic potential of fluoride in the treatment of osteoporosis, fluoride can best be characterized as a beneficial mineral element *(see* Chapter 2).

4.5. Magnesium

Magnesium is an essential intracellular cation, a co-factor of many basic cellular processes, particularly those involving energy metabolism. In the face of true magnesium deficiency, there is widespread cellular dysfunction, including the cells and tissues that control the calcium economy and bone remodeling, among others. Although slightly more than half the body magnesium is contained in the mineral of bone, it is less certain whether it plays any role there or is, like zinc, present simply accidentally, insofar as it was present in the ECF bathing the mineralizing site. On the other hand, magnesium alters the surface properties of calcium phosphate crystals, and its concentration in bone is sufficiently high to exert such an effect there. However, the physical-chemical equilibrium between bone crystals and the dissolved minerals in the ECF is itself poorly understood; hence any role of magnesium therein is correspondingly uncertain.

Magnesium deficiency clearly occurs in humans of all ages, most often resulting from severe alcoholism or intestinal magnesium leaks, as from sprue or from ileostomy losses. One well-studied manifestation is hypocalcemia, now recognized to be due both to refractoriness of the parathyroid glands to the hypocalcemic stimulus itself, coupled with refractoriness of the bone resorption apparatus to parathyroid hormone.

Low bone mass is also a common feature in these situations. But individuals with magnesium deficiency commonly have calcium deficiency as well, and for the same reasons — a combination of low intake, renal wastage, and intestinal leakage. One would expect, therefore, osteoporosis to be very common in such individuals, as is the case. How much of this bony deficit is due to the magnesium deficiency and how much to the calcium deficiency is unclear. (In a clinical sense the question is moot: both deficiencies need repairing.) Treating the underlying condition and replacing lost calcium increases bone density in these patients, but Rude et al. *(38)* have shown that even when the underlying condition is controlled and serum magnesium seemingly normal, additional magnesium supplementation will produce a further increase in bone mineral density.

This latter observation highlights one of the difficulties besetting this field — the assessment of magnesium status. Serum magnesium is recognized not to be a reliable indicator of tissue magnesium repletion. Many investigators favor the magnesium tolerance test *(39)*, i.e., measuring percent retention of an I-V infusion of magnesium. This is, of course, not practicable in clinical practice. Nevertheless the observations of Rude et al. highlight the fact that serum magnesium values within the "normal" reference range may mask a capacity to respond to further magnesium supplementation.

This is precisely the point at which magnesium intersects the arena of the pathogenesis and treatment of common postmenopausal osteoporosis. Unfortunately there is probably no segment of the osteoporosis field more beset with poorly designed, poorly executed, and inadequately powered studies than this one. For example, two small trials, one not randomized, the other with high loss of subjects during the trial, reported bone gain in postmenopausal women given a supplement containing magnesium *(40,41)*. Neither study constitutes persuasive evidence of a magnesium effect. The upshot of these and many other even weaker studies is that it is simply not possible to say with any certainty what, if any, may be the role that magnesium plays in pathogenesis or treatment.

One fact seems certain: in any unselected group of individuals with low bone mass, calcium and/or vitamin D supplementation results in clear skeletal benefits (see above), without using extra magnesium. And despite the fact that magnesium may be necessary for the functioning of such cells as those responsible for synthesizing $1,25(OH)_2D$ (the hormonally active form of vitamin D) *(42)*, there is clear proof that supplemental magnesium does not enhance calcium absorption in ostensibly healthy older adults. Spencer et al. *(43)* more than doubled daily magnesium intake in a group of volunteers and could find no effect on calcium absorption, whether from low or normal calcium intakes. Similarly, the many randomized controlled trials demonstrating efficacy of calcium supplementation in reducing age-related bone loss and fractures all achieved their effect without supplementing with magnesium.

But absence of proof is not the same as absence of effect. One cannot say, in the routine management of osteoporosis, that the results would not have been even better had extra magnesium been provided as well. Since sprue syndromes can be silent *(44)*, subtle magnesium deficiency could well exist in some individuals with otherwise typical osteoporosis (to mention only one potential cause of magnesium deficiency). Hence, lacking the ability easily to identify individuals with unrecognized magnesium deficiency, it is hard to argue against prudent attention to magnesium supplementation in individuals who have osteoporosis or are at high risk for fragility fractures.

5. CLINICAL STUDIES

The foregoing sections have concentrated mainly on the mechanisms by which minerals may affect the skeleton — a bottom-up approach, in a sense. A top-down approach is to look for mineral abnormalities in individuals who have osteoporosis, or to study the effects of trace mineral supplements on the course of osteoporosis. It will be important to make clear at the outset that osteoporosis is a distinctly multifactorial disorder. Bony fragility is the defining end point of the disease process, but there are many ways to get there. When we study a group of patients with osteoporotic fractures, we generally have no way of knowing which pathogenetic pathways each may have followed. Thus, calcium deficiency will have been important in some, but not in others; vitamin D insufficiency in some, but not in others; estrogen deficiency, thinness, or poor postural reflexes in yet others. And in some, there will have been a combination of two or more pathogenetic factors. For the most part we cannot tell. If abnormalities of micro-mineral metabolism play any role in clinical osteoporosis, it is unlikely that they will be uniformly deficient in all cases. Thus when we look for abnormalities in a group of patients with osteoporosis, average effects will be minimized or diluted by the inevitable heterogeneity of our sample.

A possibly good example of this problem is found in the randomized controlled trial of Strause et al. *(45)*. In a four-way design, postmenopausal women received placebo, a trace mineral supplement containing zinc, manganese, and copper, a calcium supplement, or calcium plus the trace minerals. The end point was change in bone mineral density. The sample sizes were relatively small, and only the calcium effect proved statistically significant. Nevertheless, the trace mineral supplement mix produced a better effect than placebo alone, and when given with the calcium supplement, a better effect than calcium alone. As already noted, even if some of the subjects were in a position to benefit from the trace minerals, it is unlikely that all of them would have been deficient. Thus lacking a priori ability to recognize those who might benefit, one would expect a small average effect, likely not to be statistically significant. The same investigators in an isolated observation in a fracture-prone athlete (Strause, personal communication), used a trace mineral cocktail and reported fracture healing where other standard therapies had failed. The athlete concerned was said to have low serum levels of copper and zinc, and completely undetectable manganese, so there was a rationale for the treatment. But whether this isolated observation was a reflection of the individual's bizarre diet or of abnormalities in his trace mineral transport, or simply happenstance, cannot be determined. And even if this observation could be confirmed, it would remain a relatively isolated occurrence with uncertain generalizability.

6. CONCLUSION

Calcium is essential for acquisition and maintenance of the genetic potential for bone mass. Diets deficient in calcium will, correspondingly, limit bone mass or lead to bone loss. Phosphorus is also essential for proper bone mineralization and for the action of bone-forming cells, but diets are not often deficient in phosphorus, and phosphorus deficiency syndromes are usually of metabolic, rather than dietary origin. By contrast, magnesium deficiency is relatively more common, though the best recognized instances involve excessive magnesium losses from the body rather than low intake. In the face of severe magnesium depletion, the control of extracellular fluid calcium ion concentration is impaired and bone mass is reduced. Magnesium supplementation is necessary to correct both defects. Whether magnesium supplementation plays any role in the average case of postmenopausal osteoporosis is unclear. Calcium and vitamin D repletion, estrogen replacement therapy, and a variety of new bone active drugs all produce fairly dramatic improvements in bone status without requiring magnesium supplementation. Nevertheless, because intestinal leaks of magnesium can be silent, it is possible that some small fraction of cases of postmenopausal osteoporosis would benefit from magnesium supplementation in addition to ensuring adequate calcium and vitamin D status and whatever other treatment may be needed. Copper, zinc, and manganese are all essential both for organism growth and for skeletal development. Whether adults develop deficiencies of these nutrients, and whether these deficiencies play a role in ordinary osteoporosis cannot be decided on the basis of available evidence. There is suggestive evidence implicating all three trace micro-minerals, with copper being perhaps the most probable; but clearly much more research needs to be done. One of the problems besetting the field is the inability to recognize marginal deficiencies of these micro-nutrients.

REFERENCES

1. Eaton SB, Nelson DA. Calcium in evolutionary perspective. Am J Clin Nutr 1991;54:281S–287S.
2. McLean FC, Urist MR. Bone (Fundamentals of the Physiology of Skeletal Tissue). The University of Chicago Press, Chicago, IL,1968.
3. NIH Consensus Conference: Osteoporosis. JAMA 1984;252:799–802.
4. NIH Consensus Conference: Optimal Calcium Intake. JAMA 1994;272:1942–1948.
5. Recommended Dietary Allowances 10th edition. National Academy of Sciences, National Academy Press, Washington, DC,1989.
6. Dietary Reference Intakes for Calcium, Magnesium, Phosphorus, Vitamin D, and Fluoride Food and Nutrition Board, Institute of Medicine, National Academy Press, Washington, DC, 1997.
7. Heaney RP. Nutrition and risk for osteoporosis. In: Marcus R, Feldman D, Kelsey J, eds. Osteoporosis. Academic Press, San Diego, CA, 1996,pp. 483–505.
8. Heaney RP. Nutritional factors in osteoporosis. Ann Rev Nutr 1993;13:287–316.
9. Schmidt H, Herwig J, Greinacher I. The skeletal changes in premature infants with copper deficiency. Rofo. Fortschritte aud dem Gebiete der Rontgenstrahlen und der Neuen Bildgebenden Verfahren 1991;155:38–42.
10. Asling CW, Hurley LS. The influence of trace elements on the skeleton. Clin Orthop 1963;27:213–264.
11. Suttle NF, Angus KW, Nisbet DI, Field A C. Osteoporosis in copper depleted lambs. J Comparative Pathol 1972;82:93–97.
12. Whitelaw A, Armstrong RH, Evans CC, Fawcett AR. A study of the effects of copper deficiency in Scottish blackface lambs on improved hill pasture. Veterinary Record 1979;103:455–460.
13. Baxter JH, Van Wyk JJ, Follis RH, Jr. A bone disorder associated with copper deficiency II. Histological and chemical studies on the bones. Bull Johns Hopkins Hosp 1953;93:25–39.
14. Buchman AL, Keen CL, Vinters HV, Harris E, Chugani HT, Bateman B, Rodgerson D, Vargas J, Verity A, Ament M. Copper deficiency secondary to a copper transport defect: a new copper metabolic disturbance. Metabolism 1994;43:1462–1469.
15. Opsahl W, Zeronian H, Ellison M, Lewis D, Rucker RB, Riggins RS. Role of copper in collagen cross-linking and its influence on selected mechanical properties of chick bone and tendon. J Nutr 1982;112:708–716.
16. Howard G, Andon M, Bracker M, Saltman P, Strause L. Low serum copper a risk factor additional to low dietary calcium in postmenopausal bone loss. J. Trace Elements Experimental Med 1992;5:23–31.
17. Oxlund H, Mosekilde Li, Ørtoft G.1996; Reduced concentration of collagen reducible cross links in human trabecular bone with respect to age and osteoporosis. Bone 19:479–484.
18. Oxlund H, Barckman M, Ørtoft G, Andreassen T T.1995; Reduced concentrations of collagen cross-links are associated with reduced strength of bone. Bone 4:365S–371S.
19. Jonas J, Burns J, Abel EW, Cresswell MJ, Strain J, Paterson CR. Impaired mechanical strength of bone in experimental copper deficiency. Ann Nutr Metab 1993;37:245–252.
20. Herzberg M, Foldes J, Steinberg R, Menczel J. Zinc excretion in osteoporotic women. J Bone Miner Res 1990;5:251–257.
21. Herzberg M, Lusky A, Blonder J, Frenkel Y. The effect of estrogen replacement on zinc in serum and urine. Obstet Gynecol 1996;87:1035–1040.
22. Devine A, Rosen C, Mohan S, Baylink DJ, Prince RL. Effects of zinc and other nutritional factors on IGF-1 and IGF binding proteins in postmenopausal women. Am J Clin Nutr 1998;68:200–206.
23. Schürch MA, Rizzoli R, Slosman D, Bonjour J-Ph. Protein supplements increase serum IGF-1 and decrease proximal femur bone loss in patients with a recent hip fracture. In: Papapoulos SE, Lips P, Pols HAP, Johnston CC, Delmas PD, eds. Osteoporosis 1996. Elsevier Science BV, Amsterdam, The Netherlands, 1996,pp. 327–329.

24. Elmstahl S, Gullberg B, Janzon L, Johnell O, Elmstahl B. Increased incidence of fractures in middle-aged and elderly men with low intakes of phosphorus and zinc. Osteoporosis Int 1998;8:333–340.
25. New SA, Bolton-Smith C, Grubb DA, Reid D M. Nutritional influences on bone mineral density: a cross–sectional study in premenopausal women. Am J Clin Nutr 1997;65:1831–1839.
26. González-Reimers E, Arnay-de-la-Rosa M. Ancient skeletal remains of the Canary Islands: bone histology and chemical analysis. Anthrop Anz 1992;50:201–215.
27. Strause L, Saltman P, Glowacki J. The effect of deficiencies of manganese and copper on osteoinduction and on resorption of bone particles in rats. Calcif Tissue Int 1987;41:145–150.
28. Strause LG, Hegenauer J, Saltman P, Cone R, Resnick D. Effects of long-term dietary manganese and copper deficiency on rat skeleton. J Nutr 1986;116:135–141.
29. Reginster JY, Strause LG, Saltman P, Franchimont P. Trace elements and postmenopausal osteoporosis: a preliminary study of decreased serum manganese. Med Sci Res 1988;16:337–338.
30. Taves DR. New approach to the treatment of bone disease with fluoride. Fed Proc1970; 29:1185–1187.
31. Turner CH, Akhter M, Heaney RP. The effects of fluoridated water on bone strength. J Orthop Res 1992;10:581–587.
32. Rich C, Feist E. The action of fluoride on bone. In: Vischer TL ed. Fluoride in Medicine. Hans Huber, Bern, 1970, pp. 70–87.
33. Bernstein DS, Sadowsky N, Hegsted DM. et al. Prevalence of osteoporosis in high- and low-fluoride areas in North Dakota. J Am Med Assoc 1966;198:85–90.
34. Simonen O, Laitinen O. Does fluoridation of drinking water prevent bone fragility and osteoporosis. Lancet ii 1985;432–434.
35. Arnala I, Alhava EM, Kivivuori R, Kauranen P. Hip fracture incidence not affected by fluoridation. Acta Orthop Scand 1986;57:344–348.
36. Sowers MR, Clark MK, Jannausch ML, Wallace RB. A prospective study of bone mineral content and fracture in communities with differential fluoride exposure. Am J Epidemiol 1991;133:649–660.
37. Kroger H, Alhava E, Honkanen R, Tuppurainen M, Saarikoski S. The effect of fluoridated drinking water on axial bone mineral density - a population based study. Bone Miner 1994;27:33–41.
38. Rude RK, Olerich M. Magnesium deficiency: possible role in osteoporosis associated with gluten-sensitive enteropathy. Osteoporosis Int 1996;6:453–461.
39. Ryzen E, Elhaum N, Singer FR, Rude RK. Parenteral magnesium tolerance testing in the evaluation of magnesium deficiency. Magnesium 1985;4:137–147.
40. Abraham GE. The importance of magnesium in the management of primary postmenopausal osteoporosis. J Nutritional Med 1991;2:165–178.
41. Stendig-Lindberg G, Tepper R, Leichter I. Trabecular bone density in a two-year controlled trial of peroral magnesium in osteoporosis. Magnesium Res 1994;6:155–163.
42. Rude RK, Adams JS, Ryzen E, Endres DB, Niimi H, Horst RL, Haddad JG, Jr, Singer FR. Low serum concentrations of 1,25-dihydroxyvitamin D in human magnesium deficiency. J Clin Endocrinol Metab 1985;61:933–940.
43. Spencer H, Fuller H, Norris C, Williams D. Effect of magnesium on the intestinal absorption of calcium in man. J Am College Nutr 1994;13:485–492..
44. Ott S, Tucci JR, Heaney RP, Marx SJ. Hypocalciuria and abnormalities in mineral and skeletal homeostasis in patients with celiac sprue without intestinal symptoms. Endocrinol Metab 1997;4:201–206.
45. Strause L, Saltman P, Smith KT, Bracker M, Andon MB. Spinal bone loss in postmenopausal women supplemented with calcium and trace minerals. J Nutr 1994;124:1060–1064

15 Trace Element and Mineral Nutrition in Ischemic Heart Disease

Leslie M. Klevay, MD

1. INTRODUCTION

Ischemic heart disease is one of the more important of the Western diseases closely associated with the Western diet. As Burkitt has noted *(1)* there is no term that is entirely satisfactory in characterizing these diseases. For example, ischemic heart disease can be found on every continent and in every racial group. There are enormous differences in risk from place to place *(2)*; generally those affected in nations with low overall risk resemble people in the industrialized parts of the world in their diet and habits.

The etiology of ischemic heart disease, the leading cause of death in the United States and much of the industrialized world, remains obscure. Hundreds of environmental and personal factors have been associated with risk of this illness *(3,4)*. Before the etiology of a disease is known, students are confronted with a bewildering array of apparently paradoxical or dissimilar observations *(5,6)*.

Deaths from cardiovascular disease were unusual in the United States early in this century; infectious diseases were predominant. Deaths from heart disease did not exceed those from tuberculosis until 1910 *(7)*.

Risk of ischemic heart disease increases with age, is greater in men, and is increased among people with hypercholesterolemia, glucose intolerance, hypertension, abnormalities of the electrocardiogram and among smokers of cigarettes. The last five of these characteristics are called risk factors; consideration of these factors can identify 20% of the presymtomatic population with 40% of the heart disease risk *(8)*.

1.1. Ischemic Heart Disease as Fat Intoxication

Keys *(9)* was among the first to notice the great variation in death rates among various nations *(2)*. In a coordinated and systematic study of seven countries *(10)*, a rather close and direct relationship was found between the heart disease death rate and the percentage of the habitual diet obtained from saturated fat. This relationship and data on migrating populations provided a powerful argument that heart disease was neither an inevitable consequence of age nor of predominantly hereditary origin.

From: Clinical Nutrition of the Essential Trace Elements and Minerals: The Guide for Health Professionals
Edited by: J. D. Bogden and L. M. Klevay © Humana Press Inc., Totowa, NJ

251

When epidemiology is done in single nations such as the United States, one generally finds no relationship between dietary fat and either risk of heart disease or the concentration of cholesterol in blood plasma or serum. I have collected approximately 50 negative articles *(2,11)* since the first one in 1959 was found *(12)*. No association between dietary fat and serum cholesterol was found in Framingham *(13)* or NHANES *(14)*. Some of the enthusiasm for a dietary fat-heart disease relationship, at least in regard to cholesterol lowering, arises from over-citation of favorable work and under-citation of unfavorable work *(15)*.

Even though the association between dietary fat and risk of heart disease is, at best, considerably smaller within nations than among nations, there have been myriad recommendations that people should eat less fat. Some of these suggestions are made following juxtaposition of apparently increasing dietary fat in the United States with increasing risk of coronary heart disease in the first half of this century. The increase in dietary fat probably is artifactual *(16)*; the increase in disease is real.

Even if an increase in dietary fat occurred, the amount of the increase was too small to account for the increase in heart disease risk *(17,18)*. It has been suggested that if nearly everyone in the United States eats too much of the wrong kind of fat, dietary fat is no longer of epidemiologic interest because only a minority of people in the U.S. die of ischemic heart disease *(2,19)* even though ischemic heart disease remains the leading cause of death. Ravnskov *(20)* reviewed ecological, dynamic population, cross-sectional, cohort, case-control studies, and randomized trials and concluded *inter alia* that "there is little evidence that saturated fatty acids...are harmful or that polyunsaturated fatty acids...are beneficial."

Recently a harmful association between coronary heart disease morbidity plus mortality and the proportion of total fat and monounsaturated fat in the diet was found for younger (but not older) Framingham men *(21)*. This finding occurred when Cox regression coefficients were calculated, but not when standard lipid scores were used. Total fat, saturated fat and monounsaturated fat were found to have a beneficial association with either completed stroke or ischemic stroke in all men in the same population *(22)*.

One can conclude that the effects of dietary fat on heart disease (if any) are subtle, are somewhat dependent on the method of study, require examination of very large numbers of people for detection *(23)*, and may have contrary effects on other illnesses. Correlations between lipids in the Framingham diet *(21)* make menu planning difficult because people select foods, not fatty acids.

Some important characteristics of ischemic heart disease have not been confirmed by experiment. Experiments showing, for example, that dietary fat can produce abnormal electrocardiograms or glucose intolerance have not been reported. Thus, although the lipid hypothesis has been helpful in understanding ischemic heart disease, we should consider the possibility that this concept has outlived its usefulness.

1.2. Unexplained Associations

There are many characteristics of ischemic heart disease and associations with ischemic heart disease that require explanation. For example, there is an increasingly close association between bone disease and either atherosclerosis or ischemic heart disease that cannot be explained either by dietary fat or by the fact that both illnesses occur increasingly with age *(24)*.

My first recognition of this association was the work of Menczel, et al. *(25)* who found that lateral roentgenograms of men and women with high degrees of aortic calcification showed greater osteoporosis (and *vice versa*). Prompted by earlier work *(26,27)*, Uyama, et al. *(28)* found lower total bone mineral density by dual-energy X-ray absorptiometry in postmenopausal women with higher carotid atherosclerosis assessed by ultrasonography. More recently Cox et al. *(29)* found excessive osteophytic lipping of the thoracic spine in people with coronary heart disease.

Periodontal disease *(30,31)* and dental disease *(32)* are associated with increased risk of coronary heart disease. Perhaps periodontal disease and other signs of poor oral health are signs of osteoporosis. Beck et al.*(33)* found that bone loss was associated with excess coronary heart disease mortality when studying this phenomenon.

Poor dental health, mainly as periodontal disease, is associated with increased risk of death from coronary heart disease *(185)*. Whalen and Krook *(186)* consider periodontal disease to be the early manifestation of osteoporosis. The increased risk of heart disease in short women has been confirmed *(187)*. Women with aortic calcification had lower femur bone density than women without calcification *(188)*.

Deformities of the thoracic spine, low ulnar mineral content as measured by a resonant frequency method and greater calcification of the aortic arch all were more frequent in men and women from a mountainous, in comparison to a seacoast, village in Japan *(27)*. The authors referred to a shift of calcium from bone to soft tissue. Bernstein et al. *(34)* found greater evidence of osteoporosis and more aortic calcification in North Dakota where municipal water was low in fluoride compared to towns where fluoride was high. Examination of their roentgenographic tabulations reveals that overall, osteoporosis and calcification are associated when data are stratified by age. A dissent to the association between osteoporosis and aortal calcification has been registered from South Africa *(26)*.

Proponents of the lipid hypothesis may explain this association between atherosclerosis and osteoporosis as evidence that diets high in fat promote osteoporosis. In fact, the opposite seems to be the case. A positive correlation between monounsaturated fat intake and bone mineral density was found among Greek men and women *(35)*.

An even greater problem with attempts to explain ischemic heart disease as a problem of fat intoxication is that many phenomena characterize this illness and most of these are not related to, or affected by, lipid metabolism. *(vide infra)* Some phenomena unexplainable by the lipid hypothesis are shown in Table 1. Many of these can be attributed to intoxication with dietary fat only in the boldest and most extravagant interpretations of the data.

Epidemiology has not revealed that women eat less, or better fat than men. Nor is there an experiment showing that women (or female animals) tolerate fat better than men (or male animals). That men with heart disease are more likely to die suddenly and women are more likely to die with thrombosis also cannot be explained by difference in dietary fat *(36)*.

It may seem surprising that ischemic heart disease can occur without risk factors *(37)*. Conversely, 69% of the men in the highest cholesterol quintile (256–514 mg/dL) were free of heart disease for 20 yr *(38)*.

The tenuous epidemiologic relationship between dietary fat and either serum cholesterol or risk of death from heart disease has been mentioned above. Neither epidemiology nor experiment has provided a relationship between dietary fat and hypertension or hyperuricemia. This latter characteristic usually is not mentioned among the risk factors, but in Framingham uric acid is so closely associated with risk that multivariate analyses are corrected for uric acid *(39)*. The associations among serum uric acid and blood pressure, cardiac enlargement, cholesterol, electrocardiograms, glucose intolerance, and heart disease also are unexplained by dietary fat *(40–43)*.

Table 1
Characteristics of Ischemic Heart Disease Unexplained by Dietary Fat

Bone disease	Male/female differences
Disease without risk factors	Risk factor associations
Electrocardiographic abnormalities	Seasonality
Glucose intolerance	Small stature
Hearing loss	Water factor
Hypertension	

Cholesterol values in plasma or serum are seasonal, being lower in summer than in winter (44). It has been suggested (45) that higher consumption of beer in summer contributes to the lowering of cholesterol.

Perhaps the increased risk of heart disease in smaller men (42,46,47) and women (42) is explained by maternal and fetal influences (48,49). It does not seem likely that these influences result in craving for, and consumption of, too much of the wrong dietary fat. Measurements of short leg length in the Boyd Orr Survey associated with adult coronary heart disease mortality by Gunnell, et al. (50) seem more related to maternal and fetal influences than to adult anthropometry because they were restricted to those younger than age eight when measured.

It has been shown repeatedly that risk of ischemic heart disease is higher where the drinking water is soft and is lower where the drinking water is hard (51,52). This phenomenon has led to the term "the water factor."

2. MULTIFACTORIAL DISEASE

It generally is agreed that ischemic heart disease is a complex phenomenon involving arterial endothelial damage, arterial spasm, connective tissue metabolism, foam cells and smooth muscle cells... thrombus formation, uric acid metabolism, vasoactive amines, and so on. (53). It seems unlikely that ischemic heart disease will disappear from among the leading causes of death in industrialized nations unless its etiology, pathogenesis, and pathophysiology become comprehensible as a whole. We must borrow from Chamberlin's method of "multiple working hypotheses" (54) to avoid neglecting important data.

Some may argue that ischemic heart disease is of multifactorial or pluricausal in origin when prompted by myriad associations and numerous phenomena noted here. With this view, inclusion of bone disease, for example, in the phenomenon of ischemic heart disease is not expected. Thus, one will experience no intellectual discomfort in excluding bone disease from consideration and will not be troubled by associations among measurements made on people with the illness. However, scientific progress often is made when theories incorporate other theories. That is, theories that explain more observations are superior to those that explain fewer (55). Theories attempting to explain important natural phenomena have been found wanting historically if they explained only limited characteristics of the phenomena (56,57). However, adherence to the idea that industrialization has led everyone to eat too much of the wrong kind of fat presents some difficulties. For example, in the United States less than half of the deaths of people over 80 years of age are from ischemic heart disease (58). People dying over the age of 90 have more atherosclerosis than people who die before 70, and are less likely to die of ischemic heart disease

(59). Similarly, atherosclerosis was the cause of death found at postmortem examination in less than one-fourth of 200 people older than 85 years *(60)*. Under these circumstances dietary fat is of neither epidemiologic nor pathophysiological interest.

2.1. Unifying Concepts

The homocysteine hypothesis of McCully *(61,62)* and the iron hypothesis of Sullivan *(63–67)* provide unifying ideas helpful in understanding some of the apparently dissimilar observations on ischemic heart disease that may lead to an answer to the question "what determines who lives long and who dies early of ischemic heart disease?" when people consume the Western diet for a lifetime. Both McCully *(189)* and Sullivan *(190)* have recently expended their unifying concepts.

The Western diet often is described as being high in fat. It also is high in animal protein, energy, refined sugars and is low in copper, dietary fiber, starch and phytic acid *(5,68)*. As these dietary components may modify risk of ischemic heart disease, overemphasis on fat is an oversimplification. Some of these modifications of risk may occur because these components alter trace element utilization, which, in turn changes metabolism.

3. TRACE ELEMENTS AND ISCHEMIC HEART DISEASE

The "water factor" (*see* Subheading 1.2.) phenomenon was one of the stimuli for my first experiments on trace elements *(69)* which led to a collection of chemical elements associated by experiment with ischemic heart disease *(6)*. This collection has grown and has been revised to include elements related to cholesterol metabolism *(70)* and atherosclerosis *(71,72)*. Currently, approximately one-third of the elements in the periodic table are included. Some of these elements, such as sodium have been studied extensively; others, such as germanium, have escaped general notice and are included mainly because of the pioneering efforts of Schroeder *(73)*. Both nutritionally essential elements, such as iron and zinc, and toxic elements, such as cadmium, and lead, are present. Approximately one-third of these seem to produce biological effects by affecting the utilization of copper. Elements considered in this volume are found in Table 2.

Magnesium has been suggested as being beneficial to all phases of the process that leads to death from ischemic heart disease. For example, Selye *(74,75)* mentioned magnesium as being protective against experimental cardiopathies. Seelig and Heggtveit *(76)* summarized some plausible, protective mechanisms. Hellerstein et al. *(77)* found a diet low in magnesium sometimes contributed to the production of aortic lipidosis in rats fed an atherogenic diet (*see* Subheading 3.1.2.2.). Elin and Hosseini *(78)* suggested that magnesium may protect Seventh-Day Adventists who eat nuts regularly from coronary heart disease. The Chipperfields *(79)* found less magnesium in the uninfarcted heart muscle of people who died suddenly in comparison to normal controls; data were related to the "water factor." There is a high correlation between magnesium in water and hardness of water (r=0.90) *(5,47)*. Intravenous magnesium seems beneficial in arrhythmias immediately after myocardial infarction *(80–82)*.

Selenium deficiency has been associated with Keshan disease, a cardiomyopathy endemic in some parts of China *(83,84)*. The main pathological feature of this disease is "multiple focal myocardial necrosis...with different degrees of cell infiltration and various stages of fibrosis" *(85)*. Although sodium selenite tablets are very effective in prophylaxis of Keshan disease *(86)*, it seems likely that there is a viral component to the illness *(87)* confirming the suggestion

Table 2
Trace Elements and Minerals Affecting the Cardiovascular System[a]

chromium	manganese
fluorine	molybdenum[c]
iodine	selenium[b]
iron	zinc[c]
magnesium[b]	

[a] Elements receiving emphasis in this book. Experimental data on these elements have been reviewed *(6,58, 70–72)*.
[b] Some effects may be from enhancement of copper (*see* ref. *71,72*).
[c] Some effects may be from inhibition of copper (*see* ref. *72*).

that infection and deficiency can cooperate to produce human illness *(88)*. Cardiomyopathy has been observed in people fed intravenously who were not supplemented with selenium *(87)*. Oster et al. *(89)* found a positive correlation between cardiac output and cardiac selenium in heart tissue of patients with coronary heart disease. Vincenti et al. *(90)* interpreted data on changes in selenium in drinking water and changes in coronary deaths in a municipal territory of northern Italy as being consistent with a beneficial effect of selenium on coronary disease.

Ascherio et al. *(91)* found that risk of myocardial infarction was greater in men who consumed a higher intake of heme iron, which is associated with higher iron stores. Total dietary intake was not associated with risk of coronary heart disease, however, and some other data collected were not consistent with the iron hypothesis (*see* Subheading 2.1.).

It will be argued here that copper deficiency is the simplest and most general explanation for the epidemic of ischemic heart disease. As in earlier articles, references will be cited here only to new work, or to older work noticed since the previous review *(72)*. Strain *(92)* has reviewed some of these concepts and has concluded that "copper status should be central to any discussion of trace elements and CVD" (cardiovascular disease).

Antimony, chromium, cobalt and gold were increased greatly in myocardia of patients with idiopathic, dilated cardiomyopathy *(191)*. Zinc was increased in urine and decreased in plasma and erythrocytes in patients with cardiomyopathy; the authors attributed these observations as being effects secondary to heart failure *(192)* .

3.1. Diet and Ischemic Heart Disease: Copper in Contrast to Lipid

Four successful copper depletion experiments with diets of conventional foods and involving more than 30 men and women have been summarized *(93)* revealing that daily copper intakes of 0.65 to 1.02 mg were insufficient. Criteria for insufficiency included hypercholesterolemia, a decrease in high density lipoprotein cholesterol and an increase in low density lipoprotein cholesterol, abnormal electrocardiograms, decreased glucose clearance, and increased blood pressure during sustained handgrip. Two of the experiments were interrupted prematurely with early repletion with copper because of abnormal electrocardiography; all of the metabolic and physiological abnormalities disappeared with copper repletion.

Some unsuccessful attempts at human copper depletion also were summarized *(93)*. Individual animals and individual people fed the same depleted diets respond with individuality. Signs of deficiency do not occur uniformly in experimental pellagra *(93,94)* or in animal experiments on biotin *(95)*, thiamin *(96)* or copper deficiencies *(97)*. It seems unlikely that one should expect men and women to respond uniformly to a diet low in copper. Our success rate in inducing copper depletion resembles that of Goldberger in inducing pellagra *(94)*.

That there is a disparity between dietary analyses and dietary reference values is becoming well-known *(93,98–100)*. As late as 1974 *(101)* it was thought that most daily diets contained 2 mg of copper. More recently, it was suggested that "the most important problem in human nutrition is determination of the degree to which this disparity affects human health" *(93)*.

Approximately one-third of daily diets in Belgium, Canada, the United Kingdom, and the United States contain daily amounts of copper in the insufficient range noted above *(102)*. Approximately 60% were less than 1.5 mg and 18% exceeded 2.0 mg/d.

The highest daily amount of copper found to be insufficient for adults to date is 20 µg/kg of body weight *(103)*. This corresponds to 1.1 mg daily for women and 1.4 for men if 55 and 70 kg are representative, respective weights. This latter value agrees rather well with the possibility that 1.4 to 1.5 mg daily may have been insufficient because of lipoprotein changes in repletion *(104)* and negative balance *(47,105)* in the depletion experiments cited above. Only 44% of diets *(102)* exceed 1.4 mg of copper daily.

3.1.1. SOME EPIDEMIOLOGY

The copper deficiency theory *(2,24,47,58,70,106)* explains some observations on populations that otherwise seem to be isolated curiosities. The increased risk of heart disease associated with chronic renal dialysis and kidney disease *(5,58,70)*, the apparently protective effects of consuming human milk in infancy *(5,70)* or of hepatic cirrhosis *(5)* are accompanied by consonant changes in copper metabolism and/or utilization (*see* Chapters 9, 16, and 17). The mortality rate for coronary heart disease and the ratio of zinc to copper in milk sold in 47 cities of the U.S. are positively correlated (r=0.354, p<0.02) *(193)*. Zinc can inhibit copper utilization (Table 2). Changes in copper status explain the low serum cholesterol values found in acrodermatitis enteropathica *(70,107)* and Wilson's disease *(47)*, the decreased cholesterol following the ingestion of calcium supplements *(5,51,70)* or the injection of ethylenediamine tetraacetate *(5,108)* and the hyperlipidemia and glucose intolerance of Menkes' disease *(11,47,58)*. The hypercholesterolemia of pregnancy *(5,108)*, the dyslipidemia associated with the ingestion of zinc supplements *(2,11,47,58)* and seasonal variations in cholesterol *(2,45)* probably are secondary to alterations in copper. One also can conclude from experiments with animals that the increased risk of heart disease associated with high serum uric acid *(11,47,58,106,109)*, with small stature *(47,106)* and with the availability of soft water *(5,6,47,51,70,107–109)* may be related to diets low in copper. Space does not permit full documentation here of these concepts; primary references including those to specific experiments are included in the theoretical references cited.

Epidemiology was emphasized in the early development of the copper deficiency theory. This theory has been criticized *(110)*, however, because "there are no prospective epidemiologic data supporting" it. Mielcarz, et al. provide supportive, epidemiologic data collected in Japanese people living in Brazil and Okinawa *(111)*.

They reviewed some migration of Japanese people and compared ischemic heart disease mortality rates. The rate for Okinawa is well below the Japanese average; emigrants from Okinawa to Brazil increase their risk nearly fourfold in a generation. Copper in leucocytes was lower in Brazil than in Okinawa; they attributed these differences to dietary change associated with immigration. More seafood (seaweed, shell fish, etc.) is eaten in Japan; more meat, in

Table 3
The Anatomy of Copper Deficiency and Ischemic Heart Disease

Aortic valve thickening[a]	Hemopericardium
Arterial	Hemothorax
Elastic degeneration	Myocardial infarction
Fibrosis	Pericarditis
Foam cells	Pleural effusion[a]
Hemorrhage (intramural)	Ruptured papillary muscle
Mucopolysaccharide increase	Small stature
Necrosis	Ventricular
Smooth muscle proliferation	Aneurysm
Atrial	Calcification
Thrombosis	Edema
Bone density decrease	Fibrosis
Coronary artery	Hemorrhage (focal)
Dissecting aneurysms	Hypertrophy
Elastic fragmentation	Infiltration
Hyalinization	(neutrophil and round cell)
Necrosis	Myocyte-myocyte struts decreased
Smooth muscle degeneration	Necrosis (myocardial cell)
Sudanophilia	Rupture
Thrombosis	Thrombosis (endocardial)

[a] Newly added, see text. The work of numerous authors is incorporated into Tables 2–4. Their work has been cited in earlier writings (2,11,46,47,53,58,106,109); citation of most primary references is omitted for the sake of brevity. All of the entries in the table have been found in both animals deficient in copper and in people with ischemic heart disease.

Brazil. These data are consonant with lower copper status in Brazil and an inverse correlation between leucocyte copper and coronary atherosclerosis found by Kinsman, et al. (112).

3.1.2. ISCHEMIC HEART DISEASE RESEMBLES COPPER DEFICIENCY

Oster et al. (89) found a positive correlation between cardiac output and copper in heart tissue of patients with coronary heart disease (in addition to the similar correlation with selenium noted in Subheading 3). Copper deficient rats resemble those deficient in selenium in some aspects of selenium metabolism (71).

Characteristics common to animals deficient in copper and people with ischemic heart disease are summarized in Tables 3–5. Tabulation began in 1980 (109); similarities between the two conditions were noted in 1987 and collection continues as new similarities are found (24).

3.1.2.1. Anatomy. The most important anatomical similarities between copper deficiency in animals and human heart disease are arterial foam cells and smooth muscle cell proliferation, which are thought to be the earliest signs of atherosclerosis, and ventricular aneurysms and myocardial infarction, which obviously are late in the clinical course (Table 3).

In a comparison between echocardiography and coronary angiography, people with thickened aortic valves had a higher incidence of luminal narrowing (113). Rats deficient in copper also have thickened heart valves as assessed by quantitative light microscopy (114). Aortic valve sclerosis, calcification, and thickening in the absence of obstruction is associated with increased risk of myocardial infarction (194). This observation complements the

Table 4
The Chemistry of Copper Deficiency and Ischemic Heart Disease

Decreased	Increased
Cardiac copper	Cardiac sodium
Cardiac iron[a]	Cholesterolemia[b]
Dihomo-γ-linolenic acid	Serum ferritin[a]
Hepatic zinc	Thiobarbituric acid reactive
Lecithin: cholesterol acyltransferase[a]	substances[a]
Leucocyte copper	Thromboxane A_2/prostacyclin
Lipoprotein lipase[a]	Triglyceridemia
Myocardial cytochrome oxidase	Uricemia
Na/K-ATPase[a]	
Plasma retinol	

Exacerbated by	Mitigated by
Homocysteine	Aspirin
Salt	Beer
	Clofibrate

[a] Newly added, see text. [b]Risk factor. See Table 3 for further explanation.

Table 5
The Physiology of Copper Deficiency and Ischemic Heart Disease

Abnormal electrocardiograms	Decreased
Blocks	Arterial dilation with acetylcholine[a]
bundle branch[b]	Blood pressure under load
first degree	Glucose tolerance[b]
second degree	Hearing[a]
third degree	Longevity
His-ventricular interval increased[a]	
Pathological Q waves	Exacerbated by
P wave morphology altered	Pregnancy[a]
QT interval increased	
R waves are tall	Increased
ST segment[b]	Blood pressure[b]
Ventricular premature beats	Euglobulin clot lysis time
	Female thrombosis
	Male sudden death

[a] Newly added, see text. [b] Risk factor. See Table 3 for further explanation.

association between valve disease and coronary artery disease *(113)* and shows the latter can lead to coronary heart disease. Boon et al. *(195)* suggest that valvular calcifications should be considered manifestations of generalized atherosclerosis because of strong associations with conventional risk factors.

Bone disease in copper deficiency, first noticed by Baxter, et al. *(115),* reviewed by Underwood *(116)* and confirmed recently in pigs *(117)* and rats *(118)* has not received much attention from nutritionists. Some related data have been collected and reviewed *(119).*

Data from the Nurses Health Study do not support the hypothesis that higher consumption of milk protects against fractures *(120)*. The only significant (*p*=0.05) trend of several sought was an increase in hip fracture risk with daily, dairy calcium; significance may have occurred from applying the laws of chance to multiple comparisons. These results are not puzzling, however, because milk and yogurt are among the more copper deficient foods *(119)*. Milk diets were used in some of the classical experiments on copper deficiency in animals *(115,121,122)*. Trochopoulu et al. *(35)* found no association between calcium intake and bone mineral density, but the association between bone disease and ischemic heart disease is becoming increasingly obvious (*see* Subheading 1.2).

Pleural effusion occurs in ischemic heart disease *(123)* and in swine *(122)*, rats *(124)*, and mice *(125)* deficient in copper. More references confirm that ventricular aneurysms occur in copper deficiency *(126,127)* and after human myocardial infarction *(128)*, respectively.

3.1.2.2. Chemistry. According to Prohaska *(129)*, hypercholesterolemia following copper deficiency is generally accepted. The first data that joined the metabolism of copper with that of cholesterol were published in 1973 *(108)*. Since the last enumeration *(47)*, several more confirmations have been noticed bringing the total of independent laboratories to twenty-two *(130–138)*.

There is a long history of adding cholesterol or cholesterol plus cholic acid to animal diets to induce hypercholesterolemia or atherosclerosis. Since these methods were found to decrease the concentration of copper in liver *(139,140)*, others have confirmed and extended these observations *(141,142)*. Vlad, et al. *(142)* also found decreased aortic copper and increased serum lipid peroxide. These experiments lengthen the list of those demonstrating increased copper in plasma or serum accompanied by decreased copper in organs *(141,142)*. The results of Hellerstein et al. *(77)* on the benefits of magnesium (*see* Subheading 3) to rats fed an atherogenic diet may require reinterpretation because the diet contained cholesterol and cholic acid. The extra magnesium might have decreased the harmful effect of the sterols on copper utilization.

Metallic elements have been measured in presumably normal heart muscle in people with ischemic heart disease. Emphasis was placed on calcium and magnesium to provide data related to the "water factor." Several studies revealed that muscular copper was low in heart disease (for review see *[47,107]*) in comparison with accident victims, etc. The Chipperfields *(79)* also found iron was decreased in ventricular muscle of people with ischemic heart disease. Because cardiac iron is decreased in copper deficiency, these data on iron support the copper deficiency theory of ischemic heart disease better than the concept that subtle degrees of iron overload are toxic *(36,63,64)*.

Salonen et al. *(66)* examined nearly 2,000 men from Kupio in Eastern Finland and found that high serum ferritin predicts risk of acute myocardial infarction in multivariate models better than low density lipoprotein cholesterol. Serum ferritin in rats doubles in copper deficiency *(143)*. Perhaps some of the people with high ferritin have low copper nutriture.

Patients with coronary heart disease *(196)* were found to have decreased activity of lecithin: cholesterol acyltransferase. Copper deficiency in rats is accompanied by decreased lecithin: cholesterol acyltransferase activity *(197)*. Lipoprotein lipase activity is decreased in Dutch men with coronary artery disease *(198)* and in rats deficient in copper *(199)*. Bruckert et al. *(200)* found low free-thyroxine levels to be associated with atherosclerosis in euthyroid patients.

Rats *(144)* deficient in copper and people with ischemic cardiomyopathy *(145)* have decreased expression of cardiac Na/K-ATPase. The former was measured in ventricular tissue and myocytes; the latter was measured in the normal-appearing regions of left ventricules obtained at autopsy. As the number of rats studied exceeds the number of people observed, more human data are needed. These findings may explain the increase in cardiac sodium noted earlier *(24,53,106)*. Rabbits fed cholesterol also have a decrease in Na/K ATPase activity *(146)*. High dietary cholesterol disrupts the copper utilization of rabbits *(140)*.

Copper deficiency produces an increase in plasma homocysteine in rats *(201)*. Brown and Strain *(202)* found that high homocysteine interferes with copper utilizations. Thus, copper and plasma homocysteine can be harmfully cooperative as too little element can produce too much amino acid and *vice versa*.

Angiogram patients with a history of acute myocardial infarction had less extracellular superoxide dismutase in plasma than similar patients without such a history *(203)*. The enzyme also was lower in men than in women and in smokers than nonsmokers.

There is growing interest in the concept that people with ischemic heart disease may have an impaired ability to defend against oxidative damage. Malondialdehyde and thiobarbituric acid reactive substances have been used as indices of peroxidation. These substances are found to be increased in serum in coronary artery disease *(147)* and angina pectoris *(148)* and in plasma of copper deficient rats *(149)*.

It has been known for decades that increases or decreases in the output of the thyroid gland can have opposite effects on the concentration of cholesterol. This realization has prompted interest in the relationship, if any, between thyroid function and atherosclerosis and ischemic heart disease. Atherogenic diets for animal experiments frequently contain antithyroid substances.

Lower thyroid status in people is associated with higher low density lipoprotein cholesterol and lower high density cholesterol *(150,151)* which, in turn, are associated with increased heart disease risk. Fewer data are available on thyroid function and heart disease. Women with severe coronary artery disease have an exaggerated response of thyroid stimulating hormone to thyrotrophin releasing hormone *(152)*. Both Allen et al. *(153)* and Lukaski, et al. *(137)* found lower thyroxine concentrations in sera of rats deficient in copper. The inability of Kralik et al. *(154)* to confirm these results may not be relevant to people because the food intakes of their rats were restricted. More studies of pituitary/thyroid hormones in copper deficiency are needed before thyroid chemistry or function can be added to the tables.

3.1.2.3. Physiology. Tomanek et al. *(155)* confirmed that increased QT intervals have been found in ischemic heart disease. The His-ventricular interval is prolonged in rats deficient in copper *(156)* and in some people with ischemic heart disease *(157)*. Mao et al. *(204)* found that high dietary fat and marginal dietary copper can cooperate to prolong the QT interval. Mice lacking copper/zinc superoxide dismutase have hearing loss secondary to choclear pathology *(205)*.

Bengtssen et al. *(158)* found that women with angina pectoris were more likely to have borne five or more children than other women in Göteborg. Ness et al. *(159)* used data from Framingham and NHANES and found that women with six or more pregnancies had increased risk of coronary heart disease. Study of this phenomenon dates at least from 1958 *(158)* and, although not all data are supportive, the association seems to be real. This increase in heart disease risk associated with multiple pregnancies may occur because of copper depletion. The near impossibility of avoiding copper depletion when eating a diet from the lowest tertile of copper content during pregnancy has been noted *(93)*.

A diet high in lard produced numerous cardiovascular abnormalities in mice *(160)* but the harmful effects were found to be the result of copper deficiency *(125)*. Mice fed this diet died earlier with more frequent thrombosis if they had been bred *(161)*. These mice generally die with very large atrial thromboses *(160)* as a result of an impaired ability to dissolve blood clots *(162)* and unfavorable prostaglandin metabolism *(163,164)*.

Thus, these experiments on copper deficiency illustrate an important feature of ischemic heart disease. When deaths are sudden, deficient males are more susceptible *(165)*, when deaths occur with thrombosis, deficient females are more susceptible *(166)*. Lerner et al. *(167)* confirmed the observation of Spiekerman et al. *(36)* that sudden death in ischemic heart disease is more common in men. Women are more likely to die with thrombosis *(36)*.

Vasodilation in response to acetylcholine is decreased in people with hypercholesterolemia *(168)*, untreated hypertension *(169)*, coronary artery disease *(170)*, and with angina pectoris and normal coronary angiograms *(171)*. This impaired response resembles that of aortas isolated from copper deficient rats *(172–174)*. In contrast, sodium nitroprusside responses were not different in hypercholesterolemia *(168)* or hypertension *(169)* but were impaired in copper deficiency *(172)*. These effects in copper deficiency probably are mediated via nitric oxide *(173,174)* because copper-zinc superoxide dismutase activity is decreased in deficiency, nitric oxide is destroyed by superoxide, and extra superoxide dismutase can restore the response.

Rubenstein may have been first to measure hearing loss in the aged and relate it to cardiovascular pathology *(175)*; loss was greater in people with "appreciable cardiovascular disturbances with signs (not defined) of impaired peripheral circulation in comparison to people matched by age and sex without these pathologies. In Framingham, people with cardiovascular events such as angina pectoris, myocardial infarction, etc., had greater hearing thresholds; impaired hearing status was greater for women than men, and more in the low than the high frequencies. Hearing loss has been associated with cardiovascular risk factors, but associations are not always consistent *(176–178)*.

Perinatal copper deficiency produces a decrease in auditory startle response in rats even after months of repletion with a diet adequate in copper *(179)*. It seems that the rats had poor hearing. Response was not impaired in rats depleted of copper at weaning. Perhaps this finding is an example of a perinatal influence on adult disease *(48)*, as pregnant women who consume diets low in copper will deplete their copper stores *(93)*. Three percent of low birth weight infants had hearing loss *(180)*.

3.1.2.4. Copper in Contrast to Fat. Table 1 contains nearly a dozen characteristics of ischemic heart disease unlikely to be the result of fat intoxication. Some may argue that bone disease or hearing loss, for example, should not be considered as part of ischemic heart disease. Exclusion of risk factors, such as abnormal electrocardiograms or glucose intolerance, is more difficult, however.

Tables 3 to 5 contain similarities between animals deficient in copper and people with ischemic heart disease. Some of these, such as foam cells and smooth muscle proliferation have been produced in experiments with dietary fat. As the diets in these experiments usually contain cholesterol (with or without cholic acid) the results may not be simply direct intoxication with dietary fat. Cholesterol with or without cholic acid interferes with the utilization of dietary copper *(139,140,181)*. These experiments may need reinterpretation; copper deficiency may have produced the effects. Major pathology of diets high in lard *(160)* was eliminated by extra copper *(125)*. Lamb et al. *(206)* added extra copper to the diets of cholesterol-fed rabbits, found less aortic atherosclerosis, and confirmed that feeding cholesterol to rabbits raises plasma copper *(140)*.

Other changes such as those in cardiac calcium, copper, iron, sodium, and zinc or in enzyme activities such as ATPase or cytochrome oxidase seem unlikely to be induced by diets high in fat and adequate in copper. Effects on heart disease of aspirin, beer, homocysteine, and salt are more likely to be direct effects on copper utilization than individual effects mediated via dietary fat. Beneficial effects in some experiments with human volunteers may have occurred because of concomitant changes in dietary copper *(182–184)* instead of changes in dietary lipid. Consideration of ischemic heart disease as a problem of copper deficiency seems more inclusive than consideration of the disease as a problem of fat intoxication. Copper deficiency might have been a hidden variable in important experiments and fat intoxication explains too few important phenomena.

4. SUMMARY

Ischemic heart disease was rare early in the century but gradually increased to be the leading cause of death in the industrialized world. Gradually it was realized that heart disease risk varies considerably from nation to nation and that national diets were quite variable in the amount and type of fat they contained. The apparently clear association between ischemic heart disease and the Western diet has led many to infer that amount and type of dietary fat are of prime importance in the etiology and pathophysiology of ischemic heart disease: the lipid hypothesis. The Western diet has other characteristics other than lipid that may alter heart disease risk.

There has been a gradual realization that the relationship between dietary fat and heart disease risk is very small or nonexistent within nations, that the cardinal risk factors identify a minority of people with the illness and that nearly everyone eats too much of the wrong fat. Also, many phenomena that are integral parts of ischemic heart disease seem unrelated to fat intake or lipid metabolism.

Three alternatives to the lipid hypothesis are being developed as being more general explanations for some of the apparently paradoxical or dissimilar observations on ischemic heart disease. Two of these, based on homocysteine and iron, have been described more thoroughly in **Subheading 2.1.**; the copper deficiency theory is being extended here. Perhaps these alternatives eventually can determine why some people tolerate the Western diet for a lifetime and others die early of ischemic heart disease and can complement the lipid hypothesis so that eventually ischemic heart disease will disappear from among the leading causes of death in the industrialized nations.

The copper deficiency theory is offered as the simplest and most general explanation of the etiology and pathophysiology of ischemic heart disease. Diets often are low enough in copper that they fall into the range proved insufficient for men and women in controlled depletion experiments in which alterations in blood pressure regulation, dislipidemia, electrocardiograms, and decreased glucose clearance have been observed. There are numerous anatomical, chemical, and physiological similarities between animals deficient in copper and people with ischemic heart disease. Few of these, particularly among those of chemistry and physiology, can be explained by an intoxication with dietary fat; fewer still have been produced in animals fed fat. Some of the other elements implicated in the process that leads to ischemic heart disease seem to produce some of their effects by modifying copper utilization.

REFERENCES

1. Burkitt DP. Western diseases and what they encompass. In: Temple NJ, Burkitt DP, Eds. Western Diseases : Their Dietary Prevention and Reversibility. Humana Press, Totowa NJ, 1994, pp.15–27.
2. Klevay LM. Some environmental aspects of ischaemic heart disease. Environ Manage Health 1990;1:9–17.
3. Hopkins PN, Williams RR. A survey of 246 suggested coronary risk factors. Atherosclerosis 1981;40:1–52.
4. Strasser T. Coronary risk factors revisited. World Health Forum 1982;3:85–88.
5. Klevay LM. Coronary heart disease: the zinc/copper hypothesis. Am J Clin Nutr 1975;28:764–774.
6. Klevay LM. Elements of ischemic heart disease. Perspect Biol Med 1977;20:186–192.
7. Klevay LM. Changing patterns of disease: some nutritional remarks. J Am Coll Nutr 1984;3:149–158.
8. Kannel WB. Some lessons in cardiovascular epidemiology from Framingham. Am J Cardiol 1976;37:269–282.
9. Keys A. Coronary heart disease—the global picture. Atherosclerosis 1975;22:149–192.
10. Keys A. Seven Countries, A Multivariate Analysis of Death and Coronary Heart Disease. Harvard University, Cambridge 1980;pp. 1–381.
11. Klevay LM. Copper and ischemic heart disease. Biol Trace Elem Res 1983;5:245–255.
12. Zukel WJ, Lewis RH, Enterline PE, Painter RC, Ralston RS, Fawcett RM, Meredith AP, Peterson B. A short-term community study of the epidemiology of coronary heart disease. Am J Public Health 1959;49:1630–1639.
13. Gordon T. Section 24: The Framingham Study-An epidemiological investigation of cardiovascular disease. US Government Printing Office, Washington, DC, 1970; p. 9.
14. Harlan WR, Hull AH, Schmouder RP, Thompson FE, Larkin FA, Landis JR. Dietary intake and cardiovascular risk factors. Part II. Serum Urate, Serum Cholesterol, and Correlates. DHHS Publication No. (PHS) 1983;83–1677 Series 11, p. 1.
15. Ravnskov U. Cholesterol lowering trials in coronary heart disease: frequency of citation and outcome. Br Med J 1992;305:15–19.
16. Call DL, S'anchez AM. Trends in fat disappearance in the United States, 1909–1965. J Nutr 1967;93 Suppl 1, Part II:1–28.
17. Kahn HA. Change in serum cholesterol associated with changes in the United States civilian diet, 1909–1965. Am J Clin Nutr 1970;23:879–882.
18. Wen CP, Gershoff SN. Changes in serum cholesterol and coronary heart disease mortality associated with changes in the postwar Japanese diet. Am J Clin Nutr 1973;26:616–619.
19. Klevay LM. Coronary heart disease and dietary fiber. Am J Clin Nutr 1974;27:1202–1203.
20. Ravnskov U. The questionable role of saturated and polyunsaturated fatty acids in cardiovascular disease. J Clin Epidemiol 1998;51:443–460.
21. Posner BM, Cobb JL, Belanger AJ, Cupples LA, D'Agostino RB, Stokes J. Dietary lipid predictors of coronary heart disease in men. The Framingham Study. Ann Intern Med 1991;151:1181–1187.
22. Gillman MW, Cupples LA, Millen BE, Ellison RC, Wolf PA. Inverse association of dietary fat with development of ischemic stroke in men. JAMA 1997;278:2145–2150.
23. Shekelle RB, Shryock AM, Paul O, Lepper M, Stamler J, Liu S, Raynor WJ, Jr. Diet, serum cholesterol and death from coronary heart disease. The Western Electric study. N Engl J Med 1981;304:65–70.
24. Klevay LM. Copper and cardiovascular disease. In: Berthon G, Ed. in Handbook of Metal-Ligand Interactions in Biological Fluids. Bioinorganic Medicine, Vol. 2 Marcel Dekker, New York, 1995, pp. 843–848.
25. Menczel J, Reshef A, Schwartz A, Guggenheim K, Hegsted DM, Stare FJ. Aortic calcification in Israel. An epidemiological study. Arch Environ Health 1971;22:667–671.
26. Dent CE, Engelbrecht HE, Godfrey RC. Osteoporosis of lumbar vertebrae and calcification of abdominal aorta in women living in Durban. Br Med J 1968;476–79.
27. Fujita T, Okamoto Y, Sakagami Y, Ota K, Ohata M. Bone changes and aortic calcification in aging inhabitants of mountain versus seacoast communities in the Kii Peninsula. J Am Geriatr Soc 1984;32:124–128.
28. Uyama O, Yoshimoto Y, Yamamoto Y, Kawai A. Bone changes and carotid atherosclerosis in postmenopausal women. Stroke 1997;28:1730–1732.
29. Cox JM, Gideon D, Rogers FJ. Incidence of osteophytic lipping of the thoracic spine in coronary heart disease: results of a pilot study. J Am Osteopath Assoc 1983;82:837–838.
30. DeStefano F, Anda RF, Kahn HS, Williamson DF, Russell CM. Dental disease and risk of coronary heart disease and mortality. Br Med J 1993;306:688–691.

31. Seymour RA, Steele JG. Is there a link between periodontal disease and coronary heart disease? Br Dent J 1998;184:33–38.

32. Loesche WJ, Schork A, Terpenning MS, Chen YM, Dominguez BL, Grossman N. Assessing the relationship between dental disease and coronary heart disease in elderly U.S. veterans. J Am Dent Assoc 1998;129:301–311.

33. Beck J, Garcia R, Heiss G, Vokonas PS, Offenbacher S. Periodontal disease and cardiovascular disease. J Periodontol 1996;67:1123–1137.

34. Bernstein DS, Sadowsky N, Hegsted DM, Guri CD, Stare FJ. Prevalence of osteoporosis in high- and low-fluoride areas in North Dakota. JAMA 1966;198:499–504.

35. Trichopoulou A, Georgiou E, Bassiakos Y, Lipworth L, Lagiou P, Proukakis C, Trichopoulos D. Energy intake and monounsaturated fat in relation to bone mineral density among women and men in Greece. Prev Med 1997;26:395–400.

36. Spiekerman RE, Brandenburg JT, Achor RW, Edwards JE. The spectrum of coronary heart disease in a community of 30,000: A clinicopathologic study. Circulation 1962;25:57–65.

37. Anonymous. Coronary heart disease without risk factors. Nutr Rev 1989; 47:18–22.

38. Kannel WB, Gordon T. The search for an optimum serum cholesterol. Lancet 1982;2:374–375.

39. Kannel WB, Castelli WP, Gordon T. Cholesterol in the prediction of atherosclerotic disease. New perspectives based on the Framingham study. Ann Intern Med 1979;90:85–91.

40. Jacobs D. Hyperuricemia as a risk factor in coronary heart disease. Adv Exp Med Biol 1977;76B:231–237.

41. Brand FN, McGee DL, Kannel WB, Stokes J, Castelli WP. Hyperuricemia as a risk factor of coronary heart disease: The Framingham Study. Am J Epidemiol 1985;121:11–18.

42. Tunstall-Pedoe H, Woodward M, Tavendale R, Brook R, McCluskey MK. Comparison of the prediction by 27 different factors of coronary heart disease and death in men and women of the Scottish Heart Health Study: cohort study. Br Med J 1997;315:722–729.

43. Ichihara Y, Sugino M, Hattori R, Anno T, Mizuno Y, Yokoi M, Kondo T, Hirai M, Kawamura T. Relation of electrocardiographic left ventricular hypertrophy with and without T-wave changes to systemic blood pressure, body mass, and serum lipids and blood glucose levels in Japanese men. Am J Cardiol 1997;80:730–735.

44. Gordon DJ, Trost DC, Hyde J, Whaley FS, Hannan PJ, Jacobs DR, Jr. Ekelund LG. Seasonal cholesterol cycles: the Lipid Research Clinics Coronary Primary Prevention Trial placebo group. Circulation 1987; 76:1224–1231.

45. Klevay LM, Moore RJ. Beer mitigates some effects of copper deficiency in rats. Am J Clin Nutr 1990;51:869–872.

46. Klevay LM. Ischemic heart disease. A major obstacle to becoming old. Clin Geriatr Med 1987,3.361–372.

47. Klevay LM. Ischemic heart disease: toward a unified theory. In: Lei KY, Carr TP, Eds. Role of Copper in Lipid Metabolism. CRC Press, Boca Raton, 1990, pp. 233–267.

48. Goldberg GR, Prentice AM. Maternal and fetal determinants of adult diseases. Nutr Rev 1994;52:191–200.

49. Godfrey K, Robinson S. Maternal nutrition, placental growth and fetal programming. Proc Nutr Soc 1998;57:105–111.

50. Gunnell DJ, Davey SG, Frankel S, Nanchahal K, Braddon FE, Pemberton J, Peters TJ. Childhood leg length and adult mortality: follow up of the Carnegie (Boyd Orr); Survey of Diet and Health in Pre-war Britain. J Epidemiol Community Health 1998;52:142–152.

51. Klevay LM. The influence of copper and zinc on the occurrence of ischemic heart disease. J Environ Pathol Toxicol 1980;4:281–287.

52. Lacey RF, Shaper AG. Changes in water hardness and cardiovascular death rates. Int J Epidemiol 1984;13:18–24.

53. Klevay LM. Ischemic heart disease: nutrition or pharmacotherapy? J Trace Elem Electrolytes Health Dis 1993;7:63–69.

54. Chamberlin TC. The method of multiple working hypotheses. Science 1965;148:754–759.

55. Kuhn TS. The Structure of Scientific Revolutions. The University of Chicago Press, Chicago, 1970;pp. 95,154,169.

56. Bancroft WD. How to ripen time. J Phys Chem 1931;35:1904–1921.

57. Neyman J. The Heritage of Copernicus: theories "pleasing to the mind." MIT Press, Cambridge, Mass, 1974, pp. 1–22.

58. Klevay LM. The role of copper, zinc and other chemical elements in ischemic heart disease. In: Rennert OM, Chan WY, Eds. Metabolism of Trace Metals in Man, Vol. 1. CRC Press, Boca Raton, FL, 1984, pp. 129–157.

59. Jonsson A, Agnarsson BA, Hallgrimsson J. Coronary atherosclerosis and myocardial infarction in nonagenarians: a retrospective autopsy study. Age Ageing 1985;14:109–112.
60. Kohn RR. Cause of death in very old people. JAMA 1982;247:2793–2797.
61. McCullyKS. Homocystinuria, arteriosclerosis, methylmalonic aciduria, and methyltransferase deficiency: a key case revisited. Nutr Rev 1992;50:7–12.
62. McCully KS. The Homocysteine Revolution. Keats Publishing, Inc, New Canaan, 1997, pp.1–242.
63. Sullivan JL. Iron and the sex difference in heart disease risk. Lancet 1981;1:1293–1294.
64. Sullivan JL. The iron paradigm of ischemic heart disease. Am Heart J 1989;117:1177–1188.
65. Sullivan JL. Stored iron and ischemic heart disease. Empirical support for a new paradigm. Circulation 1992;86:1036–1037.
66. Salonen JT, Nyyssönen K, Korpela H, Tuomilehto J, SeppanenR, Salonen R. High stored iron levels are associated with excess risk of myocardial infarction in eastern Finnish men. Circulation 1992;86:803–811.
67. Sullivan JL. Iron versus cholesterol—perspectives on the iron and heart disease debate. J Clin Epidemiol 1996;49:1345–1352.
68. Klevay LM. Can copper deficiency cause ischemic heart disease? In: Momcilovic B, Ed. Trace Elements in Man and Animals - TEMA 7. Institute for Medical Research and Occupational Health, University of Zagreb, Zagreb, 1991.
69. Klevay LM. This week's citation classic on hypercholesterolemia in rats produced by an increase in the ratio of zinc to copper ingested. Amer J Clin Nutr 26:1060-1068, 1973. Current Contents Clin Med 1987;15:20–20.
70. Klevay LM. The role of copper and zinc in cholesterol metabolism, In: Draper HH, Ed. Advances in Nutritional Research, Vol. 1. Plenum Publishing Corp, New York, 1977, pp. 227–252.
71. Klevay LM. Elements of atherosclerosis. In: Reis MF, Pereira JM, Machado AA, Abdulla M, Eds. Trace Elements in Medicine, Health and Atherosclerosis Smith-Gordon, London, 1995, pp. 9–14.
72. Klevay LM. Copper and other chemical elements that affect the cardiovascular system. In Toxicology of Metals. Chang LW, Ed. Target Organ Toxicology. Vol. 2. CRC Press, Boca Raton, 1995, pp. 921–928.
73. Schroeder HA. Serum cholesterol levels in rats fed thirteen trace elements. J Nutr 1968;94:475–480.
74. Selye H. The Pluricausal Cardiopathies. Thomas, C.C., Springfield, 1961, p. 231.
75. Selye H. Experimental cardiovascular diseases. Springer-Verlag, New York, 1970, pp. 223,348,358.
76. Seelig MS, Heggtveit HA. Magnesium interrelationships in ischemic heart disease: a review. Am J Clin Nutr 1974;27:59–79.
77. Hellerstein EE, Nakamura M, Hegsted DM, Vitale JJ. Studies on the interrelationships between dietary magnesium, quality and quantity of fat, hypercholesterolemia and lipidosis. J Nutr 1960;71:339–346.
78. Elin RJ, Hosseini JM. Is the magnesium content of nuts a factor for coronary heart disease? Arch Intern Med 1993;153:779–780.
79. Chipperfield B, Chipperfield JR. Differences in metal content of the heart muscle in death from ischemic heart disease. Am Heart J 1978;95:732–737.
80. Abraham AS, Rosenmann D, Kramer M, Balkin J, Zion M, Farbstien H, Eylath U. Magnesium in the prevention of lethal arrhythmias in acute myocardial infarction. Arch Intern Med 1987;147:753–755.
81. Teo KK, Yusuf S, Collins R, Held PH, Peto R. Effects of intravenous magnesium in suspected acute myocardial infarction: overview of randomised trials. Br Med J 1991;303:1499–1503.
82. Gurfinkel E, Pazos A, Mautner B. Abnormal QT intervals associated with negative T waves induced by antiarrhythmic drugs are rapidly reduced using magnesium sulfate as an antidote. Clin Cardiol 1993;16:35–38.
83. Anonymous. Observations on effect of sodium selenite in prevention of Keshan disease. Chin Med J Engl 1979; 92:471–476.
84. Anonymous. Epidemiologic studies on the etiologic relationship of selenium and Keshan disease. Chin Med J Engl 1979;92:477–482.
85. Chen X, Yang G, Chen J, Wen Z, Ge K. Studies on the relations of selenium and Keshan disease. Biol Trace Elem Res 1980;2:91–107.
86. Yang GQ, Chen JS, Wen ZM, Ge KY, Zhu LZ, Chen XC, Chen XS. The role of selenium in Keshan disease. Adv Nutr Res 1984;6:203–231.
87. Levander OA, Burk RF. Selenium. In: Ziegler EE, Filer LJ, Jr. Eds. Present knowledge in nutrition. ISLI Press, Washington, 1996,pp. 320–328.
88. Klevay LM. Four ways of becoming ill. Med Hypotheses 1988;27:65–70.

89. Oster O, Dahm M, OelertH. Element concentrations (selenium, copper, zinc, iron, magnesium, potassium, phosphorous) in heart tissue of patients with coronary heart disease correlated with physiological parameters of the heart. Eur Heart J1993;14:770–774.

90. Vinceti M, Rovesti S, Marchesi C, Bergomi M, Vivoli G. Changes in drinking water selenium and mortality for coronary disease in a residential cohort. Biol Trace Elem Res 1994;40:267–275.

91. Ascherio A, Willett WC, Rimm EB, Giovannucci EL, Stampfer MJ. Dietary iron intake and risk of coronary disease among men. Circulation 1994;89:969–974.

92. Strain JJ. Trace elements and cardiovascular disease. Bibl Nutr Dieta 1998;127–140.

93. Klevay LM, Medeiros DM. Deliberations and evaluations of the approaches, endpoints, and paradigms for dietary recommendations about copper. J Nutr 1996;126:2419S–2426S.

94. Klevay LM. And so spake Goldberger in 1916: pellagra is not infectious! J Am Coll Nutr 1997;16:290–292.

95. György P. The curative factor (vitamin H) for egg white injury,with particular reference to its presence in different foodstuffs and in yeast. J Biol Chem 1939;131:733–744.

96. Williams RR. Toward the conquest of beriberi. Harvard University Press, Cambridge,1961,p. 110.

97. Klevay LM, Saari JT. Comparative responses of rats to different copper intakes and modes of supplementation. Proc Soc Exp Biol Med 1993;203:214–220.

98. Anonymous. Recommended Dietary Allowances. National Academy of Sciences, Washington, DC, 1980, pp.151–154.

99. Anonymous. Recommended Dietary Allowances. National Academy Press, Washington, DC, 1989, pp. 7, 224–230.

100. Pennington. Chapter 4 in this book, 2000.

101. Anonymous. Recommended Dietary Allowances. National Academy of Sciences, Washington DC, 1974, pp. 95–96.

102. Klevay LM, Buchet JP, Bunker VW, Clayton BE, Gibson RS, Medeiros DM, Moser-Veillon PB, Patterson KY, Taper LJ, Wolf WR. Copper in the western diet (Belgium Canada, U.K. and USA). In: Anke M, Meissner D, Mills CF, Eds. Trace Elements in Man and Animals - TEMA 8.Verlag Media Touristik Gersdorf, Germany,1993, pp. 207–210.

103. Higuchi S, Higashi A, Nakamura T, Matsuda I. Nutritional copper deficiency in severely handicapped patients on a low copper enteral diet for a prolonged period: estimation of the required dose of dietary copper. J Pediatr Gastroenterol Nutr 1988;7:583–587.

104. Reiser S, Powell A, Yang CY, Canary JJ. Effect of copper intake on blood cholesterol and its lipoprotein distribution in men. Nutr Rep Int 1987;36:641–649.

105. Klevay LM, Inman L, Johnson LK, Lawler M, Mahalko JR, Milne DB, Lukaski HC, Bolonchuk W, Sandstead HH. Increased cholesterol in plasma in a young man during experimental copper depletion. Metabolism 1984;33:1112–1118.

106. Klevay LM. Ischemic heart disease as copper deficiency. In: Kies C, Ed. Copper bioavailability and metabolism (Adv. Exp. Med. Biol. Vol. 258) Plenum Press, New York, 1990, pp. 197–208.

107. Klevay LM. Ischemic heart disease: Updating the zinc/copper hypothesis. In: Naito HK, Ed. Nutrition and Heart Disease. S.P. Medical & Scientific Books, New York, 1982, pp. 61–67.

108. Klevay LM. Hypercholesterolemia in rats produced by an increase in the ratio of zinc to copper ingested. Am J Clin Nutr 1973;26:1060–1068.

109. KlevayL.M. 1980; Interactions of copper and zinc in cardiovascular disease. Ann.N.Y.Acad.Sci. 355140–151.

110. Salonen JT, Salonen R, Korpela H, Suntioinen S, Tuomilehto J. The authors reply. Am J Epidemiol 1992;135:833–834.

111. Mielcarz GW, Howard AN, Williams NR, Kinsman GD, Moriguchi E, Moriguchi Y, Mizushima S, Yamori Y. Copper and zinc status as a risk factor for ischemic heart disease: a comparison between Japanese in Brazil and Okinawa. J Trace Elem Exp Med 1997;10:29–35.

112. Kinsman GD, Howard AN, Stone DL, Mullins PA. Studies in copper status and atherosclerosis. Biochem Soc Trans 1990;18:1186–1188.

113. Lin SL, Liu CP, Chen CY, Ger LP, Chiang HT. The relation between thickened aortic valve and coronary artery disease. Chung Hua I Hsueh Tsa Chih Taipei 1997;60:92–97.

114. Medeiros DM, Bagby D, Ovecka G, McCormick R. Myofibrillar, mitochondrial and valvular morphological alterations in cardiac hypertrophy among copper–deficient rats. J Nutr 1991;121:815–824.

115. BaxterJH, Van Wyk JJ. A bone disorder associated with copper deficiency I. Gross morphological, roentgenological, and chemical observations. Bull Johns Hopkins Hosp 1953;93:1–13.

116. Underwood EJ. Trace Elements in Human and Animal Nutrition. Academic Press, New York, 1971,pp. 82–83.
117. Pond WG, Krook LP, Klevay LM. Bone pathology without cardiovascular lesions in pigs fed high zinc and low copper diet. Nutr Res 1990;10:871–885.
118. Medeiros DM, Ilich J, Ireton J, Matkovic V, Shiry L, Wildman R. Femurs from rats fed diets deficient in copper or iron have decreased mechanical strength and altered mineral composition. J Trace Elem Exp Med 1997;10:197–203.
119. Klevay LM. Lack of a recommended dietary allowance for copper may be hazardous to your health. J Am Coll Nutr 1998;17:322–326.
120. Feskanich D, Willett WC, Stampfer MJ, Colditz GA. Milk, dietary calcium, and bone fractures in women: a 12-year prospective study. Am J Public Health 1997;87:992–997.
121. Hart EB, Steenbock H, Waddell J, Elvehjem CA. Iron in nutrition. VII. Copper as a supplement to iron for hemoglobin building in the rat. J Biol Chem 1928;77:797– 812.
122. Shields GS, Coulson WF, Kimball DA, Cartwright GE, Winthrobe M. Studies on copper metabolism XXXII. Cardiovascular lesions in copper deficient swine. Am J Pathol 1962;41:603–621.
123. Sobel BE. Acute myocardial infarction. In: Wyngaarden JB, Smith LH, Jr. Bennett JC, Eds. Cecil Textbook of Medicine. W.B. Saunders Co, Philadelphia, 1992, pp. 304–318.
124. Viestenz KE, Klevay LM. A randomized trial of copper therapy in rats with electrocardiographic abnormalities due to copper deficiency. Am J Clin Nutr 1982;35:258–266.
125. Klevay LM. Atrial thrombosis, abnormal electrocardiograms and sudden death in mice due to copper deficiency. Atherosclerosis 1985;54:213–224.
126. Redman RS, Fields M, Reiser S, Smith JC, Jr. Dietary fructose exacerbates the cardiac abnormalities of copper deficiency in rats. Atherosclerosis 1988;74:203– 214.
127. Fields M, Lewis CG, Lure MD, Burns WA, Antholine WE. The severity of copper deficiency can be ameliorated by deferoxamine. Metabolism 1991;40:105–109.
128. Meizlish JL, Berger HJ, Plankey M, Errico D, Levy W, Zaret BL. Functional left ventricular aneurysm formation after acute anterior transmural myocardial infarction. Incidence, natural history, and prognostic implications. N Engl J Med 1984;311:1001–1006.
129. Prohaska JR. Biochemical changes in copper deficiency. J Nutr Biochem 1990;1:452– 461.
130. Koh ET. Comparison of copper status in rats when dietary fructose is replaced by either cornstarch or glucose. Proc Soc Exp Biol Med 1990;194:108–113.
131. Saari JT, Reeves PG, Noordewier B, Hall CB, Lukaski HC. Cardiovascular but not renal effects of copper deficiency are inhibited by dimethyl sulfoxide. Nutr Res 1990;10:467–477.
132. Gonzales FA, Elizaga IV, Klussmann FA. Copper deficiency and persistence of the ductus arteriosus. Dev Pharmacol Ther 1991;17:172–179.
133. Johnson PE, Korynta ED. Effects of copper, iron, and ascorbic acid on manganese availability to rats. Proc Soc Exp Biol Med 1992;199:470–480.
134. DiSilvestro RA, Greenson JK, Liao Z. Effects of low copper intake on dimethylhydrazine-induced colon cancer in rats. Proc Soc Exp Biol Med 1992;201:94–97.
135. Mazur A, Nassir F, Gueux E, Cardot P, Bellanger J, Lamand M, Rayssiguier Y. The effect of dietary copper on rat plasma apolipoprotein B, E plasma levels, and apolipoprotein gene expression in liver and intestine. Biol Trace Elem Res 1992;34:107–113.
136. Werman MJ, Bhathena SJ. Restricted food intake ameliorates the severity of copper deficiency in rats fed a copper-deficient, high-fructose diet. Med Sci Res 1993;21:309–310.
137. Lukaski HC, Hall CB, Marchello MJ. Body temperature and thyroid hormone metabolism of copper-deficient rats. J Nutr Biochem 1995;6:445–451.
138. Werman MJ, David R. Lysyl oxidase activity, collagen cross-links and connective tissue ultrastructure in the heart of copper-deficient male rats. J Nutr Biochem 1996;7:437–444.
139. Klevay LM. Metabolic interactions among cholesterol, cholic acid and copper. Nutr Rep Int 1982;26:405–414.
140. Klevay LM. Dietary cholesterol lowers liver copper in rabbits. Biol Trace Elem Res 1988;16:51–57.
141. Vlad M, Bordas E, Tomus R, Sava D, Farkas E, UzaG. Effect of copper sulfate on experimental atherosclerosis. Biol Trace Elem Res 1993;38:47–54.
142. Vlad M, Uza G, Zirbo M, OlteanuD. Free radicals, ceruloplasmin, and copper concentration in serum and aortic tissue in experimental atherosclerosis. Nutrition 1995;11:588–591.
143. Klevay LM. Serum ferritin doubles in rats deficient in copper. FASEB J 1994;5:A819.

144. Huang W, Lai C, Wang Y, Askari A, Klevay LM, Chiu TH. Altered expressions of cardiac Na/K-ATPase isoforms in copper deficient rats. Cardiovasc Res 1995;29:563–568.

145. Zahler R, Gilmore HM, Baldwin JC, Franco K, Benz-EJ J. Expression of alpha isoforms of the Na, K-ATPase in human heart. Biochim Biophys Acta 1993;1149:189–194.

146. Chen WJ, Lin SS, Huang HC, Lee YT. Decrease in myocardial Na(+)- K(+)-ATPase activity and ouabain binding sites in hypercholesterolemic rabbits. Basic Res Cardiol 1997;92:1–7.

147. Sakuma N, Hibino T, Sato T, Ohte N, Akita S, Tamai N, Sasai K, Yoshimata T, Fujinami T. Levels of thiobarbituric acid-reactive substance in plasma from coronary artery disease patients. Clin Biochem 1997;30:505–507.

148. Mendis S, Sobotka PA, Leja FL, Euler DE. Breath pentane and plasma lipid peroxides in ischemic heart disease. Free Radic Biol Med 1995;19:679–684.

149. Saari JT. Evidence that dimethyl sulfoxide inhibits defects of copper deficiency by inhibition of glycation. Nutr Res 1996;16:467–477.

150. Althaus BU, Staub JJ, Ryff DL, Oberhansli A, Stahelin HB. LDL/HDL- changes in subclinical hypothyroidism: possible risk factors for coronary heart disease. Clin Endocrinol (Oxf.) 1988;28:157–163.

151. Gomo Z, Ascott MB. The association of serum thyroid stimulating hormone and serum lipids and lipoproteins in patients with suspected hypothyroidism. Cent Afr J Med 1994;40:94–98.

152. Dean JW, Fowler PB. Exaggerated responsiveness to thyrotrophin releasing hormone: a risk factor in women with coronary artery disease. Br Med J Clin Res Ed 1985;290:1555–1561.

153. Allen DK, Hassel CA, Lei KY. Function of pituitary-thyroid axis in copper-deficient rats. J Nutr 1982; 112:2043–2046.

154. Kralik A, Kirchgessner M, Eder K. Concentrations of thyroid hormones in serum and activity of hepatic 5' monodeiodinase in copper–deficient rats. Z Ernahrungswiss 1996;35:288–291.

155. Tomanek RJ. Response of the coronary vasculature to myocardial hypertrophy. J Am Coll Cardiol 1990;15:528–533.

156. Kopp SJ, Klevay LM, Feliksik JM. Physiological and metabolic characterization of a cardiomyopathy induced by chronic copper deficiency. Am J Physiol 1983;245:H855–H866.

157. Pasternak. Braunwald E, Ed. Heart disease : a textbook of cardiovascular medicine. Saunders, Philadelphia, 1988,pp.1222–1313.

158. Bengtsson C. Ischaemic heart disease in women. A study based on a randomized population sample of women and women with myocardial infarction in Goteborg, Sweden. Acta Med Scand Suppl 1973; 549:75–81.

159. Ness RB, Harris T, Cobb J, Flegal KM, Kelsey JL, Balanger A, Stunkard AJ, D'Agostino RB. Number of pregnancies and the subsequent risk of cardiovascular disease. N Engl J Med 1993;328:1528–1533.

160. Ball CR, Williams WL, Collum JM. Cardiovascular lesions in Swiss mice fed a high fat-low protein diet with and without betaine supplementation. Anat Rec 1963;145:49–59.

161. Douglas BH, Clower BR, Williams WL. The effect of pregnancy on dietary-induced cardiovascular damage in RF strain mice. Am J Obstet Gynecol 1968;102:248–251.

162. Lynch SM, Klevay LM. Effect of a dietary copper deficiency on plasma fibrinolytic activity in male and female mice. Nutr Res 1993;13:913–922.

163. Nelson SK, Huang CJ, Mathias MM, Allen KG. Copper marginal and copper-deficient diets decrease aortic prostacyclin production and copper-dependent superoxide dismutase activity, and increase aortic lipid peroxidation in rats. J Nutr 1992;122:2101–2108.

164. Morin CL, Allen KG, Mathias M. Thromboxane production in copper-deficient and marginal platelets: influence of superoxide dismutase and lipid hydroperoxides. Proc Soc Exp Biol Med 1993;202:167–173.

165. Fields M, Lewis C, Scholfield DJ, Powell AS, Rose AJ, Reiser S, Smith JC. Female rats are protected against the fructose induced mortality of copper deficiency. Proc Soc Exp Biol Med 1986;183:145–149.

166. Lynch SM, Klevay LM. Effects of a dietary copper deficiency on plasma coagulation factor activities in male and female mice. J Nutr Biochem 1992;3:387–391.

167. Lerner DJ, Kannel WB. Patterns of coronary heart disease morbidity and mortality in the sexes: a 26-year follow-up of the Framingham population. Am Heart J 1986; 111:383–390.

168. Casino PR, Kilcoyne CM, Cannon RO, Quyyumi AA, Panza JA. Impaired endothelium-dependent vascular relaxation in patients with hypercholesterolemia extends beyond the muscarinic receptor. Am J Cardiol 1995;75:40–44.

169. Garcia CE, Kilcoyne CM, Cardillo C, Cannon RO, Quyyumi AA, Panza JA. Effect of copper-zinc superoxide dismutase on endothelium-dependent vasodilation in patients with essential hypertension. Hypertension 1995;26:863–868.

170. Berkenboom G, Crasset V, Giot C, Unger P, Vachiery JL, LeClerc JL. Endothelial function of internal mammary artery in patients with coronary artery disease and in cardiac transplant recipients. Am Heart J 1998;135:488–494.

171. Egashira K, Inou T, Hirooka Y, Yamada A, Urabe Y, Takeshita A. Evidence of impaired endothelium-dependent coronary vasodilatation in patients with angina pectoris and normal coronary angiograms. N Engl J Med 1993;328:1659–1664.

172. Saari JT. Dietary copper deficiency and endothelium-dependent relaxation of rat aorta. Proc Soc Exp Biol Med 1992;200:19–24.

173. Schuschke DA, Saari JT, Miller FN. A role for dietary copper in nitric oxide-mediated vasodilation. Microcirculation 1995;2:371–376.

174. Lynch SM, Frei B, Morrow JD, Roberts LJ, Xu A, Jackson T, Reyna R, Klevay LM, Vita JA, Keaney JF Jr. Vascular superoxide dismutase deficiency impairs endothelial vasodilator function through direct inactivation of nitric oxide and increased lipid peroxidation. Arterioscler Thromb Vasc Biol 1997;17:2975–2981.

175. Rubinstein M, Hildesheimer M, Zohar S, Chilarovitz T. Chronic cardiovascular pathology and hearing loss in the aged. Gerontology 1977;23:4–9.

176. Gold S, Haran I, Attias J, Shapira I, Shahar A. Biochemical and cardiovascular measures in subjects with noise-induced hearing loss. J Occup Med 1989;31:933–937.

177. Cocchiarella LA, Sharp DS, Persky VW. Hearing threshold shifts, white- cell count and smoking status in working men. Occup Med Oxf 1995;45:179–185.

178. Fuortes LJ, Tang S, Pomrehn P, Anderson C. Prospective evaluation of associations between hearing sensitivity and selected cardiovascular risk factors. Am J Ind Med 1995;28:275–280.

179. Prohaska JR, Hoffman RG. Auditory startle response is diminished in rats after recovery from perinatal copper deficiency. J Nutr 1996;126:618–627.

180. Bahado SR, Dashe J, Deren O, Daftary G, Copel JA, Ehrenkranz RA. Prenatal prediction of neonatal outcome in the extremely low-birth-weight infant. Am J Obstet Gynecol 1998;178:462–468.

181. Allen KG, Klevay LM. Copper: an antioxidant nutrient for cardiovascular health. Curr Opin Lipidol 1994; 5:22–28.

182. Klevay LM. The Lifestyle Heart Trial. Nutr Rev 1992;50:29–29.

183. Klevay LM. Copper in nuts may lower heart disease risk. Arch Intern Med 1993;153:401–402.

184. Klevay LM. Soy protein may affect plasma cholesterol through copper. Am J Clin Nutr 1994;60:300–301.

185. Morrison HI, Ellison LF, Taylor GW. Periodontal disease and risk of fatal coronary heart and cerebrovascular diseases. J Cardiovasc Risk 1999;6:7–11.

186. Whalen JP, Krook L. Periodontal disease as the early manifestation of osteropororis. Nutrition 1996;12:53–54.

187. Wamala SP, Mittleman MA, Horsten M, Schenck GK, Orth GK. Short stature and prognosis of coronary heart disease in women. J Intern Med 1999;245:557–563.

188. Banks LM, Lees B, MacSweeney JR, Stevenson JC. Effect of degenerative spinal and aortic calcification on bone density measurements in postmenopausal women: links between esteoporosis and cardiovascular disease? Eur J Clin Invest 1994;24:813–817.

189. McCully KS, McCully M. Harper Collins, New York, The heart revolution: the B vitamin breakthrough that lowers homocysteine, cuts your risk of heart disease, and protects your health 1999, pp. 1–221.

190. Sullivan JL. Iron and the genetics of cardiovasulcar disease. Circulation 1999;100:1260–1263.

191. Frustaci A, Magnavita N, Chimenti C, Caldarulo M, Sabbioni E, Pietra R, Cellini C, Possati GF, Maseri A. Marked elevation of myocardial trace elements in idiopathic dilated cardiomyopathy compared with secondary cardiac dysfunction. J Am Coll Cardiol 1999;33:1578–1583.

192. Ripa S, Ripa R, Giustiniani S. Are failured cardiomyopathies a zinc-deficit related disease? A study on Zn and Cu in patients with chronic failured dilated and hypertrophic cardiomyopathies. Minerva Med 1998;89:397–403.

193. Klevay LM. The ratio of zinc to copper in mink and mortality due to coronary heart disease: An association. Hemphill DD, Ed. In: Trace Substances in Environmental Health-VIII, University of Missouri, Columbia 1974, pp. 9–14.

194. Otto CM, Lind BK, Kitzman DW, Gersh BJ, Siscovick DS. Association of aortic-valve sclerosis with cardiovascular mortality and morbidity in the elderly. N Engl J Med 1999;341:142–147.

195. Boon A, Cheriex E, Lodder J, Kessels F. Cardiac valve calcification: characteristics of patients with calcification of the mitral annulus or aortic valve. Heart 1997;78:472–474.

196. Solajic-Bozicevic N, Stavljenic A, Sesto, M. Lecithin: cholesterol acyltransferase activity in patients with acute myocardial infarction and coronary heart disease. Artery 1991;18:326–340.
197. Lau BW, Klevay LM. Plasma lecithin: cholesterol acyltransferase in copper-deficient rats. 1981;111:1698–1703.
198. Henderson HE, Kastelein JJ, Zwinderman AH, Gagne E, Jukema JW, Reymer PW, Groenemeyer BE, Lie KI, Bruschke AV, Hayden MR, Jansen H. Lipoprotein lipase activity is decreased in a large cohort of patients with coronary artery disease and is associated with changes in lipids and lipoproteins. J Lipid Res 1999;40:735–743.
199. Lau BW, Klevay LM. Postheparin plasma lipoprotein lipase in copper-deficient rats. J Nutr 1982;112:928-933.
200. Bruckert E, Giral P, Chadarevian R, Turpin G. Low free-thyroxine levels are a risk factor for subclinical atheroslerosis in euthyroid hyperlipidemic patients. J Cardiovasc Risk 1999;6:327–331.
201. Tamura T, Hong KH, Mizuno Y, Johnston KE, Keen CL. Folate and homocysteine metabolism in copper-deficient rats. Biochim Biophys Acta. 1999;1427:351–356.
202. Brown JC, Strain JJ. Effect of dietary homocysteine on copper status in rats. J Nutr 1990;120:1068–1074.
203. Wang XL, Adachi T, Sim AS, Wilcken DE. Plasma extracellular superoxide dismutase levels in an Australian population with coronary artery disease. Arterioslcer Thromv Vasc Biol 1998;18:1915–1921.
203. Mao SM, Medeiros DM, Hamlin, RL. Marginal copper and high fat diet produce alterations in electrocardiograms and cardiac ultrastructure in male rats. Nutrition 1999;15:890–898.
205. McFadden SL, Ding D, Buckard RF, Jiang H, Reaume AG, Flood DG, Salvi RJ. Cu/Zn SOD deficiency potentiates hearing loss and cochlear pathology in aged 129, CD-1 mice. J Comp Neurol 1999;413:101–112.
206. Lamb DJ, Reeves GL, Taylor A, Ferns GA. Dietary copper supplementation reduces atherosclerosis in the cholesterol-fed rabbit. Atherosclerosis. 1999;146:33–43.

16 Trace Element and Mineral Nutrition in Renal Disease

Saulo Klahr, MD

1. INTRODUCTION

The hallmark of chronic renal disease is a decrease in glomerular filtration rate (GFR). The progressive loss of nephrons affects most of the functions of the kidney (Table 1). As GFR decreases, solutes that are excreted by the kidney preferentially by filtration (urea, creatinine) accumulate in body fluids and concentrations in plasma increase *(1)*. Indeed, the plasma concentrations of urea and creatinine provide a crude measurement of the decrease in GFR. As GFR falls to values < 25% of normal ((30 mL/min), other solutes that are filtered and either reabsorbed or secreted by the renal tubules may accumulate in body fluids *(1,2)*. These solutes include phosphate, sulfate, uric acid, magnesium, and hydrogen, the latter resulting in the development of metabolic acidosis. Finally, other compounds are retained in body fluids when renal disease is far advanced:phenols, guanidines, organic acids, indoles, a number of metabolic products, and certain peptides. Some of these compounds may be toxic above specific concentrations and could contribute to the symptoms and signs of advanced chronic renal insufficiency (uremia).

2. TRACE ELEMENTS

Changes in the plasma or serum concentration of trace elements in patients with renal insufficiency depends on many factors. However, the degree of renal insufficiency is an important determinant of the plasma or serum concentrations of trace elements. In patients on renal replacement therapy (dialysis, transplantation) changes in trace elements may differ depending on the modality of treatment. Changes in concentrations of trace elements in tissues may differ markedly from those found in plasma or serum. Tissue accumulation or depletion of certain trace elements have been described in patients with renal insufficiency. Such patients have a greater risk of developing toxicity or deficiency of trace elements due to decreased excretion in the urine, contamination of the dialysate by trace elements or loss of trace elements during dialysis. Patients with advanced renal failure subjected to protein restriction are at risk of developing iron or zinc depletion.

From: *Clinical Nutrition of the Essential Trace Elements and Minerals: The Guide for Health Professionals*
Edited by: J. D. Bogden and L. M. Klevay © Humana Press Inc., Totowa, NJ

Table 1
Principal functions of the Kidney

Excretion of metabolic waste products (i.e., urea, creatinine, uric acid)
Maintenance of volume and ionic composition of body fluids
Elimination and detoxification of drugs and toxins
Regulation of systemic blood pressure
Production of erythropoietin
Control of mineral metabolism via endocrine synthesis
    (1,25- dihydroxycholecalciferol and 24,25-dihydroxycholecalciferol)
Degradation and catabolism of peptide hormones (e.g., insulin, glucagon
    parathyroid hormone) and small-molecular-weight proteins β_2
    microglobulin and light chains)
Regulation of metabolism (gluconeogenesis, lipid metabolism)

2.1. Iron

Anemia is a frequent consequence of progressive renal disease *(3)*. The major factor underlying the development of anemia in patients with renal failure is a decrease in the levels of erythropoietin *(4)*. Retention of "uremic toxins" may also shorten the half-life of red blood cells and diminish the response of the bone marrow to erythropoietin. Other aggravating factors that contribute to the anemia of chronic renal failure are bleeding, iron or other nutritional deficiencies, bone marrow fibrosis secondary to hyperparathy-roidism, and aluminum excess *(5,6)*. In the past blood transfusions were used to maintain the hematocrit of patients with end-stage renal disease (ESRD) at levels greater than 20–25%. More recently the administration of recombinant erythropoietin has decreased markedly the need for blood transfusions in patients with ESRD. The use of erythropoietin requires the assessment of iron stores because iron depletion will impair the response to erythropoietin. Three main factors affect iron balance and metabolism:intake of iron, iron stores, and iron losses. Erythropoietin administration can cause iron deficiency. Patients treated by hemodialysis or continuous ambulatory peritoneal dialysis (CAPD) are usually given iron supplements, because of the high incidence of iron deficiency in these patients. There is some controversy about the best route of iron administration in these patients. Oral iron supplements are more commonly used than intravenous iron. The latter method of iron admin-istration may result in iron overload. Iron overload (serum ferritin greater than 300 ng/mL) can occur in patients receiving multiple blood transfusions. The clinical complications of iron overload have been well described in children *(7)*. Increased iron stores and a high intake of iron are associated with a greater incidence of myocardial infarction even in the absence of kidney disease *(8,9)*. Some patients with the nephrotic syndrome were reported to have iron deficiency anemia. Presumably, increased losses of iron and transferrin in the urine may account for the iron deficiency. The treatment of the anemia of chronic renal insufficiency has included appropriate iron supplementation to maintain a serum ferritin level greater than 100 ng/mL, oral folate supplements, and avoidance of red cell injury or loss during dialysis.

2.1.1. CLINICAL RECOMMENDATIONS

Patients with chronic renal failure or those patients on dialysis with a hematocrit below 30% should be offered recombinant erythropoietin treatment. Prior to initiating treatment attention should be focused on iron status. Patients should be given iron as necessary at the start of treatment with erythropoietin. Erythropoietin can be given intravenously or subcutaneously.

2.2. Copper

This element is particularly suited for releasing and accepting electrons. A series of oxidation-reduction reactions involving O_2 are catalyzed by copper-containing enzymes. Kidney has the highest copper concentrations in the body, followed by liver and brain. At least three copper enzymes appear to have a role as antioxidants:cytosolic superoxide dismutase, ceruloplasmin, and intracellular copper thioneins. Abnormal copper metabolism has been reported in patients with renal disease (10). Increased levels of copper have been found in patients with chronic renal failure (11), and in patients on hemodialysis (12,13). The levels of ceruloplasmin are not different in patients with renal insufficiency when compared to normal subjects. Free (unbound) copper is likely minimal due to strong protein binding. The clinical consequences of increased free copper concentrations in patients with renal failure are unknown. In patients on hemodialysis high copper levels have been reported. By contrast, patients on continuous ambulatory peritoneal dialysis (CAPD) have concentrations of copper that are within normal limits, and lower than those seen in hemodialysis patients (11). Patients with the nephrotic syndrome have a greater excretion of copper in the urine and decreased levels of copper in plasma. This may be due to losses of ceruloplasmin in the urine.

Copper sulfate poisoning can result in acute renal failure (14). Dialysis patients developed acute copper poisoning owing to the presence of this trace element in the tubing used in the heating coil (15). Increases in the levels of copper may cause fever, the Fanconi syndrome (multiple renal tubular transport defects), and myocardial infarction. Decreases in the levels of the copper may result in pancytopenia, reduced activity of superoxide dismutase, and/or ischemic heart disease (see Chapter 15). It should be noted that patients with renal insufficiency in general have an increase of copper levels rather than a deficiency of this trace element, unless the patients are severely ill or receiving prolonged parenteral nutrition.

The prototype of chronic copper excess in humans is Wilson's disease (see Chapter 12). Many patients with Wilson's disease exhibit renal involvement characterized by functional alterations in the proximal tubule, a fall in GFR and renal blood flow, and in certain instances a distal acidification defect.

2.3. Zinc

This essential trace element is present in numerous metalloenzymes. Decreased plasma levels of zinc have been reported in patients with renal insufficiency and in patients with end-stage renal disease undergoing hemodialysis or CAPD (12,13,16–18). However, other authors have reported normal or elevated levels of zinc in uremic patients (19,20). Low concentrations of zinc in plasma or serum have also been reported in patients with the nephrotic syndrome. Increased urinary excretion of zinc may account for the lower concentrations of zinc in plasma or serum. It is likely that the lower levels of zinc in plasma are because of decreases in zinc binding proteins such as albumin. Decreased levels of zinc in the plasma may lead to hypogonadism, sexual dysfunction, impaired scar formation, decreased taste and smell acuities, anorexia, and a deficiency in superoxide dismutase. Some of these symptoms may improve with the administration of zinc supplements. However, there is controversy since some investigators did not observe an improvement in sexual function after the administration of zinc supplements. Some authors have reported an improvement in nerve conduction velocity and cell-mediated immunity after the administration of zinc supplements. Since most the zinc in plasma is bound to albumin, the levels of plasma albumin should be determined before making a judgment of whether or not the levels of zinc are deficient in a given individual.

2.4. Selenium

Selenium in tissues is present in two forms:selenomethionine and selenocysteine, the latter in selenoproteins such as gluthatione peroxidase, iodothyronine deiodinase, and selenoprotein P. The consequences of selenium deficiency include susceptibility to certain types of oxidative injury, including the kidney, alterations in thyroid hormone metabolism, increased propensity to injury by mercury, alteration in the activity of biotransformation enzymes, and an increased concentration of glutathione in plasma. Selenium concentration can be determined with accuracy by several methods — (fluorometry, atomic absorption, and activation analysis). Biologically "active" selenium can be estimated by measuring glutathione peroxidase activity and selenoprotein P concentration.

The concentration of selenium in serum is decreased in patients with chronic renal failure and in patients on hemodialysis *(21,22)* or CAPD. The latter patients, tend to have the lowest concentrations of selenium *(23)*. Anorexia and restricted protein intake may contribute to the low levels of selenium in patients with chronic renal failure. In patients undergoing hemodialysis, the decrease of selenium in serum may be due to loss of this trace element during the procedure. Selenium deficiency may predispose to the development of cancer *(24)*, cardiomyopathy, anemia, skeletal muscle myopathy, immune dysfunction, cardiovascular disease, renal injury, glutathione peroxidase deficiency, and peroxidative damage to cells *(25)*. Whether or not patients with chronic renal disease require selenium supplementation remains controversial. No specific abnormalities have been ascribed to selenium deficiency in patients with chronic renal failure. The postulated association of selenium deficiency and tumor and heart disease has prompted the use of selenium supplementation in a few medical centers. However, this practice remains a controversial issue.

2.5. Aluminum

The plasma levels of aluminum are often increased in patients with chronic renal failure and in those on dialysis. The use of electrothermal atomic absorption spectrometry provides an accurate and reproducible method for the measurement of aluminum in plasma and tissues. Aluminum levels in the serum of normal individuals are generally below 10 μg/L. Levels of 20–40 μg/L of aluminum are found in patients on dialysis *(26,27)*. Values in excess of 50 μg/L suggest aluminum overload. Aluminum levels in plasma reflect either the presence of this trace element in the dialysate, or the oral administration of medications containing aluminum in an effort to bind phosphorus and prevent hyperphosphatemia. Plasma aluminum levels should be monitored at regular intervals in dialysis patients and in patients with advanced renal insufficiency ingesting preparations containing aluminum.

Deposition of aluminum in tissues particularly liver and bone occurs in patients ingesting aluminum preparations. It has been suggested that this accumulation of aluminum in tissues of patients with ESRD is due to decreased excretion in the urine and increased absorption of this trace element in the gastrointestinal tract. Aluminum accumulation may also result in encephalopathy, other neurologic syndromes, bone disease (mainly osteomalacia), myopathy, and anemia *(28,29,30)*.

Deferoxamine is a metal-chelating agent that binds aluminum. An intravenous infusion of deferoxamine can increase the plasma levels of aluminum markedly in patients with renal insufficiency and aluminum-related bone disease. Deferoxamine has been used to treat patients with aluminum intoxication *(31)*. A diagnostic test has also been developed to assess the degree of aluminum retention in patients with chronic renal failure. This test is performed as follows:patients are given a standardized intravenous dose of deferoxamine, 40 mg/kg in 100 mL of 5% dextrose solution, during a two hour interval immediately after a hemodialysis procedure. Plasma aluminum levels are measured before and 24 and 48 h after the infusion of deferoxamine. An increase in plasma aluminum greater than 300 µg/L above baseline values is a good indicator of high levels of aluminum in the skeleton *(32)*.

2.6. Other Trace Elements

2.6.1. CHROMIUM

Chromium is a transition element that can occur in a number of valence states *(33)*. Chromium potentiates the actions of insulin. Chromium levels in plasma are normal or elevated in patients with chronic renal failure. The levels of chromium are clearly elevated in plasma of patients undergoing hemodialysis or continuous ambulatory peritoneal dialysis.

2.6.2. FLUORIDE

This trace element is ubiquitous, occurring in minute amounts in all foodstuffs and water supplies. Renal excretion is the predominant route for removal of inorganic fluoride from the body *(34)*. Thus, accumulation of fluoride may occur in patients with renal insufficiency. There is no evidence that fluoride ingestion at currently recommended concentrations produces renal toxicity.

2.6.3. IODINE

This element is an essential component of the thyroid hormones. Large amounts are stored in the thyroid gland as hormone or hormone precursors. Iodine is excreted by the kidney. The disorders arising from iodine deficiency include:goiter, impaired fertility, increased embryonal and post-natal mortality, deaf-mutism, cognitive and neuromuscular impairment, and cretinism *(35)*. No specific pathophysiology due to iodine is seen in patients with renal insufficiency or those undergoing dialysis.

2.6.4. MANGANESE

An average human adult has between 200 and 400 µmol of manganese. Bone, liver, pancreas, and kidney tend to have high concentrations of manganese (20–50 nmol/gm). Manganese tends to be highest in tissues rich in mitochondria *(36)*. In chronic renal disease there is a decrease of manganese in the kidney and an increase in the liver. The plasma levels of manganese are not elevated in patients undergoing hemodialysis or peritoneal dialysis.

2.6.5. MOLYBDENUM

This trace element functions as an enzyme cofactor *(37)*. It is involved in the activation of several enzymes of the uric-acid pathway. Molybdenum deficiency causes disorders in the synthesis of uric acid. In patients with chronic renal disease molybdenum levels in kidney are decreased and hepatic concentrations of molybdenum are increased. Similar findings are found in patients on hemodialysis.

3. MINERALS

3.1 Phosphorus

Serum phosphorus concentrations range from 2.8 to 4.5 mg/dL in adults *(38)*. Approximately 80% to 85% of the phosphorus in the body is present in the skeleton. The rest is widely distributed throughout the body in the form of organic phosphate compounds. In the extracellular fluid, most of the phosphorus is present in the inorganic form. On an average diet 1 gm of phosphorus is ingested daily, of which approximately 70% is absorbed and the remainder is excreted in the stool *(39)*.

Phosphorus absorption occurs mainly in the small intestine. Most of the inorganic phosphorus in serum (85%) is ultrafilterable at the level of the glomerulus *(39)*. Approximately 7 gm of phosphorus is filtered daily by the kidney, of which 80% to 90% is reabsorbed by the renal tubules and the reminder excreted in the urine (about 700 mg on a 1 gm phosphorus diet). About 60% to 70% of the filtered phosphorus is reabsorbed in the proximal tubule. However, there is also evidence that a significant amount is reabsorbed in the distal tubule *(39)*

3.1.1. RENAL REGULATION OF PHOSPHORUS

The reabsorption of phosphorus along the nephron is regulated by several factors, of which parathyroid hormone (PTH) is the most important. However, other factors, such as growth hormone, calcitonin, glucocorticoids, vitamin D metabolites, the degree of extracellular fluid (ECF) volume expansion, the filtered load of phosphate, and the acid-base balance, also play a role in the regulation of phosphorus excretion *(40)*.

Parathyroid hormone has a phosphaturic effect. This hormone blocks the reabsorption of phosphorus in both the proximal and the distal tubule. The phosphaturic effect of PTH is mediated by the adenylcyclase system and production of cyclic Adenosine 3'5' Monophosphate (AMP). In the absence of PTH the maximal tubular reabsorptive capacity for phosphorus (TM_{PO4}) is increased. Thus patients with decreased or absent PTH characteristically have hyperphosphatemia. Extracellular fluid volume expansion is accompanied by a significant degree of phosphaturia, which may occur in the absence of PTH.

Vitamin D and its metabolites increase phosphorus reabsorption by the renal tubules. Thyrocalcitonin and growth hormone have opposite effects, the former being phosphaturic, while the latter increases phosphorus reabsorption.

There is a diurnal variation in phosphorus excretion. Most of the studies indicate that excretion is minimal early in the morning until noon, gradually increasing in the afternoon, and reaching maximum values by evening. Although many factors regulate phosphorus balance by the kidney in normal individuals, the amount of phosphorus in the diet plays a key role in the amount that ultimately will be excreted.

3.1.2. PHOSPHOROUS EXCRETION IN RENAL DISEASE

Plasma levels of inorganic phosphorus change little as GFR falls, because there is a progressive decrease in tubular reabsorption of phosphorus, mediated by increased plasma concentrations of parathyroid hormone *(38)*. However, when GFR falls below 30 mL/minute, even a marked decrease in tubular reabsorption of phosphorous is not enough to overcome the substantial decrease in the filtered load, and phosphate accumulates.

Hyperphosphatemia, therefore, is seen commonly in patients with GFRs of ≤25 mL/ minute unless dietary phosphorous intake is restricted *(38)*.

A reduction in phosphorus intake in patients with mild renal insufficiency reduces the levels of parathyroid hormone and improves the skeletal response to the hormone *(41)*. Phosphorus absorption from the gastrointestinal tract can be decreased by the use of phosphate binders. Until the past decade aluminum salts (hydroxide, carbonate) were used as phosphate binders. However, aluminum is absorbed and may accumulate in plasma and tissues *(29,30)*. Because aluminum accumulation may be toxic *(27)*, other phosphorus-binding agents, such as calcium carbonate, were introduced *(42)*. When prescribed as a phosphate binder, calcium carbonate should be administered with meals. Dietary phosphorus can be decreased to 600–900 mg/d by reducing protein intake, particularly by avoiding meats and dairy products, which are major sources of dietary phosphorus.

3.2. Magnesium

Magnesium is the fourth most abundant cation of the body and, after potassium, the second most abundant intracellular cation *(43)*. Total body magnesium in adult humans weighing about 70 kg is approximately 900 mmol, with the skeleton containing about 60% of the total magnesium, the remainder being almost equally distributed between muscle and nonmuscular tissue. Liver and muscle have high concentrations of magnesium, around 15–20 mmol/kg. Red cell magnesium is 5 mmol/liter, and the normal concentration in serum ranges from 1.6 to 2.1 mEq/liter.

Magnesium plays an essential role as a cofactor for a variety of enzymes, most of them utilizing Adenosine Triphosphate (ATP). About 300 mg of magnesium are ingested daily in a normal diet. Most of the magnesium in the diet is provided by the ingestion of green vegetables *(44)*. Roughly one third of the ingested magnesium is excreted in the urine and the rest in the feces. A minimum magnesium intake of 0.3 mEq/kg body weight is apparently necessary to maintain magnesium balance in the average person.

Animals fed low-magnesium diets can excrete urine that is practically free of magnesium. However, the gastrointestinal tract continues to secrete small amounts of magnesium, and the animals develop magnesium depletion. Most of the magnesium is absorbed in the upper gastrointestinal tract *(45,46)*. Magnesium shares with calcium similar pathways for absorption in the intestine, but whereas calcium is actively absorbed from the gastrointestinal tract, magnesium is absorbed mainly by ionic diffusion and solvent "drag" resulting from the bulk flow of water *(47–49)*. There is no good evidence to indicate that magnesium is actively transported. Small amounts of magnesium, about 15–25mg/24 h, are secreted by the gastrointestinal tract. The factors controlling the absorption of magnesium from the gastrointestinal tract are not well understood. Both vitamin D and parathyroid hormone enhance magnesium absorption *(50)*. Sodium has a similar effect. On the other hand, both calcium and phosphorus intake seem to decrease the absorption of magnesium from the intestine.

3.2.1. RENAL EXCRETION OF MAGNESIUM

Approximately 80% of the magnesium present in serum is ultrafilterable; the rest is protein-bound. Most of the ultrafilterable magnesium is present in the ionized form. Approximately 2 gm of magnesium are filtered daily by the kidney, and roughly 100 mg appear in the urine. Thus, approximately 95% of the filtered load of magnesium is reabsorbed, and 5% is excreted in the urine *(51)*. There are some similarities between calcium and magnesium transport and the administration of one of these two elements decreases the reabsorption of the other.

3.2.2. MAGNESIUM IN RENAL DISEASE

The most common cause of hypermagnesemia is renal insufficiency (Table 2). The kidney can excrete large magnesium loads; thus, even when magnesium influx is increased several times (by dietary means or in the form of laxatives or enemas), hypermagnesemia is seldom seen, unless a concomitant decrease in renal function is present. Mild hypermagnesemia, is well tolerated; however, if serum magnesium levels exceed 5–6 mg/dL, there is a decrease in tendon reflexes, and some degree of mental obtundation. If the degree of hypermagnesemia increases, arrhythmias and a fall in respiratory rate and blood pressure are frequently observed (52,53). If serum magnesium levels increase above 10 mg/dL, there is usually profound hypotension and severe mental depression. When magnesium levels increase further, to about 15 mg/dL, coma and death may occur.

In the past, large amounts of magnesium were used for the treatment of eclampsia, and some of these patients became comatose after correction of the hypertensive crisis (54). However, in those days, blood magnesium was measured in only a very few instances. In retrospect, knowing the large amounts of magnesium that these patients received, it is likely that some of the neurological symptoms observed in the women were due to marked hypermagnesemia. Severe hypermagnesemia may occur after the use of laxatives and enemas containing magnesium.

Hypermagnesemia is a manifestation of advanced renal insufficiency. Seldom does hypermagnesemia occur in patients with a GFR greater than 15 mL/min. Mild hypermagnesemia is seen in patients with GFR around 10 mL/min. However, more marked hypermagnesemia is seen usually in patients with GFR values of less than 5 mL/min.

There is a remarkable adaptive change in the excretion of magnesium per nephron in patients with renal failure. As mentioned above, hypermagnesemia is not seen until the GFR is 15 mL/min or less. This, in part, is due to an increased fractional excretion of magnesium which can reach 30% to 60% of the filtered load in patients with profound renal insufficiency as compared to 5% in individuals with GFR values of 120 mL/min. There is some evidence to indicate that the increased natriuresis per nephron occurring with chronic progressive renal disease may in part be responsible for this adaptation in magnesium excretion. The increased excretion of magnesium per nephron observed in patients with far-advance renal disease does not appear to be related to secondary hyperparathyroidism, since PTH administration has little effect on renal magnesium excretion.

3.3. Calcium

Calcium is the most abundant cation in the body and the principal mineral of the human skeleton. It has a key role in the composition of skeletal tissue and is also involved in a series of regulatory processes that are vital for life. Among the principal functions in which calcium participates are the maintenance and function of cell membranes, neuromuscular excitability, transmission of nerve impulses, enzymatic reactions, regulation of secretion of parathyroid hormone, and activation of 25-hydroxycholecalciferol-1-hydroxylase, the enzyme responsible for the conversion of $25(OH)D_3$ to $1,25(OH)_2D_3$ (55). The major regulator of extracellular calcium balance is parathyroid hormone. This hormone exerts effects on the skeleton, kidney, and small intestine and interrelates with other factors such as vitamin D to maintain the extracellular calcium concentration within narrow boundaries (see Chapter 13).

Table 2
Causes of Hypermagnesemia

I.	Decreased renal excretion	
	A.	Acute renal failure
	B.	Chronic renal disease
	C.	Adrenocortical insufficiency
II.	Administration of Magnesium	
	A.	Laxatives containing magnesium
	B.	Enemas containing magnesium
	C.	Intravenous fluids containing magnesium
	D.	Intramuscular administration of magnesium (eclampsia)

The skeleton is an important reservoir of calcium and is in dynamic equilibrium with physicochemically soluble forms of circulating calcium. Thus, alterations in calcium metabolism necessarily lead to derangements in the composition of the skeleton.

3.3.1. DISTRIBUTION OF CALCIUM

Adult humans have about 1000–1200 gm of calcium or approximately 20–25 gm/kg of fat-free body tissue. About 99% of the body calcium is in the skeleton, the remaining 1% is found in blood, extracellular fluid, and intracellular space (56). In addition, about 1% of the skeletal calcium is freely exchangeable with the extracellular fluid.

In humans, total serum calcium concentration is remarkably constant, ranging from 9 to 10.5 mg/100 mL or 4.5 to 5 mEq/liter, or 2.25 to 2.5mM/liter. Total serum calcium concentration consists of two major fractions. The first is the ultrafilterable, or diffusible, fraction, which comprises approximately 60% of the total serum calcium. This fraction is composed in turn of: 1) the ionized calcium, which plays a key role in all of the feedback and enzymatic process and represents roughly 50% of the total serum calcium; and 2) calcium complexed with citrate, phosphate, and bicarbonate which represents approximately 10% of the total serum calcium concentration. The other fraction is protein-bound calcium, which constitutes approximately 40% of the total serum calcium concentration. An easy way to remember the concentration of the different fractions of calcium in blood is as follows: ionized calcium, 5 mg/100 mL; complexed calcium, 1 mg/100 mL; and protein-bound calcium, 4 mg/100 mL. Calcium is bound to serum proteins, and 80% to 90% of this calcium is bound to albumin (57).

3.3.2. DIETARY CALCIUM

The amount of calcium ingested in the diet plays a key regulatory effect in its overall balance. Roughly, 1000 mg of calcium per day is ingested in a regular diet (58). However, this amount varies greatly from patient to patient because of the varying amounts of dairy foods that different people ingest in their diet. Milk is the most important source of calcium and contributes 50% to 60% of the total amount ingested in the diet (see Table 6 in Chapter 4). In the United States, 1 liter of milk contains approximately 800–900 mg of calcium. There are some nondairy foods that have a very high calcium content, such as parsley, spinach, and mustard; however, their contribution to the total dietary calcium is small and the calcium in them is less well absorbed than that in dairy food (59). About

10 mg of calcium per kilogram body weight is the recommended daily intake. However, during the last trimester of pregnancy, there is a greater calcium requirement, since approximately 20–30 gm of calcium enters the fetus. With age, alteration in calcium metabolism, mainly due to a progressive decline in calcium absorption, requires an increase in the amount of calcium in the diet (*see* Chapter 11).

If 1 gm of calcium is ingested in the diet, approximately 30% is absorbed from the intestine. At the same time, endogenous calcium, approximately 200 mg daily, is secreted into the bowel. Thus, of the 1000 mg ingested, approximately 900 mg is excreted in the stool and the remaining 100 mg in the urine.

Many studies in animals and humans clearly indicate that vitamin D and its metabolites play a key role in regulating calcium absorption *(60)*. If a patient is maintained on a low-calcium diet, a mild decrease in ionized calcium will trigger the release of parathyroid hormone, which enhances the conversion of $25(OH)D_3$ to $1,25(OH)_2D_3$. This metabolite increases calcium absorption from the gastrointestinal tract to reestablish calcium balance. However, if there is an excess of calcium in the diet the secretion of parathyroid hormone is turned off, the circulating levels of PTH in blood decrease, and the conversion of $25(OH)D_3$ to $1,25(OH)_2D_3$ is greatly diminished. Thus the absorption of calcium decreases and the amount of calcium in the stool increases.

3.3.3. RENAL HANDLING OF CALCIUM

Only 60% of the calcium is ultrafilterable, and this fraction will cross the glomeruli and enter the proximal tubule. Approximately 10 gm of calcium is filtered per day, but usually only 100 mg appears in the urine. Therefore, 99% of the filtered load of calcium is reabsorbed by the kidney. The reabsorption of calcium along the nephron parallels the reabsorption of sodium well *(61)*.

Several factors regulate calcium reabsorption in the kidney. However, the final regulatory control mechanism is located in the distal portion of the nephron *(62,63)*. Micropuncture experiments in animals have demonstrated that in the proximal tubule the ratio of tubular fluid calcium to ultrafilterable serum calcium is usually greater than 1. Net calcium reabsorption in the loop of Henle also parallels sodium reabsorption, and a concentration gradient for calcium has been shown from cortex to papilla. Determinations of calcium concentrations in the distal convoluted tubule suggest that further reabsorption of calcium, against a steep concentration gradient, occurs in this segment.

Many factors that modify sodium transport clearly affect calcium reabsorption. ECF volume expansion, a potent stimulus in decreasing sodium transport along the whole length of the nephron, also decreases the reabsorption of calcium. In fact, ECF volume expansion is one of the most effective and therapeutic maneuvers in the treatment of hypercalcemia.

Similarly, many diuretics such as acetazolamide, ethacrynic acid, and furosemide also block sodium and calcium transport *(64)*. However, other types of diuretics, such as thiazides, have a dissimilar effect on sodium and calcium excretion. Thiazides produce a large natriuresis and a decrease in urinary calcium excretion. It is possible that this dissociation in sodium and calcium excretion results from the fact that thiazides exert their action in the distal nephron where sodium and calcium transport are independent.

A series of hormones also play a critical role in the regulation of calcium excretion by the kidney. Among these hormones, parathyroid hormone is the most important one. Its effect seems to be different in the proximal as compared to the distal tubule. It has been shown that sodium and calcium reabsorption are greatly diminished in the proximal tubule by the administration of PTH *(65)*. However, there is a remarkable enhancement in calcium reabsorption in the distal tubule when PTH is given to experimental animals. It is known that patients with hypoparathyroidism, in whom there is a lack of PTH, have a greater amount of calcium in the urine at similar levels of filtered calcium load when compared to normal or hyperparathyroid patients. Thus, the main action of PTH is to enhance calcium reabsorption in the distal segment of the nephron *(66)*. Other hormones, such as thyrocalcitonin, growth hormone, thyroid hormone, mineralocorticoids, and glucocorticoids, seem to increase urinary calcium excretion.

Metabolic acidosis decreases renal calcium reabsorption. Several mechanisms have been implicated, including an increase in ionized serum calcium levels with suppression of parathyroid hormone release. However, experiments in parathyroidectomized animals have clearly demonstrated that acidosis *per se* blocks the reabsorption of calcium independently of the levels of parathyroid hormone.

3.3.4. CAUSES OF HYPERCALCEMIA

The causes of hypercalcemia are shown in Table 3. *(67)*.

3.3.4.1. Chronic Renal Failure. Hypercalcemia is a rare finding in patients with chronic renal failure. In fact, the majority of patients with renal disease have hypocalcemia, which accounts in part for the development of secondary hyperparathyroidism. Nevertheless, a few patients with chronic renal failure and hypercalcemia have been described.

3.3.4.2. Renal Transplantation. More common is the finding of hypercalcemia after a successful renal transplant. The patients who receive transplants usually have severe secondary hyperparathyroidism. When the transplanted graft is successful the amount of $1,25(OH)_2D_3$ produced by the new kidney may be greatly increased as a result of the excess parathyroid hormone. A synergistic effect of $1,25(OH)_2D_3$ and parathyroid hormone will increase the mobilization of calcium from bone leading to hypercalcemia. Obviously $1,25(OH)_2D_3$ also increases calcium absorption from the gastrointestinal tract. Fortunately this is a rather limited condition that does not require a specific treatment and in most of the cases subsides after 2 or 3 wk. However, in some patients, specific measures should be taken in order to prevent nephrocalcinosis. Extracellular fluid volume expansion and diuretics may easily control the mild hypercalcemia. In some patients, the hypercalcemia may be more pronounced and persists for several months and sometimes several years. Occasionally some of these patients require a subtotal parathyroidectomy.

3.3.4.3. Diuretic Phase of Acute Tubular Necrosis. Hypercalcemia also has been reported during the diuretic phase of acute tubular necrosis. This is a rather rare occurrence and most of the cases in which hypercalcemia has been reported have been patients who had rhabdomyolysis with severe hyperphosphatemia and hypocalcemia during the oliguric phase. It seems that there is sequestration of large amounts of calcium in soft tissue during the oliguric phase. During the diuretic phase, part of the calcium is now mobilized and enters the extracellular space, and the patient becomes hypercalcemic. Hypercalcemia may also result from alterations in the metabolism of $1,25(OH)_2D_3$ during acute renal failure. Again, this hypercalcemia is a rather limited condition that, in most instances, does not require any specific treatment.

3.3.4.4. Immobilization. Immobilization is a frequent and sometimes serious condition that can produce hypercalcemia and severe renal impairment. It has been shown

Table 3
Causes of Hypercalcemia

Malignancy
Hyperparathyroidism
Immobilization
Intoxication with Vitamin D or A
Use of thiazide diuretics or lithium
Carbonate
Sarcoidosis
Thyrotoxicosis
Renal Failure

that practically all patients who are immobilized for several days develop some degree of hypercalciuria. However, only some patients develop hypercalcemia. If the patient has an underlying pathological process in which there is an increase in bone turnover, like Paget's disease, severe immobilization could be catastrophic.

3.3.4.5. Diuretics. Patients taking thiazide diuretics may develop hypercalcemia. The mechanism by which thiazide administration results in hypercalcemia is not fully understood, but it has become apparent that a series of factors are involved. Thiazides decrease urinary calcium excretion, and have been used to treat one of the forms of idiopathic hypercalciuria. As mentioned before, for thiazides to reduce urinary calcium excretion, some degree of volume contraction is required as well as the presence of parathyroid hormone. It seems that a synergistic effect of PTH and thiazides occurs not only at the level of the kidney but also at the level of bone, and there is evidence suggesting that when a thiazide is administered together with parathyroid hormone, there is a greater degree of hypercalcemia. There is controversy as to whether or not thiazides *per se* increase the release of parathyroid hormone. However, most of the evidence indicates that this is not the case.

3.4. Causes of Hypocalcemia

Table 4 lists the most common causes of hypocalcemia *(68)*. In addition to clinical syndromes characterized by either a deficiency of parathyroid hormone or an end-organ resistance to parathyroid hormone, hypocalcemia is also observed in uremia, malabsorption, acute pancreatitis, and hypoalbuminemic conditions such as nephrotic syndrome and cirrhosis. The symptoms related to hypocalcemia in patients with low albumin, such as cirrhosis and nephrotic syndrome, are rather mild, since the ionized calcium usually remains within the normal range. However, in those conditions in which ionized calcium is greatly diminished, a series of symptoms may frequently be seen that are attributable to hypocalcemia.

Hypocalcemia with marked irritability and convulsions has been observed in the neonate. Neuromuscular irritability and tetany accompanying hyperventilation have been ascribed to respiratory alkalosis, which causes a remarkable decrease in ionized calcium. It is important to emphasize that laryngeal stridor, tetany, muscle cramps, and twitching could be fatal if they are not treated adequately. The electrocardiogram may show a prolongation of the S-T interval.

4. SUMMARY

In summary, changes in the concentrations of trace elements in plasma and tissues may occur in patients with chronic renal insufficiency and in patients with end-stage renal disease

Table 4
Causes of Hypocalcemia

I.	Renal failure	
II.	Endocrine disorders	
	A.	Hypoparathyroidism
	B.	Pseudohypoparathyroidism
III.	Nutritional and metabolic disorders	
	A.	Vitamin D deficiency
	B.	Magnesium deficiency
	C.	Intestinal calcium malabsorption
	D.	Hyperphosphatemia
IV.	Miscellaneous	
	A.	Hypoproteinemia
	B.	Acute pancreatitis
	C.	Drugs

requiring dialysis. Such patients have a greater risk of developing excess or deficiency of trace elements due to decreased excretion by the kidney, contamination of the dialysate by trace elements, or loss of trace elements during dialysis. Dietary restrictions and/or development of anorexia in such patients may also contribute to the development of abnormal levels of trace elements in plasma and tissues.

ACKNOWLEDGMENT

The invaluable assistance of Ms. Rosalie A. Dustmann in the writing of this manuscript is gratefully acknowledged.

REFERENCES

1. Bricker NS, Klahr S, Lubowitz H, Slatopolsky E. The pathophysiology of renal insufficiency: on the functional transformation in the residual nephrons with advancing disease. Symposium on Pediatric Nephrology. Pediatr Clin North Am 1971;18:595–611.
2. Suki WM, Eknoyan G. Pathophysiology and clinical manifestations of chronic renal failure and the uremic syndrome. In Jacobson H. Striker G, Klahr S, eds. The Principles and Practice of Nephrology, 2nd ed. Mosby, St. Louis, 1995,pp. 603–614.
3. Eschbach JW. The anemia of chronic renal failure: pathophysiology and the effects of recombinant erythropoietin. Kidney Int 1989;35:134–148.
4. Eschbach JW, Egrie JC, Downing MR, et al. Correction of the anemia of end-stage renal disease with recombinant human erythropoietin: results of a combined phase I and II clinical trial. N Engl J Med 1987;316:73–78.
5. Donnelly SM, Smith EKM. The role of aluminum in the functional iron deficiency of patients treated with erythropoietin: case report of clinical characteristics and response to treatment. Am J Kidney Dis 1990;16:487–490.
6. Donnelly SM, Ali MAM, Churchill DN. Bioavailability of iron in hemodialysis patients treated with erythropoietin: Evidence for the inhibitory role of aluminum. Am J Kidney Dis 1990;16:447–451.
7. Yip R, Dallman PR. Iron. In: Ziegler EE, Filer LJ, Jr. eds. "Present Knowledge in Nutrition" ILSI Press, Washington 1996, pp. 277–292.

8. Salonen JT, Nyyssonen K,Korpela H, Tuomilehto J, et al. High stored iron levels are associated with excess risk of myocardial infarction in eastern Finnish men. Circulation 1992;86:803–811.
9. Ascherio A, Willett WC, Rimm EB, et al. Dietary iron intake and risk of coronary disease among men. Circulation 1994;89:909–974.
10. Linder MC. Copper. In: Ziegler EE, Filer LJ, Jr. eds. Present Knowledge in Nutrition 7th ed. ILSI Press, Washington 1996, pp. 307–319.
11. Sondheimer JH, Mahajan SK, Rye DL, et al. Elevated plasma copper in chronic renal failure. Am J Clin Nutr 1988;47:896–899.
12. Mahler DJ, Walsh JR, Haynie GD. Magnesium, zinc and copper in dialysis patients. Am J Clin Pathol 1970; 56:17–23.
13. Mansouri K, Halsted JA, Gombos EA. Zinc, copper, magnesium and calcium in dialyzed and nondialyzed uremic patients. Arch Intern Med 1970;125:88–93.
14. Dash SC. Copper sulphate poisoning and acute renal failure Int J Artif Organs 1989;12:610–614.
15. Klein WJ, et al. Acute copper intoxication. A hazard of hemodialysis. Arch Intern Med 1972;129:578–582.
16. Atkin-Thor E, et al. Hypogeusia and zinc depletion in chronic dialysis patients. Am J Clin Nutr 1978;31:1948–1951.
17. Burge JC, et al. Taste acuity in patients undergoing long-term hemodialysis. Kidney Int 1979;15:49–53.
18. Gilli P, et al. Is zinc status a problem in the dietary treatment of chronic renal failure? Nephron 1985;40:382.
19. Alfrey AC. Trace element alterations in uremia. In: Zurulezoglu W, et al. eds. Proceedings of the 8th International Congress of Nephrology. Karger, Basal, 1981, pp. 1007–1013.
20. Bogden JD, et al. Elevated plasma zinc concentrations in renal dialysis patients Am J Clin Nutr 1980;33:1088–1095.
21. Dworkin B, Weseley S, Rosenthal W. Diminished blood selenium levels in renal failure patients on dialysis:correlation with nutritional status. Am J Med Sci 1987;293:6–12.
22. Kostakopoulos A, et al. Serum selenium levels in healthy adults and its changes in chronic renal failure. Int Urol Nephrol 1990;22:397–401.
23. Thomson NM, et al. Comparison of trace elements in peritoneal dialysis, hemodialysis and uremia. Kidney Int 1983;23:9–14.
24. Clark LC, Alberts DS. Selenium and cancer:risk or protection? J Natl Cancer Int 1995;87:473–475.
25. Levander DA, Burk RF. Selenium. In: Ziegler EE, Filer LJ, Jr. eds. Present Knowledge in Nutrition 7th ed. ILSI Press, Washington, 1996, pp. 320–328.
26. MacGonigle RJS, Parson V. Aluminum-induced anaemia in haemodialysis patients. Nephron 1985;39:1–9.
27. Alfrey AC. Aluminum toxicity in patients with chronic renal failure. Ther Drug Monit 1993;15:593–597.
28. Drueke TB. Adynamic bone disease, anaemia, resistance to erythropoietin and iron-aluminum interaction. Nephrol Dial Transplant 1993;8:(Suppl 1):12–16.
29. Salusky IB, Foley J, Nelson P, et al. Aluminum accumulation during treatment with aluminum hydroxide and dialysis in children and young adults with chronic renal disease. New Engl J Med 1991;324:527–531.
30. Cannata JB, Olaizola IR, Gomez-Alonso C, et al. Serum aluminum transport and aluminum uptake in chronic renal failure:role of iron and aluminum metabolism. Nephron 1993;65:141–146.
31. Maluche JJ, Smith AJ, Abreo K, et al. The use of deferoxamine in the management of aluminum accumulation in bone in patients with renal failure. N Engl J Med 1984;311:140–144.
32. Delmez JA. Renal Osteodystrophy and Other Musculoskeletal Complications of Chronic Renal Failure. In: Greenberg A,eds. Primer of Kidney Diseases, Academic Press, 1994, pp. 294–300.
33. Offenbacher EG, Pi-Sanyer FX. Chromium in human nutrition. Anna Rev Nutr 1988;8:543–563.
34. Whhitford GM, Pashley DH, Stronger GE. Fluoride renal clearance:a pH dependent event. Am J Physiol 1976;230:527–532.
35. Delange F. The disorders induced by iodine deficiency. Thyroid 1994;4:107–128.
36. Nikolova P. Effect of manganese on essential trace element metabolism. Tissue concentrations and excretion of manganese, iron, copper, cobalt and zinc. Trace Elem Med 1993;10:141–147.
37. Rajagopalan KV. Molybdenum:an essential trace element in human nutrition. Annu Rev Nutr 1988;8:401–427.
38. Kovach K, Hruska KA. Hyperphosphatemia. In: Jacobson HR, Striker GE, Klahr S, eds. The Principles and Practice of Nephrology, 2nd ed. Mosby, St. Louis, 1995, pp. 1000–1005.
39. Hruska KA, Kovach K. Phosphate Balance and Metabolism. In: Jacobson HR, Striker GE, Klahr S, eds. The Principles and Practice of Nephrology, 2nd ed. Mosby, St. Louis, 1995, pp. 986–992.
40. Mizgala CL, Quamme GA. Renal handling of phosphate. Physiol Rev 1985;65:431–466.

41. Delmez J, Slatopolsky E. Hyperphosphatemia its consequences and treatment in patients with chronic renal disease. Am J Kidney Dis 1992;19:303–317.

42. Slatopolsky E, Wurts C, Lopez-Hiller S, et al. Calcium carbonate as a phosphate binder in patients with chronic renal failure undergoing dialysis. N Engl J Med 1986;315:157–161.

43. Shils, ME. Magnesium. In: Ziegler EE, Filer LJ, Jr. eds. Present Knowledge in Nutrition 7th Ed. ILSI Press, Washington, 1996, pp. 256–264.

44. Marier JR. Magnesium content of the food supply in the modern-day world. Magnesium 1986;5:1–8.

45. Danielson BG, Johansson G, Jung B, et al. Gastrointestinal magnesium absorption:kinetic studies with 28 Mg and a simple method for determination of fractional absorption. Miner Electrolyte Metab 1979;4:195–206.

46. Brannan PG, Vergne-Marini P, Hull AR, et al. Magnesium absorption in the human small intestine:results in normal subjects, patients with chronic renal disease, and patients with absorptive hypercalciuria. J Clin Invest 1976;57:1412–1418.

47. Fine DK, Santa Ana CA, Porter JL, et al. Intestinal absorption of magnesium from food and supplements. J Clin Invest 1991;88:396–402.

48. Hardwick LL, Jones MR, Brautbar N, et al. Site and mechanism of intestinal magnesium absorption. Miner Electrolyte Metab 1990;16:174–180.

49. Kayne LH, Lee DBN. Intestinal magnesium absorption. Miner Electrolyte Metab 1993;19:210–217.

50. Krejs GJ, Nicar MJ, Zerwekh II, et al. Effect of 1,25-dihydroxyvitamin D_3 on calcium and magnesium absorption in the healthy human jejunum and ileum. Am J Med 1983;75:973–976.

51. Quamme GA, Dirks JH. The physiology of renal magnesium handling. Renal Physiol 1986;9:257–269.

52. Fassler CA, Rodriguez RM, Badesch DB, et al. Magnesium toxicity as a cause of hypotension and hypoventilation:occurrence in patients with normal renal function. Arch Intern Med 1985;145:1604–1606.

53. Mordes JP, Swartz R, Arky RA. Extreme hypermagnesemia as a cause of refractory hypotension. Ann Intern Med 1975;83:657–658.

54. Pritchard JA. The use of magnesium ion in the management of eclamptogenic toxemias. Surg Gynecol Obstet 1955;100:131–140.

55. Kumar R. Disorders. In: Kokko JP, Tannen RL, eds. Fluids and Electrolyes Third Edition. WB Saunders, Philadelphia, 1996, pp. 391–419.

56. Arnaud CD, Sanchez SD. Calcium and Phosphorous. In: Ziegler EE, Fisher LS, Jr. eds. Present Knowledge in Nutrition, Seventh Edition. ILSI Press, Washington, 1996, pp. 245–255.

57. Bringhurst FR. Calcium and phosphate distribution, turnover and metabolic actions. In: DeGroot LJ, Besser GM, Cahill GF, et al. eds. Endocrinology, vol 2, 2nd ed. WB Saunders, Philadelphia, 1989, pp. 1049–1064.

58. Pak CYC, Avioli LV. Factors affecting absorbability of calcium from calcium salts and food. Calcif Tissue Int 1988;43:55–66.

59. Heaney RP, Weaver CM, Recker RR. Calcium absorbability from spinach. Am J Clin Nutr 1988;47:707–709.

60. Holick MF. Vitamin D, biosynthesis, metabolism and mode of action. In: DeGroot LJ, Besser GM, Cahill GF, et al. eds. Endocrinology vol 2, 2nd ed. WB Saunders, Philadelphia 1989,pp. 902–926.

61. Sutton RAL. Renal Filtration and Reabsorption of Calcium. In: Col FL, Favus MJ, Pak CYC, Parks JH, Preminger GM, eds. Kidney Stones:Medical and Surgical Management. Lippincott-Raven Publishers, Philadelphia, 1996, pp. 223–238.

62. Brunette MG, Mailoux J, Lajeunesse D. Calcium transport through the luminal membrane of the distal tubule. I Interrelationship with sodium. Kidney Int 1992;41:281–288.

63. Brunette MG, Mailoux J, Lajeunesse D. Calcium transport by the luminal membrane of distal tubule II. Effect of pH electrical potential and calcium channel inhibitors. Kidney Int 1992;41:289–296.

64. Edwards BR, Baer PG, Sutton RA, Dirks JH. Micropuncture study of diuretic effects on sodium and calcium reabsorption in the dog nephron. J Clin Invest 1973;52:2418–2427.

65. Agus ZS, Gardner LB, Beck LH, Goldberg M. Effects of parathyroid hormone on renal tubular reabsorption of calcium, sodium, and phosphate. Am J Physiol 1973;224:1143–1148.

66. Costanzo LS, Windhager EE. Effects of PTH, ADH, cyclic AMP on distal tubular Ca and Na reabsorption. Am J Physiol 1980;239:F478–F485.

67. Mundy GR, Reasner II CA. Hypercalcemia. In: Jacobson HR, Striker GE, Klahr S, eds. The Principles and Practices of Nephrology. Mosby, St. Louis, MO 1995,pp. 977–986.

68. Mundy GR, Reasner II CA. Hypocalcemia. In: Jacobson HR, Striker GE, Klahr S, eds. The Principles and Practices of Nephrology. Mosby, St. Louis, MO 1995, pp. 971–977.

17 Trace Element and Mineral Nutrition in Gastrointestinal Disease

Giacomo Carlo Sturniolo, MD,
Cinzia Mestriner, MD and Renata D'Incà, MD.

1. INTRODUCTION

Trace elements and minerals are considered in this chapter, with particular emphasis on their role in gastrointestinal and liver disorders. Research on trace elements has made remarkable progress in the past three decades, and it is now known that gastrointestinal diseases can impair the metabolism of trace elements whereas, on the other hand, trace element deficiency may alter the natural history of diseases of the gastrointestinal tract and liver. So far, more trace elements than previously considered essential are now known to be crucial structural and functional components of proteins and enzymes (*see* Chapter 1). On the other hand, the presence of excessive amounts of these elements in humans may have adverse effects on their health. Trace elements are important in human nutrition: their deficiency has been documented in malnourished and starving populations and in industrialized countries, where marginal deficiency is now recognized to be fairly common, especially in children and the elderly (*see* Chapter 6). Multiple factors may also affect the gastrointestinal handling of trace elements (intake levels, bioavailability, transport, storage, and excretion). Most of the trace element are metabolized by the liver: damage to hepatic cells usually results in trace element deficiency but in some conditions an altered excretion may cause toxicity. Zinc, iron, copper, selenium, manganese, and calcium have been studied more extensively whereas the importance of other trace elements and minerals in gastrointestinal diseases and the steps in their metabolism are as yet unknown.

2. ZINC

2.1. Functions and Absorption

The total body content of zinc (Zn), which is present in all organs, amounts to about 1–2 g, although only 10% of this is readily available, most being bound to the bones and skeletal muscles. Zn, which stabilizes membranes, is a catalytic component of more than 200 enzymes and a structural component of a large number of proteins, hormones, neuropeptides, hormone receptors, and nucleotides. This trace element is crucial to vital processes, playing a unique role in growth and development.

From: *Clinical Nutrition of the Essential Trace Elements and Minerals: The Guide for Health Professionals*
Edited by: J. D. Bogden and L. M. Klevay © Humana Press Inc., Totowa, NJ

The jejunum is the major site of Zn absorption, which occurs through passive diffusion and specific carrier-mediated mechanisms. Transport across the enterocyte occurs in three phases: uptake, intracellular regulation, and discharge to the serosal site. Uptake appears to be regulated by low molecular weight intracellular ligands that can bind Zn at the brush border and transfer it into the enterocyte. Suggested ligands are picolinic and citric acid and prostaglandins *(1)*. Once in the cell, Zn binds to metallothionein and other cysteine-rich intestinal proteins (CRIP) whose synthesis is stimulated by an excess of the metal in the diet with a consequent regulation of its homeostasis *(2)*.

A diet rich in phytates can reduce Zn bioavailability whereas a diet rich in animal proteins results in a much higher absorption rate. Gastric acidity is essential for appropriate Zn absorption which is significantly reduced in healthy volunteers following the administration of drugs inhibiting gastric secretion, such as cimetidine (400 mg) or ranitidine (300 mg) *(3)*. Reduced Zn absorption has been observed in healthy elderly subjects; this may support the finding of marginal Zn deficiency in the elderly reported in several studies. Atrophic gastritis in the elderly might explain these findings.

Dr. Ananda Prasad first described the clinical manifestations of Zn deficiency in young Iranian boys, who presented with growth retardation, skin rash, hypogonadism, and alopecia *(4)*. Many more signs of deficiency have been reported since, including acrodermatitis, poor wound healing, night blindness and neuropsychiatric manifestations. The mechanisms and conditions causing a predisposition to dietary and systemic Zn deprivation and possibly leading to frank Zn deficiency are reported in Table 1.

The metal has a definite influence on immune function as a result of its role in lymphocyte proliferation and differentiation. Deficiency is often associated with a decline in enzymatic and immunological reactions. As Zn supplementation is efficacious in most of these conditions, it is considered an oriented therapeutical support rather than a simple dietary integrator. However, overt clinical deficiency is quite rare; gastrointestinal diseases are more often associated with subclinical signs of marginal deficiency. Nevertheless, zinc metabolism is still important in cellular membrane integrity, immunity, as an antioxidant and in gene expression of growth factors.

Patients with new tissue synthesis (e.g., infants, particularly preterm neonates, children, adolescents, pregnant women, and individuals in post catabolic states) are more vulnerable to Zn deprivation (*see* Chapters 8–10).

2.2. Liver Diseases

Impaired Zn metabolism has been well documented in patients with liver disease *(5)*, who can develop Zn depletion for several reasons: poor diet, impaired intestinal absorption, or excessive urinary loss. Zn may exert protective effects on liver cells through inhibiting lipid peroxidation and stabilizing cell membranes.

2.2.1. ACUTE VIRAL HEPATITIS

Acute viral hepatitis is associated with reduced plasma Zn levels; after the normalization of transaminases plasma Zn levels also return to normal. Zn reduction may be part of the acute phase response through the stimulation of cytokines, such as IL-1, IL-6, and TNFα, accompanied by redistribution of the circulating metal to the inflamed tissues *(6)*. This can lead to local immobilization of macrophages in the liver tissue and induction of antioxidant enzymes. Taste and smell alterations due to Zn deficiency may be responsible for the anorexia and dysosmia observed in acute hepatitis.

Table 1
Mechanisms and conditions which predispose to dietary and systemic deprivation of zinc

Inadequate intake and absorbability	Increased losses
Malnutrition states	Catabolic states
Enteral and parenteral nutrition	Protein-losing enteropathies
Intestinal infestation	Renal failure, dialysis and diuretic therapy
Chronic blood loss and haemolysis	
Maldigestion and malabsorption	Exfoliative dermatoses
Acrodermatitis enteropathica	Chelating agent
Surgery	Increased utilization
Inflammatory bowel disease	Rapid tissue synthesis
Exocrine pancreatic insufficiency	Post catabolic convalescence
Biliary obstruction	Neoplastic disease
Hepatic disease	Resolving anaemias

2.2.2. Chronic Liver Disease

In the rat, Zn deficiency causes a significant reduction in the microsomal enzyme P450, while Zn supplementation protects the liver from carbon tetrachloride toxicity *(7)*. Alcoholic liver disease is associated with low plasma Zn levels and low hepatic Zn concentrations *(8)*. An altered Zn metabolism may be related to the inadequate calorie and protein intake found in these patients. Alcohol-induced Zn deficiency may depend on decreased intestinal absorption by ethanol, or on liver damage. Alcoholics can consume up to 50 % of their calories in alcohol, and their poor diet may be the cause of deficiency. Sturniolo et al. studied plasma Zn levels and Zn tissue concentrations in a group of 60 alcoholics with and without liver damage *(9)*. Serum Zn was significantly reduced in both groups of patients compared with healthy controls. The hepatic Zn content was reduced, irrespective of the presence or absence of liver damage. Similar results were reported by Milman et al. *(10)*.

Further aspects evaluated for studying Zn metabolism include the measurement of metal absorption by the Zn tolerance test and urinary excretion. Significantly reduced absorption and increased urinary losses have been reported in several studies irrespective of the severity of disease or its etiology. Reduced protein synthesis may also play a role, since albumin is the main binding protein in plasma. This binding can influence Zn bioavailability, tissue distribution and the amount of the metal excreted in the urine. A significant correlation was found between plasma Zn and albumin levels in patients with cirrhosis.

Taste detection thresholds are increased in patients with liver cirrhosis *(11)*, and this may hide an increased salt introduction in the diet which can play a role in the pathogenesis of ascites or its worsening.

Hepatic encephalopathy is associated with increased ammonia levels, which depend on urea synthesis, that may be altered in the presence of Zn deficiency. Moreover, reduced Zn concentrations in the brain have been found to be related to alterations in GABA-ergic neurotransmittors and brain norepinephrine concentrations. Short term Zn supplements were found to improve psychometric performance and prevent further severe recurrent episodes of hepatic encephalopathy in a 54-yr-old woman *(12)*. No modification in the degree of hepatic encephalopathy was observed in a randomized controlled trial performed on 15 cirrhotics observed in Italy *(13)*. Marchesini et al. *(14)* demostrated that long-term oral Zn supplementation speeds up the kinetics of urea formation from amino acids and ammonia. Changes in the hormonal effects and/or the antioxidant activity of Zn might be involved in the general improvement in liver function, whereas the beneficial effects on encephalopathy might stem from decreased ammonia levels.

2.2.3. HBV Vaccination in Hemodialyzed Patients

Chronic uremic patients on hemodialysis are at high risk of hepatitis B infection with a diminished seroconversion rate after hepatitis B vaccination. In a prospective study involving 40 uremic nonresponders to a first complete hepatitis B vaccination cycle, 28 patients were randomized to receive Zn-aspartate (60 mg) after each dialytic session for 8 wk *(15)*. All patients had subnormal predialysis plasma Zn levels compared to healthy controls. Six of the 28 patients treated with Zn-aspartate developed antibodies against hepatitis B after 16 wk. This effect was attributed to the correction of the immunological deficiencies involving cellular immunity in particular.

2.2.4. Wilson's Disease

Wilson's disease, characterized by abnormal copper deposition within the liver, kidney, and brain, causes liver failure if left untreated (*see* Chapter 12). The treatment of choice is penicillamine, a copper chelator. This drug, however, has several side effects, and Zn at high doses is an effective and safe alternative *(16)*.

2.2.5. Liver Transplant

Zn deficiency is common in patients with end-stage liver failure irrespective of its etiology. During the waiting period for transplant, oral supplementation with Zn should be provided. Following transplantation, Zn levels rapidly recover, obviating the need to check levels and provide oral supplementation *(17)*.

2.2.6. Cholestasis

Phillips et al. *(18)* reported an association between severe chronic cholestatic liver disease progressing to end-stage biliary cirrhosis and the presence of excess hepatic Zn and copper in six children on the waiting list for liver transplant, who were receiving total parenteral nutrition. Zn was deposited in both hepatocytes and canaliculi. Excess hepatic Zn is unexplained, and this report is the first to suggest that Zn can cause liver disease in man. However, this association may not be a cause/effect relationship. Reduced liver weight due to weight loss may have resulted in increased liver metal concentrations.

2.3. Gastrointestinal Diseases

2.3.1. Peptic Ulcer Disease

Recognition that Zn deficiency promotes the development of a number of inflammatory conditions, including gastric ulceration, together with the recognition that Zn has a number of important antisecretory and gastroprotective functions, has led to the suggestion that Zn compounds may be useful anti-ulcer agents. The anti-ulcer activity of Zn is multifactorial: it increases mucosal resistance to acids, stabilizes plasma membranes, and has antioxidant properties. Zn may prevent histamine release from mast cells and/or reduce the permeability of gastric mucosal cells. In an experimental gastrointestinal ulcer model, Zn-gluconate administration prevented mucosal damage induced by absolute ethanol, suggesting a direct cytoprotective activity *(19)*. The mucosal defence mechanisms may also be attributed to the *de novo* synthesis of mucin, a glycoprotein from the nonparietal cells of the gastric glands. Watanabe et al. *(20)* reported a decreased cell proliferation in Zn-deficient rats with respect to controls. This decrease in cell proliferation is not surprising because Zn is a cofactor of DNA and RNA polymerase, thymidine kinase, and other enzymes involved in cell replication.

Rainsford et al. *(21)* recently reported that Zn compounds may inhibit the growth of Helicobacter pylori, a bacterium with an etiopathological importance in gastroduodenal ulcer formation.

2.3.2. ACUTE DIARRHEA

Impaired immune function and malnutrition can be associated with Zn deficiency. In developing countries, long-lasting and severe diarrhea is a serious problem in malnourished children. In a double-blind controlled trial involving 937 children, daily supplementation with 20 mg elemental Zn as an adjunct to oral rehydration resulted in a clinically important reduction in the duration and severity of diarrhea *(22)*. The possible mechanisms of action of Zn on diarrhea may include improved absorption of water and electrolytes, enhanced immunological functions, stimulated regeneration of gut epithelium, and the restoration of enterocyte brush border enzymes levels.

The efficacy of Zn supplementation on the mucosal integrity and function have also been demonstrated in another trial involving 32 children with acute shigellosis *(23)*. Supplementation with Zn in adjunct to antibiotics resulted in a significant improvement in intestinal permeability and better nitrogen absorption with respect to unsupplemented children, whereas fecal protein loss was unchanged.

Recently, a new mechanism of a Zn effect during diarrhea has been documented in rats *(24)*. Animals on a Zn deficient diet had an increased synthesis of uroguanyline compared to rats receiving a normal diet. This peptide potentially regulates water and electrolyte intestinal transport, since uroguanyline stimulates cGMP synthesis. Diarrhea in Zn deficiency may therefore result from increased chloride secretion in intestinal epithelial cells.

2.2.3. INFLAMMATORY BOWEL DISEASE

Reduced plasma Zn concentrations have been reported during acute attacks of disease. Deficiency has also been referred to reduced absorption, demonstrated both in Crohn's disease and in ulcerative colitis *(25)*. Other factors contributing to deficiency may be reduced dietary intake in the presence of significant abdominal pain or increased loss with diarrhea. A reduced Zn concentration was observed at the site of the disease (i.e., in the colonic mucosa) of ulcerative colitis patients *(26)*. A direct relationship between the presence of inflammation and decreased free radical scavengers has been suggested on the basis of a reduced plasma concentration of two antioxidant proteins, glutathione peroxidase and metallothionein. Although these data demonstrate altered Zn metabolism in inflammatory bowel diseases, overt clinical manifestations of deficiency are quite rare, and the diagnosis of marginal deficiency in each patient is still difficult to assess. Although the efficacy of Zn supplementation has been observed in the ameliorating of clinical disease, several reports have found a reversal of alterations in red blood cell lipid composition, immunological parameters of T cell activation, or impaired vision.

2.2.4. CHRONIC PANCREATITIS

Zn deficiency causes pancreatic insufficiency. Rats with marginal Zn deficiency show morphological and functional alterations in the pancreatic gland similar to those observed to rats fed ethanol chronically. Zn deficiency may play a role in ethanol induced secretory alterations, because a poor intake is often associated with chronic alcoholism.

Low plasma Zn levels are frequently found in chronic pancreatitis patients *(27)*. Zn output is significantly reduced in the duodenal juice of chronic pancreatitis patients, maximal reduction occurring after secretin stimulation. A good correlation between Zn and amylase levels in duodenal juice suggests that Zn may be an index of pancreatic function, with the advantage of more stable levels with respect to amylase after storage.

Altered Zn absorption in chronic pancreatitis, especially if the latter is alcoholic, is due to reduced concentrations of ligands in pancreatic juice. The administration of ligands such as citric acid or picolinic acid can reverse these alterations *(1)*. Zn deficiency may be the effect of reduced absorption and be a contributory factor in disease progression, via reduction in free radical scavengers and an increased collagen deposition.

3. COPPER

3.1. Functions

Copper (Cu) is an essential component of many enzymes involved in cellular respiration, free radical defense, and cellular iron metabolism. Lysyl oxidase is required for the formation and function of connective tissue throughout the body, tyrosinase is responsible for the synthesis of melanin pigment, and Cu-Zn-superoxide dismutase, cytochrome oxidase, and ceruloplasmin have antioxidant function. Cu enzymes are also involved in the production of catecholamines and neuropeptides.

Cu absorption occurs in the duodenum and jejunum. The efficiency of absorption is relatively high compared with that of other trace elements.

Cu is known to be toxic in humans with prevalent hepatic damage. Cu binding to various structural cellular proteins, such as microtubules, reduces mitochondrial enzyme activities, damages DNA-crosslinking and has a harmful effect on peroxisomes.

3.2. Genetic Disorders

Two genetic diseases involving different steps of Cu transport have been recognized in humans: Menkes syndrome due to Cu deficiency, and Wilson's disease due to Cu overload and toxicity *(28)* *(see* Chapter 12*)*.

3.2.1. WILSON'S DISEASE

This disease, inherited by an autosomal recessive gene with a prevalence of about 1 in 30,000 people in almost all populations, has a pathogenesis linked to a defect in biliary excretion, with a consequent Cu accumulation in many organs, especially the liver and the brain, where Cu exerts its most devastating effects. The gene ATP 7B, recently isolated on chromosome 13, encodes a nearly 7.5-kb transcript that is highly expressed in the liver *(29)*. A summary of key elements in Cu homeostasis in humans is given in Figure 1. The liver plays a pivotal role in Cu metabolism. Most of the metal is extracted from the portal circulation by hepatocytes via an as yet unidentified plasma membrane transporter. Once within the hepatocyte, part of the Cu binds to ligands such as glutathione and metallothionein and most of the circulating Cu is incorporated into ceruloplasmin. The major route of Cu excretion is through the bile. Cu is transferred from the hepatocytes into the bile via the canalicular membrane by at least two distinct pathways. If Cu cannot

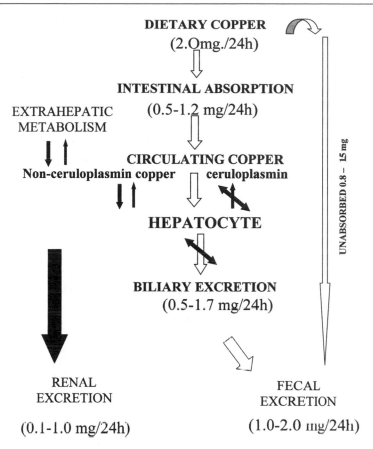

DIETARY COPPER
(2.0mg./24h)

INTESTINAL ABSORPTION
(0.5-1.2 mg/24h)

EXTRAHEPATIC
METABOLISM

CIRCULATING COPPER

Non-ceruloplasmin copper   ceruloplasmin

HEPATOCYTE

UNABSORBED 0.8 – 15 mg

BILIARY EXCRETION
(0.5-1.7 mg/24h)

RENAL
EXCRETION

FECAL
EXCRETION

(0.1-1.0 mg/24h)   (1.0-2.0 mg/24h)

Fig. 1. Copper homeostasis in normal individuals (empty arrows) and Wilson's disease patients (black arrows).

be excreted into the bile, it accumulates within hepatocytes, leading to progressive hepatic damage. There is almost no intestinal reabsorption of the metal from the bile. Under normal conditions, only a small fraction (approximately 40–50 μg/24h) is removed from the circulation and excreted into the urine.

Chelating agents such as penicillamine and trientine are first choice treatments in Wilson's disease. These drugs reduce tissue Cu levels by increasing urinary Cu excretion. Twenty per cent of patients treated with penicillamine, however, experience side effects which are occasionally severe enough to require drug withdrawal. Moreover, about 50% of Wilson's disease patients with mainly neurological manifestations worsen under penicillamine administration. Oral Zn therapy has therefore been proposed as an alternative to chelating agents. Our experience with 31 Wilson's disease patients on Zn sulphate treatment confirmed not only its safety but also the clinical amelioration of signs and symptoms, with the normalization in urinary Cu excretion *(30)*. The mechanisms underlying the action of Zn are still unclear, but evidence has been found of intestinal and hepatic metallothionein induction *(30–32)* with a blockage in Cu absorption and Cu binding in nontoxic complexes within the hepatocytes. Recently, Farinati et al. also demonstrated that Zn treatment prevents lipid peroxidation and increases glutathione availability in Wilson disease patients *(33)*. Treatment for Wilson's disease must be for life and patient compliance can easily be monitored by measuring Cu and Zn urinary excretion.

3.2.2. MENKES DISEASE

Menkes disease is a multisystemic lethal disorder with dominant neurodegenerative symptoms and connective tissue manifestations. Unlike Wilson's disease, Menkes syndrome is characterized by a normal Cu uptake with deficient Cu-dependent enzyme activity and excessive intracellular Cu intestinal accumulation. This defect causes a consequent Cu deficient state which is not amenable to current treatment *(34)*. The disease locus has been mapped on Xq 13.3, and the defective gene has been isolated by positional cloning. The protein product is predicted to be a Cu binding P type ATPase.

3.2.3. INDIAN CHILDHOOD CIRRHOSIS

This disease has been described in India, with increased hepatic Cu concentrations, an increased Cu ingestion is due to contaminated water supplies, delivered through copper pipes. It affects children with clinical, biochemical, and histological features of severe hepatic copper overload *(35)*. An underlying genetic predisposition is suspected.

3.2.4. ENDEMIC TYROLEAN INFANTILE CIRRHOSIS

The frequency of this disease, predominant in a geographically circumscribed area in northern Tyrol, increased and peaked between 1930 and 1960 *(36)*. No cases have been reported since 1974. Pedigree analysis strongly suggests that susceptibility to the disease is inherited in an autosomal recessive fashion and diets of the infants in this region during these decades were considerably enriched in Cu.

3.3. Cholestatic Conditions

Since Cu balance is greatly influenced by biliary-excretion, hepatic Cu overload is quite common in cholestatic disease, such as primary biliary cirrhosis and extrahepatic biliary obstruction.

During both primary sclerosing cholangitis and primary biliary cirrhosis, hepatic Cu concentrations are increased, and not infrequently concentrations are above 250 mg/Kg dry wt *(37)*. The disturbed Cu metabolism may play a role in the pathogenesis of the disease, as the accumulation of Cu is reported to induce formation of oxygen species and membrane lipoperoxidation, with cell necrosis and fibrosis. Cu retention results in increased serum Cu levels and the induction of ceruloplasmin synthesis. However, treatment with Cu chelators, such as penicillamine, does not improve the prognosis in primary biliary cirrhosis.

3.4. Gastrointestinal Diseases

3.4.1. INFLAMMATORY BOWEL DISEASE

Crohn's disease and ulcerative colitis patients may exhibit increased serum Cu concentrations. Elevated serum levels have been reported in patients with active disease and in those taking steroids, whereas normal Cu concentrations have been found in outpatients with Crohn's disease. Increased Cu levels may parallel increased ceruloplasmin levels during inflammation *(38)*. Other factors such as age, sex, and contraceptive consumption may, however, influence Cu levels. As yet we are unable to prove whether Cu plays a role at the inflamed sites in ulcerative colitis, since metal concentrations are not detectable in the colonic mucosa *(26)*.

3.4.2. Chronic Pancreatitis

The metabolism of Cu is altered in pancreatic diseases and the most important alteration is increased absorption with a possible pathogenetic role in increasing pancreatic damage. Experimental studies with Cu dependent antioxidant scavengers were effective in reducing the severity of acute pancreatitis *(39)*.

4. IRON

4.1. Functions

Iron (Fe) is required for the synthesis of the oxygen transport proteins, hemoglobin and myoglobin, and for the formation of heme enzymes participating in electron transfer and oxidative-reductive reactions. Fe is absorbed in the duodenum, through an active, saturable process. The regulation of Fe homeostasis is controlled by variations in absorption. The excess Fe is stored as ferritin or hemosiderin in the liver, spleen, and bone marrow. The substances controlling bioavailability are summarized in Table 2.

The liver is particularly sensitive to the toxic effects of Fe, reflecting its role in storage and metabolism. Hepatic Fe overload induces lipid peroxidation and leads to structural and/or functional alterations in various cell organelles. Fe may also enhance the cell-damaging effects of other hepatotoxic factors, such as alcohol, Cu, or viruses.

4.2. Chronic Liver Disease

4.2.1. Hemochromatosis

The most common cause of Fe overload is HLA-linked hemochromatosis *(40)* *(see* Chapter 2). Excess Fe absorbed from the gut is transported through the portal vein to the liver, where it is predominantly stored in hepatocytes. Increasing concentrations of Fe in hepatocytes play a catalytic role in the initiation of free radical mediated reactions with damage to the cellular structures such as organelle membranes, nucleic acids, protein, and carbohydrates. In humans, chronic Fe overload causes progressive fibrosis and, ultimately, cirrhosis. Kuppfer cells, stimulated to phagocyte necrotic hepatocytes, release profibrogenic cytokines such as TGFβ, leading to increased collagen synthesis. The increased collagen deposition could be counteracted by the addition of vitamin E, thus providing indirect evidence of the development of fibrosis being mediated by oxidative stress. The clinical presentation of genetic hemochromatosis has recently changed from a symptomatic constellation, often including arthropathy, weakness, lethargy, and cardiac symptoms, to an asymptomatic patient found on routine screening to have abnormal liver function tests, increased transferrin saturation, or hyperglycaemia *(41)*. Many patients are identified through family screening. Delay in diagnosis and therapy may strongly influence the course of the disease. Different studies performing long-term survival analyses demonstrated a normal survival expectation for patients diagnosed and treated to deplete total body Fe stores if the diagnosis was made before the development of cirrhosis. Cirrhotics benefited from treatment, but did not have a normal life expectancy. Nowadays, about one-third of patients die with hepatocellular carcinoma. The development of hepatocellular carcinoma correlates with the amount and duration of iron overload and, in the presence of cirrhosis, is not prevented by depletion of hepatic Fe stores by venesection therapy. A recent Italian study demonstrated *(42)* that cirrhosis was essential to the development of carcinoma, other predictors being age >55 years, hepatitis B surface antigen positivity, and alcohol abuse.

Table 2
Substances affecting iron absorption

Substances inhibiting absorption	Substances facilitating absorption
Phytic acid	Cysteine containing proteins
Polyphenols	Ascorbic acid
Calcium	
Protein	

The diagnosis of this condition is based on increased Fe concentrations in the liver. A hepatic Fe index has been constructed by measuring hepatic Fe concentration (expressed in μmoles iron /g dry liver) divided by the patient's age in years. If the index is > 1.9, in the absence of other diseases causing Fe overload (e.g., thalassemia, erythropoietic disorders) a diagnosis of hemochromatosis is likely. The suspicion, which should be clinical, can be confirmed by evaluating Fe, ferritin, and transferrin levels, whereas computed tomography, using a dual energy source can detect a fivefold increase in Fe stores in a fatty liver. Gradient echo magnetic resonance and imaging spin echocardiograms have been used to measure the excess hemosiderin; these methods have the advantage of eliminating motion artifacts, but are not widely available. Heterozygotic patients are also at increased risk of developing colorectal and gastric cancer (43). An excessive prevalence of hemochromatosis was also found in patients with type 2 diabetes with respect to a control population (1.34% vs 0.2%). The odds ratio of hemochromatosis in association with diabetes was 6.3 in comparison to nondiabetic patients. Screening for hemocromatosis with transferrin saturation has therefore been proposed for diabetic patients (44).

4.2.2. OTHER CAUSES OF IRON OVERLOAD

Fe overload may also derive from multiple transfusions to treat thalassemia major or sideroblastic anemia or from the interaction between the amount of dietary Fe and a gene distinct from any HLA-linked gene, such as found in Africa (45). In any of these conditions Fe in excess induces liver damage.

Increased hepatic Fe was observed in 10% of patients with chronic viral hepatitis and increased serum Fe and ferritin were found in 40% of the same group of patients (46). Increased Fe concentrations appear to reduce the efficacy of interferon therapy: Fe depletion increased sustained response to therapy by 15% in previously nonresponder patients.

4.2.3. FE-CU INTERACTIONS

Excess hepatic Fe concentrations may increase the liver damage seen in Long-Evans Cinnamon-rats (LEC), an experimental model of Cu toxicity (47). Increased Fe concentrations have been found together with an increased Cu content in the liver. These rats displayed hepatitis, hemolysis, and liver cancer. The administration of Fe-deficient diets to LEC rats reduced mortality and fulminant hepatitis. Moreover, the hepatic Fe concentrations and the extent of hepatic fibrosis were significantly reduced compared with littermates on a Fe-containing diet. After 65 wk, all rats on a Fe-containing diet, but none of the rats on a Fe-deficient diet, developed cancer. Liver Cu concentrations remained unchanged.

4.3. Gastrointestinal Inflammation

Fe tablets have been reported to cause esophageal and gastric lesions. Fe deposition has been found within ulcer granulation tissue, connective tissue, and blood venules of the lamina propria and within glandular and squamous epithelium. Fe may play a secondary role rather than being an initiator of ulceration and stricture formation.

Fe concentrations are typically increased in any inflamed area: the damaged inflamed mucosa of ulcerative colitis patients contains more iron than the uninflamed areas. Whatever the reason for the increased concentration, iron contributes to perpetuating and/or amplifying oxidative damage *(26)*.

5. SELENIUM

5.1 Functions

Selenium (Se) is found in both organic (selenomethionine, selenocysteine) and inorganic forms (selenite, selenate). Its distribution in the soil is variable with consequent variations in the amount present in the alimentary chain. The type of food (meat is rich in selenium) affects the bioavailability of the different chemical forms. Se is an integral part of the enzyme glutathione peroxidase, which assists intracellular defense mechanisms against oxidative damage. Other key functions may involve carcinogen metabolism, immune regulation, endocrine function, and inhibition of cell proliferation.

Se deficiency has been documented in humans in China and Antilla *(48)*, where it is responsible for a myocardiopathy, named Keshan's disease, and an endemic degenerative osteoarthropathy, named Kaschin-Beck's disease. These diseases have never been found in populations with mean Se dietary intakes greater than 19 μg/d.

Different absorption pathways (active transport or passive diffusion) and bioavailability derive from the different forms of dietary Se supplementation (organic or inorganic). This makes it difficult to compare results from different studies, and Se levels appear quite variable. The clinical manifestations of Se deficiency have a late onset, and deficiency may be present for a long time before they occur. Changes in status and kinetic modeling remain the most accurate measurements available to characterize the utilization of the different forms of Se, but from a practical point, plasma levels and platelet glutathione peroxidase seem to reflect immediate bioavailability while red blood cell and plasma glutathione peroxidase activity are used as long-term indicators of the Se status.

5.2. Se and Gastrointestinal Cancers

An inverse relationship between cancer and serum Se levels has been described. Se supplementation suppresses carcinogenesis in many different animal models. The inhibition of tumor growth is aspecific, since the effects have been shown in mammary gland, liver, skin, pancreas, esophagus, colon, and other sites.

An interventional trial of supplementation with various substances, including Se, which was performed in China, on a population living in the Linxian, an area which has a low Se concentration in the soil and a high risk of stomach and esophageal cancer, demonstrated effectiveness in reducing the mortality from both types of cancers *(49)*. The study involved 30,000 people receiving supplementation with four different pairs of substances (retinol and Zn, riboflavin and niacin, vitamin C and beta-carotene, vitamin E and Se) for five years at a dosage of about two times that of RDA. The group with beta-carotene, vitamin E and Se supplementation showed a significant reduction in total mortality (35%), starting 1 to 2 yr after beginning supplementation. The reduction was mainly due to lower rates for tumors, especially stomach cancer.

Another Chinese study addressed the issue of cancer prevention by administering supplementary multivitamin tablets, including Se, to patients with dysplastic esophageal lesions *(50)*. No differences were found in cancer mortality, although patients receiving multivitamins had less dysplasia at the end of the study.

Se supplementation (200 µg/d) was also attempted in the United States to reduce recurrent skin cancer. The results demonstrated that Se reduced total mortality from all cancers combined, and the incidence of lung, colorectal, and prostate cancers *(51)*. Few prospective studies have been undertaken to evaluate the importance of supplementing with Se and other trace elements on the subsequent risk of developing cancer. Another possible association may exist between the presence of precancerous lesions of the stomach, as in chronic atrophic gastritis, intestinal metaplasia, or dysplasia and serum Se levels *(52)*.

Wu et al., found significantly increased concentrations of various trace elements such as Fe, K, Mg, Na, Rb, Zn and Se in gastric cancer tissue *(53)*. However Fe, K, and Se were independently associated with gastric cancer. Elevated potassium levels were related to the presence of lymphatic duct metastasis. High Se tissue levels were linked to intestinal type adenocarcinoma.

In a case-control study, high dose Se supplementation was not found to have a protective effect in patients with colorectal cancer or adenomas *(54)*. On the other hand, in another case-control study, a significant association was found between low plasma Se and the occurrence of adenoma *(55)*. These reduced levels were associated with the presence of multiple adenomas.

5.3 Gastrointestinal Diseases

5.3.1. INFLAMMATORY BOWEL DISEASE

Low serum Se levels have been reported in Crohn's disease patients *(56)*. Significantly reduced serum concentrations of Se were observed both in males and females at an early-stage of Crohn's disease. Se levels were also reduced in patients with early-stage ulcerative colitis, with lower levels in extensive colitis than in proctitis *(57)*. It is also generally accepted that adenocarcinomas of the large and small bowel occur with greater frequency in Crohn's disease, but the exact risk requires better definition and the possible link between the risk and Se levels must be determined. Since Se may inhibit carcinogenesis by protecting cellular membranes against oxidative damage, by reducing the mutagenicity of cancer-causing chemicals, or by affecting carcinogen metabolism, reduced Se levels may be of importance in patients with inflammatory bowel disease. We determined Se serum levels in patients with ulcerative colitis at different stages of clinical activity and found that those with moderate disease activity had lower Se concentrations than controls. Further indirect evidence of the importance of Se is the finding of significantly reduced plasma glutathione peroxidase levels in patients with moderate disease activity with respect to controls and patients in remission *(26)*. Enzyme activity increased significantly in the inflamed vs noninflamed mucosa. The reduced plasma Se concentration may thus reflect a metal redistribution to tissues requiring antioxidant protection and/or a subclinical Se deficiency.

5.3.2. Chronic Alcoholic Pancreatitis

Increased free radical production may be important in the pathogenesis of alcohol-related chronic pancreatitis. Studies in ex vivo models of acute pancreatitis suggest that enzymatic scavengers can limit the extent of pancreatic injury. Van Gossum et al. *(58)* found low levels of antioxidants such as Se, glutathione peroxidase, vitamin E, and vitamin A in patients with chronic alcoholic pancreatitis. Se status impairment was demonstrated by both low Se levels and decreased activity of the Se-enzyme, glutathione peroxidase. Low plasma Se levels reflect increased metabolic requirements associated with long-term exposure to factors enhancing lipid peroxidation, such as alcohol consumption, rather than an insufficient oral Se intake, as described in alcoholic cirrhosis.

6. CALCIUM

6.1 Functions

Calcium (Ca) is a second messenger for all types of cells regulating signal transduction, cell proliferation and apoptosis.

Intestinal absorption of Ca occurs via two processes: the greater amount is passively absorbed in the ileum, while the remaining Ca is transported transcellularly in the duodenum and the jejunum.

Active transport is mediated by calcitriol, the active component of vitamin D. Availability for absorption requires Ca solubilization, either in a free ionic or complexed form.

A knowledge of Ca bioavailability is considered important for the prevention of chronic disease such as osteoporosis and hypertension. Factors controlling Ca bioavailability are endogenous (age, sex, pregnancy, lactation) and exogenous (amount of dietary of Ca, vitamin D, fiber, phytate, oxalate, fat, lactose, and a number of dietary food components which can influence urinary Ca excretion, for example sodium, phosphorus, proteins, alcohol, caffeine).

6.2. Gastrointestinal Diseases

6.2.1 Colorectal Cancer

Colorectal cancer incidence is increasing, being now the second most common cause of cancer deaths in Western societies. High fat, low fiber diets with low vegetable and fruit consumption are associated with the present increase in the incidence of colorectal cancer. Recent studies have emphasized the preventive role of fruit and vegetable intake. Ca, which has also received attention as a possible protective agent against colorectal cancer, may have a chemopreventive action through conjugating phosphate, soluble bile acids and intracolonic fatty acids. These substances act as secondary carcinogenic compounds, damaging the colonic epithelium and stimulating cell proliferation. However, these hypothesis are based on in vitro studies or investigations on animals, and other mechanisms may be more important in humans. Epithelial cell proliferation has recently been used as an intermediate marker of colorectal neoplasia, and results from interventional trials with Ca have produced inconsistent results *(59)*. In particular, Ca normalizes rectal but not always sigmoid epithelial proliferation.

Observational studies failed to demonstrate that Ca and vitamin supplements had a preventive effect when patients with newly diagnosed or recurrent adenomatous polyps were interviewed about their regular use of these substances *(60)*.

On the other hand, when Ca (2 g/d) was given after polypectomy for adenomatous polyps in a group of 175 patients, polyp recurrence (after a mean follow up of 3.1 yr), was lower (12.9 %) than in the untreated group (55 %) *(61)*.

The effect of oral supplementation with Ca and calciferol vs anti-inflammatory drugs (Sulindac) has been examined in 18 patients with familial adenomatous polyposis with polyps in the upper gastrointestinal tract. Ca did not have any effect on the crypt proliferation index in these patients, whereas Sulindac was effective *(62)*.

Patients with long-standing ulcerative colitis are at a high risk of colorectal neoplasia. The kinetics of epithelial crypt cell proliferation are frequently altered in ulcerative colitis. A pilot study involving 31 ulcerative colitis patients was performed to test the effect of 2.0 g Ca supplementation on cell proliferation *(63)*. Results were not clear-cut and larger studies are needed in order to give a more definitive answer.

Ca supplementation cannot, at present, be advised in the general population for colorectal cancer prevention, not only because of the inconsistency of the published results but also because of the possibility of side effects such as iron deficiency anemia, urolithiasis, increased fatty acid excretion, and constipation *(64)*.

7. MANGANESE

7.1. Functions

Manganese (Mn), an essential but potentially toxic metal, is a constituent of mitochondrial superoxide-dismutase, which catalyzes the dismutation of the superoxide anion into molecular oxygen and hydrogen peroxide. The physiological function of superoxide-dismutase is to protect oxygen-metabolizing organisms against superoxide free radicals. Mn, excreted primarily through the bile, provides protection against inflammation and ischemia-reperfusion injury to the gut.

7.2. Liver Diseases

7.2.1. CHRONIC HEPATIC ENCEPHALOPATHY

Increased whole blood Mn concentrations might lead to its accumulation within the basal ganglia in patients with end-stage liver disease. Ten patients and ten controls were studied by magnetic resonance imaging and Mn measurements were made in the brain tissue *(65)*. The study demonstrated hyperintensity on T1-weighted sections and whole blood Mn concentrations were increased in patients with respect to controls (34.4 vs 10.3 µg/l, $p = 0.0004$). Pallidal signal intensity indices correlated with blood Mn. Brain tissue samples have the highest Mn concentrations in the caudate nucleus, followed by the quadrigeminal plate and globus pallidus. Similarities between Mn neurotoxicity and chronic hepatic encephalopathy suggest that this metal may play a role in the pathogenesis of the disease. Moreover a normalization of Mn blood levels and pallidal signal intensity has been found after liver transplantation *(66)*.

7.2.2. HEPATIC CANCER

High Mn staining has been found in hepatocellular cancer tissue and in the surrounding capsule by immunohistochemistry *(67)*. Mn-superoxide dismutase activation may reflect a defense against cytotoxicity of cytokines such as TNFα or IL-1.

7.3. Gastrointestinal Diseases

7.3.1. GASTRIC CANCER

The cytotoxic effects of TNFα are closely related to the levels of intracellular oxygen radicals, and TNFα enhances the expression of Mn-superoxide-dismutase. It was assumed that Mn-superoxide-dismutase transcription prevents TNFα-mediated cytotoxicity. TNFα mRNA was found to be markedly increased in gastric carcinoma tissue with respect to normal tissue ($p < 0.005$)(68). Higher levels of Mn-superoxide-dismutase mRNA have also been found in gastric carcinoma tissue than in noncancerous tissue ($p < 0.0001$). The up-regulation of Mn-superoxide-dismutase mRNA found in gastric carcinoma tissue may have a protective effect against superoxide radicals and TNFα cytotoxicity.

7.4. Manganese Toxicity

The toxicity of Mn supplementation, observed in total parenteral nutrition (69), may play a role in the pathogenesis of cholestasis, which often occurs in the patients receiving total parenteral nutrition. Mn, at doses>0.8 µg/kg/d can also cause neurotoxicity. The data require confirmation in other studies. Supplementation must be evaluated accurately in long-term parenteral nutrition especially in patients with cholestasis (70). It is best to avoid giving Mn to such patients (see Chapter 20).

8. Other Trace Elements

Magnesium (Mg), which is involved in the utilization of energy rich ATP, is a constituent of numerous enzymes. The clinical manifestations of Mg deficiency are neuromuscular hyperexitability, cardiac arrythmia, hypotension, altered glucose metabolism, hypokalemia, hypocalcemia, and altered bone metabolism. The gastrointestinal tract may induce increased losses as occurs during malabsorption, diarrhea, and alcoholism. Mg deficiency is suspected when serum Mg concentrations are less than 1.5 mEq/l (71).

The hepato-renal syndrome, which is associated with pseudo-hypomagnescmia (72), may originate in a reduction in protein-bound Mg as is the case for calcium. Ionized unbound Mg should be assayed since it reflects active ions. In severe liver disease reduced Mg can be easily demonstrated in the absence of renal failure. When renal insufficiency is combined with liver failure, an increased Mg is expected. In the transplant era, the importance of evaluating Mg levels has become more evident: they can be lowered by cyclosporine treatment (72).

Molybdenum (Mo) deficiency is extremely rare but one case of Mo deficiency was seen after 12 months' total parenteral nutrition, with tachycardia, central scotomas, and night blindness. Reduced activities of the Mo-dependent enzymes, sulphite oxidase, and xanthine oxidase, are found in a syndrome in which children have mental retardation, dislocation of the lenses in the eyes, and xanthinuria. Preliminary studies report that tetrathiomolybdate appears useful in the initial treatment of Wilson's disease patients with primarily neurologic symptoms and signs (73). The drug is able to bind excess Cu in nontoxic compounds within the liver and, more importantly, the brain.

Chromium (Cr) is a potent carcinogen of the lung and respiratory tract in the +6 oxidation state. The digestive tract and liver play a major role in detoxification, and Cr ingestion (5,000 µg) did not modify DNA cross-links in human leukocytes, either with Cr+6 or Cr3. A very large detoxifying capacity is therefore presumed to occur in the gastrointestinal tract and/or the liver *(74)*. Increased urinary Cr excretion has been found in patients on total parenteral nutrition, but it has never been found to have clinical consequences.

Deficiency is suspected if the concentrations of Cr cannot be measured using a reliable sensitive technique and the clinical situation suggests that inadequate intake is possible. Improved glucose tolerance in response to dietary supplements would be a qualitative indication of Cr deficiency, since Cr supports insulin function.

9. SUMMARY

The main functions of trace elements are briefly reviewed, and the physiological role of the gastrointestinal tract and liver in their homeostasis is considered. Impaired homeostasis may derive from a single disease (e.g., inflammatory bowel disease) or from a genetically determined defective metabolism. Whatever its cause, an altered response to inflammation, immune function, and infections will inevitably result. It should therefore be recognized that trace element abnormalities tend to involve the entire organism, of which the gastrointestinal tract is an integral part. It is now known that an adequate intake of trace elements is crucial to human health, and the importance of the pharmacological administration of certain trace elements in specific diseases is now widely accepted. The role of supplementation in prevention has wide potential applications although any intervention to reduce the risk of deficiency must not increase the risk of toxicity by creating imbalances between trace elements. The therapeutic role of supplementation, moreover, is still often unclear. Trace element supplementation is mandatory during total parenteral nutrition, although the quality and the quantity administered should be controlled, and tailored to each clinical case. Manganese supplementation may be contraindicated, especially in the presence of cholestasis. We can now measure more trace elements and different types of biological samples using new techniques, but we still lack reliable indices for establishing marginal deficiencies at an early stage. Above all, the occurrence of these deficiencies, and their effects, which are sometimes even clinically evident, should receive more clinical attention if they are to be appropriately corrected.

Important research studies are now underway to explore the influence of trace elements in the development of impaired immunity and cancer. Other opportunities will develop in molecular medicine and the identification of new genes for abnormal trace element metabolism.

REFERENCES

1. Rossetto L, Martin A, Montino MC, et al. Effect of citric acid (CA) and picolinic acid (PA) on zinc absorption in chronic pancreatitis (CP). In: Sturniolo GC, McClain CJ, Abdulla M, eds. Essential Trace Elements in gastroenterology and clinical medicine. Smith-Gordon and Nishimura 1991, pp.111–113.
2. Hempe JM, Cousins RJ. Cysteine rich intestinal protein binds zinc during transmucosal zinc transport. Proc Natl Acad Sci USA 1991;88:9671–9674.
3. Sturniolo GC, Montino MC, Rossetto L, et al. Inhibition of gastric acid secretion reduces zinc absorption in man. J Am Coll Nutr 1991;10:372-375.
4. Prasad AS, Rabbani P, Abbasi A, Bowerson F, Fox MRS. Experimental zinc deficiency in humans. Ann Intern Med 1978;89:483–490.
5. Sturniolo GC, Mastropaolo G, Gurrieri G. et al. Zinc metabolism is severely altered in chronic liver disease. Liver 1981;1(2):155.

6. Klasing KC. Effect of inflammatory agents and interleukin-1 on iron and zinc metabolism. Am J Physiol 1984;247:901–904.

7. Camps J, Bargallo T, Gimenez A, et al. Relationship between hepatic lipid peroxidation and fibrogenesis in carbon tetrachloride treated rats: effect of zinc administration. Clin Sci 1992;83:695–700.

8. Sullivan JF, Heaney RP. Zinc metabolism in alcoholic liver diseases. Am J Clin Nutr 1983;23:170–177.

9. Sturniolo GC, Mastropaolo G, Gurrieri G, Parisi G, Martin A, Naccarato R. Zinc metabolism is severely altered in chronic liver disease. Liver 1981;1:155.

10. Milman N, Laursen J, Podenphant J. et al. Trace elements in normal and cirrhotic human liver tissue: iron, copper, zinc, selenium, manganese, titanium and lead measured by x-ray fluorescence spectrophotometry. Liver 1986;6:11–17.

11. Sturniolo GC, D'Incà R, Parisi G. et al. Taste alterations in liver cirrhosis : are they related to zinc deficiency? J Tr Elem Electr Health Dis 1992;6:15-19.

12. Van Der Rijt C, Schalm S, Schat H. et al. Overt hepatic encephalopathy precipitated by zinc deficiency. Gastroenterology 1991;100:1114–1118.

13. Riggio O, Ariosto F, Merli M. et al. Short-term oral zinc supplementation does not improve chronic hepatic encephalopathy. Dig Dis Sci 1991;36(9):1204–1208.

14. Marchesini G, Fabbri A, Bianchi G. et al. Zinc supplementation and amino acid-nitrogen metabolism in patients with advanced cirrhosis. Hepatology 1996;23(5):1084–1092.

15. Brodersen HP, Holtkamp W, Larbig D. Zinc supplementation and hepatitis B vaccination in chronic haemodialysis patients: a multicentre study. Nephrol Dial Transplant 1995;10:1780–1783.

16. Brewer GJ, Yuzbasiyan-Gurkan VA, Young AB. Treatment of Wilson's disease. Sem Neurol 1987;7:209–220.

17. Pescovitz MD, Mehta PL, Jindal RM. et al. Zinc deficiency and its repletion following liver transplantation in humans. Clin Transplantation 1996;10:256–260.

18. Phillips J, Ackerley C, Superina R. et al. Excess zinc associated with severe progressive cholestasis in Cree and Ojibwa-Cree children. Lancet 1996;347:866–868.

19. Bandyopadhyay B. Bandyopadhyay S. Protective effect of zinc gluconate on chemically induced gastric ulcer. Indian J Med Res 1997;106:27-32.

20. Watanabe T, Arakawa T, Fukuda T. et al. Zinc deficiency delays gastric ulcer healing in rats. Dig Dis Sci 1995;40:1340–1344.

21. Rainsford KD, Goldie J, Hunt RH. Inhibition of the growth of Helicobacter pylori by zinc compounds. Proceedings of the 4th international meetings of the Inflammation Research Association, Hershey, PA, 1996, pp. 27–31.

22. Sazawal S. Zinc supplementation in young children with acute diarrhea in India. N Engl J Med 1995;333:839–843.

23. Alan AN. Enteric protein loss and intestinal permeability changes in children during acute shighellosis and after recovery: effect of zinc supplementation. Gut 1994;35:1707–1711.

24. Blanchard RK, Cousins RJ. Upregulation of rat intestinal uroguanylin m RNA by dietary zinc restriction. Am J Physiol 1997;272:G972–G978.

25. Sturniolo GC, Martin A, Mastropaolo G. et al. Zinc absorption in cirrhosis and chronic inflammatory bowel disease. In: Histidine II-Laboratory and Clinical Aspects.Therapeutic Use of Histidine and Zinc. Third International Workshop, 1982,pp.119–128.

26. Sturniolo GC, Mestriner C, Lecis PE. et al Altered plasma and mucosal concentrations of trace elements and antioxidants in active ulcerative colitis. Scand J Gastroenterol 1998;33:644–649.

27. Fabris C, Farini R, Del Favero G, et al. Copper, zinc and copper-zinc ratio in chronic pancreatitis and pancreatic cancer. Clin Biochem 1985;18:373–375.

28. Linder M, Hazegh-Azam M. Copper biochemistry and molecular biology. Am J Clin Nutr 1996;63:797S–811S.

29. Schilsky M. Wilson disease : genetic basis of copper toxicity and natural history. Seminars Liver Disease 1996;16:83–95.

30. Rossaro L, Sturniolo GC, Giacon G. et al. Zinc therapy in Wilson's diseae : observations in five patients. Am J Gastroenterol 1990;85:665–668.

31. Yuzbasiyan-Gurkan V, Grider A, Nostrants T. et al. Treatment of Wilson's disease with zinc : X intestinal metallothionein induction. J Lab Clin Nutr 1992;120:380–386.

32. Hunziker PE, Sternlieb I. Copper metallothionein in patients with hepatic copper overload. Europ J Clin Invest 1991;21:466–471.

33. Farinati F, Cardin R, Mestriner C. et al. Mechanism of penicillamine and zinc in the treatment of Wilson's disease. Am J Gastroenterol 1995;90:2264–2265.
34. Harris ZL, Gitlin JD. Genetic and molecular basis for copper toxicity. Am J Clin Nutr 1996;63:836S–841S.
35. Tanner MS, Portmann B, Mowat AP. et al. Increased hepatic copper concentration in Indian childhood cirrhosis. Lancet 1979;i,:1203–1205.
36. Muller T, Feichtinger H. et al. Endemic Tyrolean infantile cirrhosis : an ecogenetic disorder. Lancet 1996;347:877–880.
37. Gross IB, Ludwig J, Wiesner RH. et al. Abnormalities in test of copper metabolism in primary sclerosing cholangitis. Gastroenterology 1985;89:282–285.
38. Fernandez-Banares F, Mingorance MD, Esteve M. et al. Serum zinc, copper and selenium levels in inflammatory bowel disease : effect of total enteral nutrition on trace element status. Am J Gastroenterol 1985;12:1584–1589.
39. Braganza JM, Klass HJ, Bell M, Sturniolo GC. Evidence of altered copper metabolism in patients with chronic pancreatitis. Clin Sci 1981;60:303–310.
40. Per Stal. Iron as a hepatotoxin. Dig Dis 1995;13:205–222.
41. Bonkovsky H, Ponka P, Bacon B. et al. An update on iron metabolism: summary of the fifth international conference on disorders of iron metabolism. Hepatology 1996;24:718–729.
42. Fargion S, Mandelli C, Piperno A, et al. Survival and prognostic factors in 212 Italian patients with genetic hemochromatosis. Hepatology 1992;15:655–659.
43. Nelson RL, Davis FG, Persky V, Becker E. Risk of neoplastic and other diseases among people with heterozygosity for hereditary hemochromatosis. Cancer 1995;76:875–897.
44. Conte D, Manachino D, Colli A. et al. Prevalence of genetic hemochromatosis in a cohort of Italian patients with diabetes mellitus. Ann Intern Med 1998;128(5):370–373.
45. Gordeuk V, Mukiibi J, Hasstedt SJ. et al. Iron overload in Africa. Interaction between a gene and dietary iron content. N Engl J Med 1992;326:95–100.
46. Riggio O, Montagnese F, Fiore P. et al. Iron overload in patients with chronic viral hepatitis: how common is it? Am J Gastroenterol 1997;92:1298–1301.
47. Kato J, Kobune M, Kohgo Y. et al. Hepatic iron deprivation prevents spontaneous development of fulminant hepatitis and liver cancer in Long-Evans Cinnamon rats. J Clin Invest 1996;98:923–929.
48. Keyou GE, Guangqi Y. The epidemiology of selenium deficiency in the etiological study of endemic diseases in China. Am J Clin Nutr 1993;57:259S–263S.
49. Blot W, Li JY, Taylor PR. et al. Nutrition intervention trials in Linxian, China: supplementation with specific vitamin/mineral combinations, cancer incidence and disease-specific mortality in the general population. J Natl Cancer Inst 1993;85:1483–1492.
50. Li Y, Taylor PR, Dawsey S. et al. Nutrition intervention trials in Linxian, China: multiple vitamin/mineral supplementation, cancer incidence and disease-specific mortality among adults with esophageal dysplasia. J Natl Cancer Inst 1993;85:1492–1498.
51. Combs GF, Clark LC, Turnbull BW. Reduction of cancer risk with an oral supplement of selenium. Biomed Environ Sci 1997;10:227–234.
52. Zhang L, Blot W, You W-C. et al. Serum micronutrients in relation to pre-cancerous gastric lesions. Int J Cancer 1994;56:650–654.
53. Wu CW, Wei YY, Chi CW, et al. Tissue potassium, selenium and iron levels associated with gastric cancer progression. Dig Dis Sci 1996;41:119–125.
54. Nelson R, Davis F, Sutter E, et al. Serum selenium and colonic neoplastic risk. Dis Colon Rectum 1995;38:1306–1310.
55. Russo MW, Murray SC, Wurzelmann JI, Woosley JT, Sandler RS. Plasma selenium levels and the risk of colorectal adenomas. Nutr Cancer 1997;28:125–129.
56. Mulder TPJ, Verspaget HW, Janssens AR, et al. Decrease in two intestinal copper-zinc containing proteins with antioxidant function in inflammatory bowel disease. Gut 1991;32:1146–1150.
57. Ringstad J, Kildebo S, Thomassen Y. Serum selenium, copper and zinc concentrations in Crohn's disease and ulcerative colitis. Scand J Gastroenterol 1993;28:605–608.
58. Van Gossum A, Closset P, Noel E. et al. Deficiency in antioxidant factors in patients with alcohol-related chronic pancreatitis. Dig Dis Sci 1996;41:1225–1231.
59. Kleibeuker JH, Welberg JWM, Mulsder NH, et al. Epithelial cell proliferation in the human sigmoid colon of patients with adenomatous polyps increases during oral calcium supplementation. Br J Cancer 1994;67:500–503.

60. Neugut AI, Horvath K, Whelan RL. et al. The effect of calcium and vitamin suppplements on the incidence and recurrence of colorectal adenomatous polyps. Cancer 1996;78:723–728.

61. Duris I, Hruby B, Pekarkova M, et al. Calcium chemoprevention in colorectal cancer. Hepato-gastroenterology 1996;43:152–154.

62. Seow-Choen F, Vijayan V. Keng V. Prospective randomized study of Sulindac versus calcium and calciferol for upper gastrointestinal polyps in familial adenomatous polyposis. Br J Surg 1996;83:1763–1766.

63. Bostick RM, Boldt M, Darif M, et al. Calcium and colorectal epithelial cell proliferation in ulcerative colitis. Cancer Epidemiol Biomarkers Prev 1997;6:1021–1027.

64. Kleibeuker JH, Cats A, van den Meer R. et al. Calcium supplementation as prophylaxis against colon cancer. Dig Dis 1994;12:85-97.

65. Krieger D, Krieger S, Jansen O. et al. Manganese and chronic hepatic encephalopathy. Lancet 1995;346:270–274.

66. Butterworth RF, Spahr L, Fontaine S. et al. Manganese toxicity, dopaminergic dysfunction and hepatic encephalopathy. Metab Brain Dis 1995;10:259–267.

67. Aida Y, Maeyama S, Takakuwa T. et al. Immunohistochemical expression of manganese superoxide dismutase in hepatocellular carcinoma, using a specific monoclonal antibody. J Gastroenterology 1994;29:443–449.

68. Izutani R, Katoh M, Asano S. et al. Enhanced expression of manganese superoxide dismutase mRNA and increased TNFa mRNA expression by gastric mucosa in gastric cancer. World J Surg 1996;20:228–233.

69. Fell JME, Reynolds AP, Meadows N, et al. Manganese toxicity in children receiving long-term parenteral nutrition. Lancet 1996;347:1218–1221.

70. Beath SV, Gopalan S. Booth IW. Manganese toxicity and parenteral nutrition. Lancet 1996;347:1773.

71. Dreosti IE. Magnesium status and health. Nutr Rev 1995;53:S23–S27.

72. Kulpmann WR, Robler J, Brunkhorst R. Schuler A. Ionized and total magnesium serum concentrations in renal and hepatic diseases. Eur J Clin Chem Clin Biochem 1996;34:257–264.

73. Brewer GJ, Johnson V, Dick RD, Kluin KJ, Fink JK, Brunberg JA. Treatment of Wilson disease with ammonium tetrathiomolybdatc. II. Initial therapy in 33 neurologically affected patients and follow up with zinc therapy. Arch Neurol 1996;53:1017–1025.

74. Kuykendall JR, Kerger BD, Jarvi EJ, Corbett GE, Paustenbach DJ. Measurement of DNA-protein cross-links in human leukocytes following acute ingestion of chromium in drinking water. Carcinogenesis 1996;17.1971–1977.

18 Immune Dysfunction in Iron, Copper, and Zinc Deficiencies

Adria R. Sherman, PhD

1. INTRODUCTION

1.1. Overview of the Immune Response

The immune response is comprised of a complex, interactive system of cells, structures, and secretory products which protect the host against invasive organisms, their toxic products, and other harmful chemical and biological substances. Unique among bodily systems, the immune system has no central organ of control. Immune response to "foreignness" is brought about by interactions of the lymphoid organs, approximately 1% of the body's 100 trillion cells which are white blood cells, and the secretory products of these cells and organs. Working together these processes mount both systemic and localized assaults on the invading organism or foreign substance. Often, a healthy individual's immune responses function efficiently killing off pathogens without symptoms of significant illness.

The skin is the most exterior component of host defense forming a barrier to penetration by foreign organisms and chemicals. The skin's barrier is less effective at body openings, which are constantly exposed to the external milieu of microorganisms and are vulnerable to invasion. The external secretory immunity response protects body orifices and is considered the first line of defense. Secretions from mucosal surfaces of the eyes, nasopharyngeal cavity, mouth, respiratory tract, gastrointestinal tract, genitourinary tract, and mammary glands contain powerful bactericidal substances which prevent entry of foreign compounds into the body. Should a foreign organism or chemical gain entry, an elaborate array of defenses of both nonspecific and specific immunity are called into action.

Nonspecific immunity includes the skin, mucosal factors, the complement system of proteins, and various circulating bactericidal scavenger cells. Recognition of a particular antigen is not required by the non-specific immune components. Specific immunity includes a variety of cellular and noncellular processes which require recognition of foreign antigens, are specific in their interaction with the antigen and have a memory of past antigenic exposure. The major effector proteins for specific immunity are antibodies or immunoglobulins produced by cloned plasma cells derived from mature B lymphocytes. Antibodies are produced specific for each antigen and comprise the major component of humoral immunity. Highly specialized classes of phagocytes, T lymphocytes, and B lymphocytes participate in the cell-mediated branch of specific immunity. Each of these

From: *Clinical Nutrition of the Essential Trace Elements and Minerals: The Guide for Health Professionals*
Edited by: J. D. Bogden and L. M. Klevay © Humana Press Inc., Totowa, NJ

components of immunity performs individual roles, but act in concert in a highly orchestrated, self-regulated manner.

1.2. Influences on Immunocompetence

Considering the complexity of the immune responses it is not surprising that it is sensitive to many internal and external influences. Indeed, there are multiple points where the processes can and do go awry. Genetic, physiological, hormonal, environmental, and developmental characteristics of the host are among the factors which influence immunity. A major environmental factor is nutrition. Although it has been appreciated for decades that protein energy malnutrition devastates immunity, only recently has attention been directed toward the trace elements and immunity. Iron, zinc, and copper have been studied the most thoroughly. Three decades of research in clinical and experimental settings has resulted in detailed descriptions of the effects of trace element deficiencies on components of the immune response. Some scant literature on overloads of these minerals is also available. However, at the end of the 20th century, our understanding of the mechanisms of action of these trace elements in immunity is rudimentary at best.

1.3. The Integrated Immune Response

To appreciate the many potential roles that trace elements might play in immunity, let us consider the events, cells, organs, and compounds of the integrated immune response. Once a foreign antigen does enter the body, contact is made with macrophages in lymphoid tissue. Phagocytic in action, the macrophage cell has the ability to consume antigen and display the antigen molecule on its surface. Released into circulation, the antigen-displaying macrophage attracts the attention of helper T cells which have receptors for that specific antigen. Among millions of helper T cells, those with the antigen specific receptor bind to the macrophages and become excited. These stimulated helper T cells in turn stimulate other T cells in the thymus to mature, under the influence of thymic hormone. Armies of stimulated helper T cells move toward spleen and bone marrow to activate B cells. Meanwhile in the thymus, additional helper T cells proliferate and are released into circulation along with killer T cells. The killer T cells begin to consume antigen as well. Activated helper T cells targeted at the bone marrow and spleen stimulate the activation and release of B cells which clone into plasma cells. The plasma cells secrete antibody capable of immobilizing the antigen. The orchestrated effects of cell-mediated (T cells and macrophages) and humoral (B cells) activities combine to destroy and consume invading foreign antigen. Once the killing has resulted in removal of the antigen, suppressor T cells are released from thymus and inhibit the processes and cellular activities involved in killing. Memory T and memory B cells, which are capable of initiating a rapid response during future encounters with the same antigen, remain in circulation and in lymphoid tissue. These processes are regulated and modulated by several hormones and by cytokines produced by immune cells.

1.4. Role of Trace Elements in Immunity

Whether taken as a whole, integrated process, or examined by individual components, the immune response reveals a myriad of potential functions in which trace elements might take part. In the prenatal and neonatal periods, nutritional status can influence the differentiation of cells and anatomic development of lymphoid tissues. Mucous production by the external secretory immune system needs an adequate nutrient supply.

Malnutrition almost always influences the ability to maintain healthy protective skin. The constant synthesis of hundreds of immunologically active proteins requires the presence of nutrients involved in protein synthesis and gene expression. Unimpaired and rapid cellular proliferation is an absolute requirement for a fully functional immune response. Any deficits in nutrients involved in cell division or differentiation will have a profound impact on immune cells. As described above, multiple cell types with numerous movements and secretions are needed to mount an effective immune response. Trace element deficits would be expected to have an obvious impact in these processes. The biochemical reactions involved in killing of microorganisms might require trace element cofactors. One can also postulate that the efficient processes of modulation and regulation of immunity which keep it in check might also involve direct or indirect participation of trace elements.

2. IRON

2.1. Increased Morbidity Seen in Iron Deficient Populations

Earliest indications that iron is involved in immunity came from field studies associating increased morbidity with iron deficiency anemia which is very prevalent in developing and developed countries worldwide (Table 1) (*see* Chapter 6). Infancy and early childhood is a period during which immunity is still developing and in which iron deficiency is common. In 1928 Mackay *(1)* first reported that infants given iron supplements had 50% fewer respiratory and gastrointestinal tract infections than unsupplemented infants. Later, Andleman and Sered *(2)* found that infants fed iron fortified formula experienced a lower incidence of both anemia and respiratory infections compared with infants fed unfortified evaporated milk with less iron. Although these and subsequent studies *(3–6)* relating iron deficiency anemia in infancy to increased morbidity are subject to criticisms based on subject number and selection, data collection methods, and statistical interpretations, taken together there is a body of literature supporting the conclusion that iron deficiency, severe enough to be diagnosed as anemia, is associated with significant morbidity during infancy. Contradicting this is a smaller body of literature reporting either no alteration of morbidity in iron supplemented infants *(7)* or an increase in neonatal sepsis in infants injected with a large dose of iron at birth *(8)*. Adding further confusion to the story, repletion of severely iron deficient subjects is sometimes accompanied by increased morbidity *(9–11)*.

2.2. Experimental Iron Deficiency Increases Infectious Morbiity in Rodents

In order to avoid confounding variables inherent to field studies such as intercurrent infections, multiple nutritional deficiencies, and psychosocial factors, rodents have been used to study the effects of uncomplicated iron deficiency on susceptibility to infection. Rats fed iron-deficient diets are significantly more susceptible to Salmonella typhimurium *(12)* and Streptococcus pneumonia *(13)* than are control rats. Parasitic infestation, prevalent in developing countries, is a common cause of iron deficiency anemia. Since dietary iron deficiency often coexists in the same individuals, it is possible that iron deficiency potentiates infestation. Host response to the intestinal parasite Nippostrongylus brasiliensis has been tested in rats made iron deficient through diet. In a series of experiments Brolin et al. *(14)* and Duncombe et al. *(15)* showed that iron deficiency produced a delay in worm expulsion which was reversed with iron repletion. Iron sufficient rats show a strong acquired resistance to infestation when infected a second time after antihelmintic treatment. Iron deficiency prevented this protective immunity.

Table 1
Effects of Deficiencies in Iron, Copper and Zinc on Measures of Disease Resistance

	Iron Deficiency	*Copper Deficiency*	*Zinc Deficiency*
Morbidity	**Increased in Humans** MacKay; 1928 (1) James & Combes; 1960 (3) Andelman & Sered; 1966 (2) Fuerth; 1971 (4) Cantwell; 1972 (5) Burman; 1972 (7) Oppenheimer; 1980 (6)	**Increased in Humans** Castillo-Duran, et al.; 1983 (45) Goyens, et al.; 1985 (139 Prohaska & Lukasewycz; 1990 (43) **Increased in Domestic Animals** Pletcher & Banting; 1983 (46) Suttle & Jones; 1986 (47)	**Increased in Humans** Prasad, et al.; 1963 (73) Moynahan & Barnes; 1973 (74)) Duchateau, et al.; 1981 (77) Wagner, et al.; 1983 (78) Hambidge, et al.; 1986 (75) Lockitch, et al.; 1987 (76) Bogden, et al.; 1988 (79)
Protection from Morbidity	Masawe, et al.; 1974 (11) Murray, et al.; 1975 (9) Murray, et al.; 1978 (10) Barry & Reeve; 1977 (8)		
Response to Infection	**Decreased In Rodents** Baggs & Miller; 1973 (12) Chu, et al.; 1976 (13) Brolin, et al.; 1977 (14) Duncombe, et al.; 1979 (15)	**Decreased in Rodents** Newberne, et al.; 1968 (48) Jones & Suttle.; 1983 (49) **Decreased in Domestic Animals** Stabel & Spears; 1989 (50)	**Decreased in Rodents** Pekarek, et al.; 1977 (80) Fraker, et al.; 1982 (81) Lee, et al.; 1983 (82) Salvin & Rabin; 1984 (83) Fraker, et al.; 1987 (84)

Reference number shown in parentheses.

312

2.3. Effects of Iron Status on Components of Immunity

Nutritional immunology has developed as a field of scientific inquiry during the past two decades. During this time and at present efforts have been directed toward identifying which components of immune responsiveness are altered by iron deficiency. Animal models and human clinical studies have been used to characterize specific defects in immunity present in the iron deficient state.

2.3.1. HUMORAL RESPONSES

Humoral immunity (Table 2) was initially thought to be protected during iron deficiency. Serum immunoglobulins were reported to be preserved in iron deficient children (16–19) and adults (20). One limitation of using serum immunoglobulin level as an indicator of humoral response is that it reflects past exposure more than present immunocompetence. This is an unavoidable, but severe limitation, which led to the erroneous conclusion that humoral immunity is not altered in iron deficient humans. However, lower serum immunoglobulin levels were found in iron deficient rats where environmental conditions were carefully controlled and dietary iron was the only variable. Nalder et al. (21) measured blood antibody following serial tetanus toxoid immunizations in rats with varying degrees of iron deficiency. Antibody titer decreased as the level of dietary iron decreased. Sheep red blood cells have been used as an antigenic challenge in rodents to study humoral responses mounted in the spleen. Kuvibidila et al. (22) found that iron deficient mice had a lowered IgM and IgG response, and lowered splenic T and B lymphocytes after challenge with sheep red blood cells.

Adequate iron status has been shown to be critical to the development of immunity during the intrauterine and neonatal period of life. Using the sheep red blood cell challenge to measure humoral response, Kochanowski & Sherman (23) found that splenic production of IgG and IgM were reduced by 50% in pups born and suckled by iron deficient dams. Importantly, repletion of the iron deficient pups after weaning did not restore antibody production to control levels. Interestingly plasma immunoglobulin levels were normal in iron deficient rats. Severe and moderate iron deficiency established after weaning, during another rapid growth phase, also impairs splenic IgM and IgG production and plasma IgM levels following antigenic challenge (24). The sheep red blood cell challenge assay allows highly sensitive measurement of immunoglobulin production by individual splenocytes. This may explain the apparent discrepancy in results of humoral immunity in humans versus the animal models. Serum immunoglobulin levels are not nearly as sensitive or timely as direct measures of antibody production to a specific antigen.

2.3.2. CELL MEDIATED RESPONSES

The earliest indication that cell mediated immunity (Table 3) is compromised in iron deficiency came from reports that the number or percentage of circulating T cells, derived from the thymus, is lower in iron deficient children (19,25). Animal models were useful in establishing that iron deficiency early in life results in morphological abnormalities in lymphoid tissues where the cells involved in cell mediated immunity differentiate and proliferate. Intrauterine and neonatal iron restriction in rat pups leads not only to smaller thymus and spleen mass, but 50% reductions in lymphopoietic areas of these immunologically vital organs (25). Further studies using the rat model of iron deficiency in early life reveal that maternal iron deficiency during reproduction alters cellular growth in rapidly dividing organs in the offspring. Smaller spleen and thymus size and at least a

Table 2
Effects of Deficiencies of Iron, Copper, and Zinc on Humoral Immunity

	Iron Deficiency	Copper Deficiency	Zinc Deficiency
Circulating Immmunoglobulins	**No Change or Increased in Humans** Chandra; 1975 (16) Macdougall, et al.; 1975 (17) Sawitsky, et al.; 1976 (20) Bagchi, et al.; 1980 (18) Krantman, et al.; 1982 (19) **Decreased in Rodents** Nalder, et al.; 1972 (21) **Increased in Rodents** Sherman; 1984 (140)	**Decreased in Rodents** Prohaska & Lukasewycz; 1989b (54)	**Distorted in Rodents** Beach, et al.; 1982 (89)
Antibody Production	**Decreased in Rodents** Nalder, et al.; 1972 (21) Kuvibidila, et al.; 1982 (22) Kochanowski & Sherman; 1985a (23) Kochanowski & Sherman; 1985b (27) Sherman; 1990 (24) Prohaska & Lukasewycz; 1989a (53) Prohaska & Lukasewycz; 1989b (54) Prohaska & Lukasewycz; 1990 (43) Lukasewycz & Prohaska; 1990 (69)	**Decreased in Rodents** Prohaska & Lukasewycz; 1981 (51) Lukasewycz & Prohaska; 1982 (68) Vyas & Chandra; 1983 (55) Kishore, et al.; 1984 (57) Blakely & Hamilton; 1987 (52) Eason, et al.; 1988 (58) Failla, et al.; 1988 (56)	**Decreased in Humans** Oleske, et al.; 1979 (91) Antilla, et al.; 1986 (90) **Decreased in Rodents** Fraker, et al.; 1977 (84) Zwickl & Fraker; 1980 (88) Jardieu & Fraker; 1990 (87) King & Fraker; 1991 (85)
Secretory Immunity	**Unchanged in Rodents** Kochanowski & Sherman; 1982a (26)		

314

Table 3
Effects of Deficiencies of Iron, Copper and Zinc on Cell Mediated Immune Responses

	Iron Deficiency	Copper Deficiency	Zinc Deficiency
Circulating T Cells	**Decreased in Humans** Chandra; 1975 (16) Krantman, et al.; 1982 (19)		**In Rodents** Fraker, et al.; 1977 (86) Fraker, et al.; 1978 (92) Fraker, et al.; 1986 (93)
Morphological Abnormalities in Lymphoid Tissues	**In Rodents** Rothenbacher & Sherman; 1980 (25) Kochanowski & Sherman; 1982b (141) Kochanowski & Sherman; 1985a (23) Mulhern & Koller; 1988 (61) Lukasewycz & Prohaska; 1990 (69)	**In Rodents** Prohaska, et al.; 1983 (60) Koller, et al.; 1987 (59) Failla, et al.; 1988 (56) King & Fraker; 1991 (85) **In Humans** Smythe, et al.; 1971 (94) Golden, et al.; 1977 (44)	
Lymphocyte Subsets	**Decreased in Rodents** Helyar & Sherman; 1992 (28)	**Decreased in Rodents** Lukasewycz, et al.; 1985 (62) Mulhern & Koller; 1988 (61) Bala, et al.; 1990 (142) Bala, et al.; 1991 (63)	
Lymphocyte Proliferation Response	**Decreased in Humans** Joynson, et al.; 1972 (29) Chandra & Saraya; 1975 (30) MacDougall, et al.; 1975 (17) Kielman, et al.; 1976 (31) **Increased in Humans** Suskind, et al.; 1977 (32) **Unchanged in Humans** Kulapongs, et al.; 1974 (33) Krantman, et al.; 1982 (19) **Decreased in Rodents** Kuvibidila, et al.; 1983 (**34**)	**Decreased in Humans** Smith. et al.; 1994 (66) **Decreased in Rodents** Lukasewycz & Prohaska; 1983 (64) Lukasewycz, et al.; 1985 (62) Blakely & Hamilton; 1987 (52) Kramer, et al.; 1988 (65) Mulhern & Koller; 1988 (61) Prohaska & Lukasewycz; 1989a (53) Prohaska & Lukasewycz; 1990 (43) Bala, et al.; 1991a (63)	**Decreased in Humans** Allen, et al.; 1981 (97) Moynahan & Barnes; 1973 (74) Bogden, et al.; 1988 (79) Chandra; 1989 (143) **No Change in Rodents** Dowd, et al.; 1986 (95) Cook-Mills & Fraker; 1993 (96)

Table 3 (cont.)
Effects of Deficiencies of Iron, Copper and Zinc on Cell Mediated Immune Responses

	Iron Deficiency	Copper Deficiency	Zinc Deficiency
Hypersensitivity Response	**Decreased in Humans** Chandra & Saraya; 1975 (30) Krantman, et al.; 1982 (19) **Decreased in Rodents** Omara & Blakely; 1994 (35) Koller, et al.; 1987 (59)	**Decreased in Rodents** Kishore, et al.; 1984 (57) **Increased in Rodents** Jones; 1984 (67) **No Change in Rodents** Fraker, et al.; 1986 (93)	**Decreased in Humans** Ballester & Prasad; 1983 (99) Bogden, et al.; 1987 (98)
Phagocyte Functon	**Decreased in Humans** MacDougall, et al.; 1975 (17) Chandra; 1975 (16) Kochanowski & Sherman; 1984 (36)	**Decreased in Rodents** Newberne, et al.; 1968 (48) Lukasewycz & Prohaska; 1982 (68) Lukasewycz & Prohaska; 1990 (69) Babu & Failla; 1990 (70) **Decreased in Domestic Animals** Jones & Suttle; 1981 (71) Boyne & Arthur; 1981 (72)	**Decreased in Rodents** Fraker, et al.; 1986 (93) **Decreased in Humans** Weston, et al.; 1977 (101) Chandra & Dayton; 1982 (100) **Increased in Humans** Allen, et al.; 1983 (102)
Natural Killer Cell Cytotoxicity	**Decreased in Rodents** Sherman & Lockwood; 1987 (37) Lockwood & Sherman; 1988 (38) Hallquist & Sherman; 1989 (40) Hallquist, et al.; 1992 (39) Spear & Sherman; 1992 (41) Hrabinski, et al.; 1995 (42) **No Change in Rodents** Helyar & Sherman, 1993 (144)	**Decreased in Rodents** Koller, et al.; 1987 (59) **Decreased in Rodents** Babu & Failla; 1990 (70)	**Decreased in Rodents** Fernandes, et al.; 1979 (103) Fraker, et al.; 1986 (93) **Increased in Rodents** Chandra & Au; 1980 (104) **Decreased in Humans** Tapazoylou, et al.; 1985 (105)
Macrophage Function	**Decreased in Rodents** Hallquist, et al.; 1992 (39)	**Decreased in Rodents** Babu & Failla; 1990 (70)	**Decreased in Rodents** Wirth, et al.; 1989 (145) **No change in Rodents** Wirth, et al.; 1984 (107)

30% reduction in cellularity, as indicated by spleen DNA content, has been found in pups of iron deficient rats (26). By changing the diet fed to dams postpartum, Kochanowski and Sherman (27) showed that reductions in lymphoid tissue cellularity occurred in pups only if the iron-deficient diet was fed during both pregnancy and lactation. Iron repletion of offspring post weaning did not correct the reductions in thymic cellularity. Splenic cell number increased with repletion but did not achieve levels found in animals fed iron adequate diets throughout life. Taken together these data indicate that iron deficiency during critical periods of development of immune responses leads to profound morphological abnormalities and suggests that "catch up" growth may not repair structural defects. These animal studies suggest that immunodeficiency due to iron deficiency early in life may be permanent.

Adequate iron status is also required for the young animal to establish the appropriate distribution of lymphocyte subsets in the spleen. Both severe and moderate iron deficiencies established after weaning result in altered populations of spleen lymphocyte subsets (28). Percentage of T-lymphocytes in spleen is lowest in severely iron deficient mice, intermediate in moderate iron deficiency, and highest in the controls. Percentages of helper/inducer T, cytotoxic/suppressor T, and B lymphocytes follow the same pattern. The surface markers which are measured by flow cytometry to identify these subsets stained positively in cells from all diet groups. These markers are associated with differentiation and function. This suggests that iron deficiency alters the quantity and percentage of the lymphocyte subsets but not the functionality of the cells.

Lymphocyte proliferation assays are functional measures of cell mediated immunity in which peripheral lymphocytes are harvested from blood and stimulated to divide in vitro with mitogens. Labeled thymidine incorporated into DNA is usually measured in stimulated and resting lymphocytes. Using this approach in the 1970s a number of investigators found that lymphocytes from iron deficient children proliferated less when stimulated in vitro (16,17,29,30,31). Three researchers report otherwise. Suskind et al. (32) reported increased proliferative responses in iron deficiency. Children studied by Krantman (19) and Kulapongs et al. (33) had normal proliferative responses. These disparate findings are most likely due to confounding variables such as intercurrent illness, small number of subjects, and assay conditions. Avoiding these variables, Kuvibidila et al. (34) established that uncomplicated iron deficiency in mice reduces in vitro lymphocyte proliferation.

A direct functional measure of cell mediated immunity is the delayed cutaneous hypersensitivity response. Since this technique measures the inflammatory responses to a skin test antigen in vivo, the criticisms often raised about in vitro measures are avoided. Iron deficient children have been found to respond less vigorously to cutaneous test antigens than well nourished children (19,30). Omara and Blakley (35) confirm that iron deficiency impairs the delayed hypersensitivity reaction in rodents.

Phagocytosis of invading bacteria by neutrophils is a component of nonspecific immunity which does not require recognition of a specific antigen. In vitro measures of phagocytosis include measurement of bactericidal activity and measurement of metabolites produced by the killing process. These measurements, made on small blood samples, are useful in both human subjects and animal models. In iron deficient children (16,17) and rat pups (36) lowered phagocytosis has been found.

Natural killer (NK) cells are large granular lymphocytes derived from bone marrow and found in spleen, lymph nodes, peripheral blood, and peritoneum. Without previous antigenic exposure, NK cells function in surveillance against virally infected cells and cancer cells. In the unstimulated host, NK cell level is low. NK cells proliferate in response to viral, chemical, and cellular agents and are cytotoxic. The effects of iron deficiency on NK cell cytotoxicity have been explored in a series of studies by Sherman and coworkers. Rat pups born and suckled by iron deficient dams and given a viral challenge had NK cytotoxicity less than half that of control rats *(37)*. In response to viral or chemical challenges, interferon stimulates the activity of NK cells. Using the neonatal rat model for iron deficiency, NK cells were harvested and stimulated with exogenous interferon in vitro *(38)*. As expected interferon treatment in vitro increased NK cytotoxicity in virally challenged control rat pups. Whereas both moderate and severe iron deficiency impaired NK cytotoxicity compared to that found in control rats, NK cells from moderately deficient rats were able to be stimulated to a small extent by interferon. In the severely iron deficient rat pups, NK cells did not significantly respond to interferon stimulation. Lowered cytotoxicity has also been found in peritoneal NK cells from iron deficient rat pups *(39)*.

Iron deficiency established in the rapid growth phase after weaning also leads to lowered NK activity in spleen *(40)*. Macrophage cells were isolated from spleens and treated in vitro to produce interferon which was subsequently added to NK cell preparations. NK cells from iron deficient rats responded with increased cytotoxicity, but still failed to achieve levels as high as those from control rats. Treatment of the NK cell preparation with anti-rat interferon antibody had the greatest effect on control cells suggesting that in iron deficiency interferon production by macrophages is lowered. Syngeneic B cells from iron deficient rats were able to compensate somewhat for the apparent lack of interferon action on NK cells. Whether the defect in NK cytotoxicity is due to less active or reactive cells or due to fewer NK cells is not known at present. However, Helyar and Sherman *(28)* have found that the percentage of null cells in spleen lymphocytes from iron deficient mice is higher than that of control mice. This population of null cells, not expressing lymphocyte surface antigens, includes NK cells. This indirect evidence suggests that the relative number of NK cells is not decreased by iron deficiency.

The compromised NK activity of iron deficiency leads to defects in the surveillance for cancer cells. Moderate iron deficiency established after weaning lowered blood hemoglobin by 14% and resulted in lower NK cytotoxicity and a greater tumor burden and incidence of DMBA induced mammary tumors in rats *(41,42)*.

As described above, macrophages function early in the immune response consuming and displaying antigen. Macrophage cytotoxicity also contributes to cell mediated actions against a variety of targets including cancer cells. Peritoneal macrophage cytotoxicity against mouse lymphoma cell targets is lowered significantly by both severe and moderate iron deficiencies *(39)*.

3. COPPER

3.1. Copper Deficient Humans and Experimental Animals Experience High Morbidity

Although dietary copper deficiency is rare in human genetic diseases, other clinical situations do lead to copper deficiencies (Table 1). Individuals with X-linked Menkes' Disease suffer from copper deficiency (*see* Chapter 12). Frequent morbidity and lethal bronchopneumonia have been reported in 29 separate reports over a 20 yr period. Prohaska and Lukasewycz *(43)* provide a critical summary of these reports. Additional evidence that copper deficiency leads to increased infectious diseases is provided by reports of infants developing copper deficiency due to clinical situations such as celiac disease *(44)* and marasmus *(45)*. Domestic animals raised on copper deficient feeds also experience increased infections *(46,47)*.

3.2. Dietary Copper Restriction Leads to Decreased Resistance to Infection

Rodents *(48,49)* and cows *(50)* with copper deficiency have little resistance to bacterial and viral challenges.

3.3. Effects of Copper Status on Components of Immunity

Specific components of the immune response have been studied during the past two decades using copper deficient animal models and cell culture methods.

3.3.1. HUMORAL RESPONSES

Antibody production (Table 2) by splenocytes following challenge with sheep red blood cells, a T-cell dependent antigen, has been reported to be decreased in experimental copper deficiency in mice *(51–54)*. Postpartum and post weaning copper deficiency in mice has a major impact on antibody production *(54)*. Sheep red blood cell challenges to copper deficient rats also result in lowered antibody response compared to control rats *(55,56)*. Copper deficient rats and mice given a variety of other antigens also fail to mount a vigorous humoral response *(57,58)*. Serum immunoglobulins have also been found to be lower in copper deficient animals *(54,58)*.

3.3.2. CELL MEDIATED RESPONSES

The gross appearance and morphology of lymphoid tissues are abnormal in experimental copper deficiency (Table 3). Splenomegaly and small thymus are typically observed in copper deficient rodents *(43,54,56,59)*. Histological examination of spleen and thymus from copper deficient mice showed lymphocytes with enlarged mitochondria and abnormally shaped nuclei *(60)*. The thymic cortex *(61)* and medulla *(59)* are both abnormal in copper deficiency. Thymic hypoplasia in copper deficient mice is reversed after only 2 wk of copper repletion *(43)*.

The presence of surface antigens on splenic mononuclear cells has been used to determine the effects of copper deficiency on lymphocyte subsets. Studies by several groups confirm that copper deficiency lowers the relative number of splenic T lymphocytes, helper T cells, and cytotoxic T cells in mice *(61,62)* and rats *(63)*. In contrast, relative numbers of B lymphocytes in spleen were found to be higher *(62)* or unchanged *(61)* in mice and higher *(63)* in rats with copper deficiency.

There is evidence that cell mediated immunity, as measured by in vitro lymphocyte proliferation assays, is diminished by experimental copper deficiency. Lukasewycz and Prohaska *(64)* used a mouse model in which copper deficiency was instituted at birth to show that mitogen induced proliferation of T cells and B cells is diminished. Depressed lymphocyte proliferation in copper deficiency in rats is also reported by Kramer et al. *(65)* and Bala et al. *(63)*. However, murine studies by Blakely and Hamilton *(52)* with post weaning copper deficiency in females and by Prohaska and Lukasewycz *(53)* in males showed normal response of lymphocytes to mitogenic stimulation. Drawing a firm conclusion from these data is further complicated by evidence that unstimulated lymphocyte proliferation *(43,61,62)* and spontaneous DNA synthesis *(61)* may be elevated in copper deficiency. Most likely differences in gender, species, timing of dietary deficiency, and in vitro culture conditions contribute to these discrepancies.

More direct evidence that copper is involved in lymphocyte proliferation comes from a report of one human subject. Occasionally a rare case of copper deficiency is brought to the attention of researchers in the field of nutritional immunology. An anemic woman, unresponsive to iron or vitamin B12 supplementation was evaluated and found to be copper deficient (66). T-cell proliferation in response to mitogenic stimulation in vitro was found to be suppressed. Copper supplementation restored in vitro mitogenic response. However, each time the woman relapsed into copper deficiency, T-cell proliferation also declined.

Hypersensitivity responses have been reported to increase in copper deficient mice (67), decrease in copper deficient rats (57), and remain unaltered by copper deficiency (59). Thus, the effect copper deficiency has on delayed hypersensitivity responses is unclear from the limited literature available.

Impairments in phagocytosis have been reported in copper deficient mice (68,69), rats (48,70), sheep (71), and cattle (72). Natural killer cell cytotoxicity appears to also depend on adequate copper status. Koller et al. (59) reported a 5–7-fold reduction in splenic natural killer cytotoxicity in copper deficient rats compared with controls. Activated peritoneal macrophages from copper deficient rats have impaired candidacidal activity and an attenuated respiratory burst compared with cells from control rats (70). Interestingly, phagocytic activity of the macrophages was preserved in copper deficiency.

4. ZINC

4.1. Increased Morbidity is Found in Zinc Deficient Humans and Animals

That zinc deficiency is accompanied by increased susceptibility to infections (Table 1) was documented in 1963 when human zinc deficiency was first characterized by Prasad et al. (73). Along with the characteristic hypogonadism and dwarfism, zinc deficient adolescent boys were very susceptible to infections. Discovery of acrodermatitis enteropathica, an inborn error in metabolism which impairs zinc absorption and produces severe zinc deficiency, provides additional evidence that zinc is involved in immunity (74). The major causes of death in this disease are all linked to immunodeficiency which can be prevented by zinc supplementation. Increased morbidity in other clinical situations involving milder zinc deficiencies has been observed. Hambidge et al. (75) reported the association of low serum zinc with increased incidence of infectious illnesses. Secondary zinc deficiencies ranging from mild subclinical states to severe states have been observed in Down syndrome, aging, sickle cell anemia, and in patients on hemodialysis or total parenteral nutrition. Down syndrome patients are at risk for autoimmune diseases and often have low serum zinc levels. Some improvements in immunologic function is found following zinc supplementation (76). Poor zinc status and immunodeficiencies are often found in the elderly. Zinc supplementation has been shown to improve cellular immunity (77,78). However, Bogden et al. (79) did not find a significant immunologic benefit to zinc supplementation.

Zinc deficient animals also show increased susceptibility to a variety of pathogenic organisms (80–84). For example, after only eight days of eating a zinc deficient diet, mice were more susceptible to the parasite Trypanosoma cruzi (81).

4.2. Effects of Zinc Status on Components of Immunity

4.2.1. HUMORAL RESPONSES

The ability of B cells to produce antibody in response to a foreign antigenic challenge is markedly impaired by zinc deficiency (Table 2). Using a dietary zinc deficiency model in rodents, Fraker's group found lowered number of B cells in peripheral blood and spleen (85) and a 50–70% reduction in antibody production in response to antigen (86–88). The ability to mount an IgM response to sheep red blood cells was restored with zinc repletion (88). Altered humoral immunity is also manifested by distortion in serum immunoglobulin profiles resulting from prenatal and postnatal zinc deficiency (89) in mice.

Few studies of human zinc deficiency have measured humoral immune components. The select few which have been reported generally have few subjects, but, are worthwhile to consider. The limited body of literature suggests that in adults with hypozincemia associated with acrodermatitis enteropathica suboptimal numbers of circulating B cells are present (90) and that in childhood acrodermatitis enteropathica, plasma immunoglobulin levels are reduced (91).

Both rodents (85,86,92,93) and humans (44,94) exhibit rapid thymic atrophy in response to zinc deficiency.

4.2.2. CELL MEDIATED RESPONSES

Lymphocyte proliferation in response to mitogens appears to be preserved in experimental zinc deficiency (Table 3). Here, in the two most convincing studies care was taken to use autologous serum in the in vitro assay medium. This best simulates the in vivo environment since it prevents normalizing influences of exogenous serum on results. Neither Dowd et al. (95) nor Cook-Mills and Fraker (96) found diminished lymphocyte proliferation in zinc deficiency under these stringent conditions.

In contrast to the animal models, evidence derived from human studies suggests that lymphocyte proliferation is reduced by zinc deficiency. Decreased proliferation was reported in patients maintained on parenteral hyperalimentation that did not contain zinc (97) and in patients with acrodermatitis enteropathica. Bogden and colleagues (98) evaluated several aspects of immunity and nutritional status in a free living elderly population. Zinc status was marginal in at least 15% of the subjects where plasma zinc concentrations were in the low end of the normal range established for healthy young subjects (98). A battery of mitogens was used to test lymphocyte proliferation in vitro using autologous serum. Subjects were classified as either normal responders or nonresponders/ suboptimal responders. Nonresponders and suboptimal responders to lymphocyte stimulation by mitogen had significantly lower platelet zinc concentrations and significantly higher mononuclear cell zinc concentrations than normal responders. The significance of these data is unclear since plasma zinc levels did not differ between responders and nonresponders/ suboptimal responders. In a subsequent clinical trial Bogden et al. (79) provided zinc supplements to 60–89-yr-old healthy subjects for 3 mo. Zinc supplements did not alter indicators of zinc status or immune measure such as in vitro lymphocyte proliferation. There were 15 subjects with poor lymphocyte proliferation prior to the supplementation. In 14 of these 15 subjects improved proliferative responses were found after the trial. Interestingly, this improvement was not due to zinc, but may have been due to components in the multi-vitamin and mineral supplement given to all study participants.

Zinc deficiency is also associated with a diminished delayed hypersensitivity response in rodents (93). Ballester and Prasad (99) reported skin test anergy in patients with sickle cell anemia and poor zinc status. In Bogden's *(98)* elderly subject population anergy to a battery of seven skin test antigens was found in 41% of subjects. Comparison of nonresponders with responders to the tests revealed significantly lower plasma zinc levels in nonresponders.

Studies of phagocytic functions in humans with zinc deficiencies give equivocal results. Whereas Chandra and Dayton *(100)* found lowered phagocytosis in patients with acrodermatitis enteropathica, and Weston et al. *(101)* found altered chemotaxis in phagocytic cells from acrodermatitis enteropathica patients; Allen et al. *(102)* noted enhanced phagocytic function in a patient with zinc deficiency due to prolonged parenteral nutrition.

Natural killer cell cytotoxicity has been reported to be lowered *(93,103)* and enhanced *(104)* by zinc deficiency in rodents. Impaired NK cell cytotoxicity in patients with sickle cell anemia was improved with zinc supplementation *(105)*. One year of supplementation with 100 mg zinc per day enhanced natural killer cell activity in elderly subects *(106)*.

Fraker's group has investigated the effects of murine zinc deficiency on macrophage functions. Peritoneal macrophages showed normal phagocytosis of polystyrene beads *(107)*. However, when Trypanosoma cruzi, the parasite which causes Chagas's disease, was incubated with macrophages from zinc deficient mice, reduced capacity to take up the parasite and kill it was found *(107)*.

5. MECHANISMS OF TRACE ELEMENT ACTION IN IMMUNITY

It is apparent from the wealth of research cited previously that deficiencies of iron, copper or zinc profoundly influence immunity. For most indicators of immune response the preponderance of evidence shows deficits in functioning during dietary or clinical deficiencies. The questions which now arise are:

- What are the mechanisms of action by which these minerals participate in immune functions?
- Are these mechanisms general functions of the nutrients or specific to immunity?
- Do the compromises in immunity observed in severe nutrient deficiencies result from a diversion of the nutrient to more "critical" functions?
- Do the lessons learned about trace elements and immunity suggest new functions for the nutrients?

At the present time definitive answers to these questions do not exist. Investigations into mechanisms are diffused in the literature and somewhat difficult to track. In this section the most well studied mechanisms are reviewed and insights to these questions gleaned.

5.1. Protein Synthesis

Immune reactions are dependent on many secretory proteins released from lymphocytes and macrophages which stimulate other branches of immunity. In addition protein synthesis is involved in cellular replication and antibody production. While a direct role of iron in overall protein synthesis is not recognized, protein synthesis has been reported to be impaired in neonatal experimental iron deficiency. Protein synthesis is impaired in spleens of both severely and moderately iron deficient rat pups and in thymus of severely iron deficient pups *(108)*. Whereas splenic protein synthesis nearly doubled in moderately iron deficient and normal pups after immunization with sheep red blood cells, protein synthesis in severely iron deficient rats did not increase significantly. Although the specific site for this impairment in protein synthesis has not been identified, a role for iron in protein synthesis provides an explanation for many of the defects in immunity observed in experimental and clinical iron deficiencies.

5.2. Cytokine Production

Cytokine assessment is becoming an important parameter on studies in nutritional immunology. Cytokines are soluble mediators of immunity secreted by activated immune cells. These mediators have a variety of actions at the local level on other immune cells and systemically. Cytokines are considered accessory molecules which transmit immune messages. Interleukin (IL) 1 is a cytokine which has numerous biological activities in cell mediated and humoral immunity as well as nonspecific immunity. IL-1 causes fever, granulocytosis, and alters mineral distribution. It also enhances lymphocyte proliferation and stimulates helper T cells to produce IL-2. IL-1 is produced by phagocytic cells including monocytes, macrophages, Kupffer cells, and polymorphonuclear cells.

Interleukin 1 production has been reported to be decreased in both severe and moderate iron deficiency *(109)* and in copper deficient rodents *(52,69)*. In contrast, Cook-Mills et al. *(110)* found that zinc deficiency does not alter IL-1 production.

Interleukin 2, produced by activated helper T cells, is a powerful cytokine which stimulates proliferation and clonal expansion of T and B cells, and the cytotoxicity of NK cells and cytotoxic T lymphocytes. Indeed, the binding of IL-2 to its receptors on cell membranes provides a signal for the activated cell to progress to the proliferative stage. Kuvibidila et al. *(111)* found that spleen cell IL-2 production in iron deficient mice was significantly lower than that in control or food restricted mice. They speculate that the deficit in IL-2 production is secondary to impaired IL-1 production in iron deficiency. French children aged 6 mo to 3 yr at high risk for iron deficiency were studied longitudinally by Thibault et al. *(112)*. IL-2 production by activated T lymphocytes was found to be lower in iron deficient children that in iron sufficient children. After a two month double blinded iron supplementation trial no overall changes in IL-2 production were attributed to iron supplementation. The study protocol precluded the separate analysis of improvements in IL-2 with iron repletion among iron deficient children.

Copper deficiency in rodents has been consistently reported to decrease IL-2 bioactivity *(69,113,114)*. Mitogen stimulated splenic mononuclear cells from copper deficient rats show a 50% reduction in IL-2 activity compared to cells from control rats *(114)*. Adding rat IL-2 or physiological levels of copper to these cultures increased DNA synthesis indicating increased cell proliferation. Addition of copper to cell cultures from copper deficient rats also increased IL-2 activity. Even marginal copper deficiency with a minimal impact of indicators of copper status, reduces IL-2 bioactivity *(115)*. These results suggest that the mechanism by which copper functions in cell proliferation is via IL-2 production. The action of copper however does not appear to be via the up regulation of IL-2 receptors on the surface of mitogen treated T lymphocytes *(113)*.

Failla's research group has developed an in vitro model of human T cell copper deficiency *(116)* to more thoroughly study the mechanisms by which copper functions in IL-2 production. Through mitogen stimulation, IL-2 synthesis is induced in Jurkat cells, from a human leukemic T-cell line. Pretreatment of the cells with a high affinity copper chelator for at least 24 hr makes the cells copper deficient, reduces the production of IL-2 by 75%, and reduces the abundance of mRNA for IL-2 by 50% *(116)*. Nonspecific chelation of iron and zinc was carefully ruled out in these studies. The decreased mRNA in these copper deficient cells suggests potential mechanisms for copper in IL-2 synthesis

(117): decreased transcription of IL-2 gene; altered processing of the primary transcript; decreased stability of the mRNA; or a combination of the preceding. Supporting evidence for these hypotheses comes from the fact that copper deficiency alters the expression of at least seven mammalian genes *(117)*.

Less research has examined zinc as a variable in IL-2 bioactivity. No changes in IL-2 activity have been found in rodent models of zinc deficiency *(95,96)*. Beck et al. *(118)* studied immune responses in five young, adult, healthy males fed a zinc restricted, high phytate diet for 4 wk. A slight decrease in IL-2 activity was found following the depletion, although statistical significance was not reached.

Interferon, produced by macrophages and helper T cells, is another soluble compound which stimulates immune cells during viral infections and in neoplasia. Changes in the ability of cells to produce interferon could provide a mechanism to explain many of the defects in cell mediated immunity observed in deficiencies of iron, copper, and/or zinc. Reduced bioactivity of interferon was found in iron deficient mice *(35,119)*. In contrast, copper deficient mice have normal levels of interferon *(120)*. Beck et al. *(89)* have reported decreased cellular production of interferon γ in experimental zinc deficiency. Since interferon is important in the maturation and activation of NK cells, lowered interferon activity may contribute to the lowered NK cytotoxicity of iron deficiency.

5.3. Endocrine Effects

Several investigators have reported that serum thymulin is lowered in human zinc deficiency *(121)*. Thymulin is a thymic hormone which reportedly requires zinc to express its biological activity *(122)*. This hormone has been reported to bind to high affinity receptors, induce T-cell markers, and promote T cell functions such as cytotoxicity, suppressor function, and IL 2 production.

Fraker's group has successfully pursued corticosteroids and apoptosis as a regulatory mechanism for zinc's action in immunity. Zinc deficient rodents activate the stress axis and have elevated levels of corticosteroid in plasma *(123)*. Adrenalectomy protects the thymus of zinc deficient mice suggesting that chronic elevation of corticosterone is immunosuppressive *(124)*. Glucocorticoid exposure induces cells to undergo apoptosis. Cells of the immune system are particularly vulnerable to death by apoptosis. Fraker's group has shown that levels of glucocorticoid similar to those found in zinc deficiency cause thymic atrophy and depletion of B cells. She proposes that there is a synergy between suboptimal zinc and elevated glucocorticoid that may intensify or prolong cell death by apoptosis *(125)*.

5.4. Mitosis vs Apoptosis

Maintenance of a normally functioning and vigorous immune response depends on two opposing cellular events: mitosis, needed for clonal expansion of lymphoid cells in response to a stimulus; and apoptosis, needed to reduce the number of active immune cells after the stimulus has been sequestered. It has been suggested that trace elements play pivotal roles in both of these cellular events.

Zalewski *(126)* proposes that zinc is required to support mitosis and suppresses apoptosis. He cites work which shows that a cellular influx of zinc accompanies mitosis whereas efflux of zinc occurs in apoptosis. In mitosis zinc is necessary for thymidine kinase, DNA polymerase, DNA-dependent RNA polymerase, terminal deoxyribonucleotidyl transferase, aminoacyl tRNA synthetase, and tubulin. Shankar and Prasad *(127)* summarize the multiple places in the cell cycle where zinc may be active. In the absence of adequate zinc, mitotic enzymes are less active and cell proliferation is impaired. At the same time, zinc deficiency is accompanied by enhanced apoptotic cell death in thymus *(15)*. The redistribution of intracellular zinc during apoptosis further implicates zinc in programmed cell death *(127)*. The net result of decreased cell division and increased cell death during zinc deficiency is that fewer immunologically competent cells remain active.

Disrupted mitosis also provides a mechanism by which iron deficiency leads to diminished immunity. Roles for iron in G1, S, and G2 phases of the cell cycle are suggested by in vivo and in vitro studies. Helyar and Sherman *(128)* found that the percentage of splenic lymphocytes in G2-M phase is lower in iron deficient mice than in controls or mice restricted in food. This suggests a delay in S phase, possibly related to the need for iron by ribonucleotide reductase. In vitro treatment of cells with transferrin receptor antibody also results in accumulation of cells in S phase *(129)*. Cultured T lymphocytes *(130)* and neuroblastoma cells *(131)* depleted of iron in vitro are blocked at or near the G1/S border. This suggests an additional role of iron before DNA replication in S phase. Cell cycle transitions are regulated by a family of serine protein kinases which are cyclin dependent. Of these proteins, p34cdc2, active in late G1 before S, is inhibited by iron depletion of cells in culture *(130)*. Iron chelation by desferrioxamine inhibits the transcription of the cdc2 gene responsible for the p34cdc2 protein *(132)*. The p34cdc2 protein is also active in M phase, suggesting an additional site for iron in the cell cycle. Reddel et al. *(133)* showed that iron and/or transferrin depletion of T47D breast cancer cells blocks at the G2 phase. The precise mechanism by which iron alters cell cycling is presently unknown.

5.5. Signal Transduction

Signal transduction is an important early event in cellular responses to stimuli. It signals and precedes initiation of protein synthesis within cells. Both zinc and iron have been implicated in signal transduction needed for lymphocyte activation. Multiple roles for zinc in signal transduction have been proposed *(127,134)* including the binding of cytoplasmic tails of CD4 and CD8 with the tyrosine kinase p56lck active in early T-lymphocyte activation. By this mechanism, zinc stimulates autophosphorylation of tyrosine residues by p56lck and the subsequent phosphorylation of the T lymphocyte receptor complex involving CD45. Next zinc is involved in the activity of phospholipase C to produce inositol triphosphate and diacylglycerol. Zinc is also involved in the phosphorylation of proteins mediated by protein kinase C. Subsequent changes via protein phosphorylation regulate cell activation and proliferation—important prerequisites to immune responsiveness.

Iron has also been implicated in signal transduction. Kuvibidila et al. *(135)* have shown that protein kinase C activity is low in splenocytes from iron deficient mice. Whereas the food restriction of iron deficiency contributed somewhat to the reduction, the correlation of iron status with activity of this important component of signal transduction was positive. Recently this group has demonstrated that this results in reduced hydrolysis of cell membrane phosphatidyl inositol -4,5-biphosphate during splenic lymphocyte activation in iron deficient C57BL/6 mice *(136)*. Activation of protein kinase C in many lymphoid and hematopoietic cells requires iron in the form of transferrin. Alcantara et al. *(137,138)* have shown that delivery of transferrin iron to cultured lymphoblastoid T cells stimulates transcription of the protein kinase C- β gene, while treatment with desferrioxamine is inhibitory. Transcription of other gene subspecies, protein kinase C- α and protein kinase C-γ were not affected by iron treatments in vitro. Transcriptional up regulation of protein kinase C- β by iron transferrin appears to be mediated by DNA sequences located between -2200 bp and -587 bp in the 5' flanking region of the human protein kinase C- β gene. Alcantara et al's in vitro studies provide evidence that iron is involved in the expression of specific genes which are central to many of the biochemical control points in cellular function including immune responses.

6. CONCLUSION

Little research has been done on the other essential trace elements (selenium, molybdenum, chromium, flouride, iodine, manganese) and immunity (*see* Chapter 19).

The past three decades have yielded a considerable body of research demonstrating that deficiencies in zinc, copper, and iron lead to marked immune dysfunction. Present knowledge of the cellular, molecular, and genetic mechanisms responsible is more rudimentary. Undoubtedly as more and more sophisticated technologies are applied to the question of trace element function in immunity answers to the questions raised herein will be forthcoming.

REFERENCES

1. MacKay HMM. Anaemia in infancy: its prevalence and prevention. Arch Dis Child 1928;2:117–147.
2. Andelman MB, Sered BR. Utilization of dietary iron by term infants. Am J Dis Child 1966;3:45–55.
3. James JA, Combes M. Iron deficiency in the premature infant. Significance and prevention by intramuscular administration of iron dextran. Pediatr 1960;102:368–374.
4. Fuerth JH. Incidence of anemia in full-term infants seen in private practice. J Pediatr 1971;79:560–562.
5. Cantwell RJ. Iron deficiency anemia of infancy. Clin Pediatr 1972;8:443–449.
6. Oppenheimer SJ. Anaemia of infancy and bacterial infections in Papua, New Guinea. Ann Trop Med Parasitol 1980;74:69–72.
7. Burman O. Haemoglobin levels in normal infants aged 3 to 24 months, and the effect of iron. Arch Dis Child 1972;47:261–271.
8. Barry DMJ, Reeve AW. Increased incidence of gram-negative neonatal sepsis with intramuscular iron administration. Pediatr 1977;60:908–912.
9. Murray MJ, Murray AB, Murray NJ, Murray MB. Refeeding malaria and hyperferraemia. Lancet 1975;i:653–654.
10. Murray MJ, Murray AB, Murray MB, Murray CJ. The adverse effect of iron repletion on the course of certain infections. Br Med J 1978;2:1113–1115.
11. Masawe AE, Muindi JM, Swai GB. Infections in iron deficiency and other types of anaemia in the tropics. Lancet 1974; ii:314–317.
12. Baggs RB, Miller SA. Nutritional iron deficiency as a determinant of host resistance in the rat. J Nutr 1973;103:1554–1560.
13. Chu SW, Welch KJ, Murray ES, Hegsted DM. Effect of iron deficiency on the susceptibility to Streptococcus Pneumoniae infection in the rat. Nutr Rep Int 1976;14:605–609.
14. Brolin, TD, Davis, AE, Cummins, AG, Duncombe, VM, Kelly JD.The effect of iron and protein deficiency on the expulsion of *Nippostrongylus brasiliensis* from the small intestine of the rat. Gut 1977;18:182–186.
15. Duncombe VM, Brolin TD, Davis A, Kelly JD. The effect of iron and protein deficiency on the development of acquired resistance to reinfection of *Nippostrongylus brasiliensis* from the small intestine of the rat. Am J Clin Nutr 1979;32:553–558.
16. Chandra RK. Fetal malnutrition and postnatal immunocompetence. Am J Dis Child 1975;129:450–454.
17. Macdougall LG, Anderson R, McNab GM, Katz J. The immune response in iron-deficient children: impaired cellular defense mechanisms with altered humoral components. J Pediatr 1975;86:883–843.
18. Bagchi K, Mohanram M, Reddy V. Humoral immune response in children with iron deficiency anaemia. Br Med J 1980;280:1249–1251.
19. Krantman HJ, Young SR, Ank BJ, O'Donnell CM, Rachelefsky GS, Stiehm ER. Immune function in pure iron deficiency. Am J Dis Child 1982;136:840–844.

20. Sawitsky B, Kanter R, Sawitsky A. Lymphocyte response to phytomitogens in iron deficiency. Am J Med Sci 1976;272:153–160.
21. Nalder BN, Mahoney AW, Ramakrishnan R, Hendricks DG. Sensitivity of the immunological response to the nutritional status of rats. J Nutr 1972;102:535–542.
22. Kuvibidila S, Baliga BS, Suskind RM. Generation of plague forming cells in iron deficient anemic mice. Nutr Rept Int 1982;26:861–871.
23. Kochanowski B A, Sherman AR. Decreased antibody formation in iron-deficient rat pups—effect of iron repletion. Am J Clin Nutr 1985;41: 278–284.
24. Sherman AR. Influence of iron on immunity and disease resistance. Ann NY Acad Sci 1990;587:140–146.
25. Rothenbacher, H, Sherman AR. Target organ pathology in iron-deficient suckling rats. J Nutr 1980;110:1648–1654.
26. Kochanowski BA, Sherman AR. Serum and secretory proteins in iron-deficient rat pups and dams. Nutr Res 1982;2:689–698.
27. Kochanowski BA, Sherman AR. Cellular growth in iron-deficient rats: effect of pre-and postweaning iron repletion. J Nutr 1985;115:279–287.
28. Helyar L, Sherman AR. Moderate and severe iron deficiency lowers numbers of spleen T-lymphocyte and B-lymphocyte subsets in the C57/B16 mouse. Nutr Res 1992;12:1113–1122 .
29. Joynson DHM, Jacobs A, Walker DM, Dolby AE. Defect of cell-mediated immunity in patients with iron deficiency anaemia. Lancet 1972;ii:1058–1059.
30. Chandra RK, Saraya AK. Impaired immunocompetence associated with iron deficiency. J Pediatr 1975;86:899–902.
31. Kielman AA, Uberoi IS, Chandra RK, Mehra VL. The effect of nutritional status on immune capacity and immune responses in preschool children in a rural community in India. Bull World Health Organ 1976;54:477–483.
32. Suskind RM, Kulapongs P, Vithayasai V, Olson RE. Iron deficiency anemia and the immune response. In: Suskind RM, ed. "Malnutrition and the immune response" Raven Press, New York, 1977, pp. 387–393.
33. Kulapongs P, Vithayasai V, Suskind R, Olson RE. Cell-mediated immunity and phagocytosis and killing function in children with severe iron-deficiency anaemia. Lancet 1974;ii:689–691.
34. Kuvibidila S, Nauss BS, Baliga BS, Suskind RM. Impairment of blastogenic response of splenic lymphocytes from iron- deficient mice: in vivo repletion. Am J Clin Nutr 1983;37:15–25.
35. Omara FO, Blakley BR. The effects of iron deficiency and iron overload on cell mediated immunity in the mouse. Br J Nutr 1994;72:899–909.
36. Kochanowski BA, Sherman AR. Phagocytosis and lysozyme activity in granulocytes from iron-deficient rat dams and pups. Nutr Res 1984;4:511–520.
37. Sherman AR, Lockwood J. Impaired natural killer cell activity in iron-deficient rat pups. J Nutr 1987;117:567–571.
38. Lockwood J, Sherman AR. Spleen natural killer cells from iron-deficient rat pups manifest an altered ability to be stimulated by interferon. J Nutr 1988;118:1558–1563.
39. Hallquist NA, McNeil LK, Lockwood JF, Sherman AR. Effect of maternal iron deficiency on peritoneal macrophage and peritoneal natural killer cell cytotoxicity in rat pups. Am J Clin Nutr 1992;55:741–746.
40. Hallquist NA, Sherman AR. Effect of iron deficiency on the stimulation of natural killer cells by macrophage-produced interferon. Nutr Res 1989;9:282–292.
41. Spear AT, Sherman AR. Iron deficiency alters DMBA-induced tumor burden and natural killer cell cytotoxicity in rats. J Nutr 1992;122:46–55.
42. Hrabinshi D, Hertz JL, Tantillo C, Berger V, Sherman AR. Iron repletion attenuates the protective effects of iron deficiency in DMBNA-induced mammary tumors in rats. Nutrition and Cancer 1995;24:133–142.
43. Prohaska JR, Lukasewycz OA. Effects of copper deficiency on the immune system. Adv Exp Med Biol 1990;262:123–143.
44. Golden MH, Jackson AA, Golden BE. Effect of zinc on thymus of recently malnourished children. Lancet 1977;ii:1057–1059.
45. Castillo-Duran C, Fisberg M, Valenzuela A, Egana JI, Uauy R. Controlled copper supplementation during the recovery from marasmus. Am J Clin Nutr 1983;37:898–9903.
46. Pletcher JM, Banting LF. Copper deficiency in piglets characterized by spongy myeopathy and degenerative lesions in the great blood vessels. J South Afr Vet Assoc 1983;54:43–46.
47. Suttle NF, Jones DB. Copper and disease resistance in sheep: A rare natural confirmation of interaction between a specific nutrient and function. Proc Nutr Soc 1986;45:317–325.

48. Newberne PM, Hunt CE, Young VR. The role of diet and the reticuloendothelial system in the response of rats to Salmonella typhimurium infection. Br J Exp Pathol 1968;49:448–457.
49. Jones DG, Suttle NF. The effect of copper deficiency on the resistance of mice to infection with Pasteurella haemolytica. J Comp Pathol 1983;93:143–149.
50. Stabel JR, Spears JW. Effect of copper on immune function and disease resistance. Adv Exp Med Biol 1989;258:243–252.
51. Prohaska JR, Lukasewycz OA. Copper deficiency suppresses the immune response in mice. Science 1981;213:559–561.
52. Blakely BR, Hamilton DL. The effect of copper deficiency on the immune response in mice. Drug Nutrient Interact 1987;5:103–111.
53. Prohaska JR, Lukasewycz OA. Biochemical and immunological changes in mice following postweaning copper deficiency. Biol Trace Element Res 1989;22:101–112.
54. Prohaska JR, Lukasewycz OA. Copper deficiency during perinatal development: effects on the immune response of mice. J Nutr 1989;119:922–931.
55. Vyas D, Chandra RK. Thymic factor activity, lymphocyte stimulation response and antibody producing cells in copper deficiency. Nutr Res 1983;3:343–349.
56. Failla ML, Babu U, Seidel KE. Use of immunoresponsiveness to demonstrate that the dietary requirement for copper in young rats is greater with dietary fructose than dietary starch. J Nutr 1988;118:487–496.
57. Kishore V, Latman N, Roberts CW, Barnett JB, Sorenson JRJ. Effect of nutritional copper deficiency on adjuvant arthritis and immunocompetence in the rat. Agents Actions 1984;14:274–282.
58. Eason S, Carville D, Strain JJ, Hannigan BM. The influence of dietary carbohydrate on antibody mediated immunity in copper deficiency. Biochem Soc Trans 1988;16:54–55.
59. Koller LD, Mulhern SA, Frankel NC, Steven MG, Williams JR. Immune dysfunction in rats fed a diet deficient in copper. Am J Clin Nutr 1987;45:997–1006.
60. Prohaska JR, Downing SW, Lukasewycz OA. Chronic copper deficiency alters biochemical and morphological properties of mouse lymphoid tissues. J Nutr 1983;113:1583–1590.
61. Mulhern SA, Koller LD. Severe or marginal copper deficiency results in a graded reduction in immune status in mice. J Nutr 1988;118:1041–1047.
62. Lukasewycz OA , Prohaska JR, Meyer SG, Schmidtke JR, Hatfield SM, Marder P. Alterations in lymphocyte subpopulations in copper-deficient mice. Infect Immun 1985;48:644–647.
63. Bala S, Failla ML, Lunney JK. Alterations in splenic lymphoid cell subsets and activation antigens in copper-deficient rats. J Nutr 1991a;121:745–753.
64. Lukasewycz OA, Prohaska JR. Lymphocytes from copper-deficient mice exhibit decreased mitogen reactivity. Nutr Res 1983;3:335–341.
65. Kramer TR, Johnson WT, Briske-Anderson M. Influence of iron and the sex of rats on hematological, biochemical, and immunological changes during copper deficiency. J Nutr 1988;118:214–221.
66. Smith D, Hopkins RG, Kutlar A, Failla, ML. Diagnosis and treatment of copper deficiency in adult humans. FASEB J 1994;8:A4754.
67. Jones DG. Effects of dietary copper depletion on acute and delayed inflammatory responses in mice. Res Vet Sci 1984;37:205–210 .
68. Lukasewycz OA, Prohaska JR. Immunization against transplantable leukemia is impaired in copper deficient mice. J Natl Cancer Inst 1982;69:489–493.
69. Lukasewycz OA, Prohaska JR. The immune response in copper deficiency. Ann NY Acad Sci 1990;587:147–159.
70. Babu U, Failla ML.Respiratory burst and candidacidal activity of peritoneal macrophages are impaired in copper-deficient rats. J Nutr 1990;120:1692–1699.
71. Jones DG, Suttle NF. Some effects of copper deficiency on leucocyte function in sheep and cattle. Res Vet Sci 1981;31:151–156.
72. Boyne R, Arthur JR. Effects of selenium and copper deficiency on neutrophil function in cattle. J Comp Pathol 1981;91:271–276.
73. Prasad AS, Miale A, Farid Z, Sandstead HH, Schulert AR. Zinc metabolism in normals and patients with the syndrome of iron deficiency anemia, hepatosplenomegaly, dwarfism and hypogonadism. J Lab Clin Med 1963;61:537–549.
74. Moynahan EJ, Barnes PM. Zinc deficiency and a synthetic diet for lactose intolerance. Lancet 1973;i:676–677.
75. Hambidge KM, Casey CE, Krebs NF. Zinc. In: Merz W, ed. Trace Elements in Human Health and Animal Nutrition, 5th ed. Academic Press, New York, NY, 1986, pp. 1–137, .

76. Lockitch G, Singh VK, Puterman ML, Godolophin WL, Sheps AS, Tingle AJ, Wong F, Quigley G. Age-related changes in humoral and cell-mediated immunity in Down syndrome children living at home. Ped Res 1987;22:536–540.

77. Duchateau J, Delepesse G, Vrijens R, Collet H. Beneficial effects of oral zinc supplementation on immune response in old people. Am J Med 1981;70:1001–1004.

78. Wagner PA, Jernigan JA, Bailey LB, Nickens C, Brazzi GA. Zinc nutriture and cell-mediated immunity in the aged. Int J Vitamin Nutr Res 1983;53:94–101.

79. Bogden JD, Oleske JM, Lavenhar MA, Munves EM, Kemp PW, Bruening KS, Holding KJ, Denny TN, Guarino MA, Krieger LM, Holland BK. Zinc and immunocompetence in elderly people: effects of zinc supplementation for 3 months. Am J Clin Nutr 1988;48:655–663.

80. Pekarek RS, Hoagland AM, Powanda MC. Humoral and cellular immune responses in zinc-deficient rats. Nutr Rep Int 1977;16:267–276.

81. Fraker PJ, Caruso R, Kierszenbaum F. Alteration in immune and nutritional status of mice by synergy between Zn deficiency and infection with *Typanosoma cruzi*. J Nutr 1982;112:1224–1229.

82. Lee CM, Humphrey PS, Abok-Cole GF. Interaction of nutrition and infection: effect of zinc deficiency on resistance to *Trypanosoma musculi*. Int J Biochem 1983;15:841–847.

83. Salvin SB, Rabin BS. Resistance and susceptibility to infection in inbred murine strains: effects of dietary zinc. Cell Immunol 1984;87:546–552.

84. Fraker PJ, Jardieu P, Cook J. Zinc deficiency and immune function. Arch Dermatol 1987;123:1699–1701.

85. King LE, Fraker PJ. Flow cytometric analysis of the phenotypic distribution of splenic lymphocytes in zinc-deficient adult mice. J Nutr 1991;121:1433–1438.

86. Fraker PJ, Haas SM, Luecke RW. Effect of zinc deficiency on the immune response of the young adult A/J mouse. J Nutr 1977;107:1889–1895.

87. Jardieu P, Fraker PJ. Influence of zinc deficiency on the magnitude, kinetics, and affinity of the response to trinitrophenylated (TNP) lipopolysaccharide in TNP-Ficoll in adult mice. J Trace Elements Exp Med 1990;3:1–11.

88. Zwickl CM, Fraker PJ. Restoration of the antibody mediated response of zinc/calorie deficient neonatal mice. Immunol Commun 1980;9:611–626.

89. Beach RS, Gershwin ME, Hurley LS. Gestational zinc deprivation in mice: persistence of immunodeficiency for three generations. Science 1982;218:469–471.

90. Antilla PH, Von Willebrand E, Simmell O. Abnormal immune responses during hypozincaemia in acrodermatitis enteropathica. Acta Ped Scand 1986;75:988–992.

91. Oleske J, Westphal ML, Shore S, Gorden D, Bogden J, Nahmias A. Zinc therapy of depressed cellular immunity in acrodermatitis enteropathica. Am J Dis Child 1979;133:915–918.

92. Fraker PJ, DePasquale-Jardieu P, Zwickl CM, Luecke RW. Regeneration of T-cell helper function in zinc deficient adult mice. Proc Natl Acad Sci USA 1978;75:5660–5665.

93. Fraker PJ, Gershwin ME, Good RA, Prasad A. Interrelationships between zinc and immune function. Fed Proc 1986;45:1474–1479.

94. Smythe PM, Schonland M, Brereton-Stiles G, Coovadra HM, Grace HJ, Loening WE, Mafoyane A, Parent MA, Vos GA. Thymolymphatic deficiency and depression of cell mediated immunity in protein-calorie malnutrition. Lancet 1971;ii:939–944.

95. Dowd PS, Kellecher J, Guillou PJ. T-lymphocyte subsets and interleukin 2 production in zinc-deficient rats. Br J Nutr 1986;55:59–69.

96. Cook-Mills J, Fraker PJ. Functional capacity of the residual lymphocytes from zinc deficient adult mice. Br J Nutr 1993;69:835–848.

97. Allen JI, Kay NE, McClain CJ. Severe zinc deficiency in humans: association with a reversible T-lymphocyte dysfunction. Ann Intern Med 1981;96:154–157.

98. Bogden JD, Oleske JM, Munves EM, Lavenhar MA, Bruening KS, Kemp FW, Holding KJ, Denny TN, Louria DB. Zinc and immunocompetence in the elderly: baseline data on zinc nutriture and immunity in unsupplemented subjects. Am J Clin Nutr 1987;46:101–109 .

99. Ballester OF, Prasad AS. Anergy, zinc deficiency, and decreased nucleoside phosphorylase activity in patients with sickle cell anemia. Ann Intern Med 1983;98:180–182.

100. Chandra RK, Dayton DH. Trace element regulation of immunity and infection. Nutr Res 1982;2:721–733.

101. Weston WL, Huff JC, Humbert JR, Hambidge KM, Nelderner KH, Walravens PA. Zinc correction of defective chemotaxis in acrodermatitis enteropathica. Arch Dermatol 1977;113:422–424.

102. Allen JI, Perri RT, McClain C, Kay NE. Alterations in human natural killer cell activity and monocyte cytotoxicity induced by zinc deficiency. J Lab Clin Med 1983;102:577–589.

103. Fernandes G, Nair M, Onoe K, Tanaka T, Floyd R, et al. Impairment of cell-mediated immunity functions by dietary zinc deficiency in mice. Proc Natl Acad Sci USA 1979;76:457–461.
104. Chandra RK, Au B. Single nutrient deficiency and cell-mediated responses. I Zinc. Am J Clin Nutr 1980;33:736–738.
105. Tapazoglou E, Prasad AS, Hill G, Brewer GJ, Kaplan J. Decreased natural killer cell activity in zinc deficient subjects with sickle cell disease. J Lab Clin Med 1985;105:19–22.
106. Bogden JD, Oleske JM, Lavenhar MA, Munves EM, Kemp PW, Bruening KS, Holding KJ, Denny TN, Guarino MA, Krieger LM, Holland BK. Effects of one year of supplementation with zinc and other micronutrients on cellular immunity in the elderly. J Am Coll Nutr 1990;9:214–225.
107. Wirth JJ, Fraker PJ, Kierszenbaum F. Changes in the levels of marker expression by mononuclear phagocytes in zinc-deficient mice. J Nutr 1984;114:1826–1833.
108. Rosch LM, Sherman AR, Layman DK. Iron deficiency impairs protein synthesis in immune tissues of rat pups. J Nutr 1987;117:1475–1481.
109. Helyar L, Sherman AR. The effect of iron deficiency on interleukin 1 production by rat leukocytes. Am J Clin Nutr 1987;46:346–452.
110. Cook-Mills J, Morford GL, Fraker PJ. Role of zinc in phagocytic function. Clin Appl Nutr 1991;1:25–34.
111. Kuvibidila S, Murthy KK, Suskind RM. Alteration of interleukin 2 production in iron deficiency anemia. J Nutr Immunol 1992;1:81–98.
112. Thibault H, Galan P, Selz F, Preziosi P, Olivier C, Baboual J, Hercberg S. The immune response in iron deficient young children: effect of iron supplementation on cell-mediated immunity. Eur J Ped 1993;152:120–124.
113. Bala S, Deshpande S, Tailla M. Exogenous IL-2 and copper restore in vitro reactivity of splenic mononuclear cells from copper deficient rats. FASEB J 1991;5:A4095.
114. Bala S, Failla ML. Copper deficiency reversibly impairs DNA synthesis in activated T-lymphocytes. Proc Natl Acad Sci USA 1992;89:6794–7697.
115. Hopkins RG, Failla ML. Chronic intake of a marginally low copper diet impairs lymphocyte and neutrophil function in male rats despite minimal impact on conventional indices of copper status. J Nutr 1995;125:2658–2668.
116. Hopkins RG, Failla ML. Copper deficiency reduces interleukin 2 production and IL-2 mRNA in human T-lymphocytes. J Nutr 1997;127:257–262.
117. Failla ML, Hopkins RG. Is low copper status immunosuppressive? Nutr Rev 1998;56:S59–S64.
118. Beck FWJ, Prasad AS, Kaplan, J et al. Changes in cytokine production and T cell subpopulations in experimentally induced zinc-deficient humans. Am J Physiol 1997;272:E1002–1007.
119. Spear AT, Sherman AR. Interferon activity is decreased in iron deficiency. FASEB J 1991;5:A1293.
120. Lukasewycz OA, Prohaska JR. Normal gamma interferon and decreased Interleukin 2 production by copper-deficient mice. FASEB J 1991;5:A 5351.
121. Keen CL, Gershwin ME. Zinc deficiency and immune function. Ann Rev Nutr 1990;10:415–431.
122. Prasad AS, Meftah S, Abdallah J, Kaplan J, Brewer GJ, et al. Serum thymulin in human zinc deficiency. J Clin Invest 1988;82:1202–1210.
123. DePasquale-Jardieu P, Fraker PJ. The role of corticosterone in the loss of immune funciton in the zinc-deficient A/J mouse. J Nutr 1979;109:1847–1855.
124. DePasquale-Jardieu P, Fraker PJ. Further characterization of the role of corticosterone in the loss of humoral immunity in zinc-deficient A/J mice as determined by adrenalectomy. J Immunol 1980;124:2650–2655.
125. Fraker PJ, King LE, Garvy BA, Medina CA. The immunopathology of zinc deficiency in humans and rodents. A possible role for programmed cell death. In: Klurfeld, DM, ed. Human Nutrition-A Comprehensive Treatise, Volume 8: Nutrition and Immunology, Plenum Press, New York, 1993.
126. Zalewski PD. Zinc and immunity: Implications for growth, survival, and function of lymphoid cells. J Nutr Immunol 1996;4:39–101.
127. Shankar AH, Prasad AS. Zinc and immune function: the biological basis of altered resistance to infection. Am J Clin Nutr 1998;68:447S–463S.
128. Helyar L, Sherman AR. Iron deficiency impairs lymphocyte activation marker expression and cell cycle shift in response to concanavalin A stimulation. FASEB J 1991;5:A1292.
129. Trowbridge, Lopez. Monoclonal antibody to transferrin receptor blocks transferrin binding and inhibits human tumor cell growth in vitro. Proc Natl Acad Sci USA 1982;79:1175–1179.
130. Terada N, Or R, Szepesi A, Lucas JJ, Gelfand EW. Definition of the roles of iron and essential fatty acids in cell cycle progression of normal human T lymphocytes. Exper Cell Res 1993;204:260–267.

131. Brodie C, Siriwwardana G, Lucas J, Schleicher R, Terada N, Szepsi A, Glefand, E, Seligman P. Neuroblastoma sensitivity to growth inhibition by desferrioxamine: evidence for a block in G1 phase of the cell cycle. Cancer Res 1993;53:3968–3975.

132. Lucas JJ, Szepesi A, Domenico J, Takase K, Tordai A, Terada N, Gelfand EW. Effects of iron-depletion on cell cycle progression in normal human T lymphocytes: Selective inhibition of the appearance of the cyclin-A-associated component of the p33 cdk2 kinase. Blood 1995;86:2268–2280.

133. Reddel RR, Hedley DW, Sutherland RL. Cell cycle effects of iron depletion on T-47D human breast cancer cells. Exp Cell Res 1985;161:277–284.

134. Csermely P, Somogyi J. Zinc as a possible mediator of signal trandsuction in T lymphocytes. Acta Physiol Hung 1989;74:195–199.

135. Kuvibidila S, Baliga BS, Murthy KK. Impaired protein kinase C activation as one of the possible mechanisms of reduced lymphocyte proliferation in iron deficiency in mice. Am J Clin Nutr 1991;54:944–950.

136. Kuvibidila S, Baliga BS, Warrier RP, Suskind RM. Iron deficiency reduces the hydrolysis of cell membrane phosphatidyl inositol -4,5-biphosphate during splenic lymphocyte activation in C57BL/6 mice. J Nutr 1998;128:1077–1083.

137. Alcantara O, Javors M, Boldt DH. Induction of protein kinase C mRNA in cultured lymphoblastoid T cells by iron-transferrin but not soluble iron. Blood 1991;77:1290–1297.

138. Alcantara O, Obeid L, Hannum Y, Ponka P, Boldt DH. Regulation of protein kinase C.PKC; expression by iron: effect of different iron compounds on PKC-b and PKC a gene expression and the role of the 5' flanking region of the PKC b gene in the response to ferric transferrin. Blood 1995;84:3510–3517.

139. Goyens P, Brasseru, D, Cadranel S. Copper deficiency in infants with active celiac discase. J Ped Gastro Nutr 1985;4:677–680.

140. Sherman AR. Immunoglobulins and lysozyme in iron-deficient and iron-overloaded rats. Nutr Rep Int 1984;29:859–868.

141. Kochanowski BA, Sherman AR. Cellular growth in iron-deficient rat pups. Growth 1982 ;46:126–134.

142. Bala S, Failla ML, Lunney JK. T cell numbers and mitogenic responsiveness of peripheral blood mononuclear cells are increased in copper deficient rats. Nutr Res 1990;10:749–760.

143. Chandra RK. Trace element regulation of immunity and infection. J Am Coll Nutr 1989;4:5–16.

144. Helyar L, Sherman AR. Cell-mediated cytotoxicity is protected in moderately iron-deficient C5BL/6 mice. Nutr Res 1993;13:1313–1323 .

145. Wirth JJ, Fraker PJ, Kierszenbaum F. Zinc requirement for macrophage function: effect of zinc deficiency on uptake and killing of a protozoan parasite. Immunology 1989;68:114–119.

19

Trace Element and Mineral Nutrition in HIV Infection and AIDS:
Implications for Host Defense

Susanna Cunningham-Rundles, PhD

1. INTRODUCTION

The essential trace elements and minerals obtained from the diet are crucial for the development and maintenance of life at every level and affect all aspects of human health from the formation of cells, tissues, and organs to the initiation and development of host defense by the immune system in response to foreign microbes and viruses. This chapter will focus on how changes in body stores of trace elements and minerals in the human immunodeficiency virus (HIV)+ host may affect the course of HIV disease and influence progression to acquired immune-deficiency syndrome (AIDS). Since HIV infection directly affects the immune system, by specifically targeting the CD4+ T cell, the fundamental nature of the immune response is intrinsically changed by this unique infection. As described below, trace elements and minerals interact and regulate the development of normal immune responses in such a way that relatively small changes in available pools may have a proportionately greater or amplified impact on immune function compared with effects on other cell systems *(1,2)*.

Nutrient changes may take place at several levels, in the context of HIV infection *(3–6)*. Replication of the HIV virus requires activation of host cell DNA. Processes associated with this require trace elements and minerals and may therefore potentially affect body stores. The HIV infected host is engaged in a continuous long term battle to suppress HIV viral replication and to prevent opportunistic infections, as well as to respond to new environmental antigenic challenges. While the recent development of new antiretroviral therapy has led to marked reduction if not irradication of the HIV virus, reconstitution of immune response appears to be incomplete and vulnerability to infections persists even in patients with little or no detectable virus *(7)*. Therefore, support of the HIV+ host continues to require maintainence of optimal levels of all of the key trace elements and minerals in the face of the continuing challenge to maintain health *(8–10)*. The balance of key nutrients is especially critical for immune defense in the vulnerable host. In addition it is likely that optimal levels of essential trace elements and minerals may be higher for the HIV+ host

From: *Clinical Nutrition of the Essential Trace Elements and Minerals: The Guide for Health Professionals*
Edited by: J. D. Bogden and L. M. Klevay © Humana Press Inc., Totowa, NJ

than those currently recommended for the uninfected host. As knowledge of how HIV affects the immune system develops, and new treatments emerge, it is likely that specific understanding of the role of trace elements and minerals in the HIV+ host will be enhanced, and more specific recommendations will emerge.

2. TRACE ELEMENT AND MINERAL INTERACTIONS IN IMMUNE RESPONSE

2.1. Nutrient Imbalance and Suppression of Immune Response

The suppressive effect of nutrient imbalance on immune response is most readily observed in states of malnutrition. Malnutrition leads to increased susceptibility to environmental pathogens, vulnerability to opportunistic infections that do not cause illness in the healthy host, and greater morbidity from all infections (11–13). This basic concept that malnutrition is a cause of immune deficiency was actually recognized many years (11) before the syndrome of unusual infections and rare tumors caused by the HIV virus became generally identified with the term "acquired immune deficiency." Atrophy of lymphoid organs is directly associated with experimental and clinical malnutrition and this leads to increased vulnerability to infections (12,14,15). Studies also suggest that overnutrition, particularly excess intake of fats, may have a suppressive effect on immune response (16–18). Similarly there is evidence that excess supplemental intake of some trace elements and minerals may have a negative effect upon immune responses, often through causing imbalance of other elements but also in some cases through toxic effects (19).

Malnutrition may occur relatively early in HIV infection, especially in children (20–22) and is a serious frequent consequence of late stage AIDS. The specific impact of undernutrition on immune response is strongly affected by stage of life (23–25). Maternal malnutrition may profoundly influence the development of the host defense system of the newborn, as has been shown for zinc in mice and rats (26,27) (see Chapter 18). Human malnutrition during weaning, early childhood, or adolescence may produce life long effects not only because of stunted growth, but also because of sequelae associated with failure to resolve infections (28). The importance of nutrients in maintaining immune responses during human aging has also been clearly demonstrated in several key investigations (29). As the lifespan of persons with HIV is prolonged and in light of these age related effects, there is reason to have particular concern for the nutrition of children with HIV infection now, and in the future for increasing numbers of older HIV+ persons.

The interaction between nutrients and the immune system takes place both systematically and regionally and there may be different nutrient requirements according to regional compartment of the body. Current studies suggest that the development and activity of the regional immune system in the gastrointestinal (G.I.) tract is relatively independent of systemic immunity (30). There are significant differences in functional response of T and B lymphocytes, cytokine patterns, and the use of activation pathways when regional immunity is compared to systemic immunity (31). Nutrients have both fundamental and regulatory influences on the immune response of the G.I. tract and therefore upon host defense. Since HIV viral load is often great in the lymph nodes in the region of the G.I. tract, (32) there may be local interactions with the regional immune system that are influenced by nutrient levels.

Nutrients influence host defense during the acute process of immune response which requires immediate mobilization of cells through activation, proliferation, and differentiation. Differentiated immune cells produce antibodies, cytokines, and may also become cytotoxic effector cells which directly kill altered cells expressing foreign antigens derived from the infecting organism or virus. All immune processes are in turn dependent upon cytokine and growth factor production and secretion. As described in Subheading 2.2., these activities appear to be especially influenced by trace element and mineral nutrient deficits and imbalances.

Current studies suggest that peripheral T-helper lymphocytes typically have a Type1, Th-1 cytokine response. The Th-1 cytokines, interleukin-2 (IL-2), interferon gamma, (INF gamma), and Tumor Necrosis Factor beta (TNF beta) promote cellular immune based host defense whereas T helper Type 2, Th-2, cytokines IL-4, IL-5, IL-6, IL-9,IL-10 and IL-13 promote B-cell antibody production and response to allergens (33,34). Induction of cytokine patterns appears to be signal specific and, furthermore, may be regionally compartmentalized (35,36). For example it seems that Th-2 type cytokines, IL-5, and IL-6 are selectively induced and signal B cells in the Peyer's patches of the G.I. tract to produce sIgA following oral immunization (37). Several studies have shown that when the HIV infected host has a relatively strong host defense system, a strong Th-1 response is produced and that if the predominating response is a Th-2 response, host defense is weaker and disease progression is faster (38,39).

Cytokines produced during host response to acute infection, or traumatic stress, are key mediators of the immune system response, but when these soluble factors are produced in high concentration in acute sepsis or over a long period of time in chronic infection, they can also cause potentially damaging side effects such as the loss of visceral protein. In acute sepsis, the syndrome of septic shock, loss of lean tissue and body fat is clearly evident. IL-1, IL-6, and Tumor Necrosis Factor (TNF alpha) are implicated in this process (40). Direct infusion of TNF alpha, also known as cachectin, into human volunteers, has been demonstrated to induce all of these effects as a single agent (41). Increased levels of TNF alpha have been observed in HIV infection, and are important because HIV can be specifically transactivated by TNF alpha (42).

Malnutrition is closely associated with mucosal atrophy and poor intestinal absorption (43). This too can be directly caused by cytokines. Studies by Probert et al. have shown that a lethal wasting syndrome can be induced in mice by introducing T-cell targeted human TNF transgenes (44). The degree of wasting seen in this study was directly related to level of TNF expression and could be blocked by antibodies directed against TNF. When IL-10, a cytokine which downregulates Th-1 cytokines was genetically eliminated in this mouse, severe inflammation and growth retardation were observed (45). Interestingly, the effect was less marked under germ free conditions. This may suggest that opportunistic infections, or bacterial overgrowth, may amplify the growth abnormalities associated with altered immune response. This situation is potentially relatively common in the HIV+ host (46).

2.2. Effect of Trace Element and Mineral Alteration on Host Defense

Critical studies suggest that micronutrient alteration, either affecting pool size or relative concentration with respect to other elements, may be the basis for many of the observed effects of protein calorie malnutrition on the immune system. Micronutrients, which include vitamins as well as trace elements and minerals, are often deficient in generalized infections and chronic viral illnesses (47). This type of alteration is highly likely to occur in the HIV+ host and therefore to influence host defense not only toward HIV but also toward the threat of opportunistic infections.

Trace elements have an important role in all redox reactions through participation in enzyme catalyzed reactions which offset potential oxidative damage caused by free radical formation. Two antioxidant enzymes, the copper/zinc cytosolic and manganese mitochondrial superoxide dismutases require trace metals for biological activity. Free radical formation occurs as a natural consequence of normal metabolic activity (48). In the healthy host the duration of the existence of free radicals is limited by antioxidant activity which neutralizes free radicals by conversion reactions. For example free radicals are transiently generated within the phagocytic cells of the immune system as a potent means whereby killing of ingested pathogens is accomplished. Inability to generate the oxygen burst is a pathological condition that leaves the host vulnerable to bacterial infections (49). The general principles of these interdigitating factors are illustrated in Fig. 1.

A number of studies have been undertaken that describe specific interactions between trace elements, minerals, and immune responses. The best studied interactions have focused on zinc, copper, selenium, iron, calcium, magnesium, and to some extent, chromium. In some instances data on these interactions are derived either from observations involving over exposure and toxicity or in settings of unusually severe deficiency. For example, excessive hexavalent chromium, fluorine, selenium, and iodine are highly toxic; some mechanisms may involve immune responses (50–53).

Metals affect immune responses in rather complex ways. Some of these interactions may affect cell viability generally rather than affecting immune cell processing. The type of system used in the study may strongly influence the results. For example, recent studies carried out using metal alloy discs (54) in in vitro culture of T lymphocytes suggest that inhibition of response in the presence of cobalt-chromium-molybdenum was related to the presence of cobalt. The fact that this was unrelated to decreased cell viability does support the concept that metals can have specific regulatory effects on immune response. Another approach has been to use controlled diets to adjust proportions of metals. Studies on copper deficiency with or without high dietary molybdenum or iron have shown that copper deficiency may have equivocal effects on immune response (55). However, when molybdenum was used to induce a low level of copper, altered acute phase response was observed as shown by reduction of ceruloplasmin and increased fibrinogen response. These changes were also associated with reduced immune cell response to the lymphocyte mitogen. Phytohemagglutinin in these studies was essentially a second challenge post infection, modeled in vitro (56). These results suggest that changes in the absolute or relative levels of metals may have a particularly sensitive effect in multiple infections and that immune response to a second pathogen is affected by cytokines still circulating from the previous challenge. This could weaken or alter the second response. This type of event could be critical in HIV infection which is characterized by waves of viral replication, followed by periods of vulnerability to opportunistic infections (57).

Studies of two congenital trace metal deficiencies have shown how crucial trace elements are to immune responses and host defense. Appreciation for the consequences of zinc deficiency has come from studies in patients with *Acrodermatitis enteropathica*, a genetically based zinc deficiency leading to intractable and even fatal opportunistic infections (58) (see Chapter 12). Zinc is essential for the development of normal immune function because it is required for the biological activity of thymic hormone needed for the maturation of T cells (59). When zinc levels are reduced temporarily (prematurity, intravenous hyperalimentation, artificial feeding, gastrointestinal disturbances) susceptibilty to opportunistic infections may be observed (60–64). Observed effects on

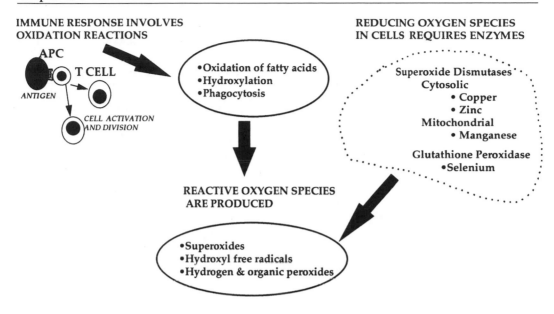

Fig. 1. Antioxident host defense: role of trace elements.

immunity range from severe thymic atrophy and profound lymphopenia to anergy to recall antigens in delayed type hypersensitivity skin testing and loss of natural killer cell activity. Studies of acquired mild or marginal zinc deficiency in chronic diseases such as beta-thalassemia and *Epidermolysis bullosa* have also shown that modest zinc depletion can lead to immune impairment (65). Zinc deficiency is associated with decreased cytokine production, specifically IL-1 alpha, IL-1 beta, and TNF alpha cytokine secretion. Zinc supplementation may have an enhancing effect on immune responses by acting as a biological response modifier, through increasing or stimulating the production of IL-2, (66) which in turn stimulates production of interferon gamma.

Zinc is also an immune stimulant. Data from our in vitro studies in HIV patients shown in Fig. 2 indicates that zinc elicited an increased response to interferon alpha even in relatively poorly responsive patients. This effect may have been mediated by direct effects of zinc on the type III Fc receptor since in related studies we observed direct triggering of interferon gamma production in vitro when zinc was added (65).

Zinc and copper compete for uptake from the gastrointestinal tract and changes in dietary intake of one will affect absorption of the other (67). Copper deficiency alone can produce immune deficiency (68). In genetic copper deficiency, Menkes syndrome (*see* Chapter 12), intractable infections may cause death (69). Copper deficiency is associated with impaired T-lymphocyte immune response, and with reduced neutrophil and monocyte activity. Short-term dietary depletion by means of a low copper diet administered to volunteers was found to cause reduced immune cell proliferative responses and IL-2 receptor secretion in response to activation in vitro (70). Reduced copper affects growth of lymphoid cell lines leading to reduced activity of the antioxidant enzyme superoxide dismutase and increased cellular damage associated with impaired mitochondrial activity and calcium efflux, thereby affecting the cell membrane (71). Copper also interacts with

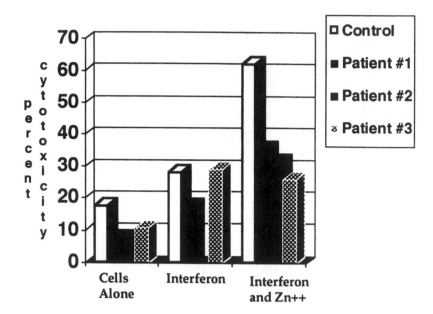

Fig. 2. Effect of Zn++ on Natural Killer Cell Activity in vitro in HIV infection
1) Patients were HIV+ hemophiliacs who were clinically asymptomatic at times of study. Control was a HIV negative, healthy person
2) Mononuclear cells were freshly isolated from peripheral blood and added to chromium labeled target cells alone, with interferon, or with interferon and Zn++
3) Data show mean percent specific cytotoxicity directed against the target cell after 18 hours under each condition at an effector to target ratio of 50:1

iron since ceruloplasmin, which contains most of the plasma copper, is a ferroxidase which facilitates release of tissue iron into plasma by oxidizing ferrous iron to ferric iron, which is then bound to transferrin for delivery to the bone marrow for hematopoiesis. High intake of iron, zinc, and manganese can interfere with copper absorption and these interactions may also have an impact on immune responses *(72)*.

Both iron deficiency and iron excess may inhibit some immune functions *(73)*. Since bacteria use iron for growth, excess iron can promote bacterial growth and even lead to infection *(74)* (*see* Chapter 18). However, although naturally occurring iron overload due to genetic causes of increased uptake in thalassemia and hereditary hemochromatosis has been temporalily linked with infections with *Vibrio vulnificus* and *Yersinia enterocolitica*, *(75)* these are uncommon events. On the other hand, low iron level can have a negative effect on immune response, especially the T-cell system, since effector functions are reduced in the absence of normal iron levels *(76,77)*. Iron deficiency has been implicated in chronic mucocutaneous candidiasis *(78)* and iron supplementation may support recovery from candidal infection secondary to primary immune deficiency *(79)*.

Selenoproteins are an important component of the antioxidant host defense system. Copper deficiency can cause reduced selenoglutathione peroxidase activity. A recent nutrient intervention study concluded that there was an overall increase in longevity in persons with genetic and environmental risk for cancer who received selenium supplementation along with beta-carotene and vitamin E after five years *(80)*. Selenium and vitamin E interact in the development of antioxidant host defense since selenium is an essential constituent of glutathione peroxidase, which catalyzes the conversion of peroxides to nontoxic alcohols and vitamin E is the major lipid soluble antioxidant in serum and cellular membranes. Host deficiency of either vitamin E or selenium may lead to a change in the viral phenotype of coxsackie B virus from nonvirulent to virulent in the mouse *(81)*. Selenium supplementation of volunteers has been shown to increase both proliferative responses and cytotoxic effector cell activity of human volunteers *(82,83)*.

Calcium and magnesium, two of the three essential minerals obtained through dietary intake have general significance for the development and expression of immune responses. Calcium and magnesium are critical for binding reactions, for example in coagulation, cell adhesion, and phagocytosis. Changes in calcium signaling have been implicated in trauma related immunosuppression *(84)*. Excess calcium will interfere with leukocyte function by displacing magnesium thereby interfering with binding reactions. It has been suggested that magnesium may also interact with vitamin D (1 alpha, 25-dihydroxyvitamin D3), but this has not been proven *(85)*.

The effect of trace elements and minerals on infections is specific to the infecting organism. Parasites which depend upon specific host cells for growth, may grow less well when essential minerals or trace elements are reduced in the host cells. For example red blood cell magnesium deficiency is protective against infections with *Plasmodium spp* and *Babesia hylomysci* but not against organisms which invade other cells *(86)*. On the other hand addition of $MgSO_4$ directly interferes with multiplication of mouse hepatitis virus (MHV) in infected cells in a stage dependent fashion *(87)*.

Interest in chromium as a potential modulator of immune response has come from observations suggesting that chromium supplementation might reduce the acute phase or "stress" response to infection in animal models *(88–90)*. However, the chemistry of chromium is complex, and under some conditions, chromium may not only modulate immune response to another antigen but may even act directly as a mitogenic trigger. Even theoretically "inert" metallic chromium may elicit an immune response. Allergic reactions may occur when chromium is released through corrosion of dental work or prostheses and in some cases antibody formation may actually lead to damage *(91)*. Supplemental chromium appears to modulate antibody response to viral immunization in cattle, promoting both a more frequent and more substantial response *(92)*. The oxidation state of chromium is also a factor. The toxic effects of lead chromate are well known. Long term human environmental exposure to chromate appears to lower immune response as demonstrated by reduced IL-6 production in response to pokeweed mitogen *(93)*. Related studies on the effect of exposure of peripheral blood mononuclear cells in vitro to chromium, as used in prostheses, also indicate that this contact causes reduced proliferative response and reduced production of IL-2 and IL-6 *(94)*.

It is crucial to recognize that supplementation with any trace element or mineral may have multiple effects. In general maintaining levels of essential trace elements and minerals through repletion is important in the HIV+ host. However, excess supplementation beyond the point of repletion may lead to overly high levels of one trace element that may suppress the uptake or relative concentration or activity of another. This could have a disproportionate effect. These considerations are important in studies involving the treatment of the HIV infected host *(95,96)*.

3. ALTERATION IN TRACE ELEMENTS
AND MINERALS IN HIV INFECTION AND AIDS

3.1. Altered Nutrient Balance in the HIV+ Host

Weight loss is a common occurrence in chronic viral illness, and in the case of HIV infection, weight loss frequently evolves into a wasting condition that may become intractable in late stage disease.

Infection-induced malnutrition, as discussed in Subheading 2.1., is primarily cytokine mediated, through the initiation of the acute phase response (97). Fever, cellular hypermetabolism, and various endocrine and metabolic changes eventually lead to catabolism and gluoconeogenesis. These are accompanied by multiple effects on metals and minerals such as fluxes of iron and zinc, and cause losses of nitrogen, potassium, magnesium, phosphate, and zinc in addition to loss of vitamins. This process is accompanied by retention of salt and water. Current work has also shown that malnutrition may occur relatively early during the asymptomatic phase of HIV infection (98,99). It seems probable that the etiology of early stage malnutrition and that of late stage malnutrition in this setting are essentially dissimilar.

Malnutrition in the late stages of AIDS is a significant clinical problem that has been approached from several points of view. Studies have shown that nutritional status is closely linked with survival (100) and is also linked with lower CD4+ T-cell level (4,101). Although response to intravenous nutrition is not impaired in the early stages of disease, (5) repletion of body mass through parenteral nutrition is effective primarily in HIV patients who have malabsorption but who have no serious ongoing systemic disease (102). Although nutritional support may not prolong life, and much gastrointestinal illness is certainly caused by recurrent opportunistic infections not directly affected by nutrient supplementation, there is increasing evidence that nutrient support can affect strength, endurance, and quality of life (103).

Among children with HIV infection, failure to thrive may occur much earlier and even be an initial manifestation (104). Children with HIV infection display certain differences in the expression of disease compared to adults and some of these differences may be associated with how HIV affects and interferes with the normal program of growth and development. Progression in children, unlike adults, may occur in the absence of significant decline in CD4+T cell number (105). Since growth abnormalities and stunting are observed among both long- and short-term survivors, studies are needed to discern what kinds of changes may influence progression. Despite the complexity of these issues and the general concern that secondary infections will often prevail over supplementation, increasing numbers of studies strongly indicate the potential value of nutritional support as a benefit to host defense in the HIV+ person (106).

Perhaps the central key to why trace elements and micronutrients may be fundamentally significant for the HIV+ host response is antioxidant defense. Antioxidant activity is needed to neutralize the harmful side effects of essential host defense in the HIV infected host. Oxygen metabolites released in the course of these reactions can damage tissues directly, if these remain unneutralized. These metabolites may also act to upregulate genes involved in the inflammatory response. One of these, NF-κ B, is an important regulator of HIV replication (107). Healthy function of the host defense system depends upon an adequate supply of antioxidative micronutrients. In the normal uninfected person, impaired host defense activity can be used as a very early and sensitive marker of marginal deficiency of antioxidant micronutrients *(108)*. Loss of antioxidant activity in HIV infection is caused by depletion in association with highly increased demand. Difficulties in attaining repletion through ordinary dietary means or supplementation as well as HIV related immune deficiency are also likely to be involved.

3.2. Trace Elements and Minerals in HIV Infection

Investigations into the significance of trace element deficiency in HIV infection and studies on whether trace element or mineral deficiency may be independent cofactors in disease progression have revealed some consistent answers *(108–112)*. Several studies have shown that micronutrient impairment is casually associated with the course of HIV infection and that there is a crucial impact on immune function.

One key to the focus and course of these interactions is reflected in the example of changes in iron status during the course of HIV disease. The anemia of chronic disease, in general, is etiologically associated with the elicitation of inflammatory cytokines, IL-1, IL-6, TNF-α, and TGF-β, which then inhibit erythroid colony formation *(113)*. The anemia of HIV infection is multifactorial, and involves effects of both cytokines and HIV on bone marrow precursor cells. This anemia is like the anemia of other chronic diseases in being characterized by iron deficiency, poor erythropoietin response, reduced number of progenitor cells of red cell colonies, and other abnormalities of reticuloendothelial iron metabolism *(113,114,115)*. It appears that low endogenous erythrypoeitin production may be a significant cause *(114)*. Interestingly, current data suggest that erthropoietin may be regulated by IL-1 and INF-γ. Both iron deficiency and iron overload may affect erthropoietin function through differential effects on T-helper function and cytokine patterns *(116)*. Whereas iron deficiency secondary to malabsorption is common in HIV infection *(117)*, iron overload also occurs frequently and is reflected in high serum ferritin and red cell ferritin *(118)*. The cytokines which mediate these effects include TNF-α, a powerful activator of NF-κB, which in turn is a critical activator of HIV replication. HIV replication leads to production of HIV-Tat protein which further shifts the cellular milieu toward a prooxidative state by downregulating the manganese dependent superoxide dismutase *(119)*. Interestingly, recent studies have shown that iron chelation can effectively block HIV replication. This may imply that iron is directly involved in the replication process and may be an important controlling element *(120,121)*.

One study has shown that fat oxidation is increased in patients with HIV infection and that whole body protein turnover is greater compared to controls *(122)*. The presence of oxidative stress has also been shown by the finding of increased lipid peroxidation in HIV infection *(122)*. This appears to be directly linked to reduction in levels of antioxidant trace elements, such as selenium and zinc *(108,109,112)*. Since increases in lipid peroxidation indices may also be related to viral replication, it is likely that these are interacting relationships. In addition trace elements interact such that an increase in one may create a deficiency of another and in a dynamic situation, these changes need to be examined longitudinally to establish key trends.

Trace element supplementation in HIV infection has been a relatively widespread practice and in many instances has been largely undirected by medically or scientifically trained persons, sometimes for fairly superficial reasons as part of a broad spectrum approach to counter suspected deficiencies *(123,124)*. In contrast measurement of blood levels of trace elements and monitoring of changes in these levels after supplementation has been considerably more rare. In some cases the basis for supplementation has been somewhat sketchy. For example, chromium has been considered for use in HIV+ persons because of reported effects on reversing loss of lean body mass, a common clinical problem that is likely to be related to cytokine activation through chronic stimulation of the immune system. Chromium is known to potentiate the action of insulin in carbohydrate, lipid, and protein metabolism and in addition chromium levels are significantly reduced during exercise. However, the possible benefit of chromium supplementation on body composition is controversial (125,126). Another reason for interest in chromium is that some studies have shown that dietary chromium from several sources (CrCl$_3$, Cr-picolinate, Cr-nicotinic acid complex) may increase immune response in animal models of cellular immune response both in vitro and in vivo (89,90). Chromium has been shown to attenuate the febrile response and reduce cortisol elevation in response to viral infection, although not in response to endotoxin (92). As noted previously, chromium can be toxic. Even trivalent chromium has been found to affect cytokine production of activated mononuclear cells in vitro when given to lactating cows in vivo (127,128). Both hexavalent and trivalent chromium levels appear to influence human peripheral blood lymphocyte subsets (93). On balance, it appears that normal levels of chromium are important in immune response but that exceeding the relatively wide 'safe' range should be avoided.

Several large studies have provided critical information about how trace element and mineral levels are affected by HIV infection and how, in turn, these changes may influence immune response and host defense. The general findings of these studies are shown in Table 1. The most commonly identified alterations in trace element and mineral levels in HIV infection involve zinc, selenium, and magnesium (106,108,109). Although many patients take supplements, supplementation may not easily replete critical stores. Skurnick et al. (108) found that taking supplements was associated with a better level of blood antioxidant micronutrients in HIV+ persons, but that almost one-third of patients on supplements showed reduced levels of at least one nutrient.

Trace elements such as zinc and selenium appear to decline in HIV disease as lipid peroxidase levels increase and this low status may persist at a later stage of disease, when polymorphonuclear leukocyte production of lipid peroxidases decreases. Low levels of both zinc and selenium have been consistently reported in HIV infected patients, and, in one study, association with increased levels of β-2 microglobulin was observed (109). Look et al. (129) found a strong correlation between stage of disease and reduced selenium such that selenium levels were positively correlated with CD4+ T cell count and negatively correlated with TNF-α levels. Furthermore, coinfection with hepatitis C virus was associated with further reduction in selenium level. Other studies have shown that there is a correlation between very low selenium levels and morbidity (106). This relationship between low selenium level and deficient immune response has also been observed in children with HIV infection (130). Furthermore, selenium is an integral part of glutathione peroxidase, and selenium supplementation in vitro can inhibit NF-κ B activation in reponse to HIV (131). Other studies have shown that selenium will suppress the enhancing effect of TNF-α on HIV replication of acutely infected monocytes but not T cells (132). The potential application of these observations was demonstrated in a supplementation study of HIV+ patients in which an increase in selenium was accompanied by enhanced glutathione peroxidase activity (133).

Since zinc is essential for many biological processes, as an essential component of more than 100 metalloenzymes, as an intracellular regulatory enzyme, in zinc dependent

Table 1
Essential Trace Elements and Minerals in HIV Disease

Nutrient	Effect of HIV	Relationship to Stage/Progression
Zinc	Reduced	Yes, some studies
Iron	Increased/Reduced	Unclear
Copper	Increased/Reduced	No
Selenium	Decreased	Yes
Calcium	Increased/Reduced	No
Magnesium	Decreased	Yes

enzymes essential for nucleic acid and protein synthesis, in "zinc" finger transcription proteins, and as a structural component of biological membranes, there are many possible reasons why zinc deficiency could be indirectly vital for immune function, including those needed for defense against HIV. More fundamentally, zinc is essential for the biological activity of the thymic hormone thymulin (59). Low thymulin levels are characteristic of zinc deficient states. In HIV infection, the virus infects the thymus and directly influences thymic maturation of T cells. Recent studies have shown that T cell maturation may shift from the thymus as a lymphoid epithelial site of true thymopoesis toward peripheral lymphoid accumulation in the perivascular space (134). Interestingly, increase in thymic mass was seen in HIV+ persons by chest computed tomography compared to adult controls where after 40 yr of age thymic mass was not detectable. And after successful antiretroviral therapy in the HIV+ host, this was further increased (135). Since the studies of Prasad and coworkers have shown that even mild zinc deficiency produced by dietary restriction of normal volunteers leads to impaired immune response (136) characterized by reduced interleukin 2 production, it is not surprising that the observation of reduced zinc levels in patients with HIV has been a cause for concern. Women who are HIV+ appear to have relatively greater micronutrient impairment, including zinc, than do men (8). It is suggested that this may be a factor in disease survival. Studies in children with congenital HIV infection have shown that zinc deficiency may be rare in this group. Interestingly, it appears that HIV+ men may require high levels of zinc intake to achieve normal plasma levels.

Although copper is an essential nutrient, clinical copper deficiency is rare. Among HIV+ persons, copper deficiency might occur in the context of high levels of zinc supplemental intake, or general malnutrition and this might be associated with reduction in the number of circulating neutrophils (137). A recent study found that copper levels were elevated among HIV+ children who had developed AIDS in comparison with HIV+ children who were asymptomatic (138). This change is likely to have occurred in the context of the acute phase response. Although copper deficiency could occur with increased supplementation of zinc, increased intake of copper containing foods might be used to offset this, safely, as long as the level of zinc supplementation did not increase plasma levels above normal limits. As noted above, copper has fundamental effects on immune response. One of these is particularly relevant to HIV infection since it appears that copper regulates a key transcription factor, NF-κ B (139), involved in both host immune response and in HIV viral replication. Under some conditions, Cu^{++} may inhibit the activation of NF-κ B by TNF alpha.

Changes in iron stores accompany the acute phase response. Studies that have directly addressed possible changes in iron status in HIV infection have reported both iron related anemia secondary to malabsorption and excess iron that tended to increase over time. Although this may appear contradictory, these findings actually reflect the complexity of iron storage pools, and the fact that there is no simple physiological means to excrete excess iron. Whereas iron supplementation has been used in HIV infection and this use was associated with increase in peripheral lymphocytes (112), other studies noted briefly above suggest that iron supplementation is potentially problematic in HIV infection. It appears that iron shifts the T-helper response toward a Th-type 2 response and this is not optimal in HIV infection although crucial for host defense in other settings. The fact that iron chelating agents have antiviral effects against HIV may be informative (119). On balance, repletion of iron deficiency could be beneficial, but unmonitored supplementation might be dangerous.

The levels of essential dietary minerals may also be affected by the course of HIV infection. In particular, a recent study has shown that magnesium levels are reduced among HIV+ persons (108). Magnesium affects the immune system at several levels including the cell cycle, stabilization of DNA/chromatin, and production of reactive oxygen species. Loss of magnesium is likely to occur in the context of the acute phase response (95). It has been suggested that low magnesium may account for some of the symptoms of HIV infection including lethargy and fatigue (108). Calcium has also been reported as reduced in HIV infection, as part of the same process (143). Calcium is crucial for cellular function and calcium influx inhibitors block proliferation and can be used to block HIV replication (140). Further, HIV fusion with the target cell is calcium dependent. Other data show that calcium pool function is involved in control of transcription of proviral HIV (142). Calcium levels may be increased or reduced in HIV infection and parathyroid hormone is reduced (143–145) for reasons that remain unclear.

4. SUMMARY

In summary, study of trace elements and mineral levels in HIV infection has suggested a pattern of losses that appear directly related to oxidative stress and to cytokine mediated initiation of the acute phase response.

The development of oxidative stress in HIV infection through increased levels of reactive oxygen species is likely to occur as a result of infection, the acute phase response, and to be related to polymorphonuclear phagocytic activation by potentially infectious agents. Cytokines elicited during the acute phase response such as TNF alpha exacerbate and drive this process. The effect of increased reactive oxygen species is twofold: 1. cellular damage will occur if this activity is not balanced by antioxidant activity. 2. HIV replication is directly promoted through the activation of NF-κ B in response to oxygen stress.

These processes are directly associated with depletion of key trace elements, specifically zinc and selenium and to altered iron metabolism (Fig.3), as well as to loss of the essential minerals, magnesium and calcium. As described, these changes in nutrients are linked through altered immune response and deficient antioxidant support which lead to increased HIV replication and susceptibility to opportunistic infections. Given strong evidence that changes in trace elements and minerals are associated with altered course of disease, it is reasonable to undertake repletion of these key nutrients. Although the use of pharmacological levels of supplements is unwarranted, there is every reason to postulate that maintaining normal levels of the essential trace elements and minerals is a vital key to host defense in HIV infection.

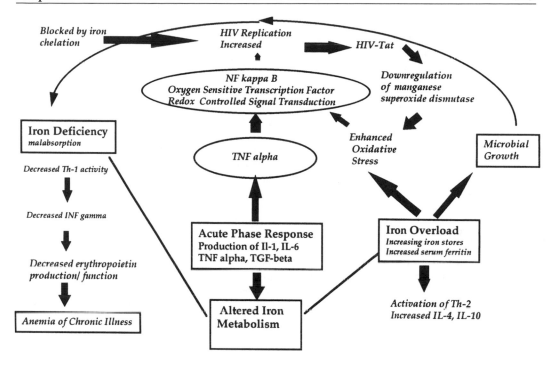

Fig. 3. Effects of altered iron metabolism in HIV infection on antioxidant host defense.

REFERENCES

1. Cunningham-Rundles S. Zinc modulation of immune function: Specificity and mechanism of interaction. J Lab Clin Med 1996;128:9–16.
2. Bendich A. Immunology functions to assess nutrient requirements. J Nutr Immunol 1995;3:47–56.
3. Baum MK, Shor-Posner G, Lu Y, Rosner B, Sauberlich HE, Fletcher MA, Szapocznik J, Eisdorfer C, Buring JE, Hennekens CH. Micronutrients and HIV-1 disease progression. AIDS 1995;9:1051–1056.
4. Allard JP, Aghdassi E, Chau J, Salit I, Walmsley S. Oxidative stress and plasma antioxidant micronutrients in humans with HIV infection. Am J Clin Nutr 1998;67:143–147.
5. Maccallan DC, McNurlan MA, Milne E, Calder AG, Garlick PJ, Griffin GE. Whole-body protein turnover from leucine kinetics and the response to nutrition in human immunodeficiency virus infection. Am J Clin Nutr 1995;61:818–826.
6. Kotler DP. Wasting syndrome: nutritional support in HIV infection. AIDS Res Hum Retroviruses 1994;10:931–934.
7. Connors M, Kovacs JA, Krevat S, Gea-Banacloche JC, Sneller MC, Flanigan M, Metcalf JA, Walker RE, Falloon J, Baseler M, Feuerstein I, Masur H, Lane HC. HIV infection induces changes in CD4+ T-cell phenotype and depletions within the CD4+ T cell repertoire that are not immediately restored by antiviral or immune-based therapies. Nat Med 1997;3:703-704.
8. Baum MK, Shor-Posner G, Zhang G, Lai H, Quesada JA, Campa A, Jose-Burbano M, Fletcher MA, Sauberlich H, Page JB. HIV-1 infection in women is associated with severe nutritional deficiencies. J Acquir Immune Defic Syndr Hum Retrovirol 1997;16:272–278.
9. Varela P, Marcos A, Santacruz I, Ripoll S, Requejo AM. Human immunodeficiency virus infection and nutritional status in female drug addicts undergoing detoxification: anthropometric and immunologic assessments. Am J Clin Nutr 1997;66:504S–508S.
10. Castetbon K, Kadio A, Bondurand A, boka Yao A, Barouan C, Coulibaly Y, Anglaret X, Msellati P, Malvy D, Dabis F. Nutritional status and dietary intakes in human immunodeficiency virus (HIV)-infected outpatients in Abidjan, Cote D'Ivoire. Eur J Clin Nutr 1997;51:81–86.

11. Smythe PM, Schonland M, Brereton-Stiles GG, Coovadia HM, Grace HJ, Loening WEK, Mafoyne A, Parent MA, Vos GH. Thymolymmphatic deficiency and depression of cell-mediated immunity in protein-calorie malnutrition. Lancet 1971;2:939–943.
12. Keusch GT. Malnutrition and the thymus gland. In: Cunningham-Rundles S, ed. Nutrient Modulation of Immune Response. Marcel Dekker, Inc., New York, 1993, pp.283–299.
13. Scrimshaw NS, San Giovani JP. Synergism of nutrition, infection and immunity: an overview. Am J Clin Nutr 1997;66:464S–477S.
14. Chandra RK.Nutrition and the immune system. Proc Nutr Soc (England) 1993;52:77–84.
15. Beisel WR. Nutrition in pediatric HIV infection: setting the research agenda. Nutrition and immune function: overview. J Nutr 1996;126(10Suppl):2611S–2615S.
16. Gillou PJ, Monson JR, Sedman PC, Brennan TG. Modification of Lymphocyte Function by fatty acids — biological and clinical implications. In: Cunningham-Rundles S, ed. Nutrient Modulation of the Immune Response. Marcel Dekker, Inc., New York, 1993, pp.369–391.
17. Garritson BK, Nikaein A, Peters GN, Gorman MA, King CC, Liepa GU. Effect of major dietary modifications on immune system in patients with breast cancer: a pilot study. Cancer Pract 1995;3:239–246.
18. Yaqoob P, Newsholme EA, Calder PC. Inhibition of natural killer cell activity by dietary lipids. Immuno Lett 1994;41:241–247.
19. Chandra RK. Excessive intake of zinc impairs immune responses. JAMA 1984;252:1443–1446.
20. Oleske JM, Rothpletz-Puglia PM, Winter H. Historical perspectives on the evolution in understanding the importance of nutrtional care in pediatric HIV infection. J Nutr 1996;126:2616S–2619S.
21. Wolf BH, Ikeogu MO, Vos ET. Effect of nutrtional and HIV status on bacteraemia in Zimbabwean Children who died at home. Eur J Pediatr 1995;154:299–303.
22. Cunningham-Rundles S, Noroski L, Cervia JS. Malnutrition as a cofactor in HIV disease. J Nutr Immunol 1997;5:33–38.
23. Prindull G, Ahmad M. The ontogeny of the gut mucosal immune system and the susceptibility to infections in infants of developing countries. Eur J Ped 1993;152:786–792.
24. Pozzetto B, Odelin MF, Bienvenu J, Defayolle M, Aymard M. Is there a relationship between malnutrition, inflammation, and post-vaccinal antibody response to influenza viruses in the elderly? J Med Virol 1993;41:39–43.
25. Bogden JD, Oleske JM, Lavenhar MA, Munves EM, Kemp FW, Bruening KS, Holding KJ, Denny TN, Guarino MA, Holland BK. Effects of one year of supplementation with zinc and other micronutrients on cellular immunity in the elderly. J Am Coll Nutr 1990;9:214–225.
26. Keen CL, Lonnerdal B, Golub MS, Uriu-Hape JY, Olin KL, Hendrickx AG, Gershwin ME. Influence of marginal maternal zinc deficiency on pregnancy outcome and infant zinc status in rhesus monkeys. Ped Resrch 1989;26:470–477.
27. Vruwink KG, Keen CL, Gershwin ME, Mareschi JP, Hurley LS. The effect of experimental zinc deficiency on development of the immune system. In: Cunningham-Rundles S, ed. Nutrient Modulation of the Immune Response. Marcel Dekker Inc., New York, 1993, pp. 263–282.
28. Beisel WR. Impact of infections disease on the interaction between nutrition and immunity. In: Cunningham-Rundles S, ed. Nutrient Modulation of the Immune Response. Marcel Dekker, Inc., New York, 1993, pp. 475–480.
29. Meydani SN, Wu D, Santos MS, Hayek MG. Antioxidants and immune response in aged persons: overview of present evidence. Am J Clin Nutr 1995;62(6 Suppl):1462S–1476S.
30. Cunningham-Rundles S. Malnutrition and gut immune function. Curr Opin Gastroenterol 1994;10:664–670.
31. Qiao L, Schurmann G, Autschbach F, Wallich R, Meuer SC. Human intestinal mucosa alters T-cell reactivities. Gastroenterology 1993;105:814–819.
32. Panteleo G, Graziosi C, Demarest JF, Butini L, Montroni M, Fox CH, Orenstein JM, Kotler DP, Fauci AS. HIV infection is active and progressive in lymphoid tissue during the clinically latent stage of disease. Nature 1993;362:355–362.
33. Yamamura MK, Uyemura RJ, Deans K, Weinberg TH, Rea B, Bloom B, Modlin RL. Defining protective responses to pathogens: cytokine profiles in leprosy lesions. Science 1991;254:277–279.
34. Barnes PF, Abrams JS, Lu S, Sieling PA, Rea TH, Modlin RL. Patterns of Cytokine production by mycobacterium-reactive human T-cell clones. Infection and Immunity 1993;61:197–203.
35. Brandtzaeg P. Humoral Immune response patterns of human mucosae: Induction and relation to bacterial respiratory tract infection. J Infectious Dis 1992;165:S167–176.
36. Mowat AM, Hutton AK, Garside P, Steel M. A role for interleukin-1 alpha in immunologically mediated intestinal pathology. Immunology (England) 1993;80:110–115.

37. Xu-Amano J, Kiyono H, Jackson RJ, Staats HF, Fujihashi K, Burrows PD, Elson CO, Pilliai S, McGhee JR. Helper T-cell subsets for immunoglobulin A responses: Oral immunization with Tetanus Toxoid and cholera toxin as adjuvant selectively induces Th2 cells in mucosa associated tissues. J Exp Med 1993;178:1309–1321.

38. Clerici M, Shearer A. Th-1/Th-2 switch is a critical step in the etiology of HIV infection. Immunology Today 1993;14:107–110.

39. Maggi E, Mazzetti M, Ravina A, Annunziato F, DeCarli M, Peirre Piccinni M, Manetti R, Carbonari M, Pesce AM, DelPrete G, Romagnani S. Ability of HIV to promote a TH1 to TH0 shift and to replicate preferentially in TH2 and TH0 Cells. Science 1994;265:244–248.

40. Moldawer LL, Lowry SF. Interactions between cytokine production and inflammation: implications for therapies aimed at modulating the host defense to infection. In: Cunningham-Rundles S, ed. Nutrient Modulation of Immune Response. Marcel Dekker, Inc., New York, 1993, pp. 511–522.

41. Tracey KJ, Beutler B, Lowry SF, Merryweather J, Wolpe S, Milsark IW, Hariri RJ, Fahey TJ, Zentella A, Albert JD, Shires GT, Cerami A. Shock and tissue injury induced by recombinant human cachectin. Science 1986;234:470.

42. Munoz-Fernandez MA, Navarro J, Garcia A, Punzon C, Fernandez-Cruz E, Fresno M. Replication of human immunodeficiency virus-1 in primary human T cells is dependent on the autocrine secretion of tumor necrosis factor through the control of nuclear factor-kappa B activation. J Allergy Clin Immunol 1997;100(6 pt 1):838–845.

43. Mata L. Diarrheal disease as a cause of malnutrition. Am J Trop Med Hyg (US) 1992;47(1 Pt 2):16–27.

44. Probert L, Keiffer J, Corbella P, Cazlaris H, Patsavoudi E, Stephens S, Kaslaris E, Kioussis D, Kollias G. Wasting, Ischemia, and lymphoid abnormalities in mice expressing T-cell-targeted human tumor necrosis factor transgenes. J Immunology 1993;151:1894–1906.

45. Kuhn R, Lohler J, Rennick D, Klaus R, Muller W. Interleukin-10-Deficient mice develop chronic enterocolitis. Cell 1993;75:263–274.

46. Nahlen BL, Chu SY, Nwanyanwu OC, Berkelman RL, Martinez SA, Rullan J. HIV wasting syndrome in the United States. AIDS 1993;7:183–188.

47. Schmidt K. Interaction of antioxidative micronutrients with host defense mechanisms. A critical review. Int J Vitam Nutr Res 1997;67:307–311.

48. Supek F, Supekova L, Nelson H, Nelson N. Function of metal-ion homeostasis in the cell division cycle, mitochondrial protein processing, sensitivity to mycobacterial infection and brain function. J Exp Biol 1997;200:321–330.

49. Ahlin A, Elinder G, Palmblad J. Dose-dependent enhancements by interferon-hamma on functional responses of neutrophils from chronic granulomatous disease patients. Blood 1997;89:3396–3401.

50. Granchi D, Ciapetti G, savarino L, Cavedagna D, Donati ME, Pizzoferrato A. Assessment of metal extract toxicity on human lymphocytes cultured in vitro. J Biomed Mater Res 1996;31:183–191.

51. Li M, Boyages SC. Iodide induced lymphocytic thyroiditis in the BB/W rat: evidence of direct toxic effects of iodide on thyroid subcellular structure. Autoimmunity 1994;18:31–40.

52. Domingo JL. Metal-induced developmental toxicity in mammals: a review. J Toxicol Environ Health 1994;42:123–141.

53. Leung FY. Trace elements in parenteral micronutrition. Clin Biochem 1995;28:561–566.

54. Faleiro C, Godinho I, Reus U, de Sousa M. Cobalt chromium molybdenum but not titanium 6alu minium-4vanadium alloy discs inhibit human T cell activation in vitro. Biometals 1996;9:321–326.

55. Ward JD, Gengelbach GP, Spears JW. The effects of copper deficiency with or without high dietary iron or molybdenum on immune function of cattle. J Animal Sci 1997;75:1400–1408.

56. Arthington JD, Corah LR, Blecha F. The effect of molybdenum-induced copper deficiency on acute-phase protein concentrations, superoxide dismutase activity, lekocyte numbers, and lymphocyte proliferation in beef heifers inoculated with bovine herpesvirus-1. J Anim Sci 1996;74:211–217.

57. Martin KA, Wyatt R, Farzan M, Choe H, Marcon L, Desjardins E, Robinson J, Sodroski J, Gerard C, Gerard NP. CD4-independent binding of SIV gp 120 to Rhesus CCR5. Science 1997;28:1470–1473.

58. Sandstrom B, Cederblad A, Lindblad BS, Lonnerdal B. Acrodermatitis enteropathica, zinc metabolism, copper status, and immune function. Arch Pediatr Adolesc Med 1994;148:980–985.

59. Dardenne M, Savino W, Borrih S, Bach JF. A zinc dependent epitope of the molecule of thymulin, a thymic hormone. Proc Natl Acad Sci USA 1985;82:7035.

60. Moynahan EM. Acrodermatitis enteropathica: A lethal inherited human zinc deficiency disorder. Lancet 1974;2:399–400.

61. Prasad AS, Miale A Jr, Farid Z, et al. Zinc metabolism in patients with the syndrome of iron deficiency anemia, hepatosplenomegaly, dwardism and hypogonadism. J Lab Clin Med 1963;61:537–549.

62. Ball C, Thompson RP. Zinc status in children with cystic fibrosis. Hum Nutr Appl Nutr 1986;40:309–310.

63. Cunningham-Rundles C, Cunningham-Rundles S, Iwata T, et al. Zinc deficiency, depressed thymic hormones and T lymphocyte dysfunction in patients with hypogammaglobulinemia. Clin Immunol Exp Pathol 1981;21:387–396.

64. Parent G, Chevalier P, Zalles L, et al. In vitro lymphocyte-differentiation effects of thymulin (Zn-FTS) on lymphocyte subpopulations of severely malnourished children. Am J Clin Nutr 1994;60:274–278.

65. Cunningham-Rundles S, Bockman RS, Lin A, Giardina PV, Hilgartner MW, Caldwell-Brown D, Carter DM. Physiological and Pharmacological effects of Zinc on immune response. Ann NY Acad Sci 1990;587:113–122.

66. Kaplan J, Hess J, Prasad AS. Impaired Interleukin-2 production in the elderly: Association with mild zinc deficiency. J Trace Elem Exp Med 1988;1:3–8.

67. Sandstead H. Requirements and toxicity of essential trace elements, illustrated by zinc and copper. Am J Clin Nutr 1995;61(Suppl):621S–624S.

68. Castillo-Duran C, Fisberg M, Valenzuela A, Egana JI, Uauy R. Controlled trial of copper supplementation during the recovery from marasmus. Am J Clin Nutr 1983;37:899–903.

69. Prohaska JR, Failla ML. Copper and immunity. In: Klurfeld DM, ed. Nutrition and immunology. Plenum Press, New York, 1993, pp. 309–332.

70. Kelley DS, Daudu PA, Taylor PC, Mackey BE, Turnlund JR. Effects of low-copper diets on human immune response. Am J Clin Nutr 1995;62:412–416.

71. Tong KK, Hannigan BM, McKerr G, Strain JJ. The effects of copper deficiency on human lymphoid and myeloid cells: an in vitro model. Br J Nutr 1996;75:97–108.

72. Johnson MA, Smith MM, Edmonds JT. Copper, iron, zinc, and manganese in dietary supplements, infant formulas, and ready-to-eat breakfast cereals. Am J Clin Nutr 1998;67 (suppl):1035S–1040S.

73. Cunningham-Rundles S, Cervia JS. "Malnutrition and Host Defense." In: Walker WA, Watkins JB, eds. Nutrition in Pediatrics: Basic Science and Clinical Application 2nd Edition. Marcel Dekker, Europe, Inc. 1996, pp. 295–307.

74. Weinberg ED. Iron withholding: defense against infection and neoplasia. Physiol Rev 1984;64:65–102.

75. Chiesa C, Pacifico L, Renzuli F, et al. Yersinia hepatic abscesses and iron overload. JAMA 1987;257:3230–3231.

76. Santos PC, Falcao RP. Decreased lymphocyte subsets and K-cell activity in iron deficiency anemia. Acta Hematol 1990;84:118–121.

77. Prema K, Ramallakshmi BA, Madhavapeedi R, Babu S. Immune status of anemic pregnant women. Br J Obstet Gynaecol 1982;89:222–225.

78. Higg JM, Wells RS. Chronic mucocutaneous candidiasis: assiciated abnormalities of iron metabolism. Br J Dermatol 1972;86(suppl):88–102.

79. Cunningham-Rundles S, Yeger-Arbitman R, Nachman SA, et al. New variant of MHC class II deficiency with interleukin-2 abnormality. Clin Immunol Immunopathol 1990;56:116–123.

80. Blot WJ, Li JY, Taylor PR, Guo W, Dawsey S, Wang GQ, Yang CS, Zheng SF, Gail M, Li GY, Yu Y, Liu B, Tangrea J, Sun Y, Liu F, Fraumeni JF Jr, Zhang YH, Li B. Nutrition intervention trials in Linxian, China: Supplementation with specific vitamin/mineral combinations, cancer incidence, and disease specific mortality in the general population. J Nat Cancer Inst 1993;85:1483–1491.

81. Beck MA. Increased virulence of coxsackievirus B3 in mice due to vitamin E or selenium deficiency. J Nutr 1997;127:966S–970S.

82. Roy M, Kiremidjian-Schumacher L, Wishe HI, Cohen MW, Stotzky G. Supplementation with selenium and human immune cell functions. Effect on lymphocyte proliferation and interleukin 2 receptor expression. Biol Trace Elem Res 1994;46:103–114.

83. Kiremidjian -Schumacher L, Roy M, Wishe HI, Cohen MW, Stotzky G. Supplementation with selenium and human immune cell functions II: Effect on cytotoxic lymphocytes and natural killer cells: Biol Trace Elem Res 1994;41:115–127.

84. Hoyt DB, Junger WG, Loomis WH, Liu FC. Effects of trauma on immune cell function: impairment of intracellular calcium signaling. Shock 1994;2:23–28.

85. McCoy H, Kenney MA. Interactions between magnesium and vitamin D: possible implications in the immune system. Magnes Res 1996;9:185–203.

86. Murios P, Delcourt PH, Gueux E, Rayssiguier Y. Magnesium deficiency protects against Babesia hylomysci and mice become resistant to rechallenge with the parasite regardless of diet fat. Parasitology1994;108(pt 3):245–248.

87. Mizutani T, Hayahi M, Maeda A, Ishida K, Watanabe T, Namioka S. The inhibitory effects of MgSo4 on the multiplication and transcription of mouse hepatitis virus. Jpn J Vet 1994;42:95–102.

88. van Heugten EV, Spears JW. Immune response and growth of stressed weanling pigs fed diets supplemented with organic or inorganic forms of chromium. J Anim Sci 1997;75:409–416.

89. Kegley EB, Spears JW, Brown TT Jr. Immune respnse and disease resistance of calves fed chromium nicotinic acid complex or chromium chloride. J Dairy Sci 1996;79:1278–1283.

90. Burton JL, Mallard BA, Mowat DN. Effects of supplemental chromium on antibody responses of newly weaned feedlot calves to immunization with infectious bovine rhinotracheitis and parainfluenza 3 virus. Can J Vet Res 1994;58:148–151.

91. Wooley PH, Nasser S, Fitzgerald RH Jr. The immune response to implant materials in humans. Clin Orthop 1996;May(362):63–70.

92. Wright AJ, Mallard BA, Mowat DN. The influence of supplemental chromium and vaccines on the acute phase response of newly arrived feeder calves. Can J Vet Res 1995;59:311–315.

92. Chang GX, Mallard BA, Mowat DN, Gallo GF. Effect of supplemental chromium on antibody responses of newly arrived feeder calves to vaccines and ovalbumin. Can J Vet Res 1996;60:140–144.

93. Snyder CA, Udasin I, Waterman SJ, Taioli E, Gochfeld M. Reduced IL-6 levels among individuals in Hudson County, New Jersey, an area contaminated with chromium. Arch Environ Health 1996;51:26–28.

94. Wang JY, Tsukayama DT, Wichlund BH, Gustilo RB. Inhibition of T and B cell proliferation by titanium, cobalt, and chromium: role of IL-2 and IL-6. J Biomed Mater Res 1996;32:655–661.

95. Oelske JM, Rothpletz-Puglia PM, Winter H. Historical perspectives on the evolution in understanding the importance of nutritional care in pediatric HIV infection. J Nutr 1996;126:2616S–2619S.

96. Stack JA, Bell SJ, Burke PA, Forse RA. High-energy, high-protein, oral, liquid, nutrition supplementation in patients with HIV infection: effect on weight status in relation to incidence of secondary infection. J Am Diet Assoc 1996;96:337–341.

97. Beisel WR. Herman Award Lecture, 1995: infection-induced malnutrition from cholera to cytokines. Am J Clin Nutr 1995;62:813–819.

98. Melchior JC, Salmon D, Riguad D, Leport C, Bouvet E, Detruchis P, Vilde JL, Vachon F, Coulaud JP, Apfelbaum M. Resting energy expenditure is increased in stable, malnourished HIV-infected patients. Am J Clin Nutr 1991;53:437–441.

99. Niyongabo T, Bouchaud O, Henzel D, Melchior JC, Samb B, Dazza MC, Ruggeri C, Begue JC, Coulaud JP, Larouze B. Nutritional status of HIV seropositive subjects in an AIDS clinic in Paris. Eur J Clin Nutr 1997;51:660–664.

100. Chlebowski RT, Grosvenor MB, Bernhard NH, Morales LS, Bulcavage LM. Nutrtional status, gastrointestinal dysfunction and survival in patients with AIDS. Comments in: Am J Gastroenterol 1990;85:476.

101. Sharkey SJ, Sharkey KA, Sutherland LR, Church DL. Nutritional status and food intake in human immunodeficiency virus infection. GI/HIV Study Group. J Acquir Immune Defic Syndr 1992;5:1091–1098.

102. Kotler DP, Tierney AR, Culpepper-Morgan JA, Wang J, Pierson RN Jr. Effect of home total perenteral nutrtion on body composition in patients with acquired immunodeficiency syndrome. J Parenter Enteral Nutr 1990;14:454–458.

103. Crocker KS. Gastrointestinal manifestations of the acquired immunodeficiency syndrome. Nurs Clin North Am 1989;24:395–406.

104. Henderson RA, Saavedra JM. Nutritional considerations and management of the child with human immunodeficiency virus infection. Nutrition 1995;11:121–128.

105. Bonagura VR, Cunningham-Rundles S, Schuval S. Dysfunction of Natural Killer cells in HIV+ children with Pnuemocystis carinii pneumonia. J Pediatr 1992;121:195–201.

106. Baum M, Cassetti L, Bonvehi P, Shor-Posner G, Lu Y, Sauberlich H. Inadequate dietary intake and altered nutrition status in early HIV-1 infec tion. Nutrition 1994;10:16–20.

107. Conner EM, Grisham MB. Inflammation, free radicals, and antioxidants. Nutrition 1996;12:274–277.

108. Skurnick JH, Bogden JD, Baker H, Kemp FW, Sheffet A, Quattrone G, Louria DB. Micronutrient profiles in HIV-1 infected heterosexual adults: J Acquir Immune Defic Sndr Hum Retrovirol 1996;12:75–83.

109. Allavena C, Dousset B, May T, Dubois F, Canton P, Belleville F. Relationship of trace element, immunological markers, and HIV1 infection progression. Biol Trace Elem Res 1995;47:133–138.

110. Sappy C, Leclercq P, Coudray C, Faure P, Micoud M, Favier A. Vitamins, trace elements and peroxide status in HIV seropositive patients: asymptomatic patients present a severe beta-carotene deficiency. Clin Chim Acta 1994;230:35–42.

111. Luder E, Godfrey E, Godbold J, Simpson DM. Assessment of nutritional, clinical and immunologic status of HIV-infected, inner-city patients with multiple risk factors. J Am Diet Assoc 1995;95:655–660.

112. Moseson M, Zeleniuch-Jacquotte A, Belsito DV, Shore RE, Marmor M, Pasternack B. The potential role of nutrtional factors in the induction of immunologic abnormalities in HIV-positive homosexual men. J Acquir Immune Defic Syndr 1989;2:235–247.

113. Bertero MT, Caligaris-Cappio F. Anemia of chronic disorders in systemic autoimmune diseases. Haematologica 1997;82:375–381.

114. Kreutzer KA, Rockstroh JK. Pathogenesis and pathophysiology of anemia in HIV infection. Ann Hematol 1997;75:179–187.

115. Means RT Jr. Cytokines and anaemia in human immunodeficiency virus infection. Cytokines Cell Mol Ther 1997;3:179–186.

116. Omara FO, Blakley BR. The effects of iron deficiency and iron overload on cell-mediated immunity in the mouse. Br J Nutr 1994;72:899–909.

117. Castaldo A, Tarallo L, Palomba E, Albano F, Russo S, Zuin G, Buffardi F, Guarino A. Iron deficiency and intestinal malabsorption in HIV disease. J Pediatr Gastroenterol Nutr 1996;22:359–363.

118. Riera A, Gimferrer E, Cadafalch J, Remacha A, Martin S. Prevalence of high serum and red cell ferritin levels in HIV-infected patients. Haematologica 1994;79:165–167.

119. Shatrov VA, Boelaert JR, Chouaib S, Droge W, Lehmann V. Iron chelation decreases human immunodeficiency virus-1 Tat potentiated tumor necrosis factor-induced NF-kapa B activation in Jurat cells. Eur Cytokine Netw 1997;8:37–43.

120. Sappey C, Boelaert JR, Legrand-Poels S, Forceille C, Favier A, Piette J. Iron chelation decreass NF-kappa B and HIV type activation due to oxidative stress. AIDS Res Hum Retroviruses 1995;11:1049–1061.

121. Boelart JR, Weinberg GA, Weinberg ED. Altered iron metabolism in HIV infection: mechanisms, possible consequences, and proposals for management. Infect Agents Dis 1996;5:36–46.

122. McCallan DC, McNurlan MA, Milne E, Calder AG, Garlick PJ, Griffin GE.: Whole-body protein turnover from leucine kinetics and the response to nutrition in human immunodeficiency virus infection. Am J Clin Nutr 1995;61:818–826.

123. Young JS. HIV and medical nutrition therapy. J Am Diet Assoc 1997;97(10 Suppl 2):S161-S166.

124. Nicholas SW, Leung J, Fennoy I. Guidelines for nutritional support of HIV-infected children. J Pediatr 1991;119:S49–S62.

125. Anderson RA. Chromium as an essential nutrient for humans. Regul Toxicol Pharmacol 1994;26(1 pt 2):S35–41.

126. Lukaski HC, Bolonchuk, WW, Siders WA, Milne DB. Chromium supplementation and resistance training: effects on body composition, strength, and trace element status of men. Am J Clin Nutr 1996;63:954–965.

127. Burton JL, Nonnecke BJ, Elsasser TH, Mallard BA, Yang WZ, Mowat DN. Immunomodulatory activity of blood serum from chromium-supplemented periparturient dairy cows. Vet Immunopatho 1995;49:29–38.

128. Burton JL, Nonnecke BJ, Dubeski PL, Elsasser TH, Mallard BA. Effects of supplemental chromium on production of cytokines by mitogen-stimulated bovine peripheral blood mononuclear cells. J Dairy Sci 1996;79:2237–2246.

129. Look MP, Rockstroh JK, Rao GS, Kreuzer KA, Barton S, Lemoch H, Sudhop T, Hoch J, Stockinger K, Spengler U, Sauerbruch T. Serum selenium, plasma glutathione and erythrocyte glutathione peroxidase levels in asymptomatic versus symptomatic human immunodeficiency virus-1 infection. Eur J Clin Nutri 1997;51:266–272.

130. Bologna R, Indacochea F, Shor-Posner G, Mantero-Atienza E, Grazziutti M, Sotomayor MC, Fletcher MA, Cabrejos C, Scott GB, Gaum MK. Selenium and immunity in HIV-1 Infected pediatric patients. J Nutr Immunol 1994;3:41–49.

131. Makropoulos V, Bruning T, Schulze-Osthoff K. Selenium-mediated inhibition of transcription factor NF-kappa B and HIV-1 LTR promotor activity. Arch Toxicol 1996;70:277–283.

132. Hori K, Hatfield D, Maldarelli F, Lee BJ, Clouse KA. Selenium supplementation suppresses tumor necrosis factor alpha-induced human immunodeficiency virus type 1 replication in vitro. AIDS Res Retroviruses 1997;13:1325–1332.

133. Delmas-Beauvieux MC, Peuchant E, Couchouron A, Constans J, Sergeant C, Simonoff M, Pellegrin JL, Leng B, Conri C, Clerc M. The enzymatic antioxidant system in blood and glutathione status in human

immunodeficiency virus (HIV)-infected patients: effects of supplementation with selenium or betacarotene. Am J Clin Nutr 1996;64:101–107.

134. Haynes B. The role of thymus in reconstituting the immune system in AIDS. 5th Conference on Retroviruses and Opportunistic Infections, Chicago, IL, 1998.

135. George A, Ritter M. Thymic involution with aging: obsolescence or good houskeeping? Immunology Today 1996;17–267–272.

136. Prasda AS, Meftah S, Adballah J, Kaplan J, Brewer GJ, Bach JF, Dardenne M. Serum thymulin in human zinc deficiency. J Clin Invest 1988;82:1202–1210.

137. Percival SS. Neutropenia caused by copper deficiency: possible mechanisms of action: Nutr Rev 1995;53:59–66.

138. Periquet BA, Jammes NM,Lambert WE, Tricoire J, Moussa MM, Garcia J, Ghisolfi J, Thouvenot J. Micronutrient levels in HIV-1-infected children. AIDS 1995; 9:887–893.

139. Satake H, Suzulki K, Aoki T, Otsuka M, Sugiura Y, Yamamoto T, Inoue J. Cupric ion blocks NF kappa B activation through inhibiting the signal-induced phosphorylation of I kappa B alpha. Biochem Biophys Res Commun 1995;216:568–573.

140. Yasui H, Butscher W, Cohen M, Spriggs N, Wersto R, Kohn EC, Liotta L, Gardner K. Selective inhibition of mitogen-induced transactivation of the HIV long terminal repeat by carboxyamidotriazole. J Biol Chem 1997;272:28762–28770.

141. Ebenbichler CF, Stoiber H, Schneider R, Patsch JR, Dierich MP. The human immunodeficiency virus type 1 transmembrane gp41 protein is a calcium-binding protein and interacts with the putative second-receptor molecules in a calcium-dependent manner. J Virol 1996;70:1723–1728.

142. Papp B, Byrn RA. Stimulation of HIV expression by intracellular calcium pump inhibition. J Biol Chem 1995;270:10278–10283.

143. Teichmann J, Stephan E, Lange U, Discher T, Stracke H, Federlin K. Elevated serum-calcium and parathormone-levels in HIV afflicted female heroin addicts. Eur J Med Res 1997;2343–346.

144. Jaeger P, Otto S, Speck RF, Villiger L, Horber FF, Casez JP, Takkinen R. Altered parathyroid gland function in severely immunocompromised patients infected with human immunodeficiency virus. J Clin Endocrinol Metab 1994;79:1701–1705.

145. Hellman P, Albert J, Gidlund M, Klareskog L, Rastad J, Aderstrom G, Juhlin C. Impaired parathyroid hormone release in human immunodeficiency virus infection. AIDS Res Hum Retroviruses 1995;10:391–394.

20

Trace Element and Mineral Nutrition in Hospital, Surgical, and Cancer Patients:
Enteral and Parenteral Nutrition

M. A. Mohit-Tabatabai, MD

1. INTRODUCTION

Most patients undergoing elective surgical operations or being admitted into intensive care units can withstand a brief period of catabolism and starvation without noticeable difficulty. However, if the expected period extends beyond 4–5 d, or if patients have preexisting weight loss or malnutrition, then nutritional support becomes a critical factor in the outcome. In fact compromised nutrition could either directly or indirectly affect patient survival.

The incidence of malnutrition in hospitalized patients can be as high as 50 % *(1)*. This malnutrition, by changing cell mediated and humoral immunity, can predispose patients to infection which, in turn, can cause increased catabolism and worsening of malnutrition (*see* Chapters 18 and 19). The malnutrition that develops in a hospitalized patient can include deficiencies of one or more trace elements.

2. CLINICAL ASSESSMENT

Nutritional assessment is necessary to determine the severity of nutrient deficiency and the need for nutritional support. An interview with the patient or family is a simple and powerful tool for identifying patients who may be malnourished or at nutritional risk. The history should include changes in oral intake, gastrointestinal symptoms, weight loss, and functional ability. Weight loss is a commonly recognized feature of malnutrition and an unintentional weight loss of 10% or more of usual weight is significant. Other findings such as recent changes in food intake, presence and severity of gastrointestinal symptoms, functional level of patient, loss of subcutaneous tissue, and muscle wasting can help to estimate the degree of malnutrition.

Anthropometric data, which include height, weight, and measurements of skin-fold thickness and mid arm muscle circumference, can help to estimate the degree of malnutri-

From: *Clinical Nutrition of the Essential Trace Elements and Minerals: The Guide for Health Professionals*
Edited by: J. D. Bogden and L. M. Klevay © Humana Press Inc., Totowa, NJ

tion. Biochemical and laboratory values, serum albumin or trasferrin, total lymphocyte count, and 24-h urinary creatinine excretion, are also helpful in assessment of nutritional status.

Metabolic cart is a reliable bedside assessment of energy requirements and it can be used to estimate resting energy expenditure and respiratory quotient. An assessment of body composition (lean body mass) can be done by bioelectric impedance analysis, although it is not accurate if the patient has significant edema.

Alternative methods of determining body composition are radiographic and ultrasound techniques, isotope dilution assays, and in vivo neutron activation analysis.

2.1. Choices of Nutritional Therapy

Over the last 30 yr, clinical studies have stressed the importance of early nutritional support in the management of surgical patients. However, the route of nutrient delivery (enteral vs parenteral) has remained a subject of discussion and clinical research.

In animal models starvation produces mucosal atrophy of the gastrointestinal tract, bacterial overgrowth, increased permeation of luminal toxins, translocation of bacteria, and atrophy of gut-associated lymphoid tissue. Early delivery of nutrients through the gastrointestinal tract can prevent or reduce the risk of these changes. Moore (2), in a meta-analysis of eight prospective randomized trials of early enteral vs parenteral feeding, have reported that the risk of complications was significantly less in the enterally fed group and septic complications were also significantly lower in this group. However, this meta-analysis showed that enteral feeding is more challenging to the patient than parenteral feeding. In the group that received total enteral nutrition there was a higher incidence of abdominal distention, gastrointestinal intolerance, and diarrhea in comparison to the group receiving parenteral feeding.

3. ENTERAL FEEDING

There are several approaches to enteral feeding. The oral approach is the preferred one, whenever it is feasible. This can be achieved by adding nutrients to the regular meal or by adding a can of formula to each meal. If the patient is not able to consume food by the oral cavity then the nutrient should be delivered by a tube in the GI tract. The options are nasogastric, nasointestinal, nasoduodenal, cervical esophagostomy, gastrostomy, and jejunostomy.

The ideal nasogastric tube is made of soft, pliable material. The tube length should be appropriate to the site of insertion and the intended feeding site of the GI tract. The tube should be strong enough to tolerate the pressure that is generated by a feeding pump or flushing the tube, and have an adequate diameter to accommodate formulas of different viscosity. These tubes are made of silicone rubber or polyurethane, and some have a weighted end with a mercury or a tungsten piece. The tube should have a different hub and adapter so as to make it compatible to intravenous tubing. This will prevent accidental misuse. The tube may have a stylet for ease of placement, although there is an increased incidence of insertion related complications from the stylet.

There is an increased risk of aspiration with the tube that passes through the gastroesophageal junction, because it causes the lower esophageal sphincter to become incompetent. For this reason a gastrostomy or jejunostomy is a better choice.

The gastrostomy can be done as an open technique or it can be inserted percutaneously with the help of a flexible gastroscope. The percutaneous endoscopic gastrostomy (PEG) is the preferred method of insertion of the gastrostomy tube and it can be done as a bedside procedure and can be utilized for feeding within 24 h of insertion.

Cervical pharyngostomy has limited usefulness. It can be inserted percutaneously, through a cervical incision or during the neck dissection. The tube can stay in place for a long period of time and it is comfortable although cosmetically most of the time is not acceptable to patients.

Stamm gastrostomy is the insertion of a gastrostomy tube through a small incision in the midline or subcostal area. The tube is inserted into the stomach through a pursestring suture, and the site of insertion will be sutured to the abdominal wall with three or four interrupted sutures.

Witzel gastrostomy is similar to Stamm gastrostomy, the difference being that a sero-muscular tunnel will be made a distance of five to eight centimeters from the insertion site.

Janeway gastrostomy is similar to Stamm gastrostomy with a difference that a gastric flap will be created to cover the tract to the skin. This type of gastrostomy is permanent, and removal of tube does not cause spontaneous closure of the gastrostomy site.

For insertion of PEG a gastroscope is passed into the stomach and stomach is filled with air. Then after transilluminating the stomach a 16-gauge catheter is inserted transabdominally through an area anesthetized with 2% lidocaine. A No. 2 silk or a guide wire is inserted into the stomach, and is then guided by grasping it with a forceps or snare and pulling it through the oral cavity by withdrawing the scope. Then a special catheter, usually some form of a Malecot, is tied to the end of the silk or guide wire and in retrograde direction is pulled into the stomach and through the skin of the abdomen. This type of gastrostomy is suitable for long term feeding and can be done at bed side. Also it is possible to insert a mercury-tipped tube through the PEG into the jejunum for feeding.

Jejunostomy is insertion of a tube in the jejunum percutaneously and is usually done under general anesthesia. There are two types of jejunostomy, one is a needle catheter jejunostomy described by Delany (3). This type of jejunostomy is used as a temporary feeding route. The other type is for a permanent jejunostomy and a larger size catheter is usually inserted in Witzel fashion.

3.1. Starter Formulas

Enteral formulas that are isosmotic can be used in full strength and do not need to be diluted. The concept of using diluted formula as starter should be reserved for hyperosmolar formulas. The starting volume is usually about 50mL/h and it can be increased up to 125mL/h as the patient shows tolerance to feeding. Absence of gastric retention is a sign that patients can tolerate a larger volume. It is recommended that a feeding pump be used for continuous trouble free enteral feedings especially if a jejunostomy is the route of feeding.

3.2. Type of Formula

The feeding admixtures that are used enterally can be classified into the following categories:

1. Blenderized formulas, made of whole food that is blenderized into liquid consistency,
2. Lactose-containing milk based formulas that can't be given to lactose-intolerant patients,
3. Lactose free formulas that are the common type used in hospitals and at home,
4. Elemental diets composed of amino acids or short chain peptides. These formulas have poor taste and should be given by tubes. They usually have an osmolarity of 600. Because these formulas are predigested, they are ideal for patients who have short bowel or pancreatic insufficiency,

5. Modular diets composed of separate modules of the basic ingredients of enteral feeding. They could be combined in different ratios in order to meet special individual dietary needs, and

6. Special formulas, commercially prepared for specific indications or situations like sepsis, stress, and pulmonary or renal insufficiency.

3.3. Nutrients for Immune Enhancement

Clinical and animal studies of specific nutrients that can produce immune-enhancing effects independent of preventing protein malnutrition have identified glutamine, arginine, omega-3 fatty acids, and exogenous nucleotides as possible immune-enhancing nutrients (4). Recently, commercially enriched formulas with one or more of these immuno modulator nutrients have become available. Although there is data suggesting that the use of these formulas can improve the clinical outcome, randomized prospective studies have failed to show significant decreases in complications or mortality. The only significant finding in the usage of these formulas was reduction in the length of hospital stay.

3.4. Complications of Enteral Nutrition

3.4.1. MISPLACED TUBE

The misplaced catheter can cause serious complications especially if nutrients are infused into the bronchus or peritoneum. This problem can be prevented by taking a chest radiograph in all patients prior to initiation of enteral feeding.

3.4.2. GASTRIC RETENTION

All patients on enteral feeding should be checked routinely for gastric residual and if it exceeds 150 mL then the feeding should be stopped or reduced.

3.4.3. ASPIRATION

Prevention of gastric retention and avoiding use of the nasogastric tube can reduce the risk of aspiration. It is also useful to keep the head of the patient's bed raised up to 30 degrees.

3.4.4. DIARRHEA, NAUSEA, VOMITING AND CRAMPS

The most common reasons for the intolerance are:

1. A formula that is not isosmotic.
2. Uncontrolled flow which could be prevented by using a pump.
3. Bacterial contamination that can be prevented by changing the feeding bag and tubing every 24 h, limiting the hanging time of the formulas to 8 h, and using aseptic technique in preparation and storage of the formulas.
4. Use of lactose based formulas in lactose intolerance patients.
5. The use of broad-spectrum antibiotics or a preexisting gastrointestinal problem.

3.4.5. METABOLIC COMPLICATIONS

Metabolic complications of enteral feeding are very similar to those seen in the course of parenteral nutrition. The type and frequency of these complications are dependent on underlying disease, route of access to the gastrointestinal tract, and type of formula. The most frequent of these complications are dehydration, hyperglycemia, hypoglycemia, hypophosphatemia, hyperkalemia, and hyponatremia.

4. TOTAL PARENTERAL NUTRITION (TPN)

The use of TPN became possible after the introduction of subclavian catheterization in Europe following the French-Vietnam war in 1959. Wilmore and Dudrick described successful long-term use of TPN in an infant with intestinal atresia in 1968 *(5)*. The use of TPN became widespread from 1970 to 1980 and the indication for use of TPN expanded. It was accepted as a safe and sometimes life-saving treatment. The use of TPN started to decrease as the complications, cost, and shortfalls of TPN became more evident, and the rediscovery of the gut as a better route of nutritional delivery limited its use further.

4.1. Indications

The decision to place a patient on TPN should be made after individual assessment. The major indications are:

1. The gastrointestinal tract cannot be used or is contraindicated.
2. Enteral feeding or a combination of enteral feeding and peripheral parenteral nutrition (PPN) cannot provide adequate nutrition.
3. PPN is unsuitable because of limited access and or anticipated length of parenteral support or required caloric need.

4.2. Interavenous Access

Administration of total parenteral nutrition formulas requires the insertion of a catheter into the venous system. It should be easily placed, short in length, and capable of remaining in place for extended periods of time. The location of the catheter should not restrict joint mobility or interfere with patient physical activity. The choices of access are peripheral vein, central vein, and through an arterio-venous fistula.

In general the high osmolarity of TPN formulas, which is usually about three to eight times serum osmolarity, requires the use of a large vein with high flow in order to avoid injury to the vein and thrombophlebitis and pain. These requirements limit the access site to the superior vena cava, and probably the subclavian insertion site is the best route because of location, lack of interference with patient's daily activities, and relative short length of catheter. It is the most commonly used access site.

4.3. Peripheral TPN

Historically, the osmolarity limitation of peripheral venous sites has limited the ability to deliver adequate amounts of calories to patients requiring parenteral nutrition. However with introduction of intravenous lipid, it becomes possible to maintain patients on peripheral parenteral nutrition for extended periods of time. When the period of starvation is predictable and short, patients can be managed with PPN. The complication of inserting a central venous catheter can be avoided by utilizing PPN. In addition, the complications associated with glucose intolerance are less frequent because fewer calories are given as glucose. Due to the hyperosmolar nature of PPN solutions, phlebitis is a problem and the catheter site should be changed every 2–3 d in order to minimize the risk of phlebitis.

4.4. Central TPN

Successful use of TPN generally depends on proper placement and management of a central venous catheter. A 16-gage catheter is introduced into the subclavian vein percutaneously and threaded into the superior vena cava. An alternative to this access is insertion through the external or internal jugular vein into the subclavian vein. This type of access is usually not comfortable to patients.

For insertion of a subclavian vein catheter, the patient is placed supine in a 15-degree head down position with a folded towel placed between the shoulder blades in order to allow the shoulder to drop posteriorly. After prepping the skin with an iodophore compound, sterile drapes are placed. Under local anesthesia, a two inch long 14-gage needle attached to small syringe is inserted at the point between the medial one-third and middle third under the clavicle and advanced into the subclavian vein although pointing toward the suprasternal notch. The needle should hug the lower surface of the clavicle and pass over the first rib.

By applying a gentle negative pressure to the syringe, the entrance into the subclavian vein can be identified and a 16 gage radiopaque catheter inserted through the needle and advanced into the subclavian vein and the superior vena cava. After fixation of the catheter to the skin with a 00 silk suture, the subclavian catheter is hooked to sterile intravenous administration tubing and the catheter insertion site is covered by a sterile occlusive dressing.

Insertion of a catheter into the inferior vena cava from the lower extremity site is not recommended due to a high incidence of complications. Insertion through a cutdown site in the cubital area of the upper extremities has proven to be unsatisfactory.

4.5. Maintenance of the Central Venous Catheter

After the insertion of a central venous catheter, a chest radiograph should be ordered to verify the location of the catheter tip and also to rule out the possibility of complications related to insertion of the central line. A common complication after insertion of a central line is infection. Potential sources of this infection are the TPN solution, administration set, TPN catheter, and the insertion site. In order to decrease the risk of infection the following guidelines are essential:

1. The TPN catheter should be used only for TPN and administration of other solutions or medication or blood products through the line is contraindicated.
2. An occlusive dressing should be used and this dressing should be changed every 2–3 d.
3. The administration set should be changed every 24 h.
4. A multiple-lumen catheter should not be used for TPN if there is no need for an additional lumen. If one has been inserted it should be changed to a single lumen catheter as soon as the need for the other port has been satisfied, because these catheters are associated with a higher rate of septic complications.
5. Routine change of catheter is not indicated.

4.6. Complications of Catheter Insertion

4.6.1. INJURY TO LUNG AND PLEURA

Pneumothorax is the most common complication of catheter insertion. It can be diagnosed easily by the chest film taken following the insertion of the catheter. If pneumothorax is symptomatic or large or enlarging on the repeated chest film then a small tube thoracostomy is indicated.

4.6.2. INJURY TO THE ARTERY OR SUBCLAVIAN VEIN

In case of injury to the subclavian artery or vein the catheter or needle should be removed immediately and direct pressure applied. However it is too difficult to apply any meaningful pressure to the subclavian artery and if there is significant bleeding it will be necessary to explore the artery by resecting the clavicular head or by a trap door approach or thoracotomy to control the bleeding and repair the artery.

4.6.3. PLEURAL EFFUSION

If the tip of the catheter lacerates the vein and enters the pleural space or is misplaced directly into the pleural space, it will cause pleural effusion and chest pain and shortness of breath upon infusion of fluid. The chest radiograph will confirm the diagnosis and it should be treated by removal of the catheter and aspiration of the pleural cavity.

4.6.4. INJURY TO BRACHIAL PLEXUS

This usually will cause severe pain in the distribution of the radial, ulnar, or median nerves and the treatment is the removal of the catheter.

4.6.5. INJURY TO THORACIC DUCT

The thoracic duct can be injured during the insertion of a left subclavian vein catheter and it may cause chylothorax. The chylothorax should be treated by removal of the catheter and tube thoracostomy. Rarely it may require ligation of the thoracic duct if the leakage persists.

4.6.6. INJURY TO MEDIASTINUM

Mediastinal hematoma is a rare complication which may need surgical intervention for hemostasis or removal of a symptomatic hematoma.

4.6.7. AIR EMBOLISM

An air embolus can occur if during catheter insertion the end of the catheter is left open to the air. The negative pressure of the superior vena cava can cause a significant air embolus. This uncommon complication is potentially fatal and requires only a small quantity of air (about 100 mL). In case of air embolism the patient should be placed in a left lateral decubitus position with the head down and an attempt to aspirate the air from the ventricle should be made.

4.6.8. CATHETER EMBOLUS

Embolus of a piece of catheter can occur if the catheter has been inserted through a needle and was pulled back although the needle is still in the vein. This will cause shredding of the tip of the catheter and embolization of it into the right heart, pulmonary artery, or the lungs. The preferred technique for removal of the embolized catheter is intravenous snaring of the broken piece by a cardiologist or invasive radiologist.

4.6.9. CARDIAC COMPLICATION

Positioning the tip of catheter in the right atrium or ventricle can cause arrhythmia. This complication can be avoided by selecting the correct catheter length and correct positioning of the catheter tip.

4.6.10. COMPLICATIONS OF CATHETER MAINTENANCE

Clotted catheter: If the catheter becomes clotted, an attempt to unplug the catheter by flushing the line with saline or instilling heparin and a thrombolytic agent should be considered.

Venous thrombosis: Venous thrombosis is usually the result of malposition of the catheter. Sometimes it occurs following long term TPN and may be associated with sepsis. The treatment is removal of the catheter.

4.6.11. SEPTIC COMPLICATIONS

Evidence of bloodstream infection and the presence of an intravenous catheter is usually an early sign of catheter sepsis. Gross evidence of site infection is not common. In most instances the infection is diagnosed by culture and a gram stain of the skin entry site or blood culture from peripheral veins or the catheter itself.

4.6.12. METABOLIC COMPLICATIONS

Metabolic complications of TPN fall into two categories: early and late. Some complications of TPN usually happen very early in the process of feeding in the first few days. These complications include volume overload, hyperglycemia, hypoglycemia, hyperosmolar nonketotic coma, hypokalemia, hypophosphatemia, hypomagnesemia, hyperchloremia acidosis, and CO_2 retention. These complications can be avoided by carefully monitoring and adjusting the formula.

Late metabolic complications of TPN are essential fatty acid deficiency, essential micronutrient deficiencies, iron deficiency anemia, vitamin K deficiency, hepatic dysfunction, and metabolic bone disease.

Hepatic dysfunction commonly occurs in patients receiving total parenteral nutrition (6) and it is the result of multiple factors. It is more common in patients with pre-TPN hepatic dysfunction (7). In this group of patients the liver function continues to deteriorate although the patient is receiving TPN. The liver function will be maintained at a normal level in most patients with normal pre-TPN liver function tests. The infection and endotoxemia of the portal circulation and gut origin infection could cause hepatic injury and keeping the patient on TPN will probably cause atrophy of the mucosa of the gut and overgrowth of bacteria and translocation of the bacteria and endotoxin. This in turn could contribute to hepatic damage and dysfunction during the administration of TPN for an extended period of time.

4.7. TPN Formulas

Parenteral alimentation is the continuous infusion of a solution containing carbohydrates, proteins, fat, electrolytes, vitamins, minerals and trace elements through an intravenous catheter inserted into a peripheral vein or the superior vena cava (Table1).

4.7.1. ENERGY

The best method of calculation of caloric need is indirect calorimetry, which permits the direct measurement of oxygen consumption. However, most studies recommend that for most patients, 25 to 30 kcal/kg per day is a reasonable goal.

4.7.2. PROTEIN

It is difficult to estimate the exact protein losses in critically ill patients. In current practice the protein requirement is calculated on the basis of 1 to 3 g/kg per day.

4.7.3. NONPROTEIN CALORIES

Nonprotein calories in TPN are provided as a mixture of carbohydrate and fat in the ratio of approximately 70:30. The advantage of this admixture are lower cost and better glucose tolerance.

Table 1
Composition per liter of formula

Volume	Formula 1 (peripheral vein) 1000 mL	Formula 2 (central vein) 1000 mL
Kcal	370	1050
Protein gm	50	50
Carbohydrate gm	50	250
Fat *		
Osmolarity	836	1819
Na mEq/L	75	25
K mEq/L	40	40
Cl mEq/L	88	33
Mg mEq/L	5	5
PO4 mM/L	14	14
Ca mEq/L	5	5
Acetate mEq/L	84	84
Zinc mg/24 h	4	4
Chromium mcg/24 h	16	16
Copper mg/24h	1.6	1.6
Mn mg/24h	.4	.4
MVI-12 Amp/24h	1	1

*500 mL of 20% lipid emulsion will be added to the formulas. This will provide 100gm of fat and an additional 1000 kcal.

4.7.4. ELECTROLYTE AND MINERAL REQUIREMENTS

All serum electrolyte and mineral requirements will be fully met by TPN formulas. The sodium requirement ranges from 80 to 100 mEq/d. This value should be adjusted for the presence of diseases such as renal failure and congestive heart failure. The chloride requirement is similar to sodium need.

Potassium can be given as a chloride, a phosphate, or an acetate salt in the amount of 80–100 mEq/ d. Calcium should be added to TPN admixture as a gluconate salt, about 15 to 20 mEq/d. Magnesium is given as magnesium sulfate, 15 to 20 mEq/d.

4.7.5. VITAMINS

Both fat and water soluble vitamins are added to the formulas. Vitamin requirements may increase in stress or trauma. Vitamins D and K usually are not added to the TPN formula.

5. TRACE ELEMENTS

Micronutrients that are important in nutritional support include the essential trace elements Iron, Zinc, Manganese, Iodine, Selenium, Chromium, Cobalt, Copper, Fluroide and Molybdenum (Fe, Zn, Mn, I, Se, Cr, Co, Cu, F, and Mo) (8,9) (see chapter 1).

Most of the enteral formulas that are used for tube feeding contain these trace elements in excess of the daily requirement and this is usually sufficient in a typical patient. For patients receiving total parenteral nutrition a commercially available combination of trace elements is usually added to the TPN admixture and these trace mineral additives usually contain Zn, Cu, Mn, and Cr. There are some formulations that in addition to these four may have Se, I, and Mo.

Measurement of trace elements in serum or other fluids by spectrophotometric analysis is the mainstay of assessing trace element nutriture. However, these measurements may not reflect the true tissue level, and changes in trace element binding proteins can affect these measurements (*see* Chapter 5).

5.1. Iron (Fe)

In adults the estimate of total daily losses of iron is about 1.0 to 2.0 mg in menstruating females and about 0.5 to 1.0 mg in males and post menopausal women. The average diet contains 10–20 mg iron a day and about 10% of this iron gets absorbed (*see* Table 3 in Chapter 4). Iron is necessary for production of hemoglobin and myoglobin. The most common reason for iron loss is usually frequent phlebotomy for monitoring patients on TPN. Typically iron is not provided during total parenteral nutrition unless the patient is receiving long-term home TPN. Limiting blood tests of patients on TPN can prevent the need for iron supplementation. Addition of iron to TPN formulas is not recommended due to the risk of allergic reactions to iron products like iron dextran (10). Parenteral administration of iron can be achieved by a series of intramuscular injections in patients who are on long-term TPN, but these injections are painful and sometimes cause discoloration of injection sites.

5.2. Zinc (Zn)

Zinc deficiency occurring in association with TPN presents itself mostly as skin lesions of the face and perineum, stomatitis, alopecia, diarrhea, abdominal pain, vomiting, psychological alteration (depression), anorexia, weight loss, and impaired growth. This element has an important role in cell mediated immune function and wound healing and it is an essential component of over 100 enzymes. Zinc deficiency is common in inflammatory bowel disease and short bowel syndrome, and it is mostly due to impaired absorption of zinc in the gastrointestinal tract.

The daily oral requirement of zinc is 10 to 15 mg per day. Adequate zinc supplementation can be achieved by the oral or intravenous route.

5.3. Manganese (Mn)

Manganese is a cofactor in many enzyme systems. Experimental manganese deficiency in animal models is associated with retarded bone growth, impaired reproductive function, discoloration of hair, and accumulation of fat *(11)*. Manganese has an important role in glucose utilization and it has been shown that manganese-deficient guinea pigs show an abnormal diabetic-like glucose tolerance test. Recommended daily dietary intake of manganese is 2.5 to 5.0 mg for adults. Since manganese is excreted primarily in the bile, provision of Mn to liver patients is contraindicated. There are reports of liver disease patients who have developed severe and sometime fatal manganese toxicity *(12)* (*see* Chapter 17).

Patients with cirrhosis usually have higher blood manganese concentrations, and it is probably the cause of hyperintensity of the T1-weighted signal on MRI of the brain of these patients. It is also possible that manganese toxicity is a contributing factor in development of encephalopathy in patients with chronic liver disease *(13)*.

5.4. Selenium (Se)

Selenium is a component of glutathione peroxidase, an enzyme that protects the cell against damage from intracellular peroxides. Keshan disease has been known for many years in China and is characterized by fatal cardiomyopathy. It has been reported in the Keshan district of China where the soil is low in selenium and can be prevented by selenium supplementation. It has been shown that long-term TPN can result in selenium depletion, and a number of cases of cardiomyopathy in patients receiving TPN have been reported (14,15). The daily requirement of selenium is 5 to 70 micrograms per day for adults.

5.5. Copper (Cu)

Copper is an essential part of several enzymes, and its deficiency in animal models has resulted in anemia, osteoporosis, loss of hair, and delays in wound healing. In adults and children it has been shown that the serum level of copper will decline in those who are on TPN without Cu supplementation (16). In humans with Cu deficiency, anemia, leukopenia, arrhythmia, hypoproteinemia, pretibial or periorbital edema, bone changes, and vascular aneurysms have been reported. The anemia associated with Cu deficiency is hypochromic normocytic with low reticulocyte count, and is usually seen when serum Cu goes below 20 µg/100 mL (17). It is unresponsive to Fe supplementation, but can be corrected by provision of Cu.

5.6. Molybdenum (Mo)

Mo is an essential element in the function of several enzymes including sulfite oxidase which is essential for the metabolism of sulfur containing amino acids.

In animals Mo deficiency appears to affect growth, but there are no defined symptoms in man. In a documented case of Mo deficiency (18), the patient developed lethargy, disorientation, tachycardia, and a very low excretion of inorganic sulfate in urine which responded to treatment with Mo supplement.

5.7. Chromium (Cr)

Chromium deficiency can cause reduced glucose tolerance and impairment of glucose metabolism, peripheral neuropathy, and weight loss (19). Cr deficiency has been reported in patients receiving long-term TPN with no supplementation (20,21), and it can be prevented by adding 10–20 µg of Cr per day to the TPN formula.

Unlike Zn or Cu deficiency, which can develop after only a few weeks of the TPN, deficiencies of Cr, Se, and Mo require months to years to become evident.

5.8. Iodine (I)

Iodine is an essential micronutrient in the diet and is a necessary element in the production of thyroid hormones which regulate the body metabolism (see Chapter 13). Iodine deficiency can cause enlargement of the thyroid gland and development of goiter. Iodine can easily be absorbed through the skin, and povidone-iodine skin preparation can probably prevent the development of iodine deficiency in patients on TPN. The daily requirement of iodine is about 150–200 µg per day.

5.9. Fluoride

Fluoride is utilized in maintenance of teeth and can produce a more acid resistant tooth structure. Fluoride stimulates bone formation and it needs calcium supplementation for these processes. The mechanism of this bone mineralization is unknown. The estimated daily requirement is 1.5–4.0 mg/d for adults. Deficiency is not a problem for TPN patients.

5.10. Cobalt (Co)

Cobalt is an element in the molecular structure of vitamin B12. The daily requirement of Co is about 1–2 μg per day and is provided in TPN solutions as vitamin B12.

5.11. Ultra-Trace Elements

In addition to the trace elements that have been discussed there is some evidence that nickel, silicon, tin, vanadium, boron, and arsenic (pentavalent) may be essential in animals, however there is not sufficient evidence that these elements are essential in man (*see* Chapter 2).

Berner *(22)* has demonstrated that a significant concentration of these ultratrace elements is often present as a contaminant in TPN solutions. These concentrations are directly related to the type of the solutions and their manufacturers *(23)*, and they are inconsistent due to variation in the degree of contamination. Aluminum is a contaminant present in TPN solution that is toxic to humans *(24)* (*See* Chapters 2 and 16) .

6. TRACE ELEMENTS AND CANCER INCIDENCE

The study of relationships between trace elements, minerals and the incidence of cancer poses difficult challenges. Epidemiological studies of minerals and trace elements in humans have been conducted and it appears that calcium, selenium, iron, and iodine are the most important of these elements, and the relationship of other minerals and trace elements with the risk of cancer is not clear. In contrast various animal studies in the laboratory have shown carcinogenic effects of many elements when administered at high levels parenterally. It is difficult to analyze these studies, because the levels of these elements in the diets of humans are different, and because of the parenteral route of administration.

Carcinogenicity of trace elements has been investigated by Schroeder and Mitchener *(26,27)* in mice and rats in detail, and they found that only rhodium and palladium in mice show carcinogenicity and other elements fail to show any increase in tumor incidence. In contrast arsenic and cadmium reduce tumor incidence in mice.

Anticarcinogenic roles of trace elements are increasingly recognized in recent years and several mechanisms have been proposed *(28)*. These proposed mechanism are antioxidant potential, induction of methallothionein, apoptosis of initiated cells, effect on immune response and DNA repair and alteration of carcinogen metabolism. However, epidemiological studies and trace element chemoprevention trials have usually not shown any benefits except for selenium *(29,30)*.

The most comprehensive assessment to date of the relationship between diet and cancer was published in 1997 by the World Cancer Research Fund and the American Institute for Cancer Research *(31)*. This authoritative monograph of more than 650 pages devotes only 4 pages to minerals and trace elements, specifically selenium, calcium, iron, and iodine, reflecting the relative paucity of definitive evidence about the influence of dietary trace elements and minerals on cancer incidence and prevention. The monograph concludes that diets deficient in iodine probably increase the risk of thyroid cancer, but diets excessive in iodine may also do so. It also suggests that selenium may decrease the risk of lung cancer. However, the limited data on dietary trace elements and cancer incidence are of little help to the clinician treating cancer patients (*see* subheading 7.1.).

6.1. Calcium

Calcium could decrease the risk of colorectal cancer by diminishing mucosal proliferation and binding with different carcinogenic compounds in the GI tract. Studies of the association of calcium intake and the incidence of colorectal polyp or cancer suggest, that increased calcium in the diet may reduce the risk (32).

6.2. Selenium

There is some evidence that suggests selenium decreases the risk of cancer *(33)*. This probably is related to antioxidant activity of selenium and it also suppresses cell proliferation. Available data has shown that there is a correlation between low tissue level of selenium and lung cancer. Several reports have been suggestive that low level of selenium may increase the risk of cancer of the stomach, thyroid gland, and liver. In addition, a placebo-controlled clinicial trial found that selenium supplements of 200 micrograms per day reduced the incidence of lung, colorectal, and prostate cancers *(34)*, and high toenail selenium concentrations were reported to be associated with a reduced risk of advanced prostate cancer *(35)*.

6.3. Iodine

There is evidence in the literature that low or high levels of iodine are associated with an increased risk of thyroid cancer (*see* Chapter 13).

6.4. Iron

A high iron diet may increase the risk of development of colorectal and liver cancer. Iron deficiency is a component of Plummer-Vinson syndrome and these patients are at increased risk for development of esophageal cancer.

7. NUTRITION THERAPY IN SPECIFIC DISEASE STATES

7.1. Cancer

Malnutrition is a common finding in cancer patients and it impacts the quality of life and survival. Very often these patients are immunocompromised with lack of appetite and weight loss. In some patients such as those with gastrointestinal malignancy and head and neck cancers, the tumors directly interfere with the use of the GI tract as a conduit for nutritional support. These malnourished patients respond poorly to treatment modalities such as radiotherapy, surgery, and chemotherapy.

Tumors can cause malnutrition indirectly by causing anorexia, changes in taste and smell perception, depression, and metabolic alteration. Also side effects of treatment modalities are the major factors in development of cancer related malnutrition. These include mucositis, zerostomia of radiation therapy, nausea, vomiting, and diarrhea related to chemotherapy, alteration of the swallowing mechanism, malabsorption and pancreatic insufficiency related to resection of a segment of the GI tract or surgical treatment.

The goal of nutritional support is reversal or prevention of malnutrition in the cancer patients. Very often nutritional support is an integral part of cancer treatment.

The route of nutritional support can be enteral or parenteral. Initially parenteral nutrition was used more often with cancer treatment. However, the available data does not support routine administration of TPN as an adjunct treatment for cancer. Klein *(25)* reviewed twenty-eight prospective randomized controlled trials in cancer patients and found no statistically significant benefit in these patients. Routine administration of TPN during chemotherapy failed to show any survival advantage or improvement in response to chemotherapy and it actually increased the risk of infection in patients who were treated with chemotherapy. Probably a useful role of TPN is in preoperative surgical management of patients with cancer if the patient is severely malnourished.

7.2. Liver Disease

Patients with hepatic failure and encephalopathy have an elevated level of aromatic amino acids in plasma. There are special formulas low in aromatic amino acids and with higher levels of branch chain amino acids. This formula has no advantage in patients who have no encephalopathy *(36)*. A particular concern in these patients is manganese toxicity, and they should not be given supplemental enteral or parenteral manganese *(see* Chapter 17).

7.3. Renal Disease

A special formula with enriched essential amino acids has been available for patients with acute tubular necrosis in oliguric phase. Studies of this special formulation have failed to show any survival advantage. Since absorbed molybdenum, fluoride, iodine, selenium, and chromium are excreted primarily in the urine, it is unwise to include these elements in TPN solutions for patients with compromised kidney function *(see* Chapter 16).

7.4. Acute Pancreatitis

Nutritional support should be given to patients with a diagnosis of acute pancreatitis on the 4th or 5th hospital day, because most of these patients have ileus and require nasogastric decompression. Total parenteral nutrition is usually well tolerated and administration of fat in the formula appears to be safe. Close observation for glucose and lipid tolerance is essential in administration of TPN in these patients. Studies of TPN use in pancreatitis have failed to show any improvement in outcome. There is also a suggestion of an increased incidence of catheter related septic complications in these patients *(37)*.

7.5. AIDS

Weight loss and malnutrition are the recognized complications of HIV infection. Malnutrition in AIDS will alter functional capacities, and quality of life and can decrease the life expectancy in these patients. Decrease of oral intake, chronic diarrhea, and intolerance limits the efficiency of enteral nutrition. TPN is an alternative to enteral feeding in these patients and can be administered safely. However TPN has no effect on survival rate or the risk of complications *(38) (see* Chapter 19 for discussion of trace elements in HIV/AIDS infection).

8. PERIOPERATIVE NUTRITION THERAPY

Perhaps the most controversial aspect of nutritional support is its perioperative use. Early aggressive preoperative nutritional support has been advocated to reduce the risk of morbidity, mortality, and the length of hospital stay in patients undergoing surgery. The relationship between nutritional support and surgery has been studied over the last 25 yr in order to define when patients undergoing operations require postoperative nutritional support, which group of patients needs preoperative support and whether it is better to use parenteral or enteral nutrition. From 1976 to 1990 most of the randomized prospective trials of perioperative TPN failed to demonstrate any improvement in overall operative morbidity or mortality in TPN-treated patients relative to controls. A meta-analysis of 11 trials in 1987 by Detsky *(39)* showed a trend suggesting that TPN reduces risk of complications from major surgery and decreases mortality.

This argument continued until the result of the randomized double-blind Veterans Affairs TPN cooperative study *(40)* showed that the rate of major complications during the first 30 days after surgery was similar in the two groups (TPN group.25.5 %; control group 24.6 %). Also the 90-d mortality rates were similar (13.4 vs 10.5). The infectious complications were more frequent in the TPN group while the noninfectious complications were more frequent in control group. The most important finding came from subset analysis of their data which showed that the noninfectious complications in severely malnourished patients were less frequent in the TPN group compared to controls, (5 vs 43 percent). This study recommended that, the use of preoperative TPN should be limited to severely malnourished surgical candidates in whom operative delay is not contraindicated. Those who are well nourished preoperatively but are anticipated to be unable to eat at least 10 d postoperatively and those who have developed postoperative complications that delay the return of gut function for more than 10 d may also benefit from receiving TPN.

9. HOME PARETERAL THERAPY

Total parenteral nutrition can be safely transferred to a home setting. Over the last two decades there have been significant improvements in ease of use and decreasing complications. In order to improve the quality of life, home TPN is usually given as a cyclic infusion during the night, and patient's understanding and cooperation is essential. The major complication of home TPN is usually catheter damage or occlusion, sepsis, and liver toxicity. With proper patient selection, and careful monitoring and education of the patient and family, it is possible to keep patients on home TPN for many years.

10. CONCLUSION

Total parenteral nutrition has remained a vital medical treatment over the last 20 yr. The use of TPN has been reduced over this period, mostly by careful definition of indications and selection criteria and improvement of enteral nutrition. Oral nutritional support by enteral feeding should be used whenever possible. The routine use of TPN is not indicated in well-nourished patients undergoing surgery, chemotherapy, or radio-therapy unless the patient cannot maintain adequate oral or enteral feeding. Current TPN formulas can deliver the recommended daily requirements of macronutrients, vitamins, electrolytes, and trace elements with minimal difficulty. However physicians, nurses, registered dietitians, and other health care providers, who use TPN must understand the requirements for each of the 9 essential trace elements. In particular, they should avoid inclusion of specific trace elements in TPN solutions where toxicity may develop (e.g., manganese for liver disease patients).

REFERENCES

1. Bistrian BR, Blackburn GL, Vitale J, et al. Prevalence of malnutrition in general medical patients. JAMA 1976;235:1567–1570.
2. Moore FA, Feliciano DC, Andrassey RJ, et al. Early enteral feeding, compared with parenteral reduces postoperative septic complications. The results of a meta-analysis. Ann Surg 1992;216:62–69.

3. Delany HM, Carnevale NJ, Garvey JW. Jejunostomy by needle catheter technique. 1973;73:786–790
4. Mainous MR, Deitch EA. Nutrition and infection. Surg Clin North Am 1994;74:659–676.
5. Wilmore DW, Dudrick SJ. Growth and development of an infant receiving all nutrients exclusively by vein. JAMA 1968;203:860–864.
6. Bowyer BA, Fleming CR, Ludwig J, et al. Does long-term home parenteral nutrition in adult patients cause chronic liver disease? JPEN 1984;9:11–17.
7. Moke KT. Etiology and outcome of total parenteral nutrition-induced hepatic dysfunction. Am Surg 1993;59:650–655.
8. Fleming CR. Trace element metabolism in adult patients requiring total parenteral nutrition. Am J Clin Nutr 1989;49:573–579.
9. Akira O, Yoji T, Richiro N, et al. Trace element metabolism in parenteral and enteral nutrition. Nutrition 1995;11(1Suppl):106–113.
10. Haamstra RD, Block MH, Schocket AL. Intravenous iron dextran in clinical medicine. JAMA 1980;243:1726–1731.
11. Leach RM. Manganese in enteral and parenteral nutrition. Bull NY Acad Med 1984;60:172–175.
12. Hauser RA, Zesiewicz TA, Martinez C, et al. Blood manganese correlates with brain magnetic resonance imaging changes in patients with liver disease. Can J Neurol Sci 1996;23:95–98.
13. Hauser RA, Zesiewicz TA, Rosemurgy AS, et al. Manganese intoxication and chronic liver failure. Ann Neurol 1944;36:871–875.
14. Fleming CR, Lie JT, McCall JT, et al. Selenium deficiency and fatal cardiomyopathy in a patient on home parenteral nutrition. Gastroenterology 1982;83:689–693.
15. Johnson RA, Baker SS, Fallon JT, et al. An occidental case of cardiomyopathy and selenium deficiency. N Engl J Med 1981;304:1210–1212.
16. Fleming CR, Hodges RE, Hurley LS. A prospective study of serum copper and zinc levels in patients receiving total parenteral nutrition. Am J Clin Nutr 1976;29:70–77.
17. Vilter RW, Bozian RC, Hess EV, et al. Manifestations of copper deficiency in a patient with systemic sclerosis on intravenous hyperalimentation. N Engl J Med 1974;291:188–191.
18. Abumrad NN, Schneider AJ, Steel D, et al. Amino acid intolerance during prolonged total parenteral nutrition reversed by molybdate therapy. Am J Clin Nutr 1981;34:2551–2559.
19. Anderson RA. Chromium and parenteral nutrition. Nutrition 1995;11:83–86.
20. Jeejeebhoy KN, Chu RC, Marliss et al. Chromium deficiency, glucose intolerance, and neuropathy reversed by chromium supplementation in a patient receiving long term parenteral nutrition Am J Clin Nutr 1977;30:531–538.
21. Freund H, Atamian S, Fischer JE. Chromium deficiency during total parenteral nutrition. JAMA 1979;241:496–498.
22. Berner YN, Shuler TR, Nielsen FH, et al. Selected ultratrace elements in total parenteral nutrition solutions. Am J Clin Nutr 1989;50:1079–1083.
23. Pluhator-Murton MM, Fedorak RN, Audette RJ, et al. Extent of trace-element contamination from simulated compounding of total parenteral nutrient solutions. Am J Health Syst Pharm 1996;53:2299–2303.
24. Klein CL. Aluminum in parenteral solutions revisited-again. Am J Clin Nutr 1995;61:449–456.
25. Klein S, Simes J, Blackburn GL. Total parenteral nutrition and cancer clinical trials. Cancer 1986;58:1378–1386.
26. Schroeder HA, Mitchener M. Scandium, chromium, gallium, yttrium, rhodium, palladium, indium in mice: effects on growth and life span. J Nutr 1971;101:1431–1438.
27. Schroeder HA, Mitchener M. Selenium and tellurium in rats: Effect on growth, survival, and tumors. J Nutr 1971;101:1531–1540.
28. Koyama H. Trace elements: mechanistic aspect of carcinogenic action. Nippon Rinsho 1996;54:52–58.
29. Kim YI, Mason JB. Nutrition chemoprevention of gastrointestinal cancers: a critical review. Nutr Rev 1996;54:259–279.
30. Bergsma-Kadijk JA, van't Veer P, Kampman J. Calcium does not protect against colorectal neoplasia. Epidemiology 1996;7:590–597.
31. World Cancer Research Fund and the American Institute for Cancer Research. Food, Nutrition, and the Prevention of Cancer: a Global Perspective. American Institute for Cancer Research, Washington, DC, 1997, pp. 417–420.
32. Garland C, Shekelle RB, Barrett-Connor E, et al. Dietary vitamin D and calcium and risk of colorectal cancer: a 19-year prospective study in men. Lancet 1985;1:307–309.

33. Schrauzer GN. Selenium and cancer: a review. Bioinorg Chem 1976;5:275–281.
34. Clark LC, Combs GF, Turnbull BW, Slate EH et al. Effects of selenium supplementation for cancer prevention in patients with carcinoma of the skin. J Am Med Assoc 1996;276:1957–1963.
35. Yoshizawa K, Willett WC, Morris SJ, Stampfer MJ, et al. Study of prediagnostic selenium level in toenails and the risk of advanced prostate cancer. J Natl Cancer Instit 1998;90:1219–1224.
36. Naylor CD, O'Rourke K, Detsky AS, et al. Parenteral nutrition with branched chain amino acids in hepatic encephalopathy: a meta-analysis. Gastroenterology 1989;97:1033–1042.
37. Sax HC, Warner BW, Talamini MA, et al. Early total parenteral nutrition in acute pancreatitis: lack of beneficial effects. Am J Surg 1987;153:117–124.
38. Melchior JC, Chastang C, Gelas P, et al. Efficacy of 2-month total parenteral nutrition in AIDS patients: a controlled randomized prospective trial. The French Multicenter Total Parenteral Nutrition Cooperative Group Study. AIDS 1996;10:379–384.
39. Detsky AS, Baker JP, O'Rourke K, et al. Perioperative parenteral nutrition: A meta-analysis Ann Int Med 1987;107:195–203.
40. Buzby GP. (Veteran AffairTotal Parenteral Nutrition Cooperative Study Group). Perioperative total parenteral nutrition in surgical patients. N Engl J Med 1991;235:525–532.

21

Trace Element and Mineral Nutrition in Diseases of the Eye

George Edwin Bunce, PhD

1. INTRODUCTION

I first became interested in the subject of nutrition and vision in 1963 when as a new PhD and Capt. in the US Army Medical Service Corps, I participated in a survey of the nutritional status of persons living in the northeast region of Brazil. This activity was sponsored by a federal office called the Interdepartmental Committee on Nutrition for National Defense or ICNND, and conducted by a joint team drawn from the United States and the University of Pernambuco in Recife, Brazil. Two observations had a striking impact upon me.

The first was our recognition and documentation of the disastrous consequences that had followed the distribution several years earlier of skimmed milk powder as a famine relief food to a population only marginally supplied with vitamin A. The stimulation of growth that followed the distribution of this protein-rich item had created a depletion of body stores of vitamin A and an outbreak of acute vitamin A deficiency including keratomalacia and xerophthalmia. We were able to call attention to this circumstance and to promote the eventual adoption of a mandatory policy of supplementation of skimmed milk powders delivered by relief agencies with water-dispersible vitamin A, thus ensuring that such tragedies would be prevented in the future.

The second was my exposure to a research project at the host laboratory in Recife. These researchers were seeking to find combinations of indigenous vegetable products that would provide a low cost source of high quality protein. They had just discovered and reported that cataract was present at weaning in 33% of the offspring of female rats fed a test diet based on one of these blends throughout gestation and lactation. When I completed my military service and joined the Department of Biochemistry and Nutrition at Virginia Tech in 1965, I began a collaboration with the Recife group aimed at discovering the cause of this phenomenon. We were able to identify this particular problem as a consequence of a simultaneous marginal intake of L-tryptophan and vitamin E and I continued to engage in the fascinating study of nutrition and cataract for the next thirty years.

In this chapter, I shall review critical papers on mineral nutrition and the most common diseases of the eye. The reader may also wish to consult previous reviews of a broader scope on nutrition and cataract *(1)* and nutrition and eye disease in the elderly *(2)*.

From: *Clinical Nutrition of the Essential Trace Elements and Minerals: The Guide for Health Professionals*
Edited by: J. D. Bogden and L. M. Klevay © Humana Press Inc., Totowa, NJ

2. The Diseases

There are three diseases of the eye which account for the vast majority of clinical concern; namely, cataract, age-related macular degeneration (AMD), and glaucoma. Each of these diseases is complex and far from fully understood. I shall first present a general description of each disease as a preface for the exploration of the possible role of mineral and trace element nutrition in their origin and maturation.

2.1. Cataract

Cataract is a general term for a clinically significant loss of vision due to the emergence of opaque regions within the normally transparent crystalline lens. The lens is an encapsulated organ without blood vessels or nerves. The anterior surface is covered by a single layer of epithelial cells. At the lens equator, these epithelial cells differentiate, lose their nuclei and organelles, and elongate into fiber cells which comprise the bulk of the lens mass. Thus the oldest cells are continually compressed to the center (nucleus) and its surrounding cortex by subsequent generations. Fiber cells are filled with structural proteins called crystallins, which are organized in a repeating lattice. Transparency occurs because the high density and repetitive spatial arrangement of these proteins produce a medium of nearly uniform refractive index with dimensions comparable to light wavelengths *(3)*. Any events that cause loss of structural order and induce abrupt fluctuations in refractive index result in increased light scattering and opacity.

Clinical cataracts may be subdivided into three categories based upon location and morphology *(4,5)*. Posterior subcapsular cataracts (PSC) are an accumulation of abnormal epithelial cells at the posterior pole of the lens. This occurs when differentiation is arrested at the equator and the epithelial cells, instead of becoming fiber cells, assume an irregular form and are displaced in a posterior direction along the interior capsular surface. This type of cataract probably arises mainly from DNA damage. Cortical cataracts are those that originate in the outer layers of the lens. They often display overhydration. Nuclear cataracts are characterized by modification and aggregation of lens structural proteins. Many patients display mixed cataract, i. e., opacities in more than one region. Cataracts may also be classified as either developmental or age-related (90%). Although age-related cataract in humans is a multifactorial disease that develops over decades, most investigators in this field believe that a primary initiating event is oxidative damage of proteins, lipids and/or nucleic acids. Diabetes is associated with a 3-5 fold increase in cataract appearance.

2.2. Age-Related Macular Degeneration

Age-related macular degeneration or AMD is a disease of the portion of the retina known as the macula. In contrast to the lens, the retina is a highly vascularized and metabolically active tissue. Light-absorbing molecules derived from vitamin A and bound to proteins called opsins, reside within membrane-enclosed discs that are constantly synthesized and shed. The discarded material is phagocytized and digested by the lysosomal apparatus within the adjacent retinal pigment epithelium (RPE). AMD is a condition of degenerative changes in the RPE followed by death of the adjacent photoreceptor rods and cones. The digestive failure of the RPE cells results in the accumulation of abnormal deposits called drusen within the extracellular space and lipofuscin within the lysosomal residual bodies *(6)*. As with cataract, chemical and light-induced oxidative damage is considered to be a critical factor in the appearance of RPE dysfunction.

2.3. Glaucoma

No precise definition of glaucoma has been put forward but ophthalmologists would agree that it is a series of conditions characterized by a particular form of progressive optic nerve damage often, but not always, associated with elevated intraocular pressure (IOP) *(7)*. The most common form (90%) of glaucoma is chronic open angle glaucoma. The pathogenesis of open angle glaucoma associated with elevated IOP is not known but the prevalent view is that blockage of the system that drains the ocular fluids occurs due to one or more of the following events; gradual loss of the endothelial cells, change in the ground substance of the trabecular meshwork or a change in the electrolyte transfer capacity of the meshwork cells. Advanced age is a significant risk factor as well as cardiovascular disease, diabetes mellitus, myopia, systemic hypertension and migraine headaches. Since oxidative damage is the common biochemical theme that unites aging and the diseases that appear with age, it is suspected to be an important factor.

The lens is a very accessible tissue and displays easily visible morphological correlates (opacities) of biochemical damage. Whole lenses can be maintained in culture and lens fiber cells can be grown in tissue culture. Consequently, the lens has been thoroughly studied and is well understood in terms of its metabolism, development, anatomy, and so on. The retina, trabecular meshwork, and optic nerve are far more difficult to study. Thus much less is known about relationships between nutrition and AMD and glaucoma than is known about nutrition and cataract.

3. SPECIFIC TRACE ELEMENTS AND MINERALS

3.1. Selenium

The recognition of the essentiality of selenium (Se) for the function of the enzyme glutathione peroxidase (GSHPx) and of the importance of oxidant challenge and defense for the maintenance of lens transparency suggests that cataract might be an outcome of selenium deficiency. Rats were fed chromium- and methionine-supplemented Torula yeast diets containing only 20 ppb Se for 9 mo and their offspring were continued on this diet for another 9 mo *(8)*. Mean selenium concentration in the lens was reduced by 10-fold and GSHPx activity declined to 15% of controls but no opacties were seen. Cai et al. *(9)* fed either selenium- and/or vitamin E- deficient diets to rats with similar results. Lens GSHPx was significantly reduced and the content of malondialdehyde, an indicator of peroxide stress, was elevated but only mild morphological changes were detected.

The risk of disease generated by oxidant stress is a function, however, of both the oxidant burden and the ability of redundant defensive mechanisms to adapt and compensate. Langle et al. *(10)* fed a hydroxytryptamine antagonist (SDZ ICT 322) with prooxidant properties to young Wistar rats. Cataracts were detected in the prooxidant-challenged rats after fourteen weeks but the time to first appearance of cataract was reduced to seven weeks if the rats were fed a diet deficient in both vitamin E and selenium for eight weeks prior to oxidant challenge. The deficient diet alone, however, was not cataractogenic within this time period.

Human studies have not established any consistent associations between cataract and selenium intake or status. Karakucuk et al. *(11)* reported lower concentrations of selenium in the sera (0.28 vs 0.32 micrograms/mL) and aqueous humor (0.19 vs 0.31 microgram/mL) but an increase in selenium in the lenses (5.43 vs 4.43 microgram/gram dry weight) in 48 patients with cataract as compared to controls. Knekt et al. *(12)* studied 47 patients with senile cataract and 94 controls with regard to serum micronutrients. This study was performed in Finland, a country known to have soils and foods low in selenium. Low serum concentrations of the antioxidant vitamins alpha-tocopherol and beta-carotene were risk factors for end stage senile cataract but no association was found for selenium. One intervention study in humans has been completed. A daily supplement of 50 µg Se for 5–6 yr in a cooperative USA/China study in Linxian, China, failed to produce a lowering of cataract prevalence *(13)*.

Selenium is not only an antioxidant but a prooxidant and under certain conditions is highly cataractogenic. Ostadalova et al. *(14)* reported that the delivery of 20–30 nmoles/ g body weight of sodium selenite by subcutaneous injection to suckling rats (10–14 d of age) produced virtually 100% bilateral nuclear cataracts within 3–4 d postinjection. This phenomenon has been studied extensively, especially by Shearer and David *(15)* and by Hess and Bunce *(16)* and their coworkers. In the presence of oxygen, selenite reacts with intracellular glutathione to produce intermediate thiyl radicals and superoxide. Within 24–48 hr, the lens Ca-ATPase pump is partially disabled concomitant with a transient increase in lens membrane permeability to Ca. The consequent 3–5-fold elevation in lens Ca stimulates the Ca-dependent protease calpain II to attack protein substrates within the lens leading to degradation and aggregation of crystallin fragments. PSC cataracts may occur at a later time as an outcome of oxidation of DNA and interference with epithelial cell differentiation.

It is remarkable to note that once rats pass the age of 18–20 d, selenite delivered by injection becomes more toxic but loses its effect upon the lens. This may be related to factors such as changes in the metabolic efficiency of selenium detoxification, maturation of the lenses or a diminished rate of delivery of selenite to the lens. I am unaware of any reported associations between excess dietary selenium exposure and cataract in human populations. The condition of "blind staggers" in selenium-intoxicated herbivores is a neurological defect rather than a visual one.

3.2. Copper, Zinc, Manganese

The enzyme superoxide dismutase (SOD) occupies a key position in the free radical defense system. Mammalian cytosolic SOD requires both copper and zinc and its mitochondrial counterpart is manganese-dependent. Even severe zinc deficiency does not inevitably lower SOD activity, but activity of this enzyme is depressed in animals fed diets deficient in copper *(17)* or manganese *(18)*. Nevertheless, lesions of the lens have not been described in mammals as part of the frank deficiency syndrome of these three minerals. Zinc deficiency has been linked to cataract in hatchery-reared salmonids. This problem emerged in the late 1970s when practical hatchery rations contained large quantities of calcium (fish filet remnants) and phytate (plant meals), components known to interfere with zinc absorption from the gut. Ketola *(19)* observed cataract in 75–85% of fingerling trout after 16–38 wk of consumption of such diets. A supplement of 150 µg zinc/kg diet completely prevented this condition. The reason for the special vulnerability of salmonid lenses to a zinc deficit has not been established but it may be related to protein phase transitions at cold ambient temperatures.

Tissue copper present as free ion may pose a cataractogenic risk as a prooxidant. Most body copper is tightly sequestered to proteins and therefore unable to catalyze Fenton-type reactions. Lin *(20)*, however, has recently reported that the concentration of unconjugated copper ion was significantly higher in cataractous lenses from human diabetics than in normal lenses from control subjects. He has proposed that the increased ion content may arise from release of copper after glycation of SOD. This would lead to a simultaneous increase in free radical burden and decrease in superoxide scavenging capability. This is certainly an interesting hypothesis that deserves further examination. Cook and McGahan *(21)* reported that copper concentration of the aqueous humor and cornea declined with age in dogs but that lens copper was significantly elevated in canine hypermature cataract. Racz and Ordogh *(22)* analyzed the concentration of several trace elements from 97 human senile cataractous lenses and 28 clear lenses from age-matched controls. Manganese and zinc were not different but total copper was moderately increased. Srivastava et al. *(23)* found both copper and zinc to be increased in both cortical and nuclear human cataracts and Rasi et al. *(24)* also reported elevated zinc, copper, and calcium in 53 human cataractous lenses compared to 10 clear lenses. So-called "sunflower cataract" observed occasionally in Wilson's disease appears to result from abnormal levels of copper deposition in the lens anterior capsular region *(25)* (*see* Chapter 12).

The importance of nutrition to the development of glaucoma has received very little attention. Fong et al. *(26)* collected aqueous humor from human glaucomatous eyes and measured its content of ascorbate. One group of samples contained a neglible amount of ascorbate and stimulated the oxidation of added ascorbate. This oxidative effect was inhibited by EDTA. The authors associated this effect with an elevated level of copper in these samples. Akyol et al. *(27)* collected both serum and aqueous humor samples from 44 patients with glaucoma and measured each for zinc and copper. No differences were detected in the serum content of these minerals but copper was elevated and zinc depressed in the aqueous humor from the subjects with glaucoma. Since ascorbate increases the outflow facility of the trabecular meshwork *(28)*, a deficit could eventually contribute to an increased intraocular pressure. These results, however, although mildly suggestive of the potential importance of ascorbate, may have no linkage to the intake of dietary copper.

A current topic of considerable interest is the potential importance of dietary zinc to retinal health. The RPE has one of the highest concentrations of zinc and copper in the body, a significant portion of which is associated with SOD. Leure-dePree and McClain *(29)* maintained weanling male Sprague-Dawley rats on a diet containing only 0.7 μgZn/g diet for seven weeks. Electron microscopic examination of the retina revealed vesiculation and degeneration of the photoreceptor outer segments and numerous large osmiophilic inclusion bodies in the retinal pigment epithelium. No such abnormalities were detected in pair-fed or weight-paired controls. Nicholas et al. *(30)* have studied AMD in a colony of cynomolgus monkeys that spontaneously develop early onset macular degeneration. They found evidence of oxidative stress (elevated albumin and decreased glyceraldehyde 3-phosphate dehydrogenase activity) and 60% lower catalase and GSHPx activities in the affected retinas. They also detected a lower than normal metallothionein content and a fourfold lower concentration of zinc relative to controls. Metallothionein expression is induced by zinc and this sulfhydryl-rich protein is believed to be able to function as a free radical scavenger. They have suggested that these events are related to the pathogenesis of AMD in this model but apparently have not yet tested the potential benefits of zinc supplements in their animals. Another group *(31)* has examined 62 elderly (> 19 years old) rhesus macaques for the presence and severity of AMD. They observed drusen in 47% of animals. The animals with the greatest number of drusen (>10) had a significantly lower activity of SOD in their red blood cells and the highest concentrations of plasma thiobarbituric acid reactive substances.

Wyszynski et al. *(32)* evaluated the effect of age upon the function of certain retinal lysosomal enzymes. They cultured human RPE cells from donors of different ages (19–80 yr) and measured the activity of six acidic glycosidases as well as acid phosphatase, lactate dehydrogenases, and citrate synthase. The zinc-dependent enzyme, alpha-mannosidase was unique among these enzymes in showing a statistically significant decline in both specific activity and V MAX (but not Km) as a function of donor age. Morever, the activity of this enzyme from older donor cells was increased almost twofold by the addition of zinc ions to the assay medium. The authors suggested that since alpha-mannosidase is probably required for the degradation of rhodopsin by the RPE, an age-dependent decrease in activity of this enzyme may be a contributing factor to the pathogenesis of AMD.

The results of clinical studies are inconsistent. Silverstone et al. *(33)* measured zinc and copper in the blood and urine of subjects with AMD and controls. Both elements were significantly elevated in the serum of the patients with AMD. Newsome et al. *(34)* conducted a clinical study designed to determine if zinc supplements might be beneficial in the treatment of macular degeneration. A total of 151 subjects with AMD including visible drusen and visual acuity of 20/80 or better in one eye were recruited. Daily supplements of 200 mg zinc sulfate (80 mg zinc) were supplied to 80 patients whereas the remainder were given a placebo. This dose is about five times the recommended daily allowance of zinc. Follow-up evaluations were performed at 6-, 12-, 18-, and 24-mo. The authors reported that zinc-treated subjects showed significantly less visual loss than controls at 12 and 24 mo. Some critics have suggested that the rate of visual loss in the placebo group was more rapid than the usual clinical experience thus generating a false positive benefit for zinc therapy. Stur et al. *(35)* tested this regimen by administering the same dosage of zinc sulfate for two years to 112 patients with exudative AMD in one eye but lacking exudative lesions and with a visual acuity of better than 20/40 in the second eye. Serum zinc was elevated in the treatment group from 79 to 108 µg/dL and hemoglobin, RBC count, and serum copper remained unchanged. They concluded that oral zinc had no apparent effect on the course of AMD in either eye.

The Eye Disease Case-Control Group has published two papers describing the results of their study on associations between nutrition and AMD *(36,37)*. They selected only the neurovascular or "wet" form of AMD which is less prevalent but much more threatening to vision loss. They found that persons with high levels of serum carotenoids had markedly reduced risks (odds ratio = 0.5) but no significant associations were seen for serum vitamin C, vitamin E, selenium, or zinc. Mares-Perlman et al. *(38)* have evaluated the relationship between AMD and dietary intake of zinc and antioxidant nutrients in Beaver Dam, Wisconsin. They concluded that the data showed no benefit associated with carotenoids but were weakly supportive of a protective effect of high dietary intake of zinc on the development of some forms of early AMD.

3.3. Calcium, Phosphorous, Magnesium

Increased membrane leakiness and swelling occurs in lenses maintained in media lacking calcium. Clinically, cataract has been well documented in subjects with hypocalcemic tetany. Delamere and Paterson *(39)* have presented a very thorough review of the chemistry and physiology of hypocalcemic cataract. Severe restrictions of dietary calcium have been found to generate cataract in experimental animals *(40,41)*. There are no recent studies of prolonged consumption of low calcium diets.

Increases in lens calcium content are often found in clinical cataract and in models for experimental production of cataract. This appears to be secondary to lens injury by other agents (see for example cataract following selenite injection). Thus, the association of increased calcium content with cataract is not likely to be a causal relationship. I have found no references to observations of cataract or other eye disorders as a direct outcome of diets high in dietary calcium or either high or low in phosphorous or magnesium.

3.4. Chromium

This is a very controversial element with regard to its nutritional significance. The reader may consult a recent paper by Nielsen (42) and chapter 2 of this book for a comphrehensive review of the evidence. The importance of chromium to diseases of the eye is related to its putative role in glucose metabolism. A number of reports have claimed beneficial effects of chromium supplements on glucose tolerance and insulin sensitivity. In addition to the specific perils of diabetic retinopathy, diabetics have a 3–5-fold higher prevalence of cataract. Thus a nutritional defict of chromium, should it exist, would indirectly enhance the risk for cataract, and probably AMD and glaucoma.

3.5. Iron, Iodine, Fluorine, Molybdenum

Iron deficiency is one of the major nutritional deficiency states in the world but there have been no reports of pathological changes in the visual organ in either chronic or acute depletion of this element (see Chapter 6). Catalase is an iron-dependent enzyme and its activity does drop under conditions of iron deficiency. Feeding aminotriazole, a catalase inhibitor, to rabbits raised the concentration of hydrogen peroxide in the lens and cataracts were seen in the treated animals (43). However, cataract has not been found in mice with an inborn deficiency of catalase.

The eye is among the organs that can be affected by thyroid insufficiency (see Chapter 13). Opacities (4.5% in a 400 patient sample) have been described in association with myxedema (44). The lenticular changes were relatively mild in that they were visible only by slit lamp microscopy and seldom interfered with vision. Thyroid hormone regulates riboflavin metabolism by increasing the activities of two enzymes responsible for the conversion of riboflavin to FAD (45,46). Endogenous glutathione reductase activity is depressed in the red blood cells of hypothyroid adults (47) and elevated five- to ten-fold in lens epithelia from adults taking daily supplements of synthetic thyroid hormone (48). Experimental riboflavin deficiency in several species results in cataract (1,2). It is possible that a combination of thyroid insufficiency and low intake of riboflavin generates a subset of human cataract patients. In my opinion, this interaction should receive further attention. I have not found any reports of visual pathology as related to fluorine or molybdenum nutrition.

4. CONCLUSION

The pivotal importance of oxidant stress in the pathogenesis of the three most prevalent diseases of the eye (cataract, AMD, and glaucoma) has stimulated an intense scrutiny of those trace elements (selenium, copper, zinc, and manganese) that participate as enzymic cofactors in the oxidant defense network. This cellular defense is a complex process comprised both of enzymes and molecular species that can act together to eliminate prooxidants and scavenge free radicals. Susceptibility to oxidant challenge damage is a function not only of the quantity and composition of the oxidant burden and the efficiency and resiliency of the entire defensive network but also factors such as the tissues under attack, the age of the animal and the period of agent exposure.

Given the large number of variables, it is hardly surprising to find conflicting or ambiguous results among the many studies on this subject. Yet it seems highly probable, if not certain, that any weaknesses in our biochemical defensive network will be exploited given the ubiquity and pervasiveness of the challenges. Thus, although no one mineral deficit (or excess) seems to play a unique role in the evolution of these diseases of the eye, the entire system will function best when none are limiting or excessive. Therefore I suggest that a prudent stance would be to assure the balanced adequacy of all of the antioxidant nutrients, both mineral and organic. This may well necessitate both wise food choices and the use of modest amounts of balanced supplements of vitamins and minerals, especially in persons wishing to maintain a healthy body mass index. Diabetes increases the incidence of cataract, AMD, and glaucoma and since obesity is a major risk factor for the development of noninsulin-dependent or type II diabetes, avoidance of obesity is highly desirable. Furthermore, one should also be wary of adding to the oxidant burden through smoking or avoidable exposure to other sources of free radicals or ultraviolet light. An additional caution would be to recognize that most substances taken in excess become hazardous. Thus, supplement usage must not be abused. Consumption of minerals in amounts in excess of minimum daily requirement levels would be unnecessary and unwise.

REFERENCES

1. Bunce GE, Kinoshita J, Horwitz J. Nutritional factors in cataract. Ann Rev Nutrition 1990;10:233–254.
2. Bunce GE. Nutrition and eye disease of the elderly. J Nutr Biochem 1994;5:66–77.
3. Benedek GB. Theory of transparency of the eye. Appl Opt 1971;10:459–473.
4. Datiles MB, Kinoshita JH. Pathogenesis of cataracts. In: Tasman W, Jaeger EA, ed. Duane's Clinical Ophthalmology, Vol. 1, Chap 72B, J.B. Lippincott Co., Philadelphia, PA, 1991.
5. Young RW. Age-related Cataract, Oxford Universtiy Press, New York, NY, 1991.
6. McDonald HR, Schutz H, Johnson RN, Madeira D. Acquired macular disease. In: Tasman W, Jaeger EA, eds. Duane's Clinical Ophthalmology, Vol 1, Chap. 23, J.B. Lippincott and Co., Philadelphia, PA, 1991.
7. Phelps CD. Glaucoma:general concepts. In: Tasman W, Jaeger EA, eds. Duane's Clinical Ophthalmology, Vol. 3, Chap 42, J.B. Lippincott and Co., Philadelphia, PA, 1991.
8. Lawrence RA, Sunde RA, Schartz GL, Hoekstra WG. Glutathione peroxidase activity in rat lens and other tissues in relation to dietary selenium intake. Exp Eye Res 1974;18:563–569.
9. Cai QY, et al. Biochemical and morphological changes in the lenses of selenium and/or vitamin E deficient rats. Biomedical and Environ Sciences 1994;7:109–115.
10. Langle UW, Wolf A, Cordier A. Enhancement of SDZ ICT 322-induced cataracts and skin changes in rats following vitamin E- and selenium-deficient diet. Arch Toxicol 1997;71:283–289.
11. Karakucuk S, et al. Selenium concentrations in serum, lens and aqueous humour of patients with senile cataract. Acta Ophthalmol Scand 1995;73:329-332.
12. Knekt P, Heliovaara M, Rissanen A, Aromaa A, Aaran RK. Serum antioxidant vitamins and risk of cataract. BMJ 1992;305:1392–1394.
13. Sperduto RD, et al. The Linxian cataract studies: Two nutrition intervention trials. Arch Ophthalmol 1993;111:1246–1253.
14. Ostadalova I, Babicky A, Obenbarger J. Cataract induced by administration of a single dose of sodium selenite to suckling rats. Experientia 1977;34:222–223.
15. Shearer TR, David LL, Anderson RS, Azuma M. Review of selenite cataract. Current Eye Res 1992;11:357-369.
16. Wang Z, Bunce GE, Hess JL. Selenite and Ca2+ homeostasis in the rat lens:effect on Ca-ATPase and passive Ca2+ transport. Current Eye Res 1993;12:213–218.
17. Taylor CG, Bettger WJ, Bray TM. Effect of dietary zinc or copper deficiency on the primary free radical defense system in rats. J Nutr 1988;118:613–621.

18. DeRosa G, Keen CL, Leach RM, Hurley LS. Regulation of superoxide dismutase activity by dietary manganese. J Nutr 1980;110:795–805.

19. Ketola HG. Influence of dietary zinc on cataracts from rainbow trout. J Nutr 1979;109:965–969.

20. Lin J.Pathophysioology of cataracts: copper ion and peroxidation in diabetics. Jap J Ophthalmol 1997;41:130–137.

21. Cook CS, McGahan MC. Copper concentration in cornea, iris, normal and cataractous lenses, and intraocular fluids of vertebrates. Curr Eye Res 1986;5:69–76.

22. Racz P, Ordogh M. Investigations on trace elements in normal and senile cataractous lenses. Activation analysis of copper, zinc, manganese, cobalt, rubidium, scandium, and nickel. Albrecht von Graefes Archiv fur Klinische und Exper Ophthalmol 1977;204:67–72.

23. Srivastava VK, Varshney N, Pandey DC. Role of trace elements in senile cataract. Acta Ophthalmologica 1992;70:839–841.

24. Rasi V, et al. Inorganic element concentrations in cataractous human lenses. Annals of Ophthalmol 1992;24:459–464.

25. Herron BE. Wilson's disease (hepatolenticular degeneration). Ophthalmic seminrs 1976;1:63–69.

26. Fong D, Etzel K, Lee PF, Lin TY, Lam KW. Factors affecting ascorbate oxidation in aqueous humor. Curr Eye Res 1987;6:357–361.

27. Akyol N, Deger O, Kcha EE, Kilic S. Aqueous humour and serum zinc and copper concentrations of patients with glaucoma and cataract. Br J Ophthalmol 1990;74:661–662.

28. Liu KM, Swann D, Lee P, Lam KW. Inhibition of oxidative degradation of hyaluronic acid by uric acid. Curr Eye Res 1984;3:1049–1053.

29. Leure-dePree AE, McClain CJ. The effect of severe zinc deficiency on the morphology of the rat retinal pigment epithelium. Invest Ophthalmol Vis Sci 1982;23:425–434.

30. Nicholas MG, Fujiki K, et al. Studies on the mechanism of early onset macular degeneration in cynomolgus monkeys. II. Suppression of metallothionein synthesis in the retina in oxidative stress. Exp Eye Res 1996;62:399–408.

31. Olin KL, Morse LS, et al. Trace element status and free radical defense in elderly rhesus macaques (Macaca mulatta) with macular drusen. Proc Soc Exp Biol Med 1995;208:370–377.

32. Wyszynski RE, Bruncr WE, et al. A donor-age-dependent change in the activity of alpha-mannosidase in human cultured RPE cells. Invest Ophthalmol Vis Sci 1989;30:2341–2347.

33. Silverstone BZ, Landau L, Berson D, Sternbuch J. Zinc and copper metabolism in patients with senile macular degeneration. Ann Ophthalmol 1985;17:419–422.

34. Newsome DA, Swartz M, Leone NC, Elston RC, Miller E. Oral zinc in macular degeneration. Arch Ophthalmol 1988;106:192–198.

35. Stur M, Tittl M, Reitner A, Meisinger V. Oral zinc and the second eye in age-related macular degeneration. Invest Ophthalmol Vis Sci 1996;37:1225–1235.

36. The Eye Disease Case-Control Study Group. Risk factors for neovascular age-related macular degeneration. Arch Ophthalmol 1992;110:1701–1708.

37. The Eye Disease Case-Control Study Group. Antioxidant status and neovascular age-related macular degeneration. Arch Ophthalmol 1993;111:104–109.

38. Mares-Perlman JA, Klein R, Klein BE, Greger JL, et al. Association of zinc and antioxidant nutrients with age-related maculopathy. Arch Ophthalmol 1996;114:991–997.

39. Delamere NA, Paterson CA. Hypocalcemic cataract. In: ed. Duncan G, ed. Mechanisms of Cataract Formation in the Human Lens. Academic Press, New York, NY, 1981, pp. 219-236.

40. Swan KC, Salit PW. Lens opacities associated with experimental calcium deficiency. Am J Ophthalmol 1941;24:611–614.

41. Chang C-Y, Chen T-T, Wu H, Luo T-H. Cause of cataract, parathyroid hypertrophy and hypocalcemia in vegetarian rats. Chinese J Physiol 1941;16:257–64.

42. Nielsen FH. Chromium. In: Shils ME, Olson JA, Shike M, ed. Modern Nutrition in Health and Diesease, 8th Ed. Lea and Febiger, Philadelphia, PA, Vol. 1, 1994, pp. 268–286.

43. Bhuyan KC, Bhuyan DK. Mechanisms of cataractogenesis induced by 3-amino 1,2,4 triazole. In: Caughey WS, ed. Biochemical and Clinical Aspects of Oxygen, Academic Press, New York, NY, 1979, pp. 785.

44. Brooks MH. Lenticular abnormalities in endocrine dysfunction. In: Bellows JG, ed. Cataract and Abnormalities of the Lens, Grune and Stratton, New York, NY, 1975; pp. 285–301.

45. Domjan G, Kokai K. The flavin adenine dinucleotide (FAD) content of the rat's liver in hypothyroid state and in the liver of hypothyroid animals after in vivo thyroxine treatment. Acta Biol Hung 1966;16:237–241.

46. Rivlin RS, Langdon RG. Regulation of hepatic FAD levels by thyroid hormone. In: Weber G, ed. Advances in Enzyme Regulation,vol. 4, Pergamon, Oxford, U.K., 1966; pp. 44–58.
47. Cimino JA, Jhangiani S, Schwartz E, Cooperman JM. Riboflavin metabolism in the hypothyroid human adult. Proc Soc Exp Biol Med 1987;184:151–153.
48. Horwitz J, Dovrat A, Straatsma BR, Revilla PJ, Lightfoot D. Glutathione reductase in human lens epithelium: FAD-induced in vitro activation. Curr Eye Res 1987;6:1249–1256.

APPENDIX

RECENT BOOKS ABOUT TRACE ELEMENT AND MINERAL NUTRITION

Notes from the Editors

RECENT BOOKS ABOUT TRACE ELEMENT AND MINERAL NUTRITION

1. Trace Elements in Human Nutrition and Health. World Health Organization, Geneva, 1996.
2. Handbook of Nutritionally Essential Minerals and Elements: BL O'Dell and RA Sunde, Eds. Marcel Dekker, 1997.
3. Preventive Nutrition: *The Comprehensive Guide for Health Professionals*. A Bendich and RJ Deckelbaum, Eds., Humana Press, Totowa, NJ, 1997.

Journals and Newsletters that often Contain Articles about Trace Element and Mineral Nutrition

American Journal of Clinical Nutrition
British Journal of Nutrition
Dairy Council Digest
European Journal of Clinical Nutrition
FASEB Journal
Food and Nutrition Research Briefs
Food Product Design
Food Technology
Free Radical Biology and Medicine
ILSI (International Life Sciences Institute) News
International Clinical Nutrition Review
International Journal of Vitamin and Nutrition Research
Journal of Bone and Mineral Research
Journal of Lipid Research
Journal of Nutrition
Journal of Nutrition Education
Journal of Nutritional Immunology
Journal of the American College of Nutrition
Journal of Trace Elements in Medicine and Biology
Nutrition
Nutrition and the M.D.
Nutrition Action Health Letter
Nutrition and Cancer, an International Journal
Nutrition Notes
Nutrition Research
Nutrition Research Newsletter
Nutrition Reviews
Nutrition Week
Nutrition Today
Tufts University Diet and Nutrition Letter
University of California at Berkeley Wellness Letter

From: *Clinical Nutrition of the Essential Trace Elements and Minerals: The Guide for Health Professionals*
Edited by: J. D. Bogden and L. M. Klevay © Humana Press Inc., Totowa, NJ

INDEX

About the Editors

John Dennis Bogden is Professor of Preventive Medicine and Community Health at the New Jersey Medical School–UMDNJ in Newark. He received MS and PhD degrees in Chemistry from Seton Hall University, South Orange, New Jersey, following a ScB degree at Brown University, Providence, Rhode Island. He has published over 90 articles in peer-reviewed journals and monographs, primarily in publications on nutrition and environmental toxicology. To support his research, Dr. Bogden has been awarded 24 grants as Principal Investigator. In 1991, he won the Labcatal First Prize for "Scientific Research in the Field of Trace Elements." Dr. Bogden is a member of several professional organizations, including the American Society for Nutritional Sci-

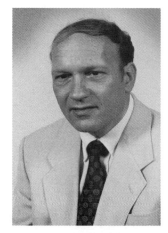

ences, American Public Health Association, and the American College of Nutrition. He is an Adjunct Professor in the Department of Nutritional Sciences at Rutgers University, New Brunswick, NJ, as well as a member of the External Advisory Board of the Core Nutrition Research Unit at Memorial Sloan-Kettering Cancer Center in New York, NY. At the New Jersey Medical School, he has been President of the Faculty and is currently the Acting Chair of the Department of Preventive Medicine and Community Health. Dr. Bogden is a Consulting Editor for *Nutrition Research* and member of the editorial board of the *Journal of Nutritional and Environmental Medicine.*

Leslie M. Klevay is a research leader at the Grand Forks Human Nutrition Research Center of the Agricultural Research Service of the USDA. He received chemistry and medical degrees from the University of Wisconsin along with degrees from the Harvard School of Public Health. He has been on the faculty of four universities, including the University of North Dakota School of Medicine, where he heads the Division of Nutrition as Professor of Internal Medicine. Dr. Klevay is a member of several societies: the American Chemical Society, the American Federation for Medical Research, the American Society for Clinical Nutrition, American Society for Nutrition Sciences, and the Society for Experimental Biology and Medicine. He has been an advisor to state, national, and international agencies and lectures

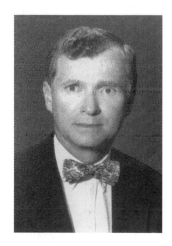

widely on his research on the epidemiology and pathophysiology of atherosclerosis and ischemic heart disease. Dr. Klevay's work has been published in over 60 scientific journals, receiving favorable review in the national and international press; he is a member of the editorial board of the *Journal of Trace Elements in Medicine and Biology.*

DATE DUE

JUN 19 01			